Rhinoplastic Surgery

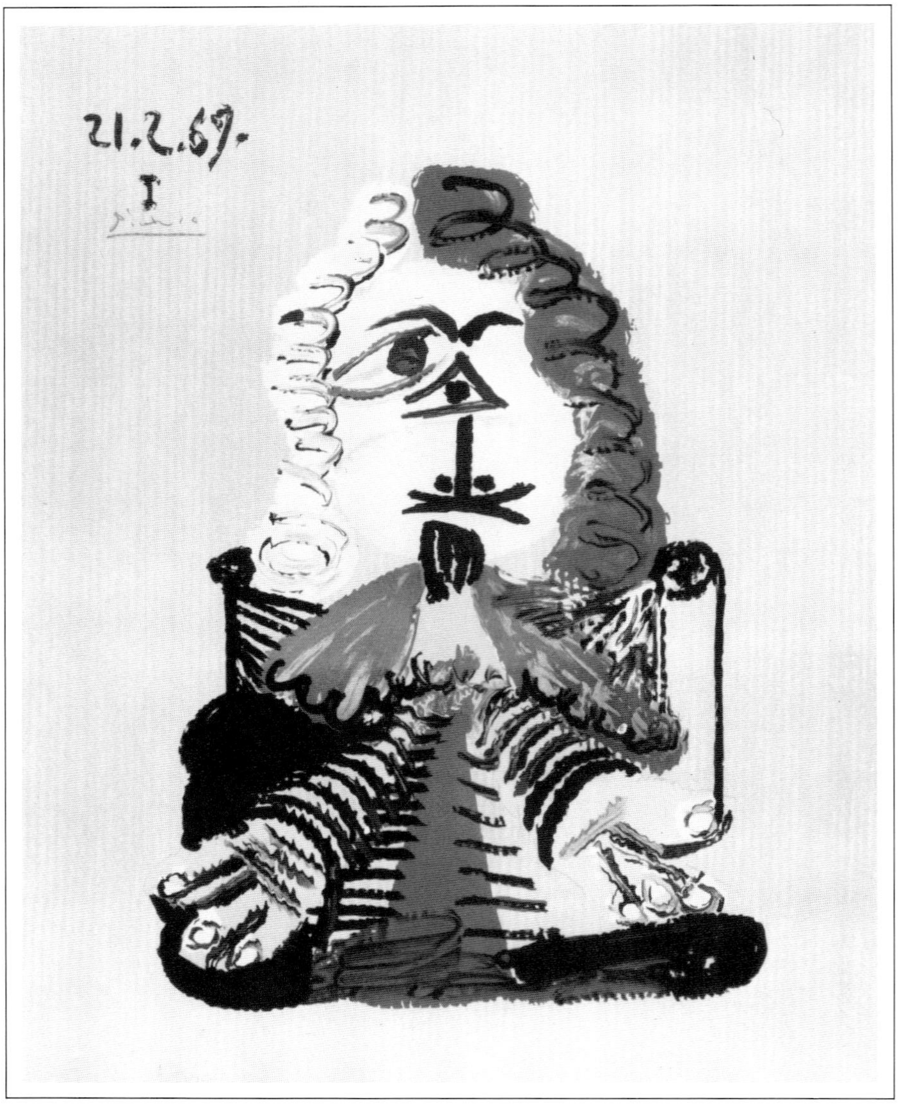

"Imaginary Portraits"

The image that appears on the cover is one of a series of 29 limited edition lithographs executed by Pablo Picasso in 1969, at the age of 88. In this series, prominent personalities from Picasso's life are rendered in the guise of Renaissance court jesters decked out in Elizabethan ruffs and harlequins in multicolored costumes.

RHINOPLASTIC SURGERY

Walter E. Berman, M.D.
Clinical Professor of Head and Neck Surgery,
Director of Facial Plastic Surgery,
University of California, Los Angeles,
Los Angeles, California
President, Beverly Hills Wilshire-Beverly Surgi-Center,
Beverly Hills, California,
Past President, American Academy of Facial Plastic and Reconstructive Surgery,
Past President, American Academy of Cosmetic Surgery

with* 18 *contributors

with 828 *illustrations,*
and 12 four-color plates

The C. V. Mosby Company
ST. LOUIS • BALTIMORE • TORONTO • PHILADELPHIA 1989

Mosby

Editor: Eugenia A. Klein
Assistant Editor: Barbara S. Menczer
Project Manager: Carlotta Seely
Production Editor: Radhika Rao Gupta
Design: Liz Fett
Production: Cynthia A. Miller, Jeanne Genz, Mary P. Tait
Cover Art: Imaginary Portraits by Pablo Picasso
Copyright © ARS, N.Y./Spadem 1988

Printed in the United States of America

The C.V. Mosby Company
11830 Westline Industrial Drive, St. Louis, Missouri 63146

Library of Congress Cataloging-in-Publication Data

Berman, Walter E.
Rhinoplastic surgery.

Includes index.
1. Rhinoplasty. I. Title. [DNLM: 1. Rhinoplasty. WV 312 B516rb]
RF350.B47 1989 617′.5230592 88-31262
ISBN 0-8016-0623-3

C/W/W 9 8 7 6 5 4 3 2 1

Contributors

Jack R. Anderson, M.D.
Clinical Professor,
Departments of Otolaryngology, Head and Neck Surgery and Ophthalmology,
Louisiana State University Medical School,
Clinical Professor,
Department of Otolaryngology, Head and Neck Surgery,
Tulane University Medical School,
New Orleans, Louisiana

W. Douglas Appling, M.D., F.A.C.S.
Assistant Professor,
Department of Otorhinolaryngology and Communicative Sciences,
Baylor College of Medicine,
Houston, Texas

David A. Behrman, D.M.D.
Associate Attending Oral and Maxillofacial Surgeon,
Assistant Professor of Surgery, Oral and Maxillofacial Surgery, Department of Surgery,
Division of Dentistry, Oral and Maxillofacial Surgery,
The New York Hospital–Cornell Medical College,
New York, New York

Stanley J. Behrman, D.M.D.
Attending Oral and Maxillofacial Surgeon-in-Charge,
Clinical Professor, Oral and Maxillofacial Surgery,
Department of Surgery,
Division of Dentistry, Oral and Maxillofacial Surgery,
The New York Hospital–Cornell Medical College,
New York, New York

Louis O. Boileau, M.D., F.R.C.S. (C)
Consulting Plastic and Reconstructive Surgeon,
Department of Surgery,
Vancouver, British Columbia, Canada

Nabil S. Fuleihan, M.D.
Assistant Professor,
Department of Otolaryngology,
Boston University School of Medicine,
Boston, Massachusetts

Usama S. Hamdan, M.D.
Clinical Instructor,
Department of Otolaryngology,
Boston University,
Boston, Massachusetts

Rodolphe Meyer, M.D.
Postgraduate Professor ISAPS (IPRS),
Former Associate Professor,
Department of ENT and Plastic, Reconstructive and Aesthetic Surgery,
University Clinic,
Lausanne, Switzerland

Nathan E. Nachlas, M.D.
Clinical Instructor,
Department of Otolaryngology/Head and Neck Surgery,
University of Miami, Private Practice,
Boca Raton, Florida

Milton Perlow, M.D.
Medical Director,
Chief, Department of Anesthesia,
Beverly Hills Wilshire Surgi-Center & Medical Group, Inc.,
Beverly Hills, California

Dominique M. Rheims, M.D.
Department of ENT Facial Plastic and Reconstructive Surgery,
Hospital Robert Debre,
Paris VII University, Paris, France

Howard W. Smith, M.D.
Clinical Professor of Surgery,
Department of Otolaryngology,
Yale University,
New Haven, Connecticut

Richard C. Smith, M.D.
Research Director,
Plastic, Aesthetic, and Cosmetic Surgery, P.C.,
Brookline, Massachusetts

Robert A. Stern, M.D.
Lecturer, Department of Head and Neck Surgery,
University of California at Los Angeles,
Los Angeles, California

Claus Walter, M.D.
Professor, Department of Hals-Nasen-
Ohrenklinik, Univrsitat Bonn,
Bonn, West Germany,
Head of Department,
Abteilung fur plastische Chirurgie und
Hals-Nasen-Ohrenkrankheiten,
Klinik am Rosenberg,
Heiden, Switzerland

Richard C. Webster, M.D.
Professor, Department of Otolaryngology,
Boston University School of Medicine,
Boston, Massachusetts

Mary Ruth Wright, Ph.D.
Clinical Assistant Professor of Psychology,
Department of Otorhinolaryngology and
Communicative Sciences,
Baylor College of Medicine,
Houston, Texas

William K. Wright, M.D., F.A.C.S.
Clinical Professor, Department of
Otorhinolaryngology and Communicative Sciences,
Baylor College of Medicine,
Houston, Texas,
Clinical Professor, Department of Otolaryngology,
Head and Neck Surgery,
University of Texas Medical School
Houston, Texas

Foreword

It is an important event when a master surgeon directs his energies to the writing of a book on a subject that has involved the major portion of his professional life. This book is a splendid reward to us of the efforts of Dr. Walter Berman and his collaborators in presenting the essence of their experience in a well structured and practical text that not only fulfills the academic and scientific aspects of the subject, but richly fills their enterprise with an illumination of experience and wisdom.

Dr. Berman has been recognized for years as a leading plastic surgeon in the world. His stature is measured by his accomplishments, his character, and his style. He is identified by all as a surgeon who has something worthwhile to say, and now we have the verification of this truth in this publication.

This book has a definite approach and orientation to the condition of rhinoplasty. It begins with the basic positions of primary and secondary rhinoplasty in a way that will enhance surgical expertise and create a feeling of security in dealing with revisions and complications.

The art of photographic documentation and esthetic competence and the management of nasal abnormalities that are associated with cleft lips, craniofacial deformities, and septal perforations are approached in a practical and realistic manner that links those situations with the rhinoplasty concept and also suggests rational principles to manage these related problems. This book concludes with a review of the psychological principles that motivate individuals to opt for rhinoplasty; the review includes warnings, precautions, and suggestions to render this procedure as effective and humane as possible.

John Conley, M.D.

Preface

Nasal surgery, certainly a most rewarding and gratifying experience, is also beset with frustrations. The best planning, meticulous surgery, and careful postoperative care do not guarantee a perfect result. The vagaries of tissue healing, condition of the tissues preoperatively and postoperatively, postoperative care, and the surgeon's skill all influence the outcome. The final result may not be known for several years, and it depends primarily on the thickness of the nasal tip skin and the factors affecting nasal tip projection.

The purpose of this text is to provide an in-depth discussion of rhinoplasty procedures. I have purposely included various points of view in an effort to present multiple pathways to the same end. A knowledge of multiple techniques will result in a more thorough understanding of nasal surgery.

In this book we will discuss why certain results are achieved, the anatomical reasons for postoperative imperfections, preoperative and postoperative care of the patient, as well as adjunctive nasal care. Rhinoplastic surgery should not be a static procedure, but rather an evolutionary process that I trust can be built upon the basic facts that are presented in this book.

I have been fortunate in that *Rhinoplastic Surgery* has as co-authors an outstanding cast of internationally respected rhinoplastic surgeons. To this I have added my own views. Together this accounts for almost two hundred years of experience with thousands of patients.

In our ever-changing field, there are still basic rules that must be followed. I hope that this text will be both pragmatic and provocative as a framework for rhinoplastic surgery and care of our patients.

I would like to thank my wife, Dee, my colleague, Robert Stern, M.D., our editor, Eugenia A. Klein, and Assistant Editor, Barbara S. Menczer, and the contributing doctors for valuable contributions that each has made to the book. I greatly appreciate the outstanding artwork done by Suzanne E. Merrick for my chapters and the illustrations done by David Bolinksy for Dr. Smith's chapters and Kathryn Sisson for one of Dr. Meyer's chapters.

Walter E. Berman

Contents

PART IV RECONSTRUCTIVE NASAL SURGERY

Part I

PREPARATION

1

Nomenclature

Walter E. Berman

Communication is the key to opening the doors of knowledge. The ability to relate thoughts to one another is the basis of learning. Unfortunately, because of the host of contributors to nasal surgery and physiology, nasal terminology has evolved into a morass. Some years ago, Drs. Jack Anderson, Richard Webster, and I devised a rather simplistic group of terms that were applicable to the nose (Fig. 1-1). We used the prime directions of *anterior* for dorsal, *posterior* for the floor of the nose, *superior* for the glabellar or forehead direction, and *inferior* for the caudal or columellar direction. This rationale, the four cardinal direction approach to nasal anatomy, has proved to be most helpful in communication.

For clarity, I have substituted the phrase *between the cartilage incisions* for the term *intercartilaginous*, which refers to the area between the upper and lower cartilages. The *nasal tip* is where the medial and lower lateral cartilages meet. The term *split incision* has also been substituted for the term *intracartilaginous* (Fig. 1-2). *Junction tunnels* are the elevations of the mucosal coverings on the undersurfaces of the upper lateral cartilages and nasal bones at their junction with the septum (Fig. 1-3). These elevations make it possible to separate the upper lateral cartilages from the nasal septum without cutting through the mucosa. This also keeps the mucosal envelope intact when decreasing the bony hump. These simple but effective terms should help to broaden our understanding.

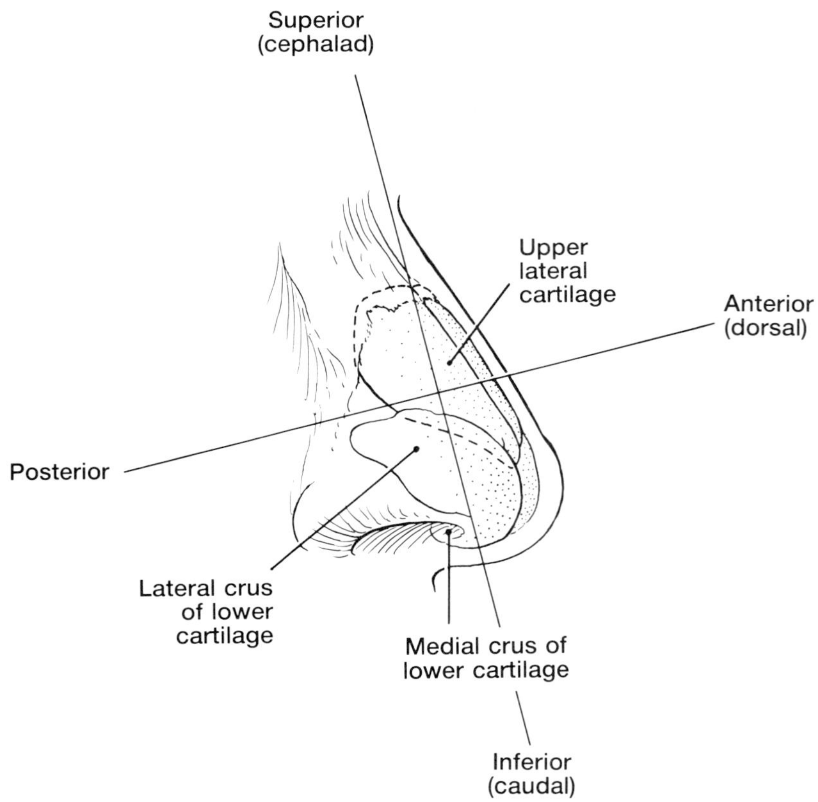

Fig. 1-1. Simplified nasal nomenclature. (From Berman, WE: Rhinoplasty, ed 2, Washington DC, 1984, American Academy of Otolaryngology-Head and Neck Surgery Foundation, Inc.)

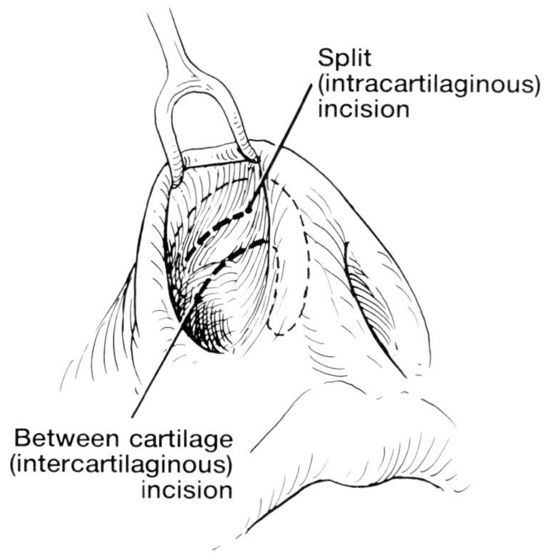

Fig. 1-2. Terms used in describing lower lateral cartilage incisions. (From Berman, WE: Rhinoplasty, ed 2, Washington DC, 1984, American Academy of Otolaryngology-Head and Neck Surgery Foundation, Inc.)

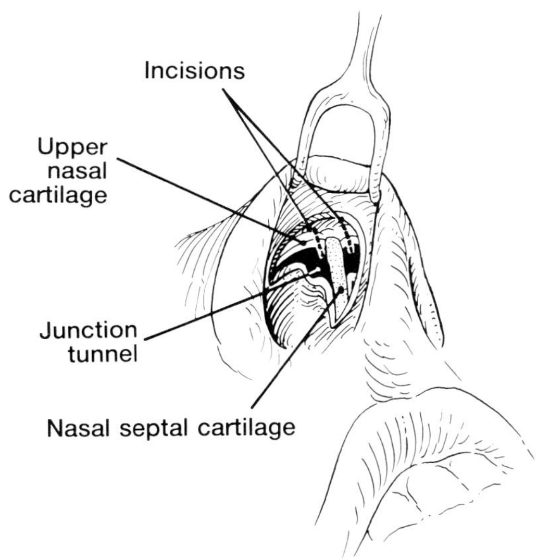

Fig. 1-3. Junction tunnel. (From Berman, WE: Rhinoplasty, ed 2, Washington DC, 1984, American Academy of Otolaryngology-Head and Neck Surgery Foundation, Inc.)

2

Applied Anatomy of the Nose

Robert A. Stern

It is said that nasal surgery is a surgery of millimeters. To effect these exacting surgical changes, a thorough knowledge of nasal anatomy is necessary. This study is based on fresh, unembalmed, cadaver dissection as well as on live operative procedures. It is assumed that the surgeon has a working knowledge of rhinoplastic anatomy. This chapter will discuss some of the detailed and complex relationships that make a difference in the final surgical result.

It is helpful to think of the nose as being like any other projecting structure: it is composed of framework and its support, and is finished with an external covering. The framework of the nose consists of skeletal components of cartilage and bone. Support is provided by ligaments and connective tissue that hold the framework together, as well as by the skeleton's inherent strength. Skin and soft tissue provide the covering for the structure of the nose. As with any well-conceived design, all of the components are interrelated.

External Coverings

Skin, subcutaneous tissue, and muscle comprise the covering of the nose. The nature of these individual components significantly affects the appearance of the nose.

Skin and Subcutaneous Tissue

Skin may be light or dark in color. Dark skin is often thicker, and may possess a greater amount of subcutaneous tissue. Thicker skin adapts to changes beneath it less readily than thinner skin does, and thus changes in the framework are less apparent in a thick-skinned nose. Stated another way, a greater change in the nasal skeleton is necessary in order to change the appearance of the nose in a thick-skinned individual.

Although thick skin can be a limiting factor in rhinoplasty and can hide modifications of the framework, it can be helpful too. Thick skin may hide small imperfections in the nasal skeleton that might otherwise be apparent in the thin-skinned nose.

In secondary rhinoplasty, a firm subcutaneous scar often makes it very difficult to modify the shape of the nose. Indeed, the subcutaneous scar may be so firm and thick that it may become its own framework, making it necessary to remove or weaken this scar before attempting to modify the true skeleton. However, such a scar may at times be used for framework when there is a deficiency of true skeletal support.

The thickness of the skin and subcutaneous tissue varies throughout the length of the nose (Plate 2-1). This is of critical importance. These tissues are thickest in the supratip area. They are somewhat less thick at the nasion (nasofrontal angle), and much less thick at the tip—specifically in the area over the nasal domes. The skin and its subcutaneous tissue is thinnest at the *rhinion* which is the junction of nasal bones with upper lateral cartilage. These factors have important applications.

First, it becomes apparent that the rhinion should be left higher (more anterior) than the adjacent upper lateral cartilage and nasal bone in order to prevent the appearance of a depressed or weak dorsum.

Second, the cephalic border of the lower lateral cartilage, the upper lateral cartilage, and the caudal septum must be on a lower (more posterior) plane than the nasal tip in order to prevent a high supratip, i.e., a "pollybeak deformity." The subcutaneous tissues here also tend to form more scarring than those in the rhinion and tip. This must be taken into account when lowering this area.

Third, as mentioned before, there is less margin for error with thin skin than with thick. After surgery, the rhinion must be free of any bony spicules or sharp angles because they may show. The nasal domes must be symmetrical and without bossae. However, the thick skin of the supratip will probably hide some unevenness of the upper lateral cartilages and septum.

Finally, the soft triangles should be mentioned. These triangles, also known as facets, are the only areas of the nose that are made up of primarily cutaneous tissue, with scant intervening subcutaneous tissue (Plate 2-2). The maintenance of these fine structures during and after rhinoplasty is extremely important. Violating them with an incision can lead to scarring and subsequent distortion. Marginal incisions for delivery of the lower lateral cartilages should not be created at the line of the vibrissae as suggested by some texts; often, this will cause the facets to be broached (see plate).

Muscle

Of the various paired muscles of the nose, only three have any significant effect on rhinoplasty: the *depressor septi,* the *procerus,* and the *transverse nasalis.*

The depressor septi is the only muscle whose function makes a difference in nasal appearance. It has its origin in the incisive fossa of the maxilla and inserts in the area of the caudal septum (Plate 2-3). If hyperactive, the depressor septi may produce pronounced tip drop during facial animation through its action on the feet of the mesial crura. If the septum is transfixed, the depressor septi may contribute to postoperative tip drop through its unopposed action on the mesial crural feet. Cutting the depressor septi helps to prevent this problem.

The procerus arises from the glabella and inserts at the upper lateral cartilage (Plate 2-4). It spans the nasion and can contribute to a shallow nasofrontal angle. Careful removal of a portion of this muscle may help to deepen the nasion, provided organizing hematoma does not later fill the cavity with cicatrix.

The transverse nasalis is important because it helps to form a covering across the mid-portion of the nose superficial to the skeleton (Plates 2-4 and 2-5). Together with the procerus, it forms a musculo-aponeurotic sheath over the dorsum of the nose that is much easier to elevate than the tightly adherent periosteum (see Plate 2-8). This musculo-aponeurotic sheath is helpful in hiding irregularities of the skeleton, and provides some support for the nasal components adhering to its deep surface.

Septum

The nasal septum is the cornerstone of the nose. It is of paramount importance in external rhinoplasty as well as in functional respiration. The dorsal and caudal borders of the septum are the portions that impact on the external nose and will be discussed with the nasal tip and mid-nose. The remaining bulk of the septum is of primary importance to respiration and support.

Framework

The septum is composed of cartilage and bone. The quadrilateral plate is the only cartilaginous portion. The bony portion is composed of the ethmoid plate and vomer, and is tucked away beneath the nasal bones. The septum rests on the nasal spine and the maxillary and palatine crests. Lateral support is provided by the structures of the external nose and their investing membranes.

The soft tissue integuments of the septum are of critical importance. The perichondrium of the cartilaginous septum and periosteum of the bony ethmoid plate are continuous and allow fairly easy elevation of flaps throughout their lengths. The perichondrium of the cartilaginous septum and the periosteum of the bony spine, crests, and vomer are not continuous. Each wraps around its own member. Sharp dissection is necessary to open these planes.

Support

Firm ligaments attach the posterior margin of the septum to the spine and crests. These ligaments, along with their investing membranes, maintain the ventral septum in approximation with its bony support. Of course, the cartilaginous septum itself provides support, either directly or indirectly, for the tip and mid-nose.

Nasal Tip

The nasal tip contains perhaps the most delicate structures and complex interrelationships of the nose.

Framework

The lower lateral cartilages provide the framework for the nasal tip. Their shape is the most varied of any of the nasal skeletal structures. They may be thick or thin, strong or weak, broad or narrow, and have various angles of sweep. The tip cartilages themselves may be divided into the areas comprising the mesial crura, the domes, and the lateral crura. The feet of the mesial crura flare laterally from the midline and superiorly, so that they straddle the posterior aspect of the caudal septum. The mid-portion of the mesial crura then narrows, only to flare again anteriorly, providing for the hourglass configuration of what we call the columella. The hourglass shape of the columella is aesthetically pleasing, and although surgically narrowing this structure is sometimes necessary, its basic curves should be maintained.

It is of interest to note that the mesial crura are immediately deep to the skin at the waist of the hourglass. An external rhinoplasty incision should be placed in this thin skin for optimal healing.

The dome area is shaped like a triangle. Medially, the anterior flaring of the mesial crus becomes the first leg of what, when perfect, is an equilateral triangle. The high point, or apex of the triangle, is the actual anatomical dome. Laterally, a portion of the lateral crus completes the triangle. The relationship of two equilateral triangles, touching at one base angle, provides for the finely sculpted tip lobule, and demonstrates desirable highlights (Plate 2-1).

It is very important to maintain, or if necessary, to create this desirable relationship. Excess morselization, tight intracrural sutures, or tip struts projecting above the domes may produce only a single tip defining point instead of the two defined by the apices of the triangles. This leads to the unappealing "tent pole deformity."

The lateral crura broaden quickly from the domal area. They soon flare posterosuperiorly away from the nostril rim (Plate 2-6). The most lateral aspect of the flaring crura usually marks the end of the relatively thin nasal tip and begins the thicker, wider nasal ala. In some noses, an accessory cartilage between the lateral aspect of the lateral crus and the pyriform aperture may be present; this is called the *sesamoid cartilage*

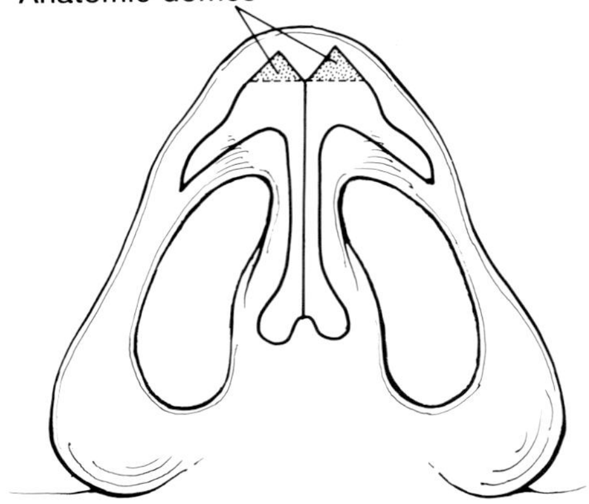

Fig. 2-1. Equilateral triangles providing two tip defining points.

(Plate 2-6, *E*). This cartilage almost never requires surgical manipulation.

At the cephalic border of the lateral crura, the ventrally curving scroll forms a hinge with the dorsally curved scroll of the upper lateral cartilage (Plate 2-6, *A* and *B*). This region is thus thicker, and provides for some supratip fullness. This fullness is removed upon trimming the cephalic border of the lower lateral cartilage in routine rhinoplasty.

Support

The tip unit, composed of the paired medial crura and posterosuperior flaring of the lateral crura, forms a tripod and is potentially a very stable structure. There are eight supports for this structure, four of them critical.

Main support. The strength of the tripod-like tip cartilages provides significant support. The ligamentous attachments of the mesial crural feet to the caudal septum, and the lateral crura to the pyriform aperture are critical to three-point support of the tripod feet. Additionally, a ligamentous attachment between the scrolls of the upper lateral and lower lateral cartilages helps prevent anterior and inferior rotation. This last support, upper lateral to lower lateral, weakens with age, and contributes to downward drooping of the tip sometimes seen in older individuals.

Additional support. Binding the mesial crura of the tip complex into one structure and strengthening the central leg of the tripod unit, intracrural fibers run from mesial crus to mesial crus (Plate 2-7, *A*). These fibers are very thick and strong, and are critical for rigidity of the central segment of the tip, or columella, which provides the tripod-like stability.

Fibers from the anterior aspect of the caudal septum attach just below the dome and contribute to the prevention of posterior and inferior tip rotation (Plate 2-7, *B*).

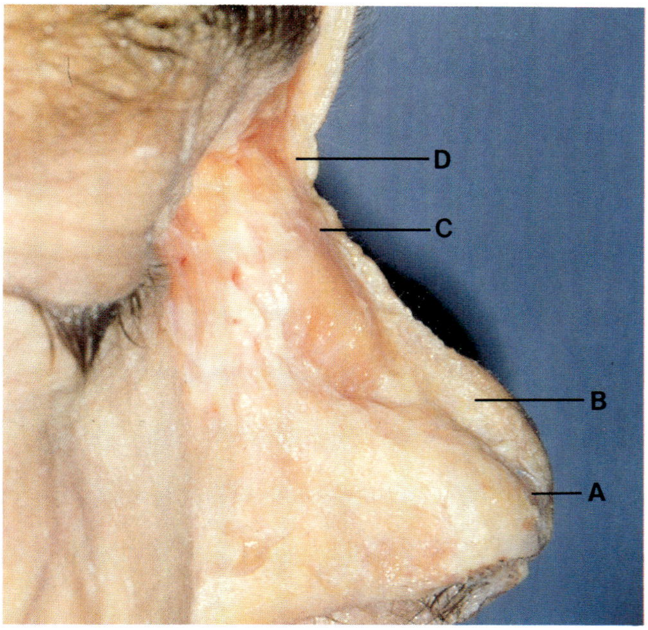

Plate 2-1. Thickness of nasal skin and subcutaneous tissue varies throughout the length of the nose: *A*, Tip. *B*, Supratip. *C*, Rhinion. *D*, Nasion.

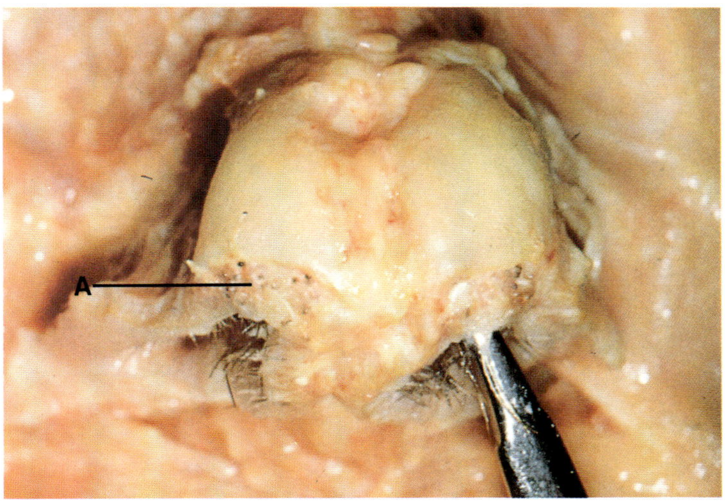

Plate 2-2. Nasal tip. Soft triangle with hair follicles, *A*.

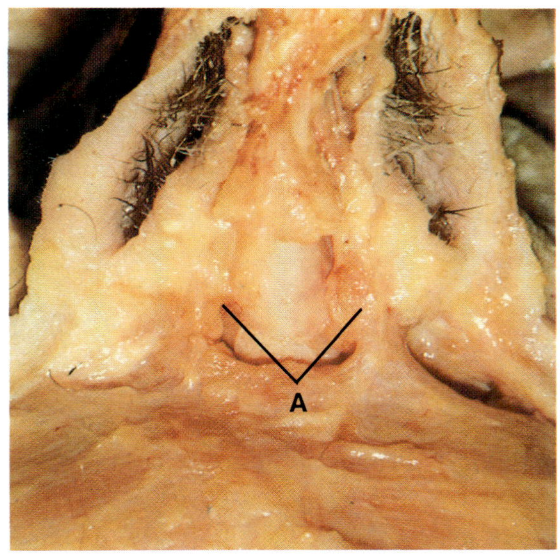

Plate 2-3. Nasal tip, basal view. Depressor septi muscle inserts in the area of the caudal septum and mesial crural feet, *A*.

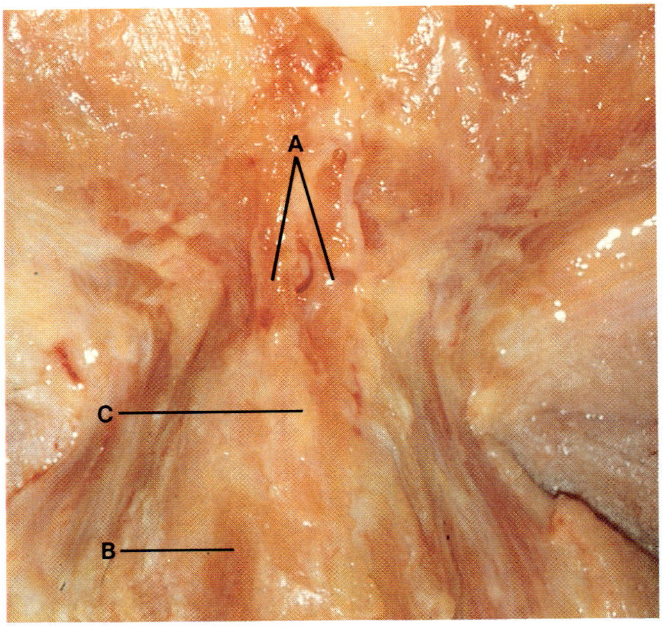

Plate 2-4. Nasal muscles and aponeurosis, frontal view. *A,* Procerus muscle. *B,* Nasalis muscle. *C,* Aponeurosis between the procerus and nasalis forming the musculo-aponeurotic sheath.

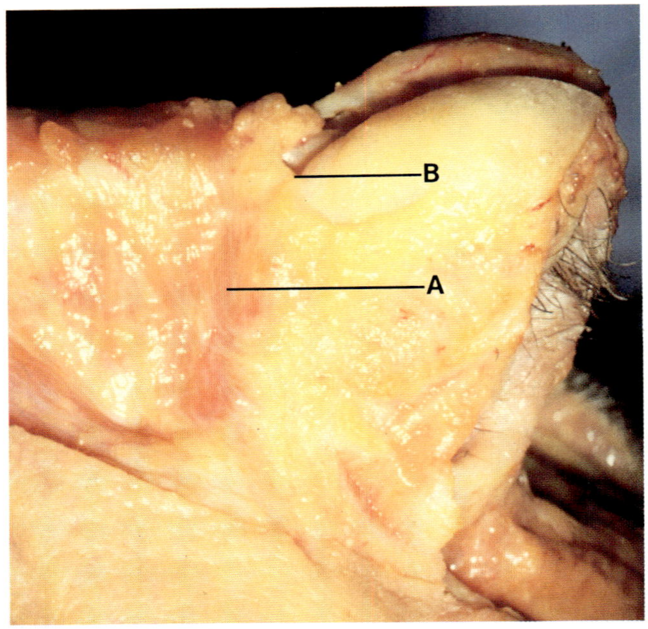

Plate 2-5. Nasal muscles and aponeurosis, lateral view. *A,* Nasalis muscle. *B,* Beginning of the musculo-aponeurotic sheath.

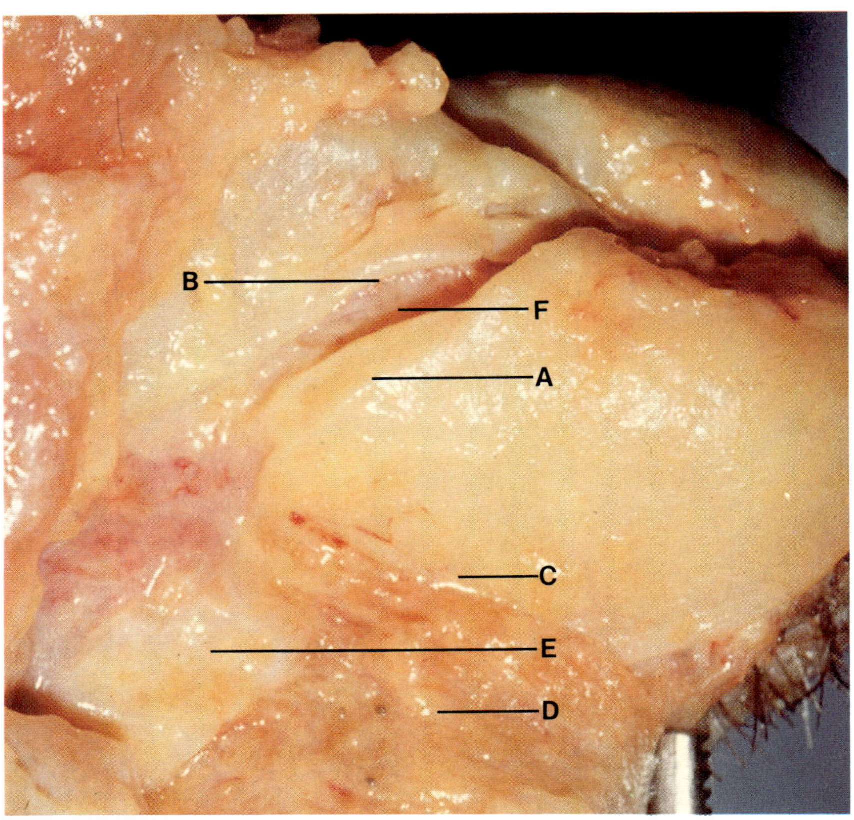

Plate 2-6. Lateral crura of the nasal tip and associated structures. *A,* Ventrally curving scroll of the lower lateral crura. *B,* Dorsally curving scroll of the upper lateral crura. *C,* Sweep of the lateral crus (posterior-superior). *D,* Fibrofatty tissue of thick alae, area of ligament between lateral crus and pyriform aperture. *E,* Sesamoid cartilage. *F,* Mucosal support.

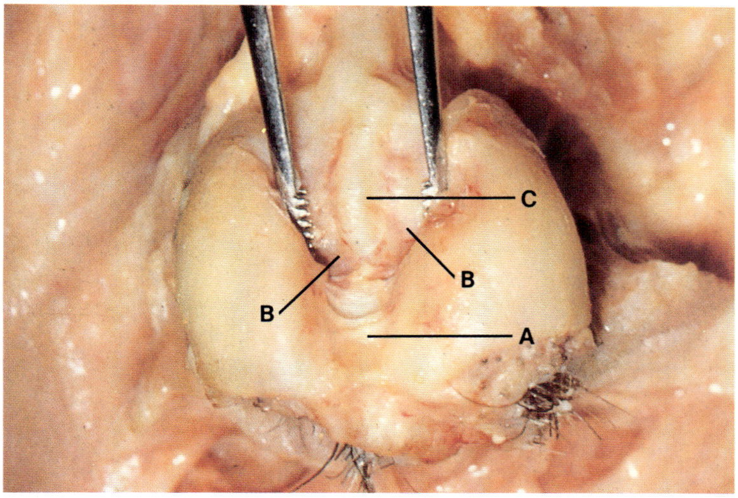

Plate 2-7. Nasal tip. *A,* Intracrural ligament. *B,* Ligaments between caudal septum and lower lateral cartilages. *C,* Caudal septum tongue-in-groove with tip.

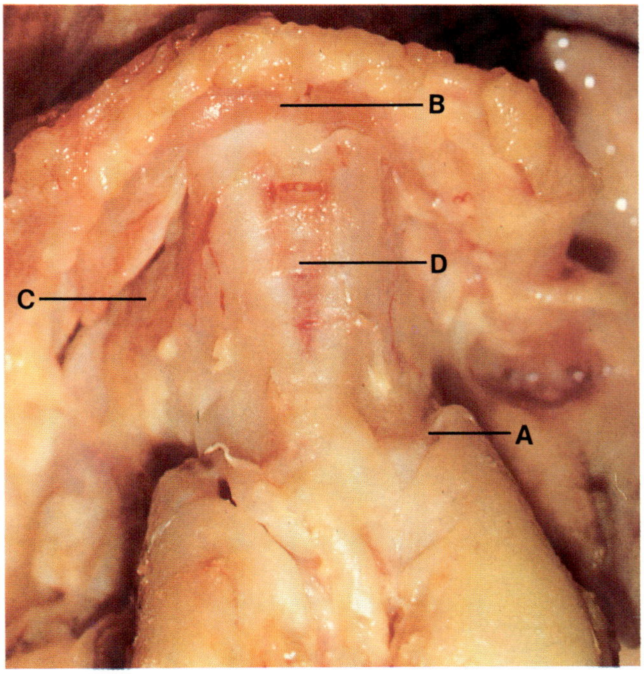

Plate 2-8. Mid-nose. *A,* Ligaments between upper and lower lateral scrolls. *B,* Musculo-aponeurotic sheath elevated. *C,* Upper lateral cartilage displaced from nasal bone. *D,* Septal platform.

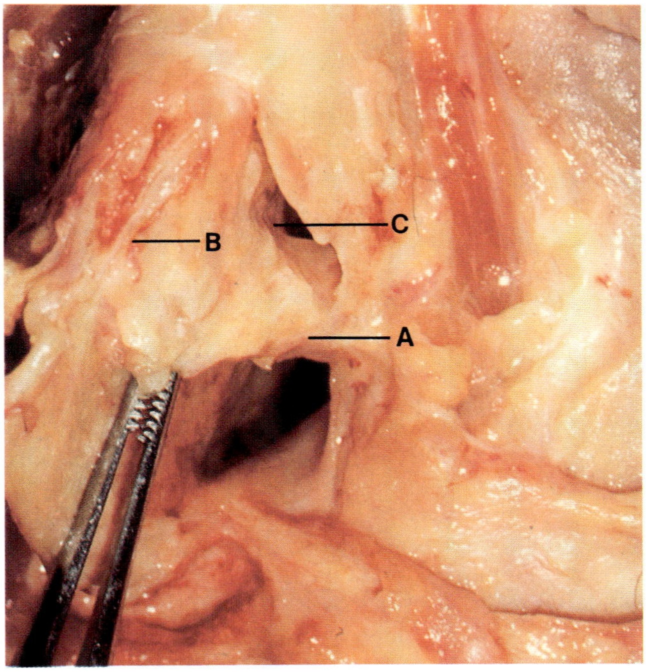

Plate 2-9. Upper lateral cartilage support. *A,* Ligament from upper lateral cartilage to pyriform aperture. *B,* Base of upper lateral cartilage articulating with septal platform. *C,* Upper lateral cartilage runs under nasal bone for approximately ¾ cm.

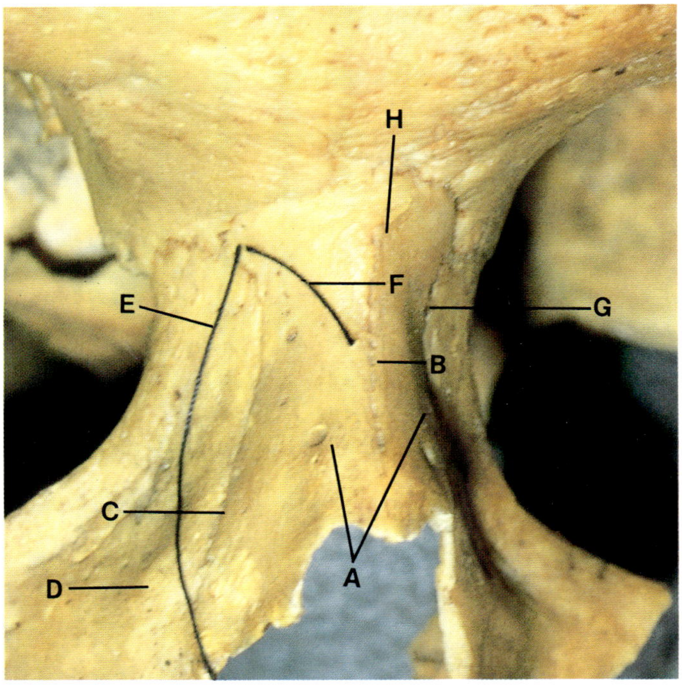

Plate 2-10. Bony vault. *A,* Nasal bones. *B,* Midline suture. *C,* Lateral suture. *D,* Frontal process maxilla. *E,* Line of lateral osteotomy. *F,* Line of medial osteotomy. *G,* Beginning of nasal bone curve. *H,* Nasal spine of frontal bone lies deep to nasal bones.

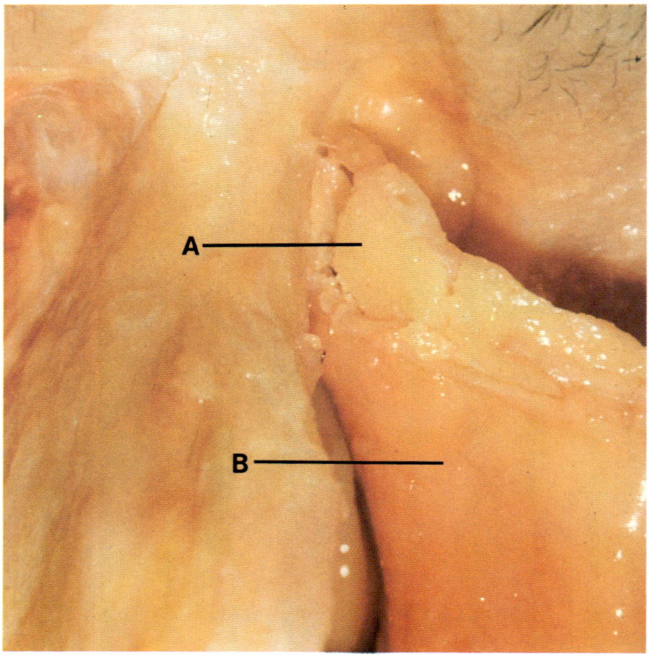

Plate 2-11. Nasal bones. *A,* Thick nasal bone superiorly. *B,* Mucosal lining.

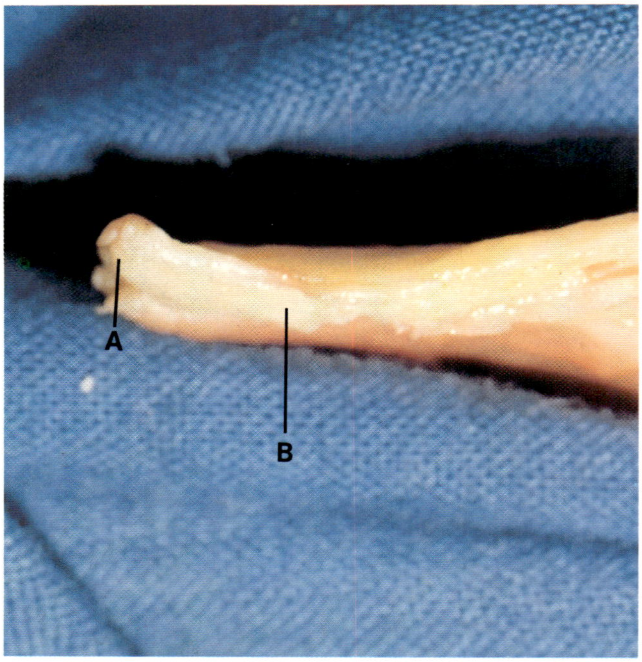

Plate 2-12. Nasal bones. *A,* Curved nasal bone. *B,* Pivot point for rocker deformity.

The skin and mucosa of the nose also provide support for the tip. With thicker-skinned individuals, this support may be considerable (Plate 2-6, *E*).

The sesamoid cartilages located between the lateral crura and pyriform aperture provide some support for the lateral legs of the tripod (Plate 2-6, *E*).

Finally, it should be said that most of the tip is suspended, either directly or indirectly, from the septum. Caudally, the septum helps determine the position of the tip complex. It fits tongue-in-groove fashion between the two lower lateral cartilages (Plate 2-7, C). If the septal cartilage is deformed, has slipped off the spine, or if the spine-cartilage complex is off the midline, it must be straightened.

Mid-nose

The mid-nose is composed of the upper lateral cartilages and their septal platform (Plate 2-8).

Framework

The upper lateral cartilages are triangular in shape. Their bases are laid along the septum, and their apices connect to the pyriform aperture. The mid-nose portion of the dorsal septum broadens to form a platform for the upper lateral cartilages. If the septum is deviated, so will be the upper lateral cartilages and, therefore, the mid-nose. The anterior septal angle is formed by the junction of dorsal and caudal septum. Its curve downward (inferiorly and posteriorly) helps establish the important supratip dip. This dip breaks up the straight line appearance of the dorsum, and is aesthetically pleasing.

The mid-nose is the area where the "pollybeak" deformity arises. In addition to excess soft tissue or scar, a "pollybeak" may consist of mid-nose septum, upper lateral cartilage, or even lower lateral cartilage that is too anterior relative to the nasal domes. This might be caused by not removing enough cartilage. It may also be caused by destroying enough tip support to allow the tip to drop postoperatively.

Support

The septal platform provides essential medial support for the upper lateral cartilage (Plates 2-8 and 2-9). Lateral support for the upper lateral cartilage is provided by a thick, firm, ligamentous attachment between the apex of the upper lateral cartilage and the pyriform aperture (Plate 2-9, *A*). This support structure is crucial because it provides for the width of the angle that describes a critical area of respiration: the internal nasal valve. This valve is located at the junction of the caudal upper lateral cartilage with the septum. If the internal valve's supporting ligament is destroyed by lateral osteotomy, it can narrow the valve and impair respiration. By beginning the osteotomy more anteriorly and superiorly, this ligament may be spared.

Superiorly, the upper lateral cartilage runs beneath the nasal bones for about a centimeter, and is held fast to the bone by a fibrous attachment (Plate 2-9, C). This attachment must be held inviolate as damage here is irreparable. Disturbing the integrity of this ligament may cause the upper lateral cartilage to be depressed into the nose on inspiration, or to actually fall into the nose if its other supports are disturbed during rhinoplasty.

Bony Vault

The bony vault is composed of the paired nasal bones, frontal processes of the maxilla, and nasal spine of the frontal bone (Plate 2-10).

Framework

The nasal bones run from a midline suture where they meet the thin bony septum and underlying nasal spine to the sutures connecting them with the frontal processes of the maxilla. They are narrow at their glabellar root and widen as they approach the pyriform aperture. The nasal bones may be gently or acutely curved along their horizontal (short) axes. If very curved, intermediate osteotomies may be required to adequately narrow the nose. These is usually no need to carry any osteotomy into the nasal root, as narrowing here is rarely necessary.

The nasal bones themselves are thick and strong at the root (Plate 2-11) and thin and fragile at the pyriform aperture. Each bone describes a gentle S shape along its vertical (long) dimension. For these two reasons, as well as the fact that the root is already narrow, osteotomy should avoid the nasion area. This thick bone is difficult to infracture, cannot be narrowed much because its width prevents it, and when coupled with the curve of the nasal bone, can lead to the *rocker deformity*—the rocking of the nasal bone on its medial support after osteotomy (Plate 2-12).

The bones of the frontal processes of the maxilla are much thicker than those of the nasal bones. The frontal processes also extend more laterally than the nasal bones (see Plate 2-10). Osteotomies must be carried into these thick bones to satisfactorily narrow the nose.

Support

Support is just as critical for the nasal bones as for any other nasal structure. The thick, heavy nasal spine of the frontal bone provides medial support for the nasal bones. Lateral support is, of course, provided by the maxilla. Minimal support is provided by the thin, fragile, bony septum.

After medial osteotomy or transverse back fracture, the important support given by the spine is lost. Lateral osteotomies destroy the maxillary support. At times, it may be very helpful to "greenstick" fractures (keep them incomplete) as some support may thus be maintained. Use of the sutures as "hinge areas" may also allow increased support. It may be possible to spare medial or intermediate osteotomies by using the lateral (nasomaxillary) or medial (nasoseptal) hinges to narrow the nose and maintain support.

Although the thin bony septum only provides a modicum of support for the nose, a deviated dorsal bony septum can prevent appropriate and symmetrical infracture of the nasal bones. If the bony septum has internal deformities that cannot be straightened, it may be lowered (e.g., with a gouge) below the level of the dorsal aspect of the nasal bones as it provides little significant support.

When medial and lateral osteotomies are completed, all bony support for the nasal bones may be temporarily lost. It is then especially crucial to maintain soft tissue support for the nasal bones. This support consists of the periosteal attachments to the superficial aspect of the bones, and the mucosal attachments to the deep aspect. Thus, it is important to limit any undermining of the periosteum and to keep the nasal mucosal lining intact.

3

Preoperative Evaluation

Walter E. Berman

Asymmetries of the Nose and Face

In discussing rhinoplasty surgery with the patient during a preoperative evaluation, it is very important that facial asymmetries be mentioned. As we all know, placing a nose exactly in the middle of an asymmetrical face will exaggerate various disproportions of the other facial features. The surgeon must recognize this and the patient must be made aware of it.

I have found it invaluable to take Polaroid photographs (seen in one minute) at the time of my first meeting with the patient. A dark eyebrow pencil, used on the photo, readily shows what tissues are to be removed or straightened. A pink eyebrow pencil shows what tissues are to be added. At this time, asymmetries of the face and nose can be pointed out and their consequences explained to the patient (Fig. 3-1). A computerized analysis may also be used in a similar fashion.

Culture and Individual Preference

It is also necessary to delve into the patient's background and culture to determine what the patient will find most acceptable. All surgical changes that are anticipated must be charted and shown to the patient. I do this at two different times before the surgical procedure. This is obviously important from a medical-legal standpoint, but it is more important from the standpoint of the doctor-patient relationship.

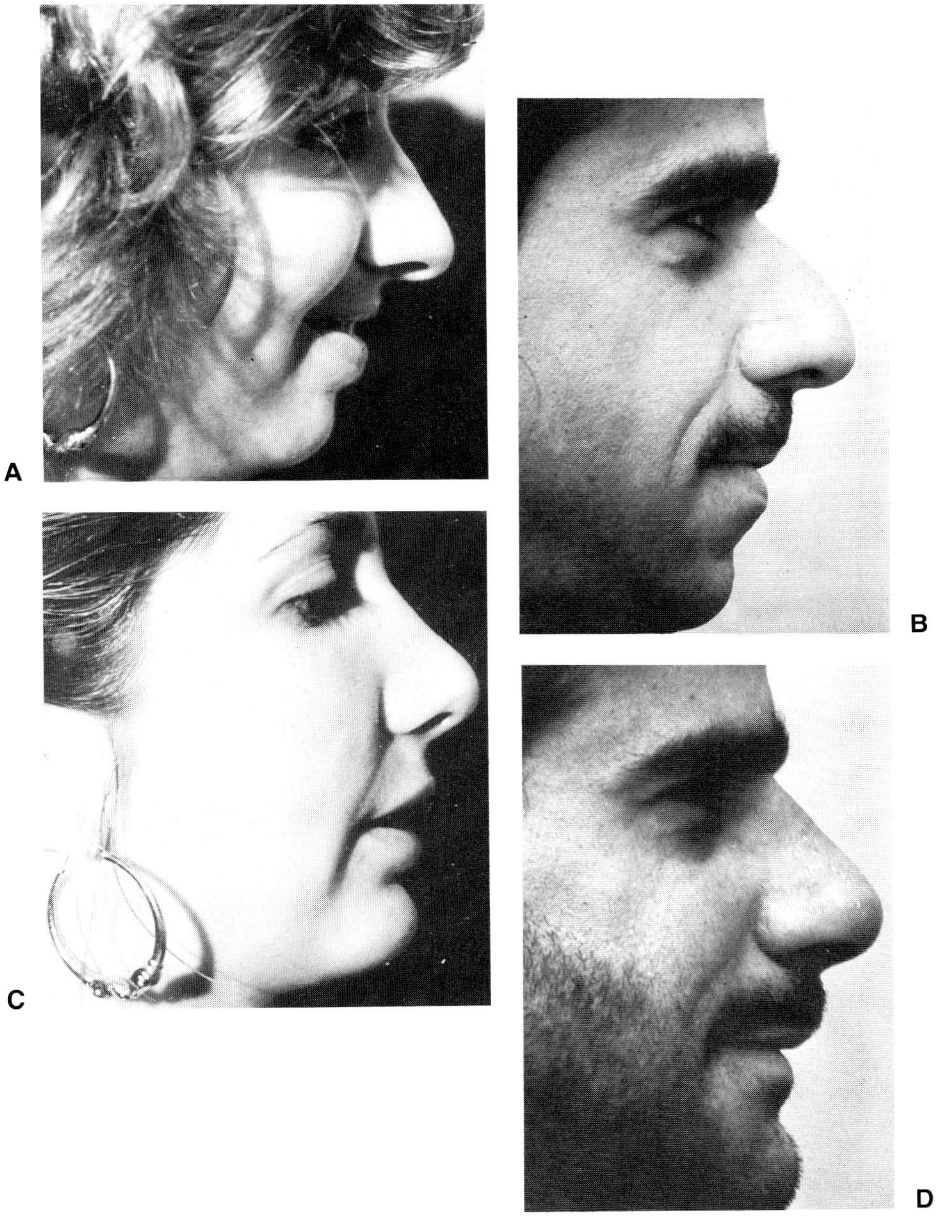

Fig. 3-1. A and B, Preoperative and C and D, postoperative photos showing the necessity of balancing the face with a chin implant.

Anatomy of the Nasal Tip

Much can be learned about the nasal tip before surgical intervention takes place. The physician's use of his two thumbs placed superiorly and inferiorly to the lower lateral cartilage while gentle pressure is exerted on this cartilage will delineate the width of the cartilage and provide him with some idea of the cartilage's thickness and firmness. The firmer the cartilage, the thicker it is.

Any bifidity of the nasal tip can be further tested with pressure between thumb and forefinger on the nasal tip. If the two domes come together readily, there is interdomal fat. If they do not, there are very strong cartilages in that region.

Fig. 3-2. Testing for a hard or soft central segment. (From Berman, WE: Rhinoplasty, ed 2, Washington DC, 1984, American Academy of Otolaryngology-Head and Neck Surgery Foundation, Inc.)

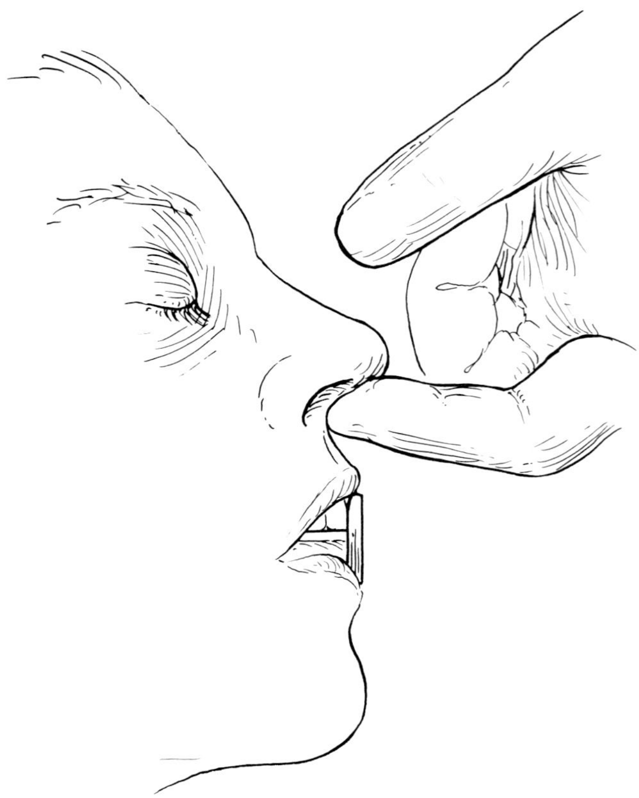

Skin Thickness

An example of this hypothesis is when there is very thick skin overlying the nasal tip. Little cartilaginous resistance is felt, so the chances of achieving an optimal tip result are fewer than in the case of thinner skin. Thick nasal tip skin usually manifests thin cartilage. Therefore, less visible changes can be expected with thicker nasal tip skin.

Length of the Nose

One of the most important considerations when planning this surgical procedure is determining if there is a hard or soft central segment. Gentle digital pressure on the columella in a superior direction will either meet with firm or soft resistance (Fig. 3-2). In a long nose with firm resistance, the classical procedure of removing cartilage from the inferior aspect of the quadrilateral cartilage works well for shortening the nose. When there is a soft central segment, particularly with heavy skin, removing the same cartilage may result in a retracted columella (Fig. 3-3). Therefore, other means of shortening or rotating the nasal tip must be used (see secondary rotation).

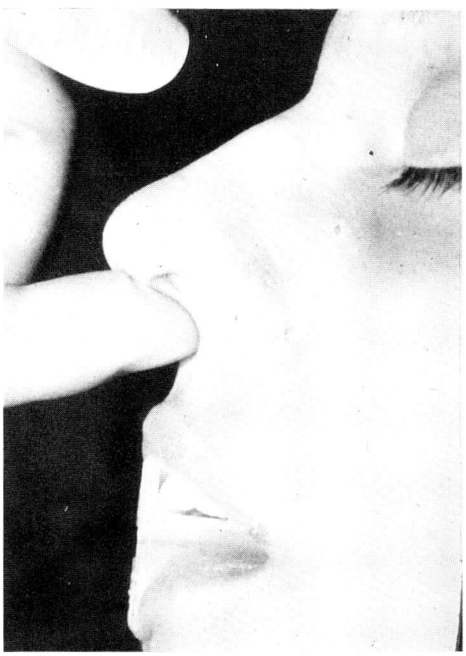

Fig. 3-3. Soft central segment. Shortening should only be done through a lateral approach as with a secondary rotation procedure.

Evaluation

Tip Support Structures

Weak tip support is evident when the forefinger exerts pressure in a posterior direction above the nasal spine. A weak tip will drop towards the lip. This will alert the surgeon that some type of compensatory procedure should be done to protect that tip support during the rhinoplasty, e.g., placement of permanent sutures, grafts, etc.

Nasal Septum

Careful examination of the nasal septum, both cartilaginous and bony, must be done (Fig. 3-4). Since we frequently narrow the external framework of the nose during a rhinoplastic procedure, even a rather moderate deviation may cause postoperative breathing problems. Explicit notes on the septal problem will make for a more efficient septoplasty.

Turbinates

Enlargements of the inferior turbinates should be noted by the examiner and told to the patient. Not only should they be reduced in size and fractured laterally, but the patient must be informed that future turbinate hypertrophy might occur.

Nasal Base

When a wide nasal base is evident, pressure between the thumb and forefinger is used to narrow the base clinically. The degree of narrowing can be determined with the patient observing the changes in a mirror. I have found this very helpful in determining what the patient is trying to achieve. This will be discussed in greater detail later in Chapter 18.

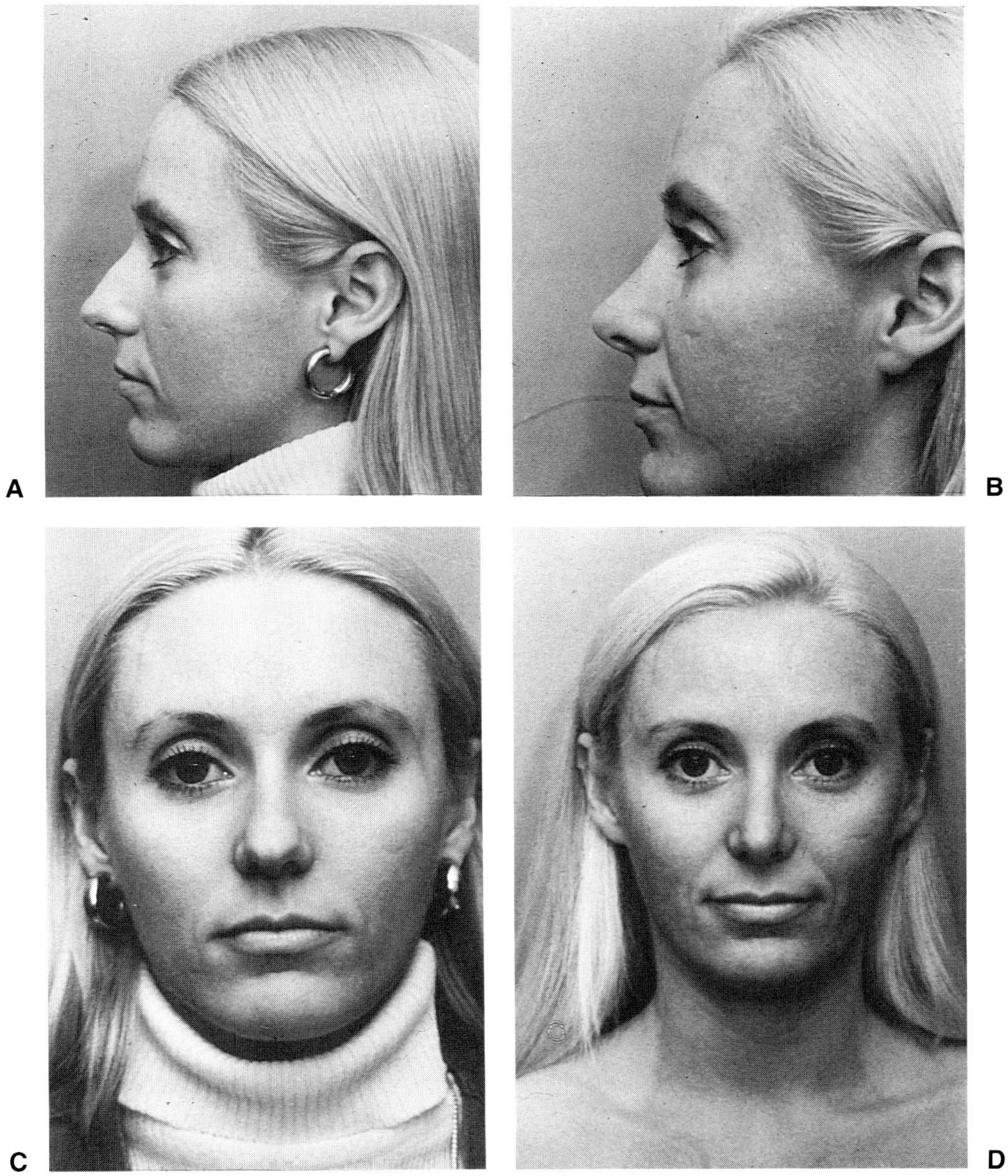

Fig. 3-4. Pre- and postoperative; a high anterior composed of bone and cartilage with a wide nasal tip. **A,** Preoperative side view. **B,** Postoperative side view. **C,** Preoperative frontal view. **D,** Postoperative frontal view.

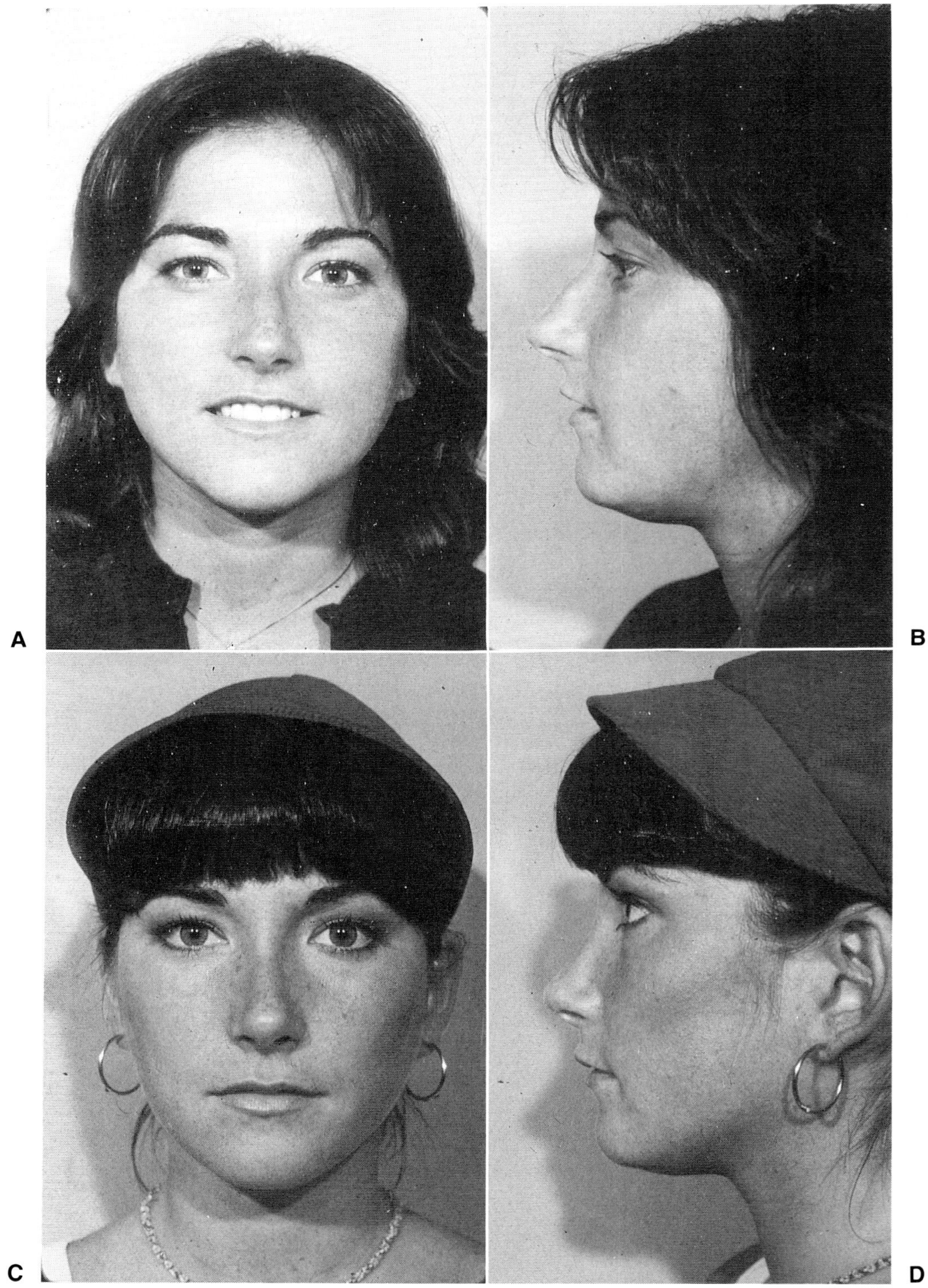

Fig. 3-5. **A** and **B**, Preoperative: irregular anterior following fractures. **C** and **D**, Postoperative: reduction of nasal fractures and rasping anterior.

Nasal Pyramid

When irregularities are felt on the anterior or lateral surfaces of the nasal bones and nasomaxillary processes, it is probable that trauma has taken place (Fig. 3-5). Often, the patient has no history of such trauma. This knowledge alerts the surgeon to the possibility that osteotomies may not fracture as desired or as expected in a nontraumatized nose. The suture line between the nasal bone and the nasomaxillary process may be used as a "hinge" in the nontraumatized nose of a person under the age of 40 (Fig. 3-6). This procedure is useful when there is a wide nasal pyramid without a bony hump. The lateral osteotomy is performed low on the face of the maxilla. This type of infracturing with a lateral osteotomy may not be possible if the nasal framework has been previously traumatized. This is an elegant technique in that it reduces surgical trauma to the anterior nose.

Prejudgment of the lateral osteotomy depends on how far the lateral cut should be made with the osteotome. Most people's noses have a thin root, which often widens in a more inferior or caudal direction. Therefore a partial osteotomy is all that is necessary rather than carrying the predetermined fracture farther superiorly than is warranted.

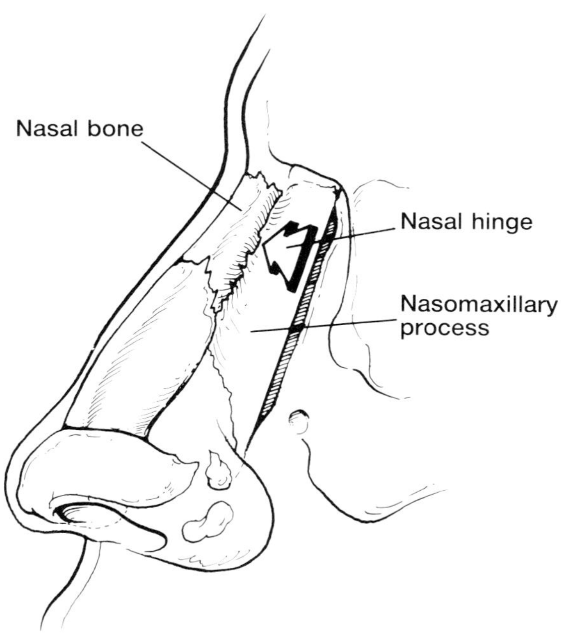

Fig. 3-6. Use of the suture line between the nasal bone and the nasal process of the maxilla as a "hinge." (From Rees TD, Baker DC, and Tabbal N: Rhinoplasty: problems and controversies: a discussion with the experts, St. Louis, 1988, The CV Mosby Co.)

4

Psychological Aspects of Rhinoplasty

Mary Ruth Wright

Rhinoplasty, probably the most intriguing of all cosmetic procedures, involves far more than restoring, repairing, and enhancing one's appearance. It alters one of the most symbolic structures of the body, the nose. Because of this important focus, a rhinoplasty can revive early identity conflicts, disturb a somatic fixation, and even cause a patient to react to his surgeon in a hostile or litigious manner. However, we must not throw up our hands in despair because once a problem is recognized, it usually can be controlled.

In terms of patient satisfaction, rhinoplasty runs a close second to rhytidectomy.[4] However, the grounds for satisfaction all too often are an enigma to the aesthetic surgeon. Although one patient might be happy with a minor improvement, or even with what might be termed an unsatisfactory result, another patient might be dissatisfied or even distressed with what might be viewed as a dramatic improvement in appearance. It is my premise that the unpredictable reactions to rhinoplasty surgery are most often caused by emotional factors. Thus, in this chapter, I will discuss the psychological manifestations of rhinoplasty, focusing on one question: why is the rhinoplasty patient more of a psychological risk than other surgery patients?

Modern technological advancements and changes in attitude toward cosmetic surgery have caused aesthetic surgery to rise in popularity and to become an accepted medical specialty. However these very advancements have brought to light the vicissitudes of psychological problems. Outstanding studies have observed more emotional sequelae following rhinoplasty surgery than other surgery.[8,9,10,16] Furthermore, studies have noted that the male rhinoplasty patient demonstrates more psychopathology than his female counterpart.[8,9,10,15] This latter finding is especially important as cosmetic surgery is no longer limited largely to women. Men are also seeking cosmetic surgery and are open about it. Although formerly only 2% to 4% of cosmetic patients were male, Goldwyn[10] in 1981 defined the female majority as 85%. In a more recent poll conducted in 1986 by Cash, Winstead, and Janda[5], 45% of the women interviewed indicated that they would have cosmetic surgery while 33% of the males stated that they would consider it.

Most authorities agree that the preponderance of female cosmetic patients stems from cultural, social, and psychological factors. Goldwyn [10] states that "our culture places a higher value on the attractive appearance of the woman than of the man; and the woman, deprived of many sources of gratification available to the man, has learned to use and value her body consciously and unconsciously to please herself and other." Kurtz[18] points out that women have a clearer body concept than men, a greater awareness of their physical appearance, and a more articulated notion of what they do and do not want from surgery. Kurtz also notes that a man is often more aware of his wife's aging than of his own and is quite critical of his wife's surgical results. Prosen and Prosen [22] explain this phenomenon in terms of psychoanalytical theory by stating that the man, who is looking for the idealized woman—his mother—in his wife, will never be satisfied with the results of his wife's cosmetic surgery. Men, society, and industry have reinforced the female's focus on physical appearance; however, this concentration is changing as sex roles become less differentiated.

As the incidence of rhinoplasty surgery increases for both sexes, the surgeon's task is becoming more complex. Not only must he defferentiate the male and female motivation for surgery, he must also be aware of the psychological dynamics that influence either or both sexes.

Psychological Dynamics

Before discussing the psychological dynamics that may cause the rhinoplasty patient to be more unstable than other surgery patients, I want to point out that the majority of rhinoplasty patients are happy with their surgical results. Also, from a practical point of view, if we did not operate on patients with psychological problems, we would not operate on many patients.

The Johns Hopkins Group[15,16] relates the psychological instability of a rhinoplasty patient to an identity conflict. The group bases its theory on the belief that early in life a child identifies with one of his parents, and focuses this identification on the parental nose. Later, usually as an adolescent, the child has ambivalent feelings about breaking this identification. For example, a male may identify with his father and, unconsciously focus this identification on his father's nose. Later, when growing up, he may want to disassociate himself from his father but not want to lose his masculine symbol of identity. Likewise, he may have ambivalent feelings about his identification with his mother, and when these conflicting feelings are expressed, he may want to rid himself of a primitive rage against his mother, but not want to give up the pleasurable, erotic feelings that accompany the rage. In order to resolve his conflict, he may want to relieve his disturbing symptoms without wanting to disturb his family symbol. These identification conflicts are usually resolved during adolescence, but they can be repressed and reactivated later in life. Jacobson, Edgerton et. al.[15] associate these identity conflicts primarily with the male patient, but other authorities relate them to both sexes.[8,10,17]

Goldwyn[10] agrees with the Hopkins Group[15] that the basic problem is one of sexual identity and that this problem is more prominent in the male because of the midline protruding structure of the nose and its sexual symbolic association. He advises the surgeon to be wary of the older neurotic male who is afraid to face natural aging, the male who is in a crisis situation, the male who suffers from unresolved grief, and the male who is seeing a psychiatrist or has a psychiatric history. Finally, Goldwyn warns the surgeon against the male who is hostile during the initial interview, stating that despite the surgical results, the hostile patient is most likely to sue the surgeon.

Knorr[17] notes a loss of identity in the female rhinoplasty patient and expounds on how the dissatisfied female patient often seeks additional surgery on the grounds that the surgeon has done too much, made too big a change or not corrected a basic problem such as a breathing difficulty. He describes how the patient's need for additional surgery can lead to surgical addiction—an insatiable desire for surgery. He warns the surgeon against the patient, male or female, who did not dislike his or her nose as a teenager and the patient who shows a hostile attitude toward the surgeon. Knorr describes the surgeon's reaction to a rhinoplasty patient as "The Exhausted Surgeon's Syndrome".

In his study of 5,019 rhinoplasty cases, Bruck[3] found that the patient's acceptance of a physical change was inversely related to his or her age. He found that "type changing," i.e., nasal changes that alter the appearance of the entire face, are usually unacceptable in older rhinoplasty patients, especially those of a higher economic and social status. Bruck had a cut-off age of 35 for "type changing," based on his theory that older patients do not tolerate change well.

Gifford[8] describes how young girls who have rhinoplasties with their mothers' consent, or at their suggestion, usually are quite satisfied with the results and often even gain personality functioning. He attributes this positive reaction to a mother and daughter alliance, possible against the father, and interprets it as a "magical gift" from a mother with "narcissistic power", a gift that can be used to obtain admiration and to control men.

Gifford defines the risk patient as a person who attributes a lifelong history of inadequacies to a "single physical defect," who continually seeks additional surgery, and who has a blaming, or in extreme cases, paranoid or persecutory attitude toward doctors. He stresses the danger of operating on a patient who has a fixation on a visible body part. Gifford's theory is that the fixation on a body part may psychologically serve the patient, i.e., as representing a reason for failure or as a focus for anxiety. If this is the case, when a surgeon operates on and alters the somatic focus, he may unwittingly disturb the patient's focus for failures, and that consequently the surgeon may receive the patient's resentment and persecutory attitude that previously was focused on the body part. Although he acknowledges more unfavorable results in the male patient, Gifford does not stress the sex differences as much as the basic personality structure of the patient. He especially warns the surgeon against the patient who has had "previous unsuccessful cosmetic operations," the patient who has had "disappointing experiences with previous physicians," and the patient who is currently in a crisis or state of bereavement.

Gifford's [8] evaluation or prognosis of the male homosexual patient differs from those of other surgeons in that Gifford feels that homosexuals are most likely to be dissatisfied with or even resentful of their surgery. Here I argue with Gifford as I think that he failed to differentiate between the patient who acknowledges his homosexuality and the patient who denies it. It is my opinion that the man who owns up to his homosexuality tends to know what he wants, such as a more feminine nose, and is usually satisfied with the surgical results, while the man who is in conflict about his sexuality or has latent homosexual tendencies is not certain what he wants and therefore is more likely to be dissatisfied.

Goldwyn,[10] whom I quoted previously, agrees with Gifford[8] that young adolescent girls are usually quite happy with the results of their rhinoplasty, but advises the surgeon to be conservative when operating on the older woman, explaining that "the older woman usually does not want a significant change in the appearance of her nose, because after several decades she has grown accustomed to her face." For lack of a better definition of the "older woman," I shall use Bruck's[3] cut-off age of 35.

Goin and Goin[9] stress the sexual symbolism of both the male and female nose, and point out that a delusion about the nose is a contraindication to rhinoplasty and may cause major psychological decompensation following surgery. For example, I recently saw a male rhinoplasty patient who decompensated following a rhinoplasty and was hospitalized with the diagnosis of psychosis. Despite the favorable results of his rhinoplasty, he felt that this operative procedure had caused his career to crater. Diagnostically, Goin and Goin relate psychological symptoms such as shyness, reclusiveness, aloofness, and a strange feeling about one's body to schizophrenic processes. An unexplained finding of Goin and Goin is that "Jewish men may be a lower risk than their non-Jewish counterparts."

In his research on body image Schilder[23] focuses on the fear of losing a body part, particularly an appendage. Based on this premise, he implies that the male penis-nose association engenders more fear than the female vagina-nose association. Schilder points out how surgery can resurrect early childhood fears about castration, and may inadvertently cause the rage and resentment that long ago was directed at the parent to be directed toward the surgeon.

Lynn and Goldman[19] work on the assumption that all cosmetic patients are "in effect, psychiatric patients." They find that the most disturbed patients are males who concentrated on the nose. To describe this exaggerated nasal focus, they coined the term *psychiatric syndrome of the rhinoplasty patient*. Lynn and Goldman, like Goin and Goin,[9] relate many of the disturbing psychological symptoms of the rhinoplasty patient to basic schizophrenic processes.

MacGregor,[20] a pioneer in psychosexual studies, documents the sexual symbolism of the nose and warns the surgeon about the patient who attempts to hide his desire for appearance improvement by saying that he wants a rhinoplasty for reasons such as nose bleeding, difficulty in breathing, or a traumatic injury.

In studying the psychological aspects of the rhinoplasty patient, only Hay[11,12] and Wright and Wright[28] used control groups. Both Hay and the Wrights found that the rhinoplasty group, both male and female, were more disturbed than the control group. The Wrights found specific characteristics associated with the rhinoplasty patient. Although these patients tended to be interesting, intelligent, likable, imaginative, enthusiastic, and energetic, and they were also prone to be restless, impulsive, immature, self-critical, and self-centered. As far as psychic pathology goes, both Hay and the Wrights found that there was a direct correlation between the personality disorder category of mental disorders and the rhinoplasty patient. The Wrights' study indicated that the patient with a personality disorder is most likely to sue his surgeon for medical malpractive. Patients with personality disorders tend to act out, to be manipulative, to have their pleasure at the expense of others, to disregard social mores, and to be lacking in emotional depth.

In his study of 45 rhinoplasty patients Hay[11] observes that the male patients are more psychologically disturbed than the female group, but he does not find the difference to be statistically significant. Most important, Hay does not find the degree of deformity to be a relevant factor in the patient's satisfaction with the postoperative outcome. Other studies support this finding.[8,9,16] Also, Hay[12] does not find, as the Hopkins' group does,[16] a strong identification with the parental nose. In the Wrights' study of 90 rhinoplasty patients,[28] the 25 patients who were re-evaluated 18 to 25 months postoperatively showed an improvement in the psychological clinical scales. However, this improvement was not of statistical significance. Only one patient in the Wrights' group, a single male with schizophrenic symptoms, had a psychotic break following surgery.

Freud's outstanding work in the early 1900s provides the basis for the current awareness of the prevalence of emotional disturbances in the rhinoplasty patient. Freud[7] was probably the first physician to recognize the sexual symbolism of the nose. From a broader context, i.e., a fixation on any visible body part, Freud in his classic study, "The Wolfman"[25] portrayed how a surgeon who removed a mole from a man's face later received the patient's blame, hostility, and accusations.

Later, based on Freud's work, Updegraff, a plastic surgeon, and Menninger, a psychiatrist, (1934)[26] published case studies describing how unconscious fears and wishes, (for example, of castration) can be acted out in surgery. They also reveal how the surgeon, especially the plastic surgeon, can become the recipient of the patient's latent hostility, resentment, and even death wish. Helen Deutsch[6] extends Freud's theory by showing that all patients have separation anxiety as well as castration fears.

Last, and most profound, two of the four recorded acts of homicide that I have reviewed, where the patient postoperatively murdered his surgeon, were performed by male rhinoplasty patients. Dissatisfied with the results of surgery, one rhinoplasty patient killed his surgeon, a Dr. Alexander,[13] which was the first recorded case. The second rhinoplasty patient killed Dr. Vaquez Anon,[14] a Spanish surgeon, after Dr. Anon's staff refused to let him see the surgeon following a rhinoplasty revision. The third assassin killed two Australian doctors after being accused of malingering a back injury.[21] (On autopsy the man did not have a back injury—proving the doctors "dead right.") In my opinion, these three patients were all paranoid schizophrenics. More important, two out of three of these assassins are rhinoplasty patients—a finding that smacks at the emotional stability of the rhinoplasty patient.

Summary of Findings

Authorities generally agree that the rhinoplasty patient is more unstable than other surgery patients, and that the male rhinoplasty patient is more unstable than the female patient. However, we must keep in mind that as cultural patterns change and male aesthetic surgery increases, we may see fewer disturbances in the male patient. In fact, Goldwyn[10] finds that in some cases the male is easier to please and not "as psychologically ill" as other studies[15] have reported. This observation raises the question: could the prominence of psychological disturbances in the male patient be because formerly society only sanctioned aesthetic surgery for the female, and only the psychologically disturbed male dared to have cosmetic surgery?

Still, we must go with what findings support. Summarizing observations from literature, four findings prevail: (1) The rhinoplasty patient, especially the male patient, is more psychologically disturbed than other surgery patients. (2) These psychological disturbances are usually long-term and tend to reflect an identity conflict or the somatic manifestation of a conflict. (3) The degree of deformity cannot be equated with postoperative satisfaction. (4) The surgeon often becomes the recipient of the patient's repressed hostility.

I have documented that rhinoplasty patients are more psychologically disturbed than other surgery patients. I have offered speculative theories as to why rhinoplasty patients may have more psychological manifestations or more emotional repercussions such as depression, hysteria or dissatisfaction, than other surgery patients. As to why the degree of deformity cannot be equated with postoperative satisfaction, the literature has little to say. However, we must remember that meaning comes from within, not from without. It is the patient's perception of the deformity, not its physical dimensions, that counts. As to the surgeon's vulnerable position, every aesthetic surgeon must realize that when he operates on the nose, he may unknowingly revive an early identity conflict or disturb or destroy a patient's somatic displacement, and consequently may become the recipient of the patient's hostility and blame.

Why the Nose

The question can only be answered by deductive theories. The nose is the most prominent midline protruding structure of the body. For the male, it is the landmark of masculine identity. For both sexes, it is a structure that has long played a part in celebratory and punitive rites. We are all familiar with the nose studded with diamonds, rings, or other jewels. We are also familiar with the punitive treatment of the woman "who strayed"—that is, cutting off her nose as punishment for her infidelity. Over time, the nose has been associated with character strengths or weaknesses. As Laurence Olivier is supposed to have said, "I don't know how to play a character until I know what kind of nose he has." The nose is composed of erectile tissue and is a sense organ that responds to fear, danger, and pleasure. It is the passageway for air—the maintenance of life. The nose is a natural site for somatic conversion. When performing a rhinoplasty, the surgeon is often faced with the difficult, sometimes impossible task of relieving disturbing symbolic symptoms without disturbing the meaningful symbol.

Recently, I saw a young maladjusted man who had a psychotic break following a rhinoplasty and two revisions. Postoperatively, he felt hostile toward the surgeon, blaming him for taking away his "Roman heritage," and later he sued him for medical malpractice. Actually, this man wanted the surgeon to relieve his ambivalent sexual feelings toward his mother who was openly seductive with him; he did not want the surgeon to mar what he thought of as his phallic symbol. This case study aptly describes the patient who has both a fixation and an identity crisis.

Counseling

Prevention is still the best treatment for psychological disturbances that may result from rhinoplasty surgery. Realizing that the rhinoplasty patient is a psychological risk, the surgeon must be aware that he requires thoughtful and careful counseling, both preoperatively and postoperatively. It is most important that the surgeon bear in mind that an understanding relationship between the surgeon and the patient is the best insurance against postoperative psychological complications and against litigation. Although the surgeon need not delve into the psychological dynamics of the disturbed rhinoplasty patient, he should accept that these psychological dynamics exist and are not just "strange Freudian concepts". It is possible to treat and respect psychic pathology without actually understanding its origin.

Psychopathological Conditions

Actually, the rhinoplasty surgeon must practice psychiatry as far as recognizing, not treating, psychic pathology. There are five psychopathological conditions that the surgeon needs to be able to recognize and differentiate: the psychoneurotic disorder, the psychotic disorder, the personality disorder, the polysurgical syndrome, and the decisional conflict. The first three, the neuroses, psychoses, and personality disorders are major psychogenic categories listed in the *Diagnostic and Statistical Manual of Mental Disorders.*[1] The polysurgical syndrome and decisional conflict are psychological disturbances that relate specifically to surgical cases.

A. The Psychoneurotic Patient

The *psychoneurotic patient* is characterized by his worry, anxiety, and somatic complaints. These symptoms serve the neurotic well, as they are his defenses against stress. With adequate counseling, the neurotic usually makes an excellent rhinoplasty patient. However, without such counseling, the neurotic is likely to become more anxious and miserable, and subsequently makes the surgeon miserable. It is well to remember that the neurotic can handle only a limited discussion about postoperative complications.

B. The Psychotic Patient

The *psychotic patient* does not have the capacity to meet the ordinary demands of life. One might say that the psychotic has given up struggling with the conflicts of life and has escaped to his own psychological island, free of stress. Since the psychotic patient may not have the emotional reserves to handle rhinoplasty surgery, psychiatric consultation is recommended as a preoperative procedure. However, it should be noted that the dangers of operating on a psychotic have been exaggerated. Studies have shown that the psychotic is often able to withstand cosmetic surgery, and in some cases, seems to gain psychological benefits from it.[4]

Schizophrenia is the most common category of psychotic disorders. The schizophrenic patient is recognized by his disorganized thoughts and flat emotional responses. He is not necessarily out of touch with reality, delusional, or hallucinatory; he is, however, unable to relate empathetically or display a genuine sense of humor. The most obvious symptom of the schizophrenic patient is his confusion, and the projection of this confusion is the key to diagnosing the schizophrenic patient. For example, if a surgeon feels unduly confused after interviewing a patient, he may have been interviewing a schizophrenic. Although the schizophrenic is not necessarily dangerous, most surgeons are uncomfortable relating to him, and therefore psychiatric consultation is recommended for any patient who reveals schizophrenic tendencies.

The paranoid schizophrenic patient is an exception to the above; he is a dangerous patient. The paranoid individual is characterized as one who is suspicious, feels persecuted, and is extremely concerned with himself. Any patient who exhibits paranoid tendencies should be referred to a psychiatrist. If, however, a surgeon unknowingly operates on a paranoid patient, he must remember that the paranoid patient requires meticulous counseling and frequent postoperative visits.

C. The Personality Disorder

The patient with a *personality disorder* has a different type of pathology from that associated with psychoneurosis and psychosis. He reveals his symptomatology in maladaptive behavior rather than in mental or emotional disturbances. Unfortunately, he is quite talented in disguising his inadequate personality and in persuading the surgeon to operate on him. However, to operate on a patient with a personality disorder under the guise of relieving his personality problem is a serious mistake, as surgery cannot mend what is missing from this patient's personality—the ability to feel deeply or sincerely. Personality disorders are manifested in infantile-narcissistic or manipulative-controlling behavior. Both types of patients seek control and shun responsibility. The patient with a personality disorder must be counseled in a different way from the neurotic or psychotic patient. The surgeon must maintain control, stick with the facts, and be alert to manipulative moves. As stated previously, it is the patient with a personality disorder who is most prone to suing his surgeon for medical malpractice.[28]

Secondary conditions can occur under any of the three major psychongenic conditions. I shall discuss three of these conditions: *depression, obsessive-compulsive tendencies* and *hysteric manifestations.*

D. The Depressed Patient

The *depressed patient* is recognized by his feelings of helplessness, hopelessness, and low self-esteem. Generally speaking, depression should be treated prior to cosmetic surgery. However, this axiom is somewhat paradoxical, because although surgery can exacerabate acute depression, it often seems to alleviate chronic depression.[9]

E. The Obsessive-Compulsive Patient

The *obsessive-compulsive patient* is recognized by his exaggerated use of rationalization, explanations, and justifications. He does not look his listener in the eye or listen to what he has to say. The obsessive-compulsive patient is not necessarily dangerous, but he will exhaust the surgeon with his logical and theoretical interpretations.

F. The Hysteric Patient

The *hysteric patient* is recognized by his somatization and flighty impulsive behavior. While he or she may not outrightly portray these attention-getting characteristics, his dramatization and physical symptoms are just too much. On the other hand, he does not necessarily portray these attention-seeking characteristics.

How does the surgeon determine whether secondary conditions are neurotic or psychotic? The distinction depends upon the degree of symptomatology and the patient's response to counseling. For example, the neurotic depressed patient will respond to reassurance while the psychotic depressed patient will become more depressed. The neurotic obsessive-compulsive can be reasoned with, while the psychotic obsessive-compulsive will become more argumentative and sophistic. The neurotic hysteric's symptoms often improve dramatically during counseling while the psychotic hysteric's symptoms become more manifest, sometimes even to the point of lapsing into a mild catatonic state.

G. The Polysurgical Syndrome

The *polysurgical syndrome* describes the surgical addict who has an insatiable desire for surgery. The surgical addict has usually suffered childhood abuse and is full of feelings of persecution and guilt. He demands surgery and usually gets it, but the gratifications of surgery are short lived. The surgical addict has a history of failures in work, marriage, and luck, and portrays an outlook of futility. His psychic pain is deeper than that of the narcissistic patient and more prolonged than that of the hysteric patient. Surgery is a fantasy to the surgical addict, a fantasy that he hopes will resolve his deep psychic conflicts, but alas, when the fantasy does not resolve his psychic conflicts, the patient becomes more desperate and demands more surgery. It is every surgeon's responsibility to recognize and resist the addict's pleas for surgery.

H. The Decisional Conflict

The *decisional conflict* usually results from one of two causes: (1) a disagreement concerning the decision for surgery, as when a wife desires a rhinoplasty and her husband opposes it, or (2) a lack of understanding about who is to be the beneficiary of the surgery, as when a wife unknowingly requests surgery for herself in order to satisfy her husband's needs or to regain his affection. Since both of these attempts usually have disastrous results, decisional conflicts must be exposed and resolved prior to surgery.

Although I do not routinely recommend psychiatric or psychological consultation for the rhinoplasty patient, I do recommend it for any patient who reveals disturbing psychological symptoms or for any patient with whom the surgeon feels intuitively uncomfortable. Actually, being aware of feeling intuitively uncomfortable is the most important diagnostic symptom of psychic pathology. "Being aware" of feeling uncomfortable is the surgeon's primary indication of disturbing psychopathology.

Patient Rejection

It is generally agreed that there are four criteria for refusing a patient rhinoplasty surgery: (1) The presence of a delusional fixation on a body part; (2) The existence of paranoid thoughts; (3) A history of surgical insatiability; and (4) A strong suggestion of malingerering.

Patients with delusional fexations and patients with paranoid thoughts do not have the emotional reserve to withstand cosmetic surgery. They are likely to decompensate or, as described in psychological terms, to have a "psychotic break" postsurgically—i.e. to depart from reality, and consequently, to bring harm to themselves or to their surgeon. Surgery is a fantasy for the surgical addict and it may destroy his meager means of coping with his shaky life and encourage him to seek repetitive surgery. The malingerer, who overplays his hand by pretending to be a legitimate candidate presurgically, is quick to turn on his surgeon after surgery, either refusing to pay him or suing him for monetary gains. Although the patient with a personality disorder is also prone to sue his surgeon, he should not be rejected outright, but his manipulative ways must be recognized and controlled preoperatively.

The litigious patient haunts every experienced rhinoplasty surgeon. Still, it is wise to remember that most patients come to their doctor for help, not with the intention of suing him. It is my belief that most malpractice suits get started in the middle of the doctor-patient relationship. What happens? Something goes wrong and the patient becomes emotional and the surgeon reacts defensively. What can the surgeon do? First, he must be secure enough, or appear to be, so as not to take the patient's hostility personally. Second, he must refrain from reasoning or arguing with the patient. Third, he must try to understand the patient and make himself understood by the patient. An understanding patient will not sue his surgeon. Even if the patient's point of view is not legitimate, the surgeon must refrain from reacting emotionally or defensively. The surgeon must rely on his intuitive judgement to recognize the patient's character flaw, and if he missed diagnosing it before surgery, he may have to rely on his malpractice insurance or on the jury. It is comforting to remember that most patients are still on the doctor's side and that the jury is made up of the public, your patients.

In summary, some specific danger signs or symptoms that must be recognized or controlled in the rhinoplasty patient are as follows:

- A fear of the loss of a defect that has served a long-standing defensive purpose.

- An identity or sexual conflict.
- A tendency to hide the desire for surgery behind other physical reasons.
- Low self-esteem and a history of feeling inadequate in relationships.
- Unresolved grief or a crisis situation.
- A history of failures or an outlook of futility.
- Being unmarried or homosexual.
- Being older or concerned about aging.
- A sudden dislike for the nose that was not present during adolescence.
- A accusatory attitude toward authority.
- A history of seeing many doctors and of being dissatisfied with them.
- A pushy or desperate approach toward the surgeon.
- A tendency to flatter the surgeon and persuade him to be the "rescuer".
- A resistance to psychiatric consultation.

The Aftermath

It should be pointed out that psychological symptoms per so do not predict a poor psychological prognosis.[9,15,28] In fact, some studies[10,16] have observed an improvement in personality functioning in many of their postsurgical rhinoplasty patients. Also, it has been noted that cosmetic patients seem to develop fewer emotional sequelae than other surgical cases.[8] Finally, let us not forget that the healthy rhinoplasty patient does exist and is usually quite satisfied and gratified with the results of surgery.

As to patient dissatisfaction, which will occur despite astute counseling, evaluation, and surgery, research lists three primary causes: 1) a physical complication or disappointment with the anatomical change, 2) an unrealistic psychological expectations, and 3) a lack of rapport between the surgeon and the patients.[2]

A. Physical Complications

A *physical complication* is a shock to the rhinoplasty patient, because no matter how well he has been counseled, he does not expect such a development.[9] Thus a complication is especially distressing to the rhinoplasty patient and may even cause him to feel guilty about having had cosmetic surgery. When a complication occurs, the surgeon must face and handle his own feelings of disappointment and realize that complications are not synonymous with mistakes. In most cases, physical complications can usually be handled quite smoothly after the surgeon has resolved his own feelings of disappointment and alleviated the patient's emotional reactions.

B. Unrealistic Expectations

Unrealistic expectations cannot be dealt with directly. If the surgeon missed handling this situation prior to surgery, postsurgically he must accept the patient's right to have had unrealistic expectations and leave the responsibility of resolving them to the patient. Listening to the patient is the best treatment for patient dissatisfaction. Listening does not necessarily mean agreeing with the patient, but it does mean that you, the surgeon, are willing to pay credence to the patient's pain—be it physical or psychic. As Shakespeare said in Macbeth,[24] "Therein the patient must minister to himself." Most patients who have complications resulting from unrealistic expectations do not continue to be unhappy, nor do they tend to decompensate emotionally. They do require numerous postoperative visits over an extended period of time, which can last from one to five years.

C. Lack of Rapport

Lack of rapport has been documented as the major cause of medical malpractice suits; therefore, it is essential that the cosmetic surgeon establish rapport with the patient. Although there is no way to tell one how to establish rapport, I recommend that the surgeon listen sensitively as well as intellectually. More importantly, the surgeon must remember to respond affirmatively rather than defensively. Patients do not want facts and figures—they want you to care and stand by. Rapport derives from care, concern, and awareness. It is an active, not a passive process.

The most important factor for the surgeon to remember about patient dissatisfaction with the result of any cosmetic procedure is that most dissatisfactions are resolved with time and return visits.[27] This means that you the surgeon must stand by until dissatisfactions are resolved, bearing in mind that the patient's primary fear is desertion.

D. Conclusion

Rhinoplasty patients have a hidden psychological agenda that can not be described in definitive terms. However, the astute cosmetic surgeon can recognize and control most psychological manifestations and alleviate most patient dissatisfaction.

Presently we must accept that the rhinoplasty patient represents a psychological risk. Still I recommend that this condition be viewed as a challenge—as a fascinating area to be explored rather than as an inevitable danger. After all, it is the mystery of rhinoplasty that makes it the most intriguing and precarious specialty of cosmetic surgery.

REFERENCES

1. Diagnostic and statistical manual of mental disorders, ed 4, Washington DC, American Psychiatric Association, 1987.
2. Baker TJ: Patient selection and psychological evaluation. In Clinics in plastic surgery: the aging face. Philadelphia, 1978, WB Saunders Co.
3. Bruck HC: Corrective rhinoplasty, Arch Otolaryngol 97:441-446, 1973.
4. Cash TF and Horton CE: Aesthetic surgery: effects of rhinoplasty on social perception of patients by others, Plas Reconstr Surg 76(4):543-548, 1985.
5. Cash TF, Winstead BA, and Janda LH: The great american shape up, Psychol Today 30-37, April 1986.
6. Deutsch H: Some psychoanalytic observations in surgery, Psychosom Med 4:115, 1942.
7. Freud S: From the history of an infantile neurosis. In Strachey J, Freud A, Strachey A, et. al., editors: The standard edition of the complete works of Sigmund Freud, London, Hogarth Press and Institute of Psycho-Analysis, 1955, 17:8-122, 1918.
8. Gifford S: Cosmetic surgery and personality change: a review of some clinical observations. In Goldwyn RM, editor: The unfavorable results in plastic surgery: avoidance and treatment, Boston, 1972, Little, Brown & Co Inc.
9. Goin JM and Goin MK: Rhinoplasty. In Goin JM and Goin MK, editors: Changing the body psychological effects of plastic surgery. Baltimore, 1981, Williams and Wilkins.
10. Goldwyn RM: The patient and the plastic surgeon, Boston, 1981, Little, Brown & Co Inc.
11. Hay GG: Psychiatric aspects of cosmetic nasal operation, Br J Psychiatry 116:85-97, 1970.
12. Hay GG and Heather BB: Changes in psychometric test results following cosmetic nasal operation, Br J Psychiatry 122:89-90, 1973.
13. Editorial, Hazards of cosmetic surgery, Br Med J 1:381, 1967.
14. Hinderer UT: Dr. Vazquez Anon's last lesson, Aesthetic Plast Surg 2:375-382, 1978.
15. Jacobson WE, Edgerton MT, and Meyer E: Psychiatric evaluation of male patients seeking cosmetic surgery, Plast Reconstr Surg 26:356, 1960.
16. Jacobson WE, Meyer E, Edgerton MT, Canter A, and Slaughter R: Screening of rhinoplasty patients from the psychological point of view. Plast Reconstr Surg 28:279-281, 1961.
17. Knorr NJ: Feminine loss of identity in rhinoplasty, Arch Otolaryngol 96:11-15, 1972.
18. Krutz RM: Sex differences and variations in body attitudes, J Consult Clin Psychol 33:528-529, 1969.
19. Lynn L and Goldman IB: Psychiatric observations concerning rhinoplasty, Psychosom Med 11:307-315, 1949.
20. MacGregor FC and Shaffner B: Screening patients for nasal plastic operations: some sociological and psychiatric considerations, Psychosom Med 12(5):227-291, 1980.
21. Parker N: Malingering: a dangerous diagnosis, Med J Aust June 1:568-569, 1979.
22. Prosen H and Prosen M: The remembered mother and the fantasized mother: a crisis of middle age, Arch Gen Psychiatry 27:791-794, 1972.
23. Schilder P: The image and appearance of the human body, New York International Universities Press, New York, John Wiley & Son (ed.), 1950.
24. Shakespeare W: Macbeth, Act 5, Scene 3, line 37.
25. Sulloway FS, editor: Freud, Biologist of the Mind, New York, 1979, Basic Books, Inc.
26. Updegraff HD and Menninger RA: Some psychoanalytic aspects of plastic surgery, Am J Surg 3:554-558, 1934.
27. Wright MR: Management of patient dissatisfaction with results of cosmetic procedures, Arch Otolaryngol Head Neck Surg 106:466-471, 1980.
28. Wright MR and Wright WK: A psychological study of patients undergoing cosmetic surgery, Arch Otolaryngol 101:145-151, 1973.

5

Photography

Nathan E. Nachlas

Photographic documentation for the aesthetic surgeon is as critical as an accurate staging system is for the head and neck oncologist. Such documentation carries a sixfold purpose: First, a careful analysis of preoperative and postoperative photographs provides a critical *self-assessment* for the facial plastic surgeon. Second, it facilitates careful *preoperative planning* of the surgery. Third, photographs displayed in the operating room make it possible for the surgeon to *refer* to them during surgery. Fourth, any attempt to describe one's results to *colleagues and students* is greatly hindered if photographic documentation is not available. Fifth, in today's *medico-legal* climate, it is vital to be able to produce preoperative photographs for every patient undergoing cosmetic or reconstructive surgery. And finally, photographic documentation is useful for the patient who notices an asymmetry or unrelated defect only postoperatively.

The key to photographic success is reproducibility. The ability to take clear photographs at the same angles and with the same skin tones of patient at various stages in the clinical course is essential. Proper scientific journalism will result in preoperative and postoperative photographs under identical photographic conditions. We will outline our approach for rhinoplasty photography, and will include a brief discussion on choosing the right equipment for this.

When one is dealing with medical photography, a distinction must be made between portrait photography, which would include the preoperative and postoperative photographs as discussed above, and "action shots," the intraoperative pictures taken to demonstrate a particular technique. The optimal photographic setup for each is different.

Portrait Photography

Portrait photography is ideally performed in a "studio." This might involve a room specially designated for photographs (Fig. 5-1). If this is not feasible, any area of an office may be used. It is important, however, to provide an area where standardization in terms of distance and lighting is possible. The goal is to provide a photographic setup that is reliable. Although ideally the physician should personally obtain all photographs, this is often not practical, and the photographic setup should be easily understood by the office staff.

Camera Equipment

For versatility, it is suggested that a 35 mm SLR camera be chosen; many excellent ones are currently available. The camera body itself does not need to be elaborate, as the critical feature determining picture quality is the lens. A tripod with fixed legs that is adjustable in height enables the photographer to make the necessary adjustments for each patient with minimal maneuvering.

For facial photography, a long focal length lens (100 mm to 135 mm) is used to minimize distortion. Closer lenses introduce a *parallax* error because of the different angles made by different regions of the face with the lens. It is generally recommended that a patient-to-camera distance of 40 to 60 inches be used.[2]

Standardization of distances with floor markings for the chair and tripod is helpful. In addition, the same facial landmark must be used for focusing.

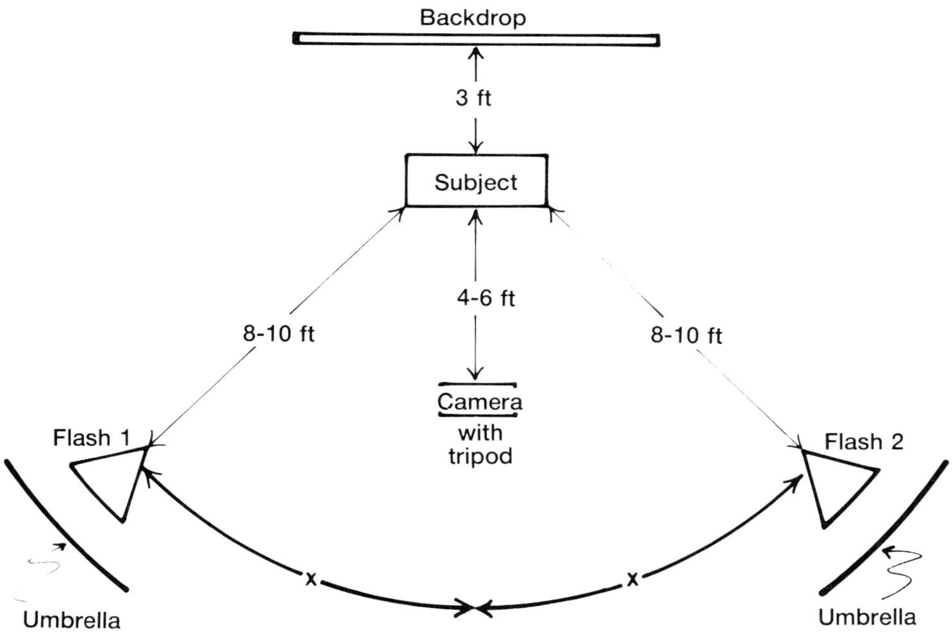

Fig. 5-1. Proposed photographic studio. There is no ideal arrangement for the studio. Rather, it must accommodate available space and lighting. The subject is placed approximately 3 to 4 feet in front of the background to eliminate shadows. The camera and tripod are situated 4 to 6 feet from the subject depending on the view obtained and the focal length of the lens. The most variable feature of the studio is the lighting. This varies from a camera-mounted flash to symmetrically placed units positioned to bounce light off the ceiling or umbrella.

Lighting

Illumination is most commonly achieved with one or more synchronized flash units. By varying the intensity, the number of lights, and the angles between the lights and the subject, the photographer may achieve contour lighting, flat lighting, or texture lighting. For preoperative and postoperative facial views, it is important to maintain symmetry. Therefore a lighting arrangement that includes symmetrically positioned flash units is optimal. By "bouncing" the light off a white reflector or a neutral ceiling, the light may be diffused, minimizing glare.

Alternate light sources have been described. Natural light may be used, but it is discouraged because of the difficulty in standardization. Tungsten light sources are available, but can only be used with tungsten films.

Whichever illumination system is used, standardization must be precise. Dickason and Hanna[1] describe "photographic rhinoplasty," "photographic blepharoplasty," "photographic face lift," and other photographic procedures accomplished by changes in lighting and patient position. The lighting conditions, if not standardized, may simulate chemical peels, scar revision, and dermabrasion.

Background

A neutral background is optimal. If the wall coloring is unsuitable, large rolls of grey or blue background paper may be purchased from a photography store. Blue backgrounds have pleasing results in color photography. It is best to avoid overly dark or light backgrounds because their light absorption and reflection properties will lead to distortion of skin tones. Again, standardization is the most important factor, and preoperative and postoperative pictures should be obtained with identical backgrounds.

Film

The choice of film depends upon the intended use for the photographs. Color negative film offers versatility and accurate skin tone reproduction. We routinely use 100 ASA film (Kodacolor or its equivalent), which gives excellent color match. These negatives are used to produce 4″ x 5″ photographs for the operating room and patient record.

Color slide film may also be used. This has the advantage of requiring less storage space. If slides are to be used in the operating theater, however, some means of projection is required. The two popular systems of color slide film are Kodachrome (ASA 64) and Ektachrome (ASA 100). The former produces extremely fine grain and accurate color. The major advantage of Ektachrome is the speed with which it can be processed—within hours in most labs. Also, Ektachrome films with speeds up to ASA 400 are available and are useful in situations requiring increased depth of field.

Black-and-white negative film is used in situations where portraits will be reproduced in black and white for publication. Several excellent films are available. The finest grain black-and-white film is Panatomic-X (Kodak). The pictures are extremely sharp. The disadvantage of this film is its low ASA (32), which reduces depth of field compared to standard color print film. As the film speed increases to Plus-X (ASA 125) and Tri-X (ASA 400), the versatility with respect to depth of field increases, while the fineness of the grain decreases. An alternative to the use of these black-and-white films is the color print or slide film as discussed above. Black-and-white prints may be obtained from either. Producing an internegative of sufficient quality for publication is a difficult task.[2] It requires photographing the color slide or negative onto black-and-white film, and subsequently enlarging this negative onto black-and-white paper. Maintaining standardization throughout these steps truly is a photographic challenge.

The Rhinoplasty Portrait

Six poses are a minimum for rhinoplasty photography (Fig. 5-2). The full face view should have the patient's head fill the frame. The camera is turned vertically, and the tripod is adjusted so that the central view is at the level of the nasal tip. The patient should be positioned such that a vertical line is present from the glabella to the lower lip vermilion border for all views except the basal view. The Frankfort line, or the line connecting the top of the tragus with the infraorbital rim, should lie in the horizontal plane. The hair should be brushed behind the ear in order that the Frankfort line may be established.

The left and right lateral views are taken with the patient's head and torso turned 90 degrees away from the camera. Midway between the frontal and lateral views are the oblique views. By turning the patient until the tip of the nose is aligned with the cheek, the left and right oblique views are obtained. Finally, the patient looks towards the ceiling for the base view, in which the nasal base is viewed with regard to its geometric structure and its relationship to the eyes. The photographer should be significantly closer to the patient for this view, which is often taken at a 1:3 magnification.

All views are taken in repose except the right lateral view, which is taken with the patient smiling. The smiling view is useful in the analysis of tip dynamics.

These views are readily explained to office personnel and are reproducible. Additional views may be desired by the surgeon, but the views above should be available preoperatively and postoperatively for every rhinoplasty.

Fig. 5-2. Rhinoplasty portrait photography.

A, The full face view should be taken with the camera at the vertical height of the nasal tip. The patient should be in repose and should be looking directly into the camera. **B,** The left lateral view is demonstrated. The Frankfort line is horizontal. A vertical line from the glabella to the anterior border of the lower lip is present. Only one eyebrow should be visible. **C,** The right lateral view is identical to the left view. In our office, we routinely have this view taken with the patient smiling. **D** and **E,** The oblique view is taken with the patient oriented halfway between the frontal and lateral views. One useful landmark is to have the patient oriented so that the nasal tip is aligned with the far cheek. **F,** The basal view should be taken closer than the other views. The tripod should be clearly outlined and seen in relation to the eyebrows and eyes.

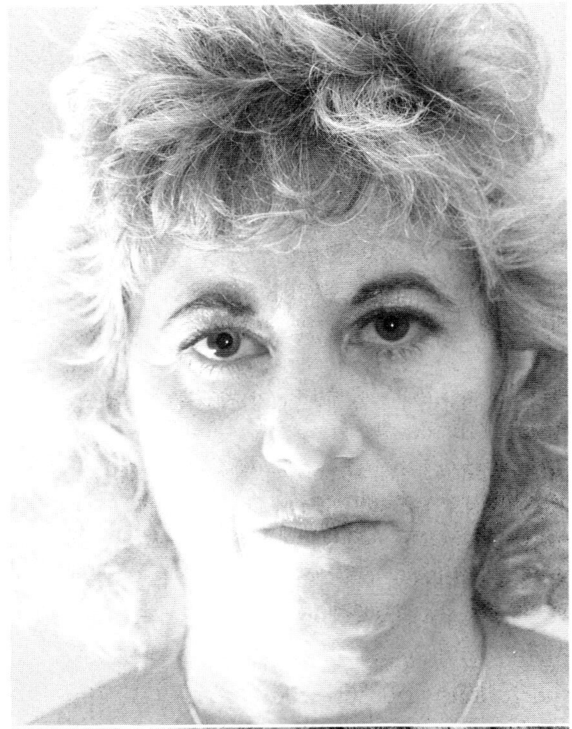

A

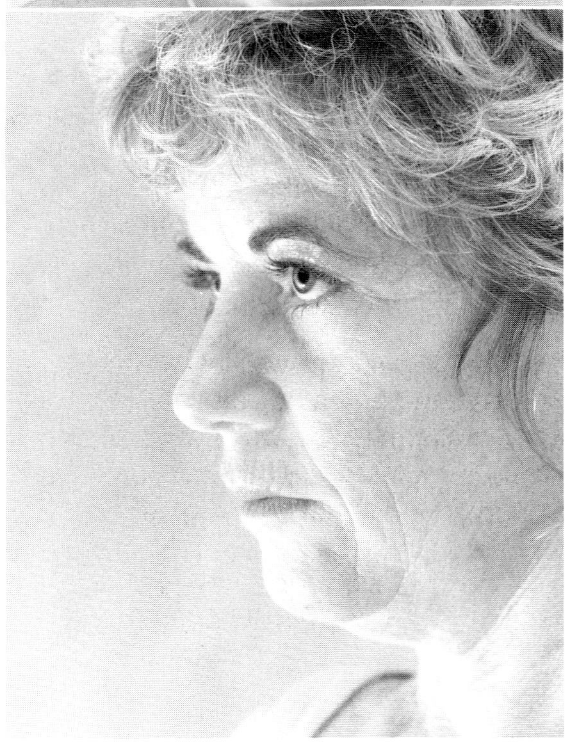

D

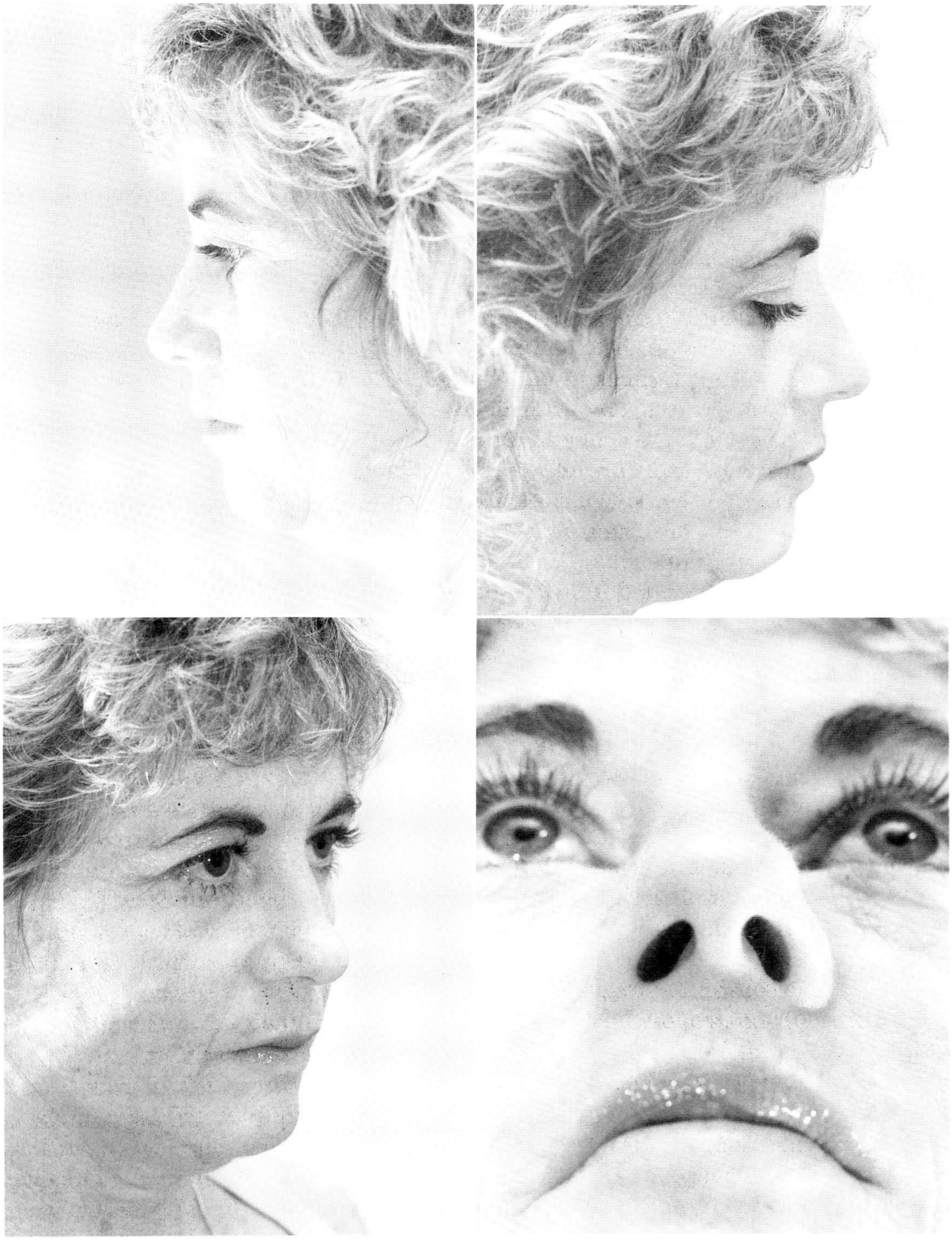

B C E F

Action Photography

Taking intraoperative photographs requires somewhat different gear. Versatility for nasal photography demands the capacity to take close-up photographs at 1:2 to 1:3 magnification. A 105 mm macro lens is well suited for this purpose. Accurate photographs may be taken encompassing the full face or focused in on the nasal tip (Fig. 5-3).

Ideally, light should be metered by an automatic through-the-lens device. This feature is available in multiple lines. For photographs taken of the full face, most standard electronic flash units will suffice. For those special close-up photographs, however, a point source at the end of the lens is optimal. Many facial plastic surgeons desire a flash that has the versatility to accommodate intraoral lesions as well. For this purpose, a ringlight is desired. However, when used for facial photography, the latter produces flat lighting that lacks depth. A ringlight system with both features is available in the Minolta Macro Ringflash. This system features a ring that is comprised of a series of 4 quadrant lights that can individually be turned on or off. In this way, the ringlight doubles as a point source with better texture definition in appropriate situations. The Medical Nikkor ringflash system does not have the point source option, but does produce extremely sharp high-quality photographs. The main feature to look for is automatic through-the-lens metering and compatibility with the rest of the camera equipment.

Color slide film is generally used for surgical photography. Black-and-white prints may be obtained from these slides after an internegative is produced. Film choice is usually determined by the surgeon's preference and is the same as discussed previously. With electronic flash photography a daylight film is required.

Demonstrating any particular technique requires taking a series of pictures from the same distance and from the same vantage point. Otherwise, the photographic series may be very confusing to the viewer. It is helpful to have a landmark in the background of the photograph for orientation.

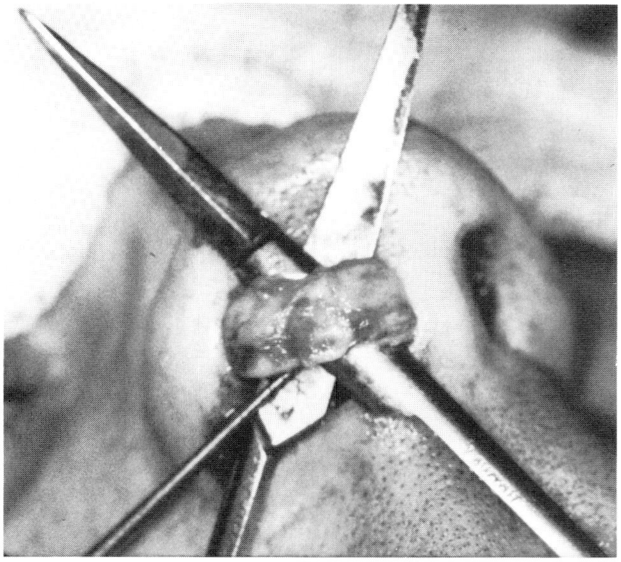

Fig. 5-3. Photographic demonstration of a technique for correcting a bulbous lower lateral cartilage. **A,** The right lower lateral cartilage is delivered. **B,** A cephalic strip is resected. **C,** Morselization of the lateral crus is performed. The photographer has made an attempt to achieve the same angle and distance in all photographs. In addition the upper lip and left nares are included for orientation. The photographs were taken with color slide film (Ektachrome 100), and an internegative was used to produce black and white prints.

A

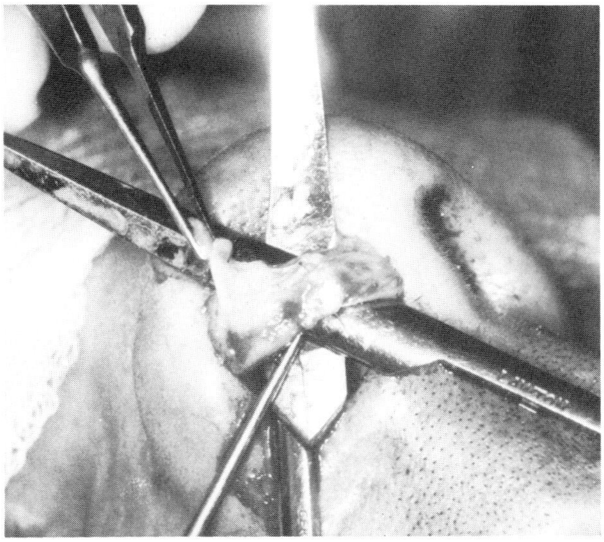

B

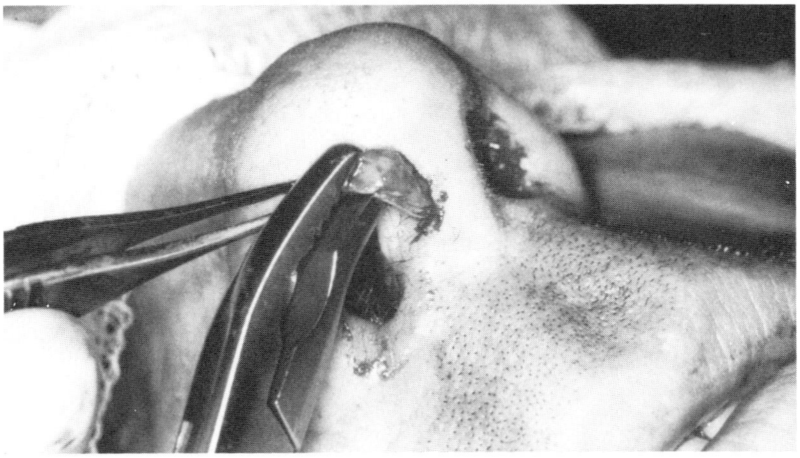

C

Computer Photography

This is an interesting new addition to the rhinoplasty photographic armamentarium. Computer systems are currently available that obtain an image of the patient by video camera and project this image onto a computer monitor. Software systems then allow the operator to alter the facial features, including the nasal profile, nasal width, tip rotation, etc., until a pleasing shape is obtained (Fig. 5-4, A). Adjustments simulating facial rejuvenation techniques may likewise be made. The latest addition to these systems allows direct cephalometric analysis of the face, with precise calculation of the appropriate angles and lengths of facial features (Fig. 5-4, B). A standard Red-Green-Blue (RGB) monitor is used, and a 19-inch screen provides a facial image in a 1:1 scale. Once the modified image is completed, it may be transferred from the Random Access Memory of the computer to a floppy disk for later reference. Future horizons of computer imaging include three-dimensional systems, analagous to those currently used in craniofacial reconstruction and facial trauma.

Computerized simulation of aesthetic surgery may become an important marketing tool for the facial plastic surgeon. It is crucial, however, that the surgeon not mislead the patient into believing such results are as readily obtained as the computer manipulations suggest. The exact role of this exciting new technology has yet to be established.

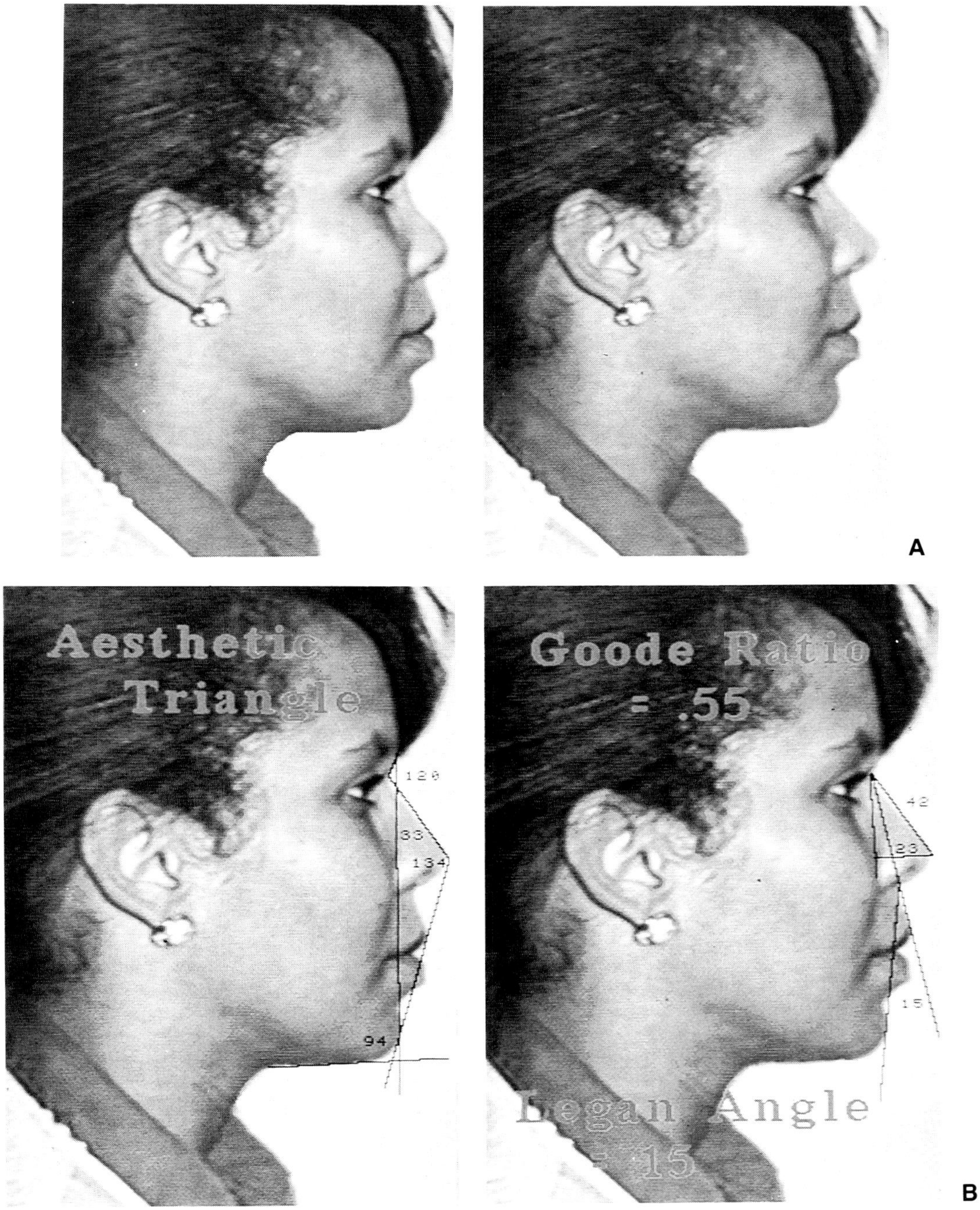

Fig. 5-4. Computer photography. **A,** Computerized rhinoplasty is performed in a patient desiring profileplasty. The patient is analyzed with respect to anatomic landmarks, and pertinent cephalometric measurements are obtained. **B,** Computerized preoperative and postoperative views are demonstrated to the patient. This facilitates communication between the surgeon and the patient. (A and B courtesy Dr. Ira Papel.)

Summary

Photography is an important tool of the aesthetic facial surgeon. Clear, reproducible photographs are essential to the surgeon's critical analysis of his results, as well as to the presentation of those results to his colleagues. Equipment currently available permits high-quality photography to be performed at reasonable cost.

REFERENCES

1. Dickason WL and Hanna DC: Pitfalls of comparative photography in plastic and reconstructive surgery, Plast Reconstr Surg 58:166-175, 1976.
2. McDowell F: On the necessity of precision photographic documentation in plastic surgery, Plast Reconstr Surg 58:214-215, 1976.

ADDITIONAL READINGS

Davidson TM: Photography in facial plastic and reconstructive surgery, Photogr Assoc 47:59-67, 1979.

Hund D: The photography of patients. In Hansell P, editor: A guide to medical photography, University of Baltimore, 1979.

Hurtgen TP: Understanding photographic parameters: guides to film selection and use, Rochester, New York, 1972, Eastman Kodak.

Karlan MS: Photographic documentation techniques, Ear Nose Throat J 58:21-29, 1979.

Morello DC, Converse JM, and Allen D: Making uniform photographic records in plastic surgery, Plast Reconstr Surg 59:366-372, 1977.

Surgnier J: Computer assisted imaging in plastic and cosmetic surgery, ENTech, 12-18, 1986.

Thomas JR, Tardy ME, and Przekop H: Uniform photographic documentation in facial plastic surgery, Otolaryngol Clin North Am 13:367-381, 1980.

6

Dynamics of Nasal Surgery

Walter E. Berman

The dynamics of nasal surgery involve the dependent relationships of the nose's anatomical parts. Nasal dynamics more specifically refers to the stress factors operating between the various nasal structures and to the realization that any alteration of one nasal structure will have an effect on other structures or on the physiological functioning of the nose. Understanding this concept will prevent unfortunate results. The interrelationships between muscles, ligaments, bone, cartilage, and skin are the keys to a natural appearing rhinoplasty. These surgical techniques will be discussed in greater depth in Part II.

Nasal Tip

The greatest interaction of nasal dynamics takes place at the tip. An incision on the inferior aspect of the quadrilateral cartilage will lyse the medial crural attachments to the septum. This type of incision will usually cause the medial crura to re-attach closer to the floor of the nose after healing. This in turn will decrease the projection of the nasal tip, which is how far the nasal tip protrudes from the floor of the nose.

In turn, reparative reconstruction will compensate for the change in the dynamics of the nasal structures. Tip projection may be increased by sutures, grafts, and rotation. Conversely, there are times when the preoperative underprojected tip is held down by these ligaments. An inferior septal incision is necessary to release these tethering ligaments to allow more tip projection and/or supporting grafts, etc. This mechanism often causes apparent "pollybeak" after complete healing and retraction of the incisional scar (see Chapter 20).

Secondary Shortening of the Nose

The nasal framework may be shortened from an inferior to a superior direction by a variety of procedures. Some may be inadvertent (see Chapter 14).

A. Debulking the Nasal Tip

Debulking or thinning the nasal tip includes removing a portion of the superior aspect of the lower lateral nasal cartilage (Fig. 6-1). Consider that normally the upper lateral cartilages fit under the lower lateral cartilages, which contribute to the overall length of the nose.

Normally, the cartilages tend to approximate each other when cartilaginous tissues are removed. This would shorten the length of the nose. An undesirable shortening of the nose may be a side effect of debulking the nasal tip. This may be avoided by doing a debulking procedure as follows: the cartilage removed on the superior aspect of the lower lateral cartilage must be restricted to a fairly thin triangle that is based superiorly. This technique is useful with a wide nasal tip and short nose (Fig. 6-2). The inferior rim is left intact. Morselization is then performed on the adjacent cartilages of the lower lateral cartilages. *Morselization* involves breaking up the single strip of lower lateral cartilage into many smaller pieces that are still in continuity with each other. Continuity is generally supplied by the perichondrium. These smaller pieces, though still providing a continuous strip, break the cartilage spring and allow

Fig. 6-1. Removal of superior lower lateral cartilage may shorten the length of the bone.

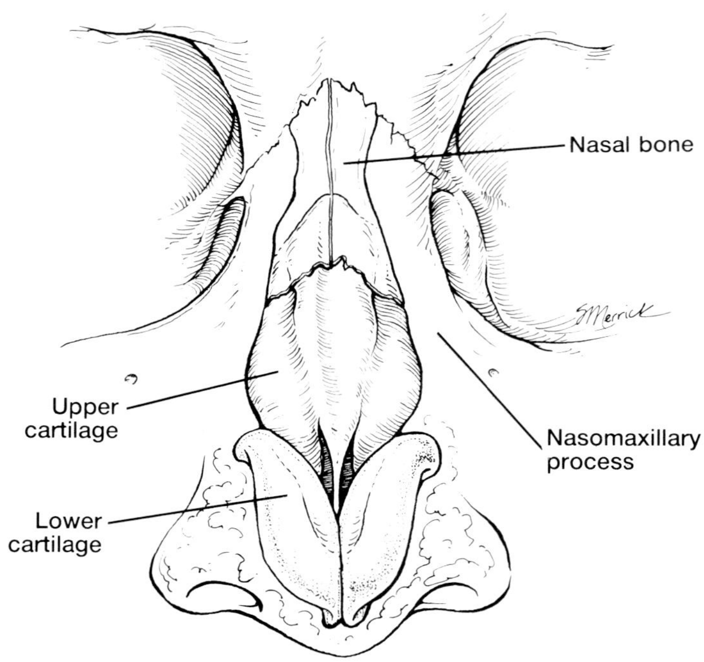

for gentle molding of the tip. I use the Rubin tip morselizer for this delicate work and am careful not to squeeze the morselizer so hard as to disrupt the perichondrium (Fig. 6-3, A and B).

This procedure thins the nasal tip without shortening the length of the nose. Removal of excessive superior aspect of the lower lateral cartilage causes insufficient cartilaginous support between the superior aspect of the lower lateral cartilage and the inferior aspect of the upper lateral cartilage. This condition may cause an inward collapse of the intervening epithelial tissues. Both the lining and the external epithelial layers may be affected, producing a "pince nez" effect.

The errors caused by removing excessive cartilage are compounded when epithelial lining is also removed. Disastrous postoperative results are caused by such overzealous tissue removal.

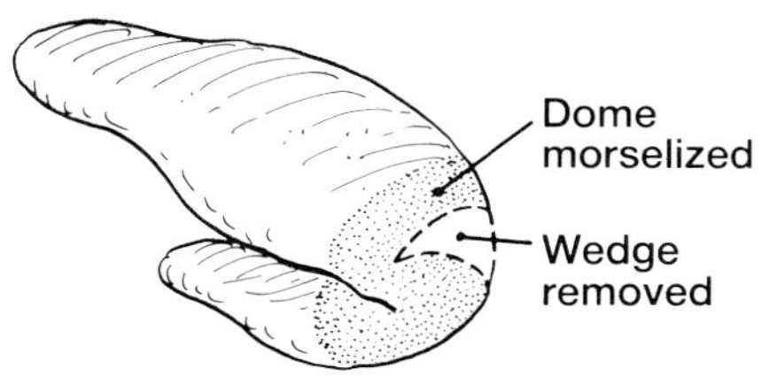

Fig. 6-2. Wedge removal to thin a wide tip of a short nose. The main body of cartilage is left in place. (From Berman, WE: Rhinoplasty, ed 2, Washington DC, 1984, American Academy of Otolaryngology-Head and Neck Surgery Foundation, Inc.)

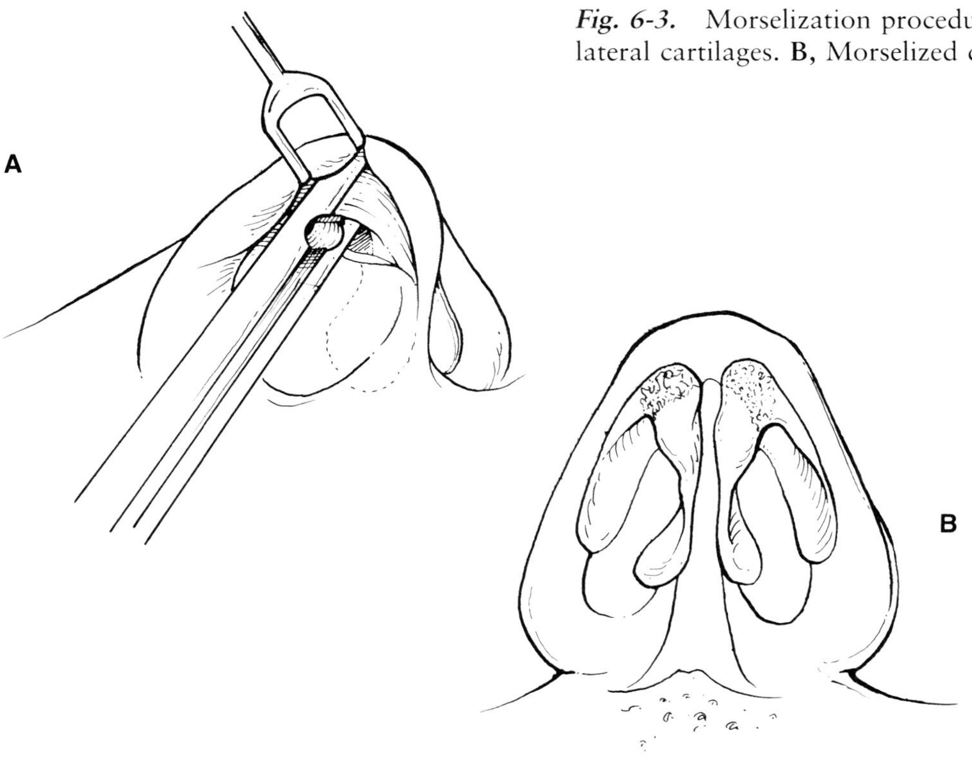

Fig. 6-3. Morselization procedure. **A,** Thinning of the lower lateral cartilages. **B,** Morselized domes creating a thinner tip.

I firmly believe in leaving intact a 5 mm rim of lower lateral and dome borders of the lower lateral cartilages. Leaving a very thin border (less than 5 mm) of lower lateral cartilage will allow the same postoperative vagaries to occur as if the inferior border of the cartilage was actually cut into two parts.

Occasionally, an exception such as a secondary rotation procedure, must be made. This is done in the case of a long nose and soft central segment. One of the forerunners and early masters of rhinoplastic surgery told me, "It doesn't matter what cartilage is removed, it's what is left."*

B. Upper Lateral Cartilage Surgery

When it is deemed advisable to separate the upper lateral cartilages from the nasoseptal cartilages, a variety of dynamic changes may follow. The lateral cartilage-septal complex may be the main anterior nasal support (Fig. 6-4). Separation and weakening of this support can cause a saddle deformity. This depends on the inherent support of the underlying septal cartilage. Conversely, separation of these cartilages, in instances when their union was holding down the upper lateral cartilages, may cause an increase of the upper lateral cartilages on the anterior surface of the nose.

*Feit L, MD; Personal communication, 1959.

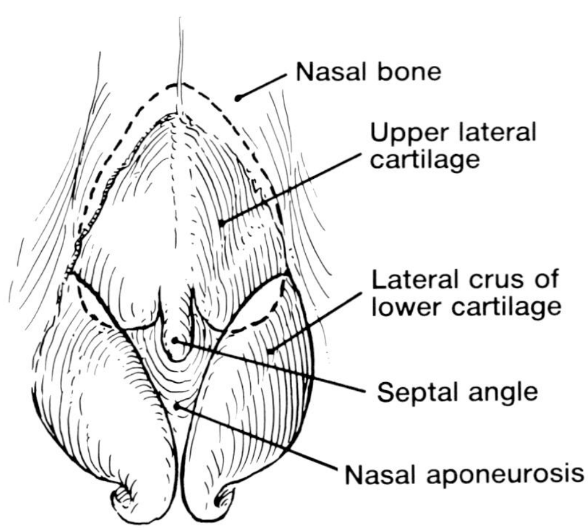

Fig. 6-4. Upper lateral cartilages attached to septal cartilage before separation. (From Berman, WE: Rhinoplasty, ed 2, Washington DC, 1984, American Academy of Otolaryngology-Head and Neck Surgery Foundation, Inc.)

When decreasing the cartilaginous profile line of the nose, it is often necessary to lower the anterior aspect of the upper lateral cartilages. Redoing this profile line will also shorten the anterior length of these cartilages, thus shortening the length of the nose.

The upper lateral cartilages are basically triangular in shape with the base in an anterior or dorsal position. When a section of the anterior base is excised, the length of the base is decreased. The new base being shorter will normally cause the lower lateral cartilage to rotate superiorly and thus shorten the nose. In other words, excessive decrease in the cartilaginous profile line of the nose as regards the upper lateral cartilages will also shorten the overall length of the nose (Fig. 6-5).

C. Secondary Rotation of the Nasal Tip

Normally, in rotation of the nasal tip for shortening, the pivotal point is the most lateral extent of the lower lateral cartilage. When this inferior border of the lower lateral cartilage is interrupted, a new pivotal point is created. Such is the case in secondary rotations. The latter shortens the nose more than the former. The secondary rotation is ideal for a long nose with a soft central segment (see Chapter 14 on Nasal Shortening).

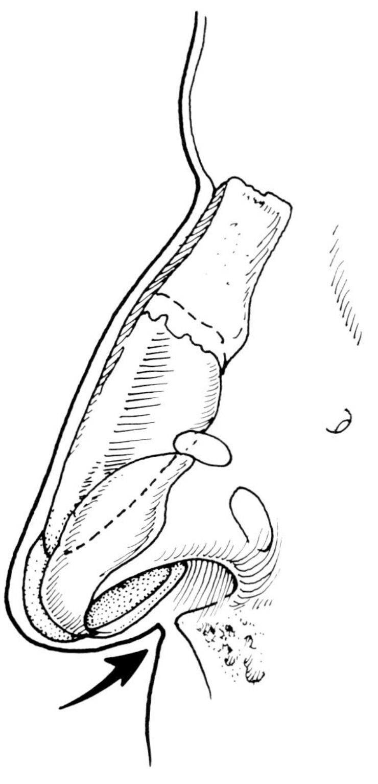

Fig. 6-5. Removal of the anterior aspects of the upper nasal cartilage in the anterior-posterior direction will shorten the base of the upper lateral triangle and may shorten the overall length of the nose.

7

Anesthesia for Nasal Surgery

Milton Perlow

The administering of anesthetics, whether general or local, for nasal surgery, whether performed as an inpatient or as an outpatient procedure, must meet the same basic criteria—a proper pre-anesthetic evaluation, a smooth intraoperative course and a pleasant postoperative experience.

Since most nasal surgery is elective in nature, it is easy to assume that the patient is healthy and free of all medical problems. These assumptions must be laid aside. The anesthesiologist must be certain that a complete medical history is taken, a thorough physical examination has been performed, all necessary laboratory tests completed and the results reported prior to the administration of an anesthetic.

A knowledge of the patient's history, including previous anesthetic experiences, along with the physical and laboratory findings enables the anesthesiologist to determine the patient's acceptability as a candidate for elective surgery.[6] Even with the history provided by the surgeon, the anesthesiologist should supplement this with his or her own history and examination. Any significant difference in findings may require an anesthetic-surgical conference or may even necessitate a postponement of the surgery.

When questioning the patient regarding any prior anesthetic experiences, it is important that the exact nature of the previous anesthetics be described. Many times patients will not mention certain procedures because they do not think of them as surgical procedures. We must direct the patient toward these "forgotten anesthetics." One must always inquire about the dental, obstetrical, and "minor procedures," e.g., lacerations, fractures, etc. It is not unusual for patients to omit mentioning childhood operations.

In soliciting information about the operations, ask questions in lay terms—e.g., were you asleep or awake? Did you tend to drift in and out? Was your anesthetic induced by the placing of needles in your back? In addition, we feel that it is important to know the patient's emotional and physical response to earlier anesthetics. Did the patient do well or poorly? Was the experience painful or pleasant? From the answers to such questions we have become properly armed to explain and administer a comforting form of anesthesia.

Once the patient is considered a satisfactory surgical candidate, a detailed explanation of the procedure chosen should be described and discussed with him. Questions should be encouraged and fully answered. In our opinion, the anesthesiologist must have an interview with the parents of young children before the latter go into surgery.

When interviewing older children and teenagers in the presence of parents, we prefer to direct all questions to the patient because that prevents excessive parental participation. The child feels, maybe for the first time, that he or she is an important player in the events that are about to happen. This helps us to build rapport and to proceed with a more relaxed and agreeable patient.

When reviewing the chart prior to interviewing the patient, it is important to note not only the patient's history, physical exam, and laboratory results, but also the surgery that is proposed and the consent that is signed. When first meeting the patient, we like the patient to describe the surgery anticipated. Occasionally what the patient describes, what the surgeon proposes, and what the consent states are not always in agreement. Most of the time this can be resolved during the pre-anesthetic visit. However, if this is not possible, suggest postponing the procedure until the surgeon and patient can redefine what is to be done.

Anesthetic Agents and Techniques

In the interests of practicality, we will discuss only a few anesthetic agents. We will divide this portion of the chapter into general inhalation anesthesia, local anesthesia, and intravenous sedation associated with local blocks.

General Inhalation Anesthesia

Historically, the most widely used approach to nasal surgery was via the nitrous oxide-narcotic-muscle relaxant use of general anesthesia. This has shifted almost universally to the use of the halogenated agents. These have been combined with nitrous oxide, narcotics, or just oxygen and with the use of muscle relaxants, the concept of balanced anesthesia has evolved.[2]

The most common anesthetic agents used today are halothane, enflurane, and isoflurane. Halothane, which is still popular in pediatric circles, is being replaced to a great extent by enflurane and its isomer isoflurane. Although the latter two are often used in combination with nitrous oxide, on questioning a number of operators we have found a preference for only the agent and oxygen and a conservative use of some narcotic.

The narcotics that are most commonly used at present are fentanyl and meperidine. Fentanyl, it seems, is fast becoming the dominant drug. This may be because of its short-acting nature and its extensive use in cardiac surgery.

We have noticed few patients being induced with the inhalation agent itself and so thiopental sodium continues to maintain its preferential role as the most significant inducting agent used.

The use of muscle relaxants is evolving rapidly. Since nasal surgery in general is not an extensive procedure that requires muscle relaxation, short-acting agents such as succinylcholine chloride or other depolarizing agents were and may still be the most widely used relaxants. Today, with the advent of the new intermediary nondepolarizing agents, namely atracurium, the entire muscle relaxant picture is changing.

It is our belief that with all general inhalation techniques, and especially in head and neck surgery, an anticholinergic is necessary. We have seen too many bradycardias result from an avoidance of anticholinergics. The form administered whether it be glycopyrolate or atropine, will vary from operator to operator and is an individual choice. Both meet the necessary criterion required.

When using a general anesthesic for nasal surgery, we approach the procedure with the philosophy that all cases are outpatient in nature because they involve little or no premedication and a rapid recovery.

All premedication is given intravenously and generally consists of atropine alone or atropine and fentanyl. The dosage of atropine is fairly consistent: 0.4 mg. It may vary on occasion from 0.2 mg to 0.8 mg, depending on the patient's preoperative vital signs. Fentanyl is administered from 0.05 mg to .1 mg and, rarely, .15 mgs, but it never exceeds the latter amount. The use of fentanyl should act as a relaxant and not as a hypnotic or a depressant. We believe the preoperative interview to be the single most important aspect to premedication.

After evaluating the effects of the intravenous drugs administered, we are ready for induction. We induce all our adult patients with thiopental sodium, given in increments to render the patient asleep and not apneic. It is important to maintain spontaneous respirations. A large bolus given rapidly will produce an apneic patient, as has been our experience many times.

We now apply a face mask and begin to administer an inhalation agent which, in the case of a nonbreathing patient, is managed by controlled respirations. Induction should be based on the patient's response and not on some dose-weight formula to which we have all been conditioned. Application of a face mask with an inhalation agent can now be a smooth continuum of the induction until a proper level of anesthesia is reached. The agent the author feels most comfortable with is enflurane in combination with nitrous oxide, but it must be emphasized that the agent of choice is the one that the operator is most familiar.

Intubation should be accomplished with soft cuffed moderate sized tubes. Those we use most commonly are the 7 mm and occasionally 7.5 mm in size. We never have found it necessary to use larger tubes. In our experience, preparation of the cords with a topical agent has helped us in reducing the incidence of postoperative sore throat. We prefer the applications via a spray; the agent to be used depends on operator preference.

Since nasal surgery does not require the need for continual muscle relaxation, the author prefers to set up a succinylcholine drip that is used for intubation and may be given in small increments if the need arises. This way we avoid having to reverse with the longer agents or scurry around for more agent if the patient is allowed to become too light and "bucks." We have found that preloading with a small dose of curare is very satisfactory in the prevention of muscle fasciculations and bradycardia.

Monitoring during nasal surgery should not be any different or any less than monitoring during more extensive procedures. The most important single aspect of monitoring is to be in constant touch with the patient by means of a chest or esophageal stethoscope.

The other modalities that we feel must be present are those that are continuous in their monitoring and include a cardioscope, a blood pressure instrument, e.g., a Dinamap®, a pulse-oximeter, and a temperature probe. There seems to be a constant debate on invasive versus non-invasive approaches to proper monitoring. In our opinion it has become fashionable to use invasive monitoring even when it is unnecessary, despite the fact that invasive techniques, as we all know, are not without the potential for serious complications. Their use in any procedure must be carefully weighed. We find no justification for the use of invasive techniques in nasal surgery.

There is no doubt that new techniques, drugs, and equipment have improved and will continue to improve the practice of anesthesia and we will be able to follow every nuance of a patient's physiology. A well-trained, dedicated anesthesiologist who is in constant contact with the patient is the bulwark of a successful anesthetic and surgical procedure.

From an anesthetic point of view, the ending of successful nasal surgery may be one of the most difficult aspects of the entire procedure. The "new" nose should not be touched or traumatized, the airway should be protected, and adequate respirations should be maintained.

When the surgery is completed and the operator is applying the dressings, there is a tendency to reduce the level of anesthesia and "over-lighten" the patient. We may now have a patient straining and "bucking" on the endotracheal tube, beginning to have spontaneous and uncoordinated movements of the body and extremities, an increase in bleeding from the surgical site, a hysterical surgeon, and a panicky anesthesiologist. The endotracheal tube is removed, usually before the dressing is applied. Ventilation is attempted via a face mask; this is sometimes easy but is generally accompanied by patient regurgitation, laryngospasm, wild gesticulations, or, more commonly, all three.

An approach we have found that has served us well is to continue administering the anesthesic at a surgical level until everything, including the nasal dressings, has been completed. The oral pharyngeal area is flushed with saline or water and is thoroughly suctioned. The anesthetic gases are now discontinued, the system is flushed with oxygen, and the patient is allowed to breathe 100% oxygen. In order to facilitate a smooth transition from intubation to extubation without disrupting spontaneous respirations, we administer intravenous lidocaine, generally in a single 100 mg dose.

Extubation is accomplished in two stages. The first is to lower the cuff and allow the patient to continue to breathe with the tube in place for a short period of time. We have found that 2 to 3 minutes are adequate. The oral cavity is gently suctioned again and on an expiratory phase the endotracheal tube is removed. Our experience has demonstrated an almost constant smooth extubation and recovery. Patients are sent to the recovery room only after they are able to respond to verbal commands in the surgical suite.

Local Anesthesia

Historically, because of its safety, ease in handling, and the minimal amount of necessary equipment it required, a local anesthesic was and in many situations still is the method of choice.[1]

These procedures are more often than not performed without the use of an anesthesiologist. Although the surgeon assumes the hats of both practitioners, the principles outlined earlier must not be overlooked. A proper history-taking and physical examination, necessary laboratory work, adequate monitoring equipment, and a thorough knowledge of the agents to be used are still essential.

Even with a strictly "local" approach to nasal surgery, the surgeon should establish a satisfactory intravenous line and "hook" the patient to the necessary monitors before any surgery is started. Many surgeons wish to medicate their patients prior to surgery with either tranquilizers, hypnotics, narcotics or a combination of these. If this is the case, minimal quantities of the drugs should be used. Relaxation and/or mild sedation of the patient, not depression, must be the watchword for proper premedication.

Since an intravenous line will have been established, it may be an easier and more efficacious route to premedication. In general the amounts of drug needed are smaller, are more quickly induced, and are more rapidly metabolized. Once the intravenous line is in place, arrival at the entire premedication encounter becomes less painful and more pleasant. Lastly, control of agents used is more exact and allows a greater prediction of their effect.

Technique. Proper preparation of the nose with a topical agent will ease the pain caused by the inevitable local injections. Topical agents must be applied in a slow, sequential manner. Start at the nasal entry with small packs or light spraying, then gradually increase the extent of the packing. One should not hurry this part of the procedure by cutting short the time the packs are left in the nose. As was stated before, adequate knowledge of the drugs will permit the surgeon to anesthetize the mucosa properly and, depending on what one uses, to achieve good vasoconstriction. Once the nose is suitably prepared, it is necessary to be verbally in contact with the patient to make it easier to "talk" one's way through the necessary injections.

After injecting the nose, we should take a leaf from our dental colleagues by allowing the agent plenty of time to reach its full effect. There is a tendency to hurry and get on with the surgery. The old adage, more hurry less speed, is especially applicable to local anesthesia.

It is necessary to discuss the emergency equipment and drugs that are necessary during the performance of any local procedure. Even though thousands of nasal blocks are done without mishap, a single event where resuscitative equipment and medication are unavailable can lead to disaster.

Everyone agrees that oxygen is as much a part of an office operating setting as a syringe and needle. However, merely having oxygen available is not enough—there must be a means to deliver it. Many offices have oxygen in every room, but absolutely no way to ventilate a patient.

If surgery is to be performed in an office, the surgical area should be treated as if it were in a hospital environment. It is essential to be able to deliver oxygen properly, the most proper way being via an anesthetic machine. The machine should be simple in nature and easily mobile. It must be routinely serviced and not permitted to gather dust in some lost corner. If no machine is available the minimal ventilatory equipment necessary is an ambulance bag that is capable of being attached to a "full" tank of oxygen.

The surgical area must have available, at easy access, a container with emergency drugs and equipment. The most convenient is a movable multiple-drawer hospital "crash cart." Emergency kits in the form of luggage sets are available but, in our opinion, are not quite satisfactory because they have a tendency to be placed in out-of-the-way cupboards, never to be seen again.

A good "crash cart" is one that is well organized; there is no best way to organize one. The easiest way is to have the hospital recovery room nurse demonstrate their cart and to set up a similar one for office surgery. Besides all the other equipment, it is useful for the office surgeon to have a defibrillator and to know how to use it.

Intravenous Sedation

As procedures became more sophisticated and therefore longer, nasal surgery has turned more and more to the use of general anesthetics.[1] Because of this increased use the surgeon has been forced out of the office and into a hospital setting. As a result of the ever-burgeoning cost of hospital care, today we see a reverse migration—a return to office surgery, which is being accompanied by a new tool: the general anesthetic.[1]

Ideally, a technique that can combine the positive aspects of general anesthesia with the safety and ease of local anesthesia would be the method of choice. The technique used in our office is one such approach. We direct ourselves in all cases to what is called the *triad of anesthesia*—amnesia, analgesia, and sedation—all under a local umbrella.[1]

Preoperative evaluation of the patient is not any different than when using other techniques. The description of the anesthetic procedure requires more time and explanation than with other approaches. Patients knowing that they will receive some sort of anesthetic can only relate to the concept of being "out." Therefore, an explanation of intravenous sedation combined with local block must be handled with care and an understanding of the patient's apprehension.

Proper preparation for intravenous sedation begins with the surgical consultation at which a discussion about the anesthetic that will be used can take place. This technique is an ideal illustration of surgical and anesthetic team work.

Rarely is a preoperative medication given. When it is used, our preference is for an amnesic given orally at least two hours preoperatively. We have chosen the two-hour period to allow for maximum gastric absorption and systemic effect. I'm sure everyone has administered oral medication, rushed the patient to surgery, and had the drug take effect sometime during the procedure, thereby losing all knowledge of its effect.

After the intravenous line is in place, the first drug administered is one that will produce a pleasant amnesia, is non-irritating, relatively long acting (and therefore one that does not have to be repeated) with minimal or no depressant effects on the cardiopulmonary system and one that will impart a feeling of well-being to the patient.

A number of agents have been tried and evaluated. We have settled on one of the benzodiazepines—lorazepam. The amount used will vary between 2 to 3 mg; we have never had to exceed 3 mg. The drug is always diluted two or three times. Although the manufacturer reports a 1% to 2% chance of a painful intravenous injection site, so far we have not experienced any patient pain on infusion.

Within a short time after injection the patients report feeling pleasantly relaxed. Much of their apprehension tends to recede. As a matter of protocol, we follow recommended suggestions about time. The drug is given 15 to 20 minutes before we progress with the rest of the preparation for local injection.

Although still cooperative and communicative, the patient has achieved a very significant plane of amnesia; this has been borne out by postoperative interviews, which are conducted with all patients.

We next administer an analgesic preparation. The agent should, in our opinion, be one that is most familiar to the operator. We have evolved, generally, to the use of fentanyl for a number of reasons. First, we have not had a problem with venous irritation. Second, it very rapidly produces the desired effect. Lastly if used in judicial amounts, it is relatively short acting.

The administration of the analgesic used (fentanyl) is in small amounts—.05 to .1 mg at a time. This rule is never waived. Properly given in conjunction with our amnesic can allow proper packing of the nose to proceed without patient discomfort.

After satisfactory analgesia, both intravenous and topical, we continue with the local injections. Again, the agent should be the one that is most familiar to the operator. In most centers the blocks are usually performed by the surgeon. However, by having the anesthesiologist conduct the block the entire surgery can be expedited, the use of the intravenous medication can be reduced, the postoperative time can be reduced, and the patients allowed to leave for home sooner.

Sedation of the patient with the use of hypnotics raises the most interesting and puzzling questions that face the anesthesiologist when using this technique. Should hypnotics be used at all? If they are used, when and how should they be used to achieve the desired effect? Hypnotic sedation by itself will not, unless used in large and dangerous quantities, remove or reduce pain. In reality the threshold of pain may well be lowered and patient responses may be exaggerated.

We approach the hypnotic as an adjunct, a supplement. Some observers visiting our clinic have described it as an afterthought. The principle we follow is that the hypnotics are agents that are to be used after analgesia. If approached in this way, proper sedation can be achieved even with minimal amounts. On occasion, hypnotics are not necessary, since everything done earlier to produce a satisfactory anesthesia has been successful. The hypnotic we prefer is thiopental sodium given in small increments of 25 to 50 mg, while monitoring the patient's response.

The cornerstone of proper intravenous anesthesia is to depart from the conventional use of medication. Traditionally, we have all been conditioned to administer medication on a dose-weight relationship. Experience has shown us that patients do not necessarily react in this way. People of slight build who weigh less often require more drug than others who weigh more and are bigger built.

We are not attempting to reach a state of anesthesia where the patient is rendered unconscious and the reflexes obtunded. The entire technique must allow a continual verbal exchange between patient and anesthesiologist. Anything less defeats the purpose. Therefore discussions of the pharmacokinetics of narcotic and non-narcotic compounds is of no value at this time. We leave that to standard texts that delve into general anesthesia with the use of narcotic agents.

Since the method is based on the introduction of medication intravenously, results are seen almost immediately and therefore the patient's reaction should be assessed on a moment-to-moment basis. Because of this, the dispensing of the agents is built around the concept of *dose-patient response* relationships, not, and we emphasize this, on a dose-weight relationship. In this way problems, which will be discussed later, can be controlled or prevented. Also, intravenous introduction of the anesthetic in many instances allows lower quantities of drugs than might otherwise be used. We are also in a better position to allow the patient to control his or her basic reflexes. It is preferable to be in the position of being required to administer more drug rather than wishing that some could be retrieved.

Agents

We will divide this discussion into two parts. One, the local anesthetics and two, the intravenous agents. Since a large number of local anesthetics are available, for the sake of brevity we have decided to restrict the discussion to the most commonly used agents. Assigning agents to this category is somewhat arbitrary and is based on a number of interviews conducted by the authors and on various conferences attended by them.

The Local Anesthetics

As far as nasal surgery is concerned, the local anesthetics are topicals and injectables. The two most extensively used topicals are cocaine hydrochloride and tetracaine.

Cocaine hydrochloride is a naturally occurring alkaloid that produces excellent surface anesthesia and a rather intense vasoconstriction when applied to a mucosal surface. The onset is rapid (1 to 2 minutes) and the duration may last an hour or in some cases as long as an hour and a half, depending upon dose and concentration. In our clinic we generally apply 2 to 3 cc of a 5% solution.

Because cocaine can potentiate the actions of epinephrine or norepinephrine, cardiovascular symptoms, e.g., tachycardia, hypertension, or even ventricular fibrillation may occur. Therefore the use of cocaine on patients who have hypertension or who exhibit cardiac problems must be done most judiciously. Toxic symptoms appear more often when there is an excess dosage given. Remember that cocaine should be used for anesthesia and vasoconstriction, not for a social "high."

Some practitioners prefer to add epinephrine to the cocaine that is to be applied, because it delays absorption and make a greater vasoconstriction obtainable. Whether this is so or not does not justify the increased risk of a potential catastrophe.

Tetracaine hydrochloride is a very potent topical anesthetic agent. Its potency may be 3 to 5 times that of cocaine. Unfortunately it lacks the vasoconstricting effects of cocaine, as do the other topical agents.

The onset of its effectiveness is slower than cocaine, taking 5 to 10 minutes to be totally effective. Our experience has shown that the length of action of tetracaine is as long if not longer than cocaine. Because of its lack of vasoconstrictive and epinephrine effects, the toxicity of tetracaine is sometimes overlooked. Actually, its toxicity may be up to 5 times that of cocaine and therefore it should be used with caution. We apply 20 mg of a 2% solution prior to the injection of local agents.

The Injectables

Today, probably the two most widely used injectable agents are lidocaine and bupivacaine. Although other local anesthetics are used, we are going to limit our discussion to the above two drugs in order to streamline this discussion.

Lidocaine hydrochloride is still the most popular and widely used local anesthetic agent. A general pharmacological discussion of the chemical makeup of lidocaine is beyond the scope of this chapter and may be obtained from any standard text on anesthesia or pharmacology. Here it should suffice to merely describe techniques, amounts, and possible complications.

In "tender" areas such as the nose, proper topical preparation (already discussed), small needles, and slow injections are essential. In general, a 1% solution with epinephrine 1:100,000 is most adequate. 2% solutions (1:100,000) are used in some settings. We are not yet sure whether there is an advantage and this aspect is under investigation in our clinic. The 0.5% solution that contains only 1:200,000 epinephrine may not be adequate for most operators. With the toxic dose (when used with epinephrine) in the range of 500 mg one has a great deal of leeway in properly blocking a nose for surgery. We have found that between 8 to 12 cc is adequate in almost all cases.

I would like to digress for a moment to discuss epinephrine concentration. We have observed a number of surgeons over the years who have used concentrations varying from 1:50,000 to 1:300,000, each claiming victory in the war against bleeding and for vasoconstriction. Most writers contend that there is no difference between 1:50,000 and 1:200,000, and for a long time, we held the same opinion. In evaluating cases more recently, I feel that there *is* a difference. We have definitely noticed a decrease in bleeding and a greater vasoconstriction with concentrations of 1:100,000 as opposed to 1:200,000, but will reserve a definite opinion for a later date. We have no experience with concentrations greater then 1:100,000 and are therefore unable to comment on these stronger solutions.

Bupivacaine is becoming increasingly common to use for nasal surgery. Its popularity is based on the increased length of its action, which obviates the need for repeat injections in cases that require longer surgery. The drug comes in three concentrations: 0.25%, 0.5%, and 0.75%—all with and without epinephrine. When supplied with epinephrine the solutions are limited to only 1:200,000 concentrations.

When using bupivacaine in areas other than nasal surgery, the concentration that has been the most efficacious—having increased longevity without complications—has been the 0.5% solution. Unfortunately, the manufacturers do not recommend greater than a 0.25% solution when the drug is to be used for local infiltration. They contend that the risk factor for tissue damage is high with concentrations above 0.25%. This potential complication has obviously restricted our use of the greater concentrations in nasal surgery. Experience with the 0.25% solution has produced variable results.

Complications of Local Agents

Problems arising from the use of local anesthetics generally arise from one (or both) of two conditions—either an overdose or an inadvertent intravenous administration of the drug, especially if epinephrine is used. Allergic reactions in the day of the amides are rare.

As Lalli and Amarnath point out in their review of fifty three deaths caused by local anesthesia, "There appears to be no evidence in this series to implicate allergy, hypersensitivity, or idiosyncrasy. The untoward effects seem to be the consequence of inadvertent intravenous injection, overdosage, improper technique, and inadequate management of toxic reactions.[5] de Jong noted "now that mostly amide-type local anesthetics are used, allergic effects . . . have become extremely rare."[4]

We have never seen a reaction that can be described as allergic or even idiosyncratic. Descriptions thought to have been allergic have, after evaluation, turned out to be responses that can be associated with an epinephrine effect. When adverse symptoms do arise, they manifest themselves in either the cardiovascular or central nervous systems.

Central nervous symptoms may produce excitation or apprehension, sometimes with a concomitant episode of nausea and/or vomiting. Many times this may be interpreted as patient hysteria. If allowed to continue, the patient may begin to have tremors or twitching and eventually may convulse. Depression of the nervous system response is immediately necessary. Many surgeons prefer the use of intravenous diazepam. Our experience with small amounts of a rapid-acting barbiturate, e.g., thiopental sodium has been most satisfactory. Whatever approach one uses, it is most important to treat the symptoms at once.

Cardiovascular symptoms may manifest themselves in a number of ways: rapid pulse, a sharp rise in blood pressure, the possibility of myocardial infarction or stroke or total cardiovascular collapse, shock, and even death.

Techniques that we have all learned and practiced, which may at times slip a bit, must always be observed: inject slowly, aspirate continually, be aware of the amounts used, and maintain an uninterrupted observation of the patient and his or her vital signs.

Problems and Complications of Intravenous Sedation

The great danger in all anesthesia is excessive use. This becomes most apparent when one uses the technique of intravenous sedation recklessly. Each step must be organized properly and undertaken slowly. Every drug and every aspect must be evaluated adequately before other drugs are administered. The tendency to hurry the procedure must be avoided.

When applying the concept discussed earlier—dose related to patient response—the susceptibility to overdose is greatly reduced. It is easy technique to add drugs; it is impossible to remove them, once administered.

With intravenous sedation the anesthesiologist must rely on spontaneous and adequate patient respirations. Without strict attention and without the proper administration of the agents used, hypoventilation may occur. This results in either one or both (usually both) of its offspring, hypoxia and hypercarbia.

Hypoxia. One of the most reliable signs of early hypoxia is an increase in the pulse rate. However, if oxygen is given, measured, shown to be adequate, and the pulse continues to be rapid, we must look elsewhere for the cause. At this point the respirations may not show any changes (increased respirations appear as the oxygen deficit becomes more acute). Central nervous symptoms, the most significant being restlessness, may be noted early in hypoxia. This is often mistakenly treated with more sedatives which results in an increase in the hypoxia. Restlessness and apprehension in any patient should suggest hypoxia and therefore oxygen therapy should be tried before any more depressant drugs are given.[3]

As oxygen deficit becomes more acute, the pulse becomes slow and bounding; the respirations, which may have been rapid and shallow, now become depressed and irregular. Cyanosis, which may have been only slight, will become severe. There is no question of the need for oxygen in this situation, but there should not have been a question for the need of oxygen earlier. We must remember that cyanosis is a late sign of hypoxia. Once cyanosis has set in we are only a step away from convulsions and possible arrest.

Hypoxia changes from mild to severe in the following stages: tachycardia—mental changes—air hunger—bradycardia—cyanosis—convulsions.[3] We must be ever vigilant to its presence and even in the very worst situations, never allow anything but the most mild manifestations to appear.

Hypercarbia. In order to explain this problem properly, we shall refer to Cullen's description of carbon dioxide retention and its effects. "The recognition of carbon dioxide retention is difficult especially in the presence of depressant drugs. This may be due in part to the fact that carbon dioxide may in ways act as an anesthetic agent. The development of its effects is often insidious. Moreover they merge so imperceptibly with the effects of depressants and anesthetic drugs that pronounced untoward responses are often misinterpreted. The anesthetist therefore must ever be aware of the possibility of carbon dioxide retention as a cause for unexplained undesirable responses in the patient and take suitable steps to eliminate the possibility.

Elevation of the blood pressure and acceleration of pulse rate are associated with hypercarbia. It is emphasized, however, that these changes usually appear early in the development of the hypercarbia. They also may be masked entirely by the concomitant use of depressant and anesthetic drugs. It may seem paradoxical to speak of hypercarbia in the presence of hypoventilation because of the common concept that an elevated carbon dioxide level always results in hyperventilation. Carbon dioxide may act as a depressant and in states of hypoventilation induced by anesthetic drugs, carbon dioxide may accumulate without evident increase in ventilation and may contribute to the state of hypoventilation.

"Muscular rigidity is not uncommon with carbon dioxide retention. During anesthesia this lack of relaxation may be ascribed erroneously to insufficient depth of anesthesia. Through such misinterpretation the patient is often subjected to increased concentrations of anesthetic agent, increased hypoventilation and accentuation of carbon dioxide retention . . . ."[3]

The prior passage most vividly describes the relationship between the patient, the anesthetic agents, and carbon dioxide. When the technique of intravenous sedation is improperly applied, the patient's restlessness and increased blood pressure and pulse rate make it clear that hypercarbia is present. When this problem is present as an isolated entity, it is easily solved. No more infusion of agents, application of oxygen, and stimulation of ventilation until the situation is corrected.

In reality, however, this does not occur as an isolated phenomenon. It usually occurs in the middle of a surgical procedure. Remember the prior description of restlessness, increased blood pressure, and an increased pulse. Surgically this becomes a "moving target" with a rather significant increase in bleeding, which results in a totally impossible situation.

The most common anesthetic response is to increase the sedation. This only intensifies the level of restlessness, the bleeding, and the lack of communication with the patient and causes more confusion. If this is continued, the potential of airway compromise and/or obstruction and the possible occurrence of a true anesthetic tragedy may easily occur.

As pointed out by Perlow[1] in his description of this very complication, the most efficacious approach is merely to stop the surgical procedure, apply oxygen, and allow the medication to metabolize. Do not hurry, take time to ensure a return to normalcy, and when all is ready, the surgeon, anesthesiologist, and staff may proceed to a successful and happy conclusion.

Procedure

On the morning of surgery, after a thorough review of the medical history, consent and all other pertinent information, the material, instruments, and drugs to be used are properly arranged and labeled. In order to adequately prepare for the surgery ahead, it is recommended that the anesthesiologist arrive at the surgical area at least 1 hour prior to the anticipated arrival of the patient. This will prevent the need to hurry and make for an orderly period of preparation.

The intravenous solution used are all of the soft plastic bag type. Glass or hard containers are no longer used. The reasons for this are patient safety and ease of storage.

Next, the medications are prepared. All syringes are marked and size-coded. For example, the amnesic used (lorazepam) is available in TUBEX® containers; the analgesic (usually fentanyl) is always in a 3 cc syringe; thiopentol Na is always in a 10 cc syringe; the local anesthetic agent(s) to be used are placed in 5 cc syringes. We have found that by using this double control, drug error has been reduced almost to zero.

Ancillary and emergency drugs are placed at hand but left in their containers until they are actually needed. Since these drugs and their appropriate syringes, needles, etc., are within easy reach, it is not necessary to prepare multitudes of emergency drugs and agents. The oxygen delivery system is checked to be sure the oxygen supply is adequate and the means to administer it are functioning. We are now ready for the patient.

When the patient arrives, he or she is ushered into a treatment room. We allow patients to be accompanied by relatives or friends. In our experience this helps most patients feel more at ease in what is at best an anxious moment.

At this time the proposed surgery and the consent are reviewed with the patient. A medical, surgical, and anesthetic history is obtained and the patient is given a thorough description of the proposed anesthetic. The patient is now allowed to gown and then is brought into the surgical suite.

We have all of our patients sit upon the surgical table. At this time the chest is auscultated and percussed and the heart sounds are evaluated. The patient is placed supine and a manual sphygmomanometer is applied. The instrument serves a double purpose: one, it allows an initial blood pressure reading, and two, it acts as a tourniquet for the introduction of the intravenous infusion.

After securing the venous catheter in place (usually #18 gauge), the first of our medications (an amnesic) is introduced and the time noted. As has been stated before in our general description of the procedure, between 2 and 3 mg of lorazepam will be administered. The actual amount given will depend on the age, not the size of the patient. Older patients obviously receive a smaller dose.

At this time we "hook" our patient to the various monitors to be used. These will include a cardioscope, an automatic blood pressure recorder, a pulse-oximeter, and an axillary temperature probe. All of the modalities used are non-invasive.

Between 15 to 20 minutes after the administration of the amnesic, we slowly begin the infusion of an analgesic (at this time fentanyl has replaced all other analgesics). We start with .05 to 0.1 mg (never more than 0.1 mg) depending on the patient response to the lorazepam. Within 5 minutes the patient is ready for our initial packing, which consists of small pieces of cotton mildly prepared with 2% topical tetracaine. These are placed superficially in the nasal cavity and left in place for at least 5 minutes.

The patient is now evaluated for level of sedation. Our approach is first to observe the battery of monitors. Secondly, we request the patient to carry out a few simple physical tasks, e.g., raising of the chin and performance of some deep respirations. Depending on the patient response, we may administer more analgesia (in doses of .05 mg) or proceed with the nasal block. If at any time during the block it becomes necessary to administer more analgesia, an evaluation of the patient's response is always performed before continuing with the nasal injections.

The Nasal Block

Using a 5 cc syringe and a #27, 1¼ inch needle, we begin by injecting along the anterior (dorsal) aspect to the glabella. We then follow along the lateral wall including the lateral osteotomy sites. We continue by blocking the inferior turbinate area, attempting to adequately infiltrate the posterior, inferior, and lateral branches of the anterior palatine nerve. We follow with an infraorbital nerve block. The same procedure is performed on the opposite side. The block is completed by infiltrating the septum, tip, and rim.

The patient is now prepared and draped and ready for surgery. It must be noted that during the entire procedure patient and anesthesiologist should be able to communicate at any time. We have found that during the surgery, small quantities of a hypnotic allow the patient to doze and help to allay any fears. Most commonly, thiopental Na is administered intermittently in increments of 25 to 50 mg during the operation and is based strictly on need.

In almost all cases, at the completion of surgery patients are usually very responsive. All patients are kept for evaluation for one to two hours postoperatively before being discharged.

REFERENCES

1. Berman WE: Rhinoplasty, ed 2, Continuing Education Program, American Academy of Otolaryngology (Head and Neck Surgery), 9-10, 1984.
2. Brown BR Jr: Contemp Anesth Prac 7:113, 1983.
3. Cullen SC: Anesthesia in general practice, Chicago, 1954, Year Book Medical Publishers Inc.
4. de Jong RH: Toxicity of local anesthetics, Reg Anaesth, 8, 1977.
5. Lalli AF, Amarnath L: A critique on mortality associated with local anesthetics, Anesthesiology Review, 29, 1982.
6. Schmidt KF: Evaluation of candidates for out patient anesthesia and surgery, Int Anesth Clin, 14:9-13, 1976.

Part II

SYSTEMATIC NASAL SURGERY

8

Turbinate and Septal Surgeries

Walter E. Berman

Septo-rhinoplasty embodies a host of particular procedures to enhance the nose and other facial features while protecting or improving nasal physiology. The basic structural problems of the nasal interior are usually treated first.

Cauterization and Outfracturing of the Inferior Turbinates

If indicated, I prefer decreasing the bulk of the inferior turbinates as the first procedure. This in turn will allow greater room and ease in any septoplastic surgery that may be necessary. The extra room provided is especially helpful when repairing severely deviated nasal septums.

Debulking the inferior turbinate may be handled in a variety of ways. The best of these will decrease the size of the turbinates and cause little, if any, postoperative bleeding and crusting. After trying many techniques for some years, I have found that a double-needle electrocautery, inserted into the entire length of the inferior turbinate in the medial and or inferior aspects, is best (Fig. 8-1). Usually this is necessary on the medial aspect, but often it is helpful on the inferior part of the turbinates as well. A heavy Boies' fracture elevator is then used to outfracture the inferior turbinate bone towards the naso-antral wall (Fig. 8-2). Care must be taken to ensure lateral displacement of the inferior turbinate throughout its length, including the posterior portion of the inferior turbinate. This procedure allows a marked increase in nasal respiration.

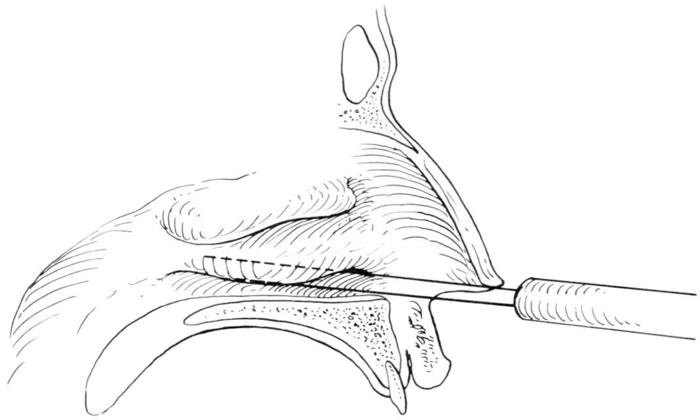

Fig. 8-1. Submucosal bipolar coagulation of the inferior turbinate. (From Berman, WE: Rhinoplasty, ed 2, Washington DC, 1984, American Academy of Otolaryngology-Head and Neck Surgery Foundation, Inc.)

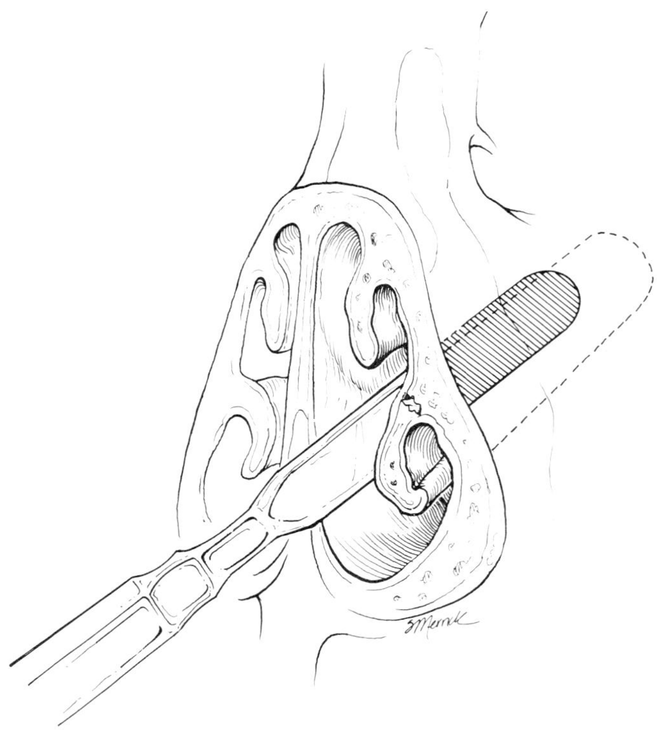

Fig. 8-2. Outfracture of inferior turbinate with a fracture elevator.

Septoplasty

Septal surgery is done in the majority of rhinoplasties, and almost always in the case of a twisted nose. This surgery corrects external nasal deviations and improves breathing as well.

When there is bony septal pathology, it is helpful to use an Ash forceps for the nasal crest or more posterior portions of the bony septum. Obviously, there is great danger at the more anterior part of the perpendicular plate of the ethmoid. I have known of two cases where cerebrospinal leaks occurred when an Ash forcep was used in this area. A closed reduction of a displaced bony part of the posterior septum does not take the place of septal surgery. It merely enhances the actual surgery by allowing greater access and straighter planes for the following septal surgery. Using an Ash forceps on the quadrilateral cartilage is wishful thinking at best because the cartilage will rapidly return to its original position.

Many of the postoperative septal "ills" of septoplastic surgery revert to excessive septal surgery that weakens the septal supports. This is an obvious problem when a saddle deformity results. A less obvious postoperative septal deformity is the retracted columella and, often, excessive columellar retraction and foreshortening of the nose.

To accomplish a straight septum while maintaining anterior to posterior as well as inferior to superior septal support, I propose the steps on the following pages.

A. Raise One Side of Mucosal Flap

Raise only one side of the perichondrium and periosteum except where it is necessary to remove some septal tissue. The contralateral elevation of the perichondrium and/or periosteum is restricted to the exact area of the tissue to be removed.

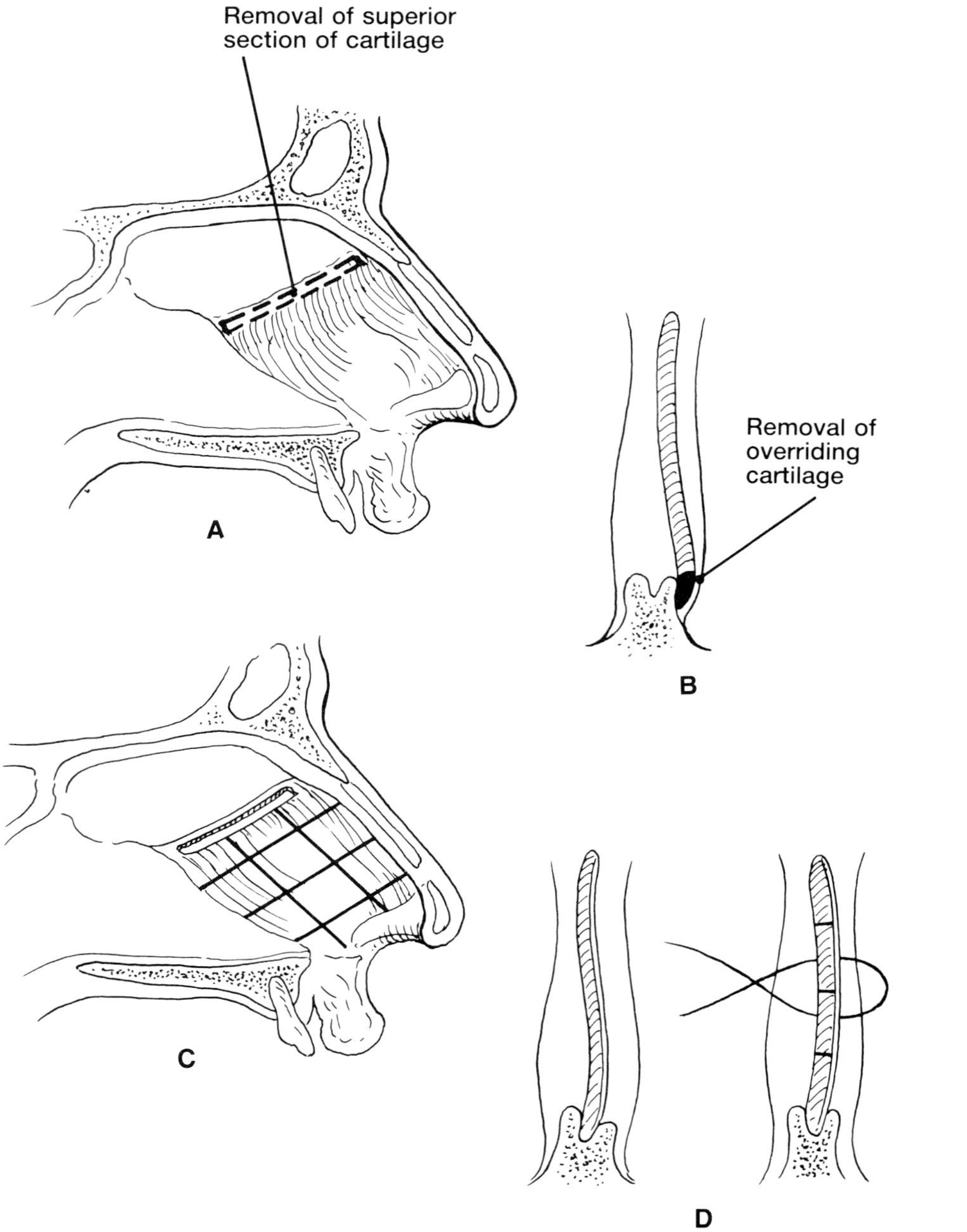

Fig. 8-3. Septoplasty without loss of support. **A,** Quadrilateral septal cartilage that overlaps vomer is removed. **B,** Cartilage is removed at the quadrilateral-ethmoid junction. **C,** Thin segments of cartilage are removed in angles of deviation. Crosshatched incisions through cartilage, forming building blocks, are made as required. **D,** Septum is splinted with 4-0 Vicryl sutures. (From Berman, WE: Rhinoplasty, ed 2, Washington DC, 1984, American Academy of Otolaryngology-Head and Neck Surgery Foundation, Inc.)

B. Remove Least Amount of Septal Support

Remove the least amount of septal framework to preserve support. Both these conditions preserve support by maintaining attachments of the perichondrium and periosteum on the other side of the septum.

I am right-handed and have found it most convenient to make a vertical incision through the septal mucosa immediately inferior to the septal pathology on the patient's right. A one-sided septal mucosal elevation is then completed. About 90% of the time the quadralateral cartilage is displaced from the nasal crest. This overlapping section of the cartilage is then excised as a horizontal strip. When possible, the quadralateral cartilage is replaced on the nasal crest. At times, this simple excision of overlapping cartilage is sufficient to straighten the septum (Fig. 8-3, A and B). However, if the bony septum is off the midline, the cartilaginous septum must be freed from it to release its deforming influence (Fig. 8-4).

If there is excessive septum, either cartilage or bone, there will necessarily be buckling of the septal tissues. This buckling of the residual septum may be congenital or traumatic.

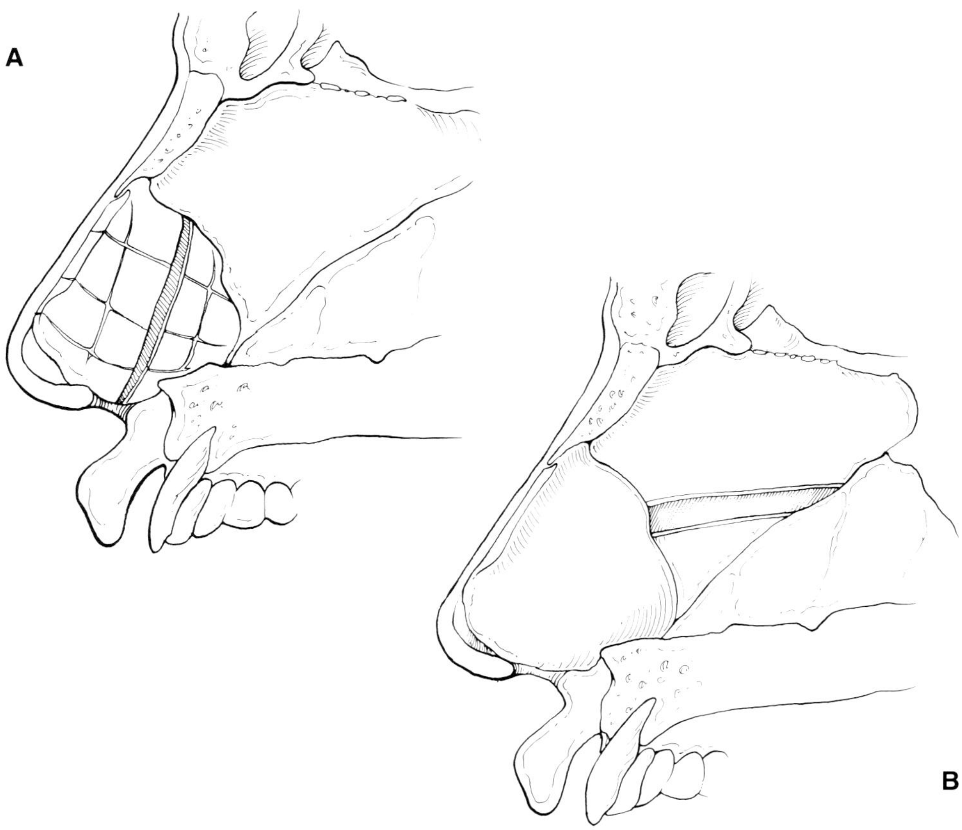

Fig. 8-4. **A,** Cartilage removal for a horizontal bowing. Residual cartilage has been stripped. **B,** Bony removal for deflection.

C. *Removal of Thin Strips at Apex of Buckled Septum*

Thin strips of septal tissue are then removed at the apex of the buckled area. This is done in any direction that the septal bowing takes. Because only thin strips are removed, sufficient support is left to prevent collapse of the septum in any direction. These thin strips may be removed to the anterior or the inferior surfaces (dorsal and caudal) (Fig. 8-5).

D. *Building Blocks Through Strippling*

After the above strips, we are essentially left with fairly straight pieces of cartilage still attached to the perichondrium on one side. If minor bowing or displacement is still evident, cross-hatching of the remaining cartilage is done in both cardinal directions. The cuts must be deep enough to transverse the cartilage to the attached periosteum of the other side. We thus end up with a series of building blocks that cannot fall down (Fig. 8-3, C). This technique leaves a solid wall of cartilage, which forms the new septum. This will also make it almost impossible to cause a septal perforation, saddle deformity, or retracted columella. Cartilage touches cartilage or bone throughout the septum.

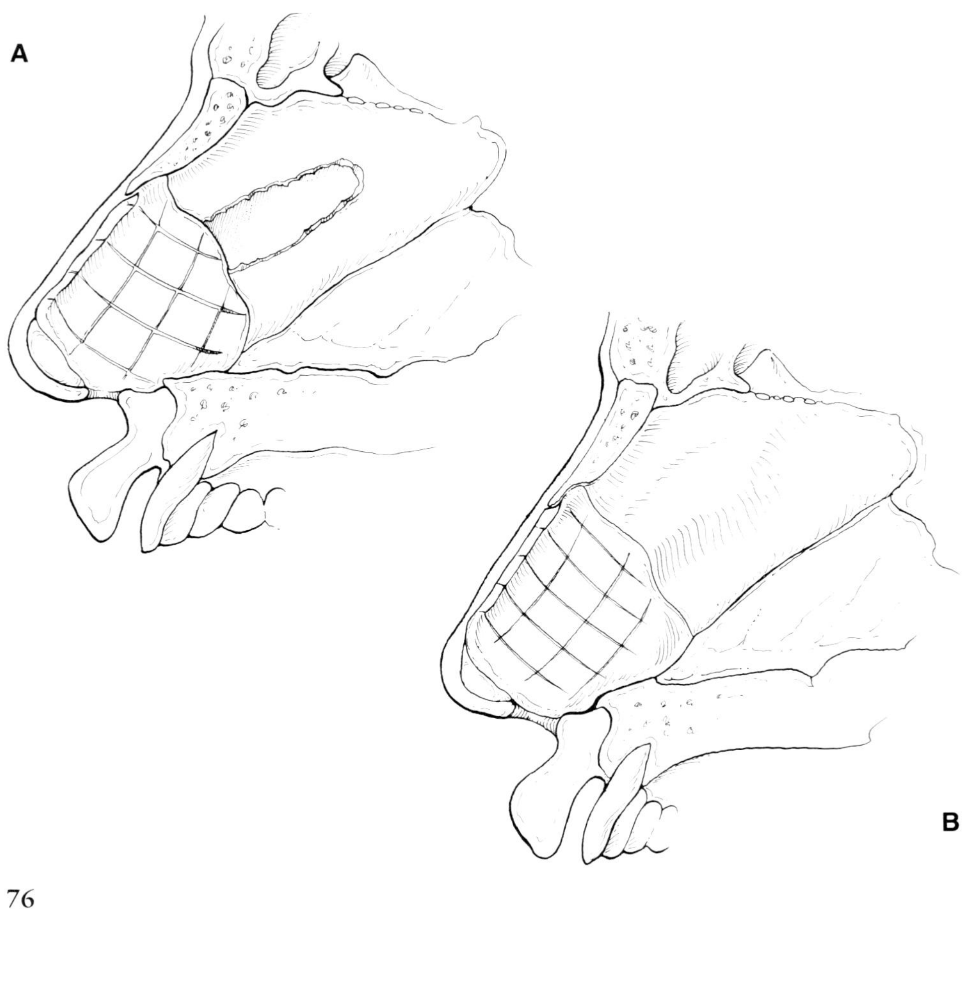

Fig. 8-5. **A,** Bony removal and cartilage stripping before suture splinting. **B,** Cartilage stripping before suture splinting.

E. Straightening Bony Component

A wide or flared nasal crest can usually be treated with a 3 to 4 mm chisel. A postage stamp or multiple perforation effect is achieved with multiple cuts as necessary. This is done on the convex side, whether it be the elevated flap side, or directly through the overlying mucosa of the undissected side. When the perpendicular plate of the ethmoid has severe problems of buckling and/or thickening, other measures must be taken. Portions of bone may be removed with the Takhahashi forceps, or a gentle fracture of the posterior areas may be performed. If the problem is severe, a heavy scissors may be used to cut anterior to the bony pathology. This will protect the cribriform plate area when working on the more posterior bony deformities.

These procedures do not affect nasal support because they affect structures posterior to the nasofrontal angle and do not contribute to the support of the external nose.

F. Splinting Sutures

In closing the septal incisions, I prefer suturing with long-acting soluble sutures like 4-0 Vicyrl. This same suture is often used as a splinting suture going from side to side about halfway back in the septum (Fig. 8-3,D). This suture should be tied on the more concave surfaces of the septum as it may help advance the septum to that side (Fig. 8-6). If packing is desired for bleeding or a difficult septal problem, a flex straw wrapped in telfa is inserted.

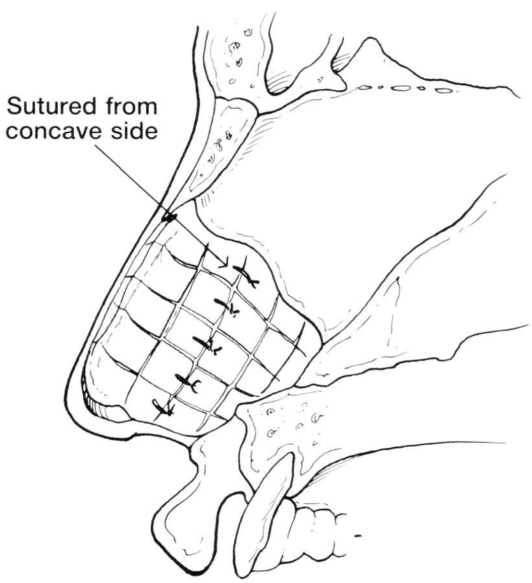

Fig. 8-6. Sutures placed at excisional site through both layers of mucosa.

One of the obvious advantages of this method of septal reconstruction is that removal and replacement of septal tissues does not have to take place (Fig. 8-7). Since there is a practical solid septum left, the stripping incisions may be made through the anterior and/or inferior surfaces with impunity (Fig. 8-8). This procedure does not introduce any risk of septal support loss, absorption or movement of a newly placed septal graft, or perforation.

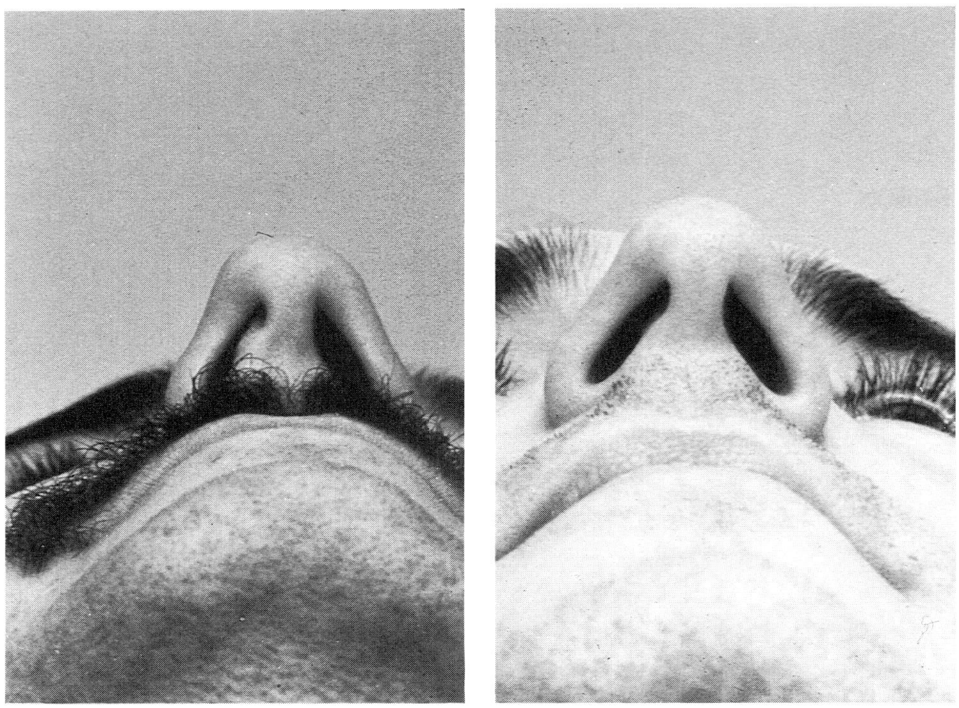

Fig. 8-7. Deviated columella secondary to inferior septal deviation treated with repositioning; no grafts.

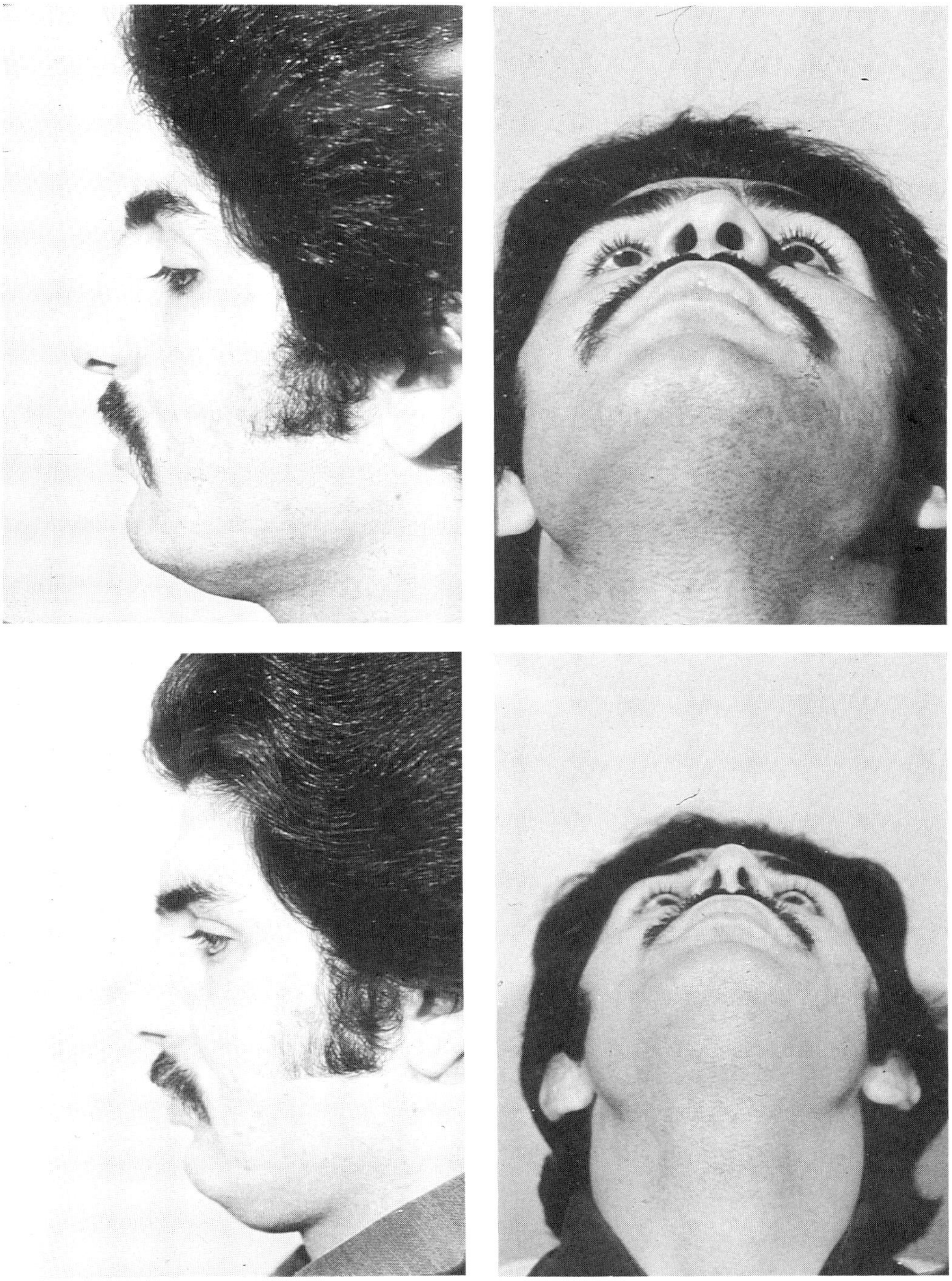

A B C D

Fig. 8-8. Tip asymmetry corrected with an inferior septal stripping and repositioning. A and B, Preoperative. C and D, Postoperative.

From a practical point of view, deflected columellas and anterior septal torsions can also be safely and effectively treated in this manner (Figs. 8-9 and 8-10). The most difficult septum and external rhinoplastic reconstruction may be done concurrently in a one-stage procedure (Fig. 8-11).

The airway is now established except in those cases where osteotomies must be completed before an optimal airway is achieved. Osteotomies are left to a later stage in the procedure because of bleeding that might ensue, interfering with surgical procedures on the nose.

Fig. 8-9. **A,** Deflected inferior nasal septum. **B,** Deflected bone and cartilage. Both **A** and **B** treated by linear excisions of bone and cartilage at the angle of bowing.

A

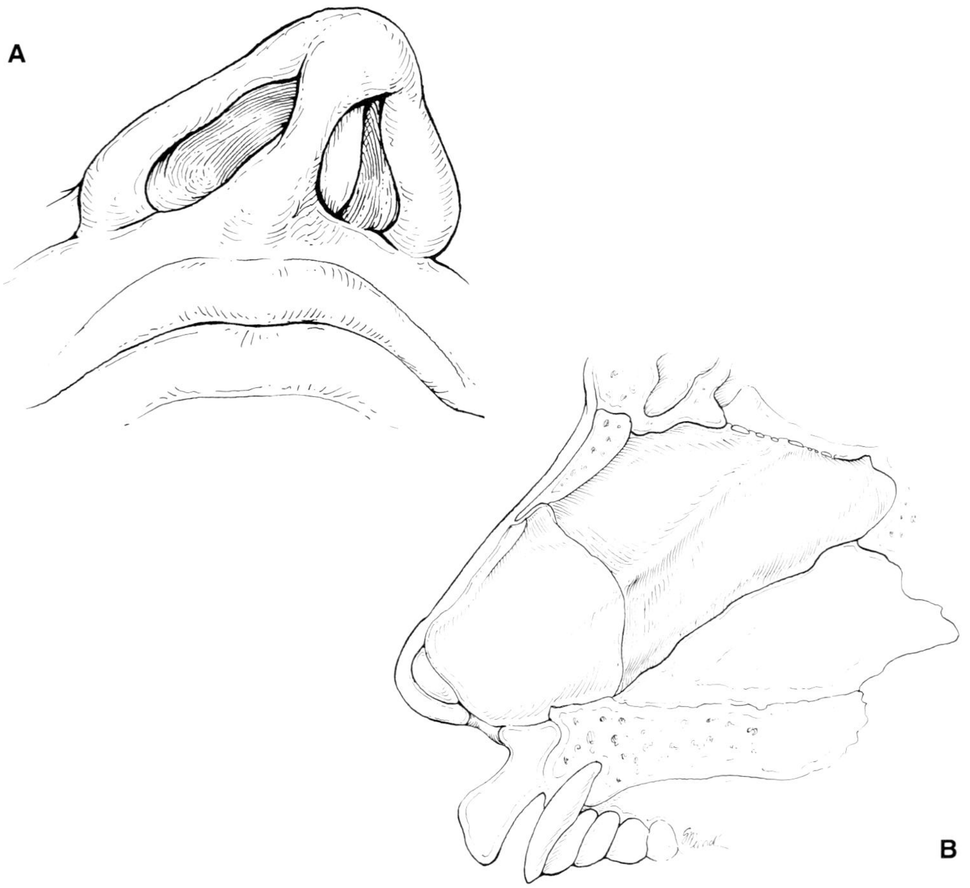

B

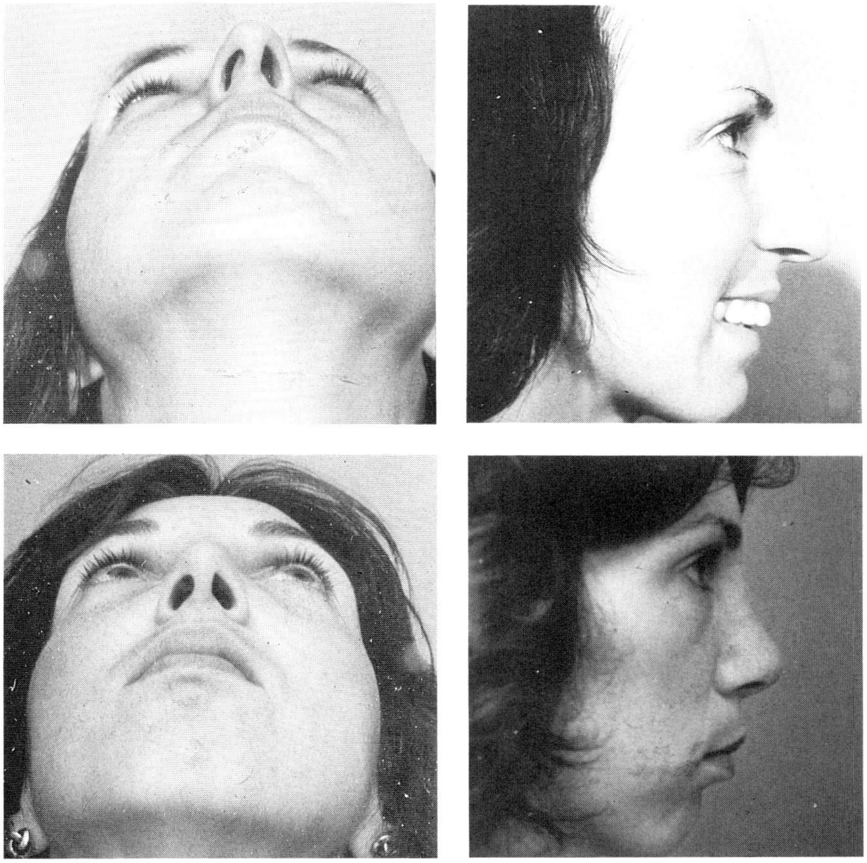

A B C D

Fig. 8-10. A and B, Preoperative: inferior septal deflection caused by tension septum. C and D, Postoperative: treated by stripping and repositioning.

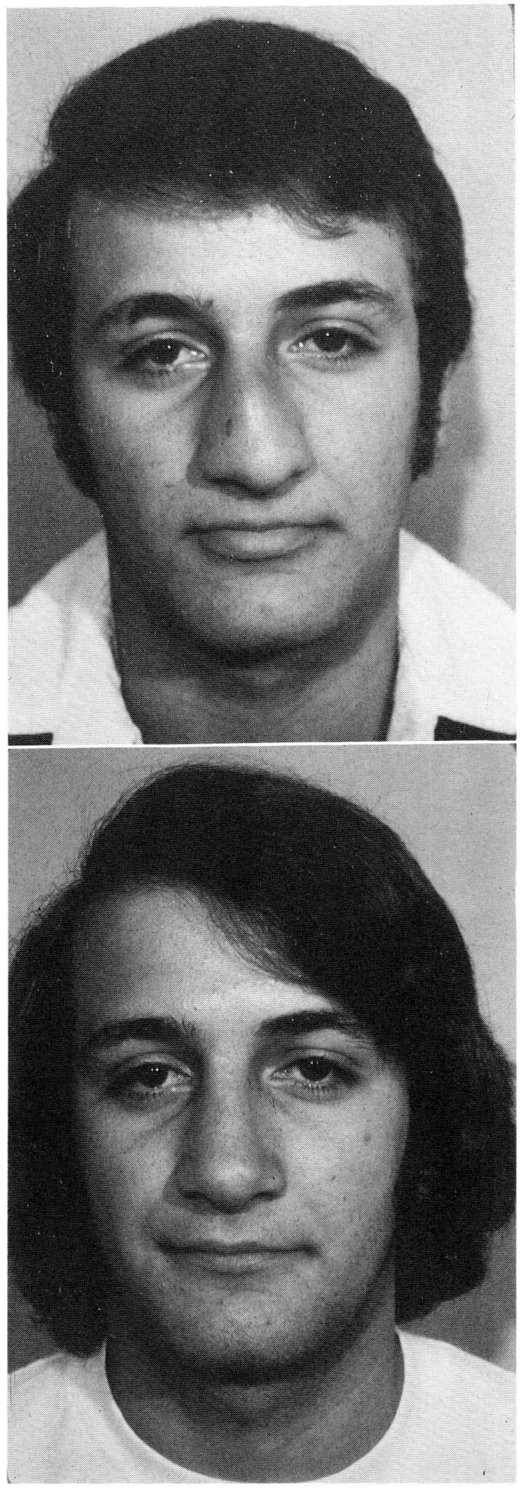

A

B

Fig. 8-11. **A,** Preoperative combined septoplasty. **B,** Reduction of nasal fractures and rhinoplasty, postoperative.

9

Inferior Septal Incisions

Walter E. Berman

Indications

Inferior septal (or caudal) incisions should only be done in specific instances. If the lip-tip angle is fine, no incision is necessary. If the lip-tip angle is fine but there is a deflection of the inferior septum, a one-sided incision should be made to correct the septum. If the anterior part of the columella is dependent, the incision should be made only on the anterior part of the inferior septum. Conversely, if the problem only involves the area of the nasal spine and if complete mobility of the nasal tip and inferior surface of the cartilage is needed, a complete inferior septal or transfixion incision should be done.

Hazards

How to separate the medial crura from the inferior or caudal septum is the question. As always, an understanding of the anatomy of the nose is the key to manipulating its components. The feet of the medial crura are wrapped around the inferior septum. There are also various ligaments holding the medial crura to the septum. If these attachments are separated from each other, support is lost and may cause a drop in tip projection.

Secondarily, as with any incision, there will be some contraction. This latter possibility may cause retraction of the columella. When studying the relationship of the feet of the medial crura to the septum, the normal relationship is approximately the mid-portion of the septum prior to a complete transfixion procedure. Postoperatively, when an inferior septal incision is done, the crural feet are often on the anterior nasal spine.

Since the medial crura are the main support of the nasal tip, this change in anatomical relationships may be imperative in producing the final tip projection. When separation of the medial crura from the inferior septum is necessary (as in the case of a long nose with a hard central segment) and maintenance or increasing tip projection is indicated, appropriate measures must be taken to maintain such. (See section Increasing tip projection).

Extent

In any inferior septal incision, care must be taken not to injure the medial crura. Therefore inferior traction of the medial crura should be applied with a Brown-Adson forceps. This maneuver will expose the inferior septum so that an incision can be accomplished on the inferior border of the quadrilateral cartilage without the possibility of amputating the medial crural feet.

Depending on the anatomical problem, a partial and not a complete incision may be indicated, i.e., if there is a mild overhang of the nasal tip with a good columellar lip angle and a firm central segment, an incision from the septal angle partway posteriorly towards the spine may be all that is necessary. This may be any proportion of the length of the inferior border of the quadrilateral cartilage. A complete incision down to the inferior nasal spine is indicated when some tip projection decrease is desirable, or when the above crural-to-septal attachments are very firm, preventing tip projection by other means: e.g., cartilaginous struts, permanent placement sutures, etc. (Fig. 9-1).

Remember, if there is a soft central segment, no inferior septal incision should be done, or a columellar retraction may result.

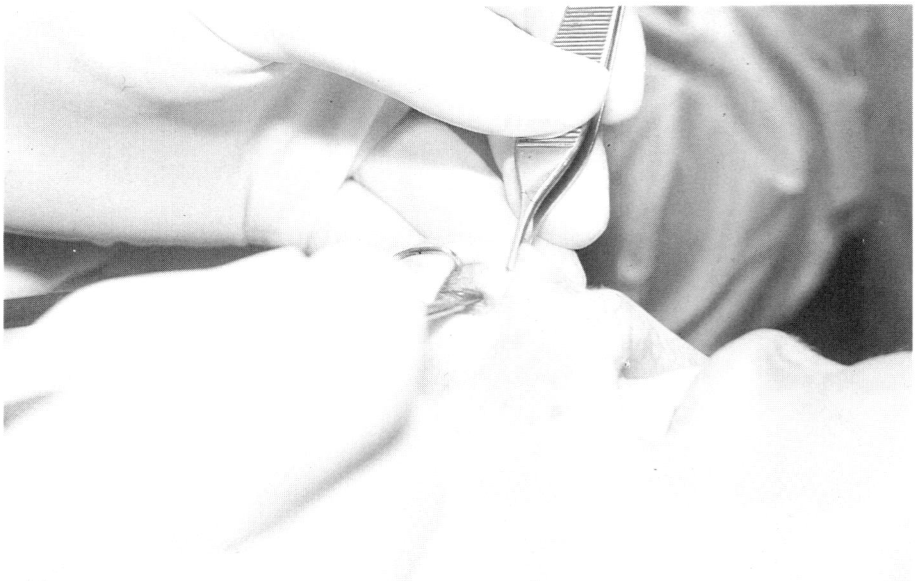

Fig. 9-1. The extent of the inferior septal incision will vary with the problem.

10

Nasal Tip

Walter E. Berman

In essence, the nasal tip sets the stage for what can be done with the other parts of the nose. It is the focal point of the nose and is paramount in determining what relationships are necessary to create a harmonious balance with other facial features. There are four possible approaches to the nasal tip as well as four types of procedures to modify tip architecture. The approaches to the tip must provide the surgeon with as much visualization and room for manipulation as necessary.

Approaches

Delivery

I prefer to deliver the lower lateral cartilages in most cases. This delivery technique allows exact comparisons between the two sides. It also completely separates the domes and lower lateral cartilages from their attachments to the overlying skin. It allows much more complete removal of fibrofatty tissues, both on the lower lateral cartilages and the undersurface of the tip skin. The only exception is the open rhinoplasty, which can have other hazards. This delivery technique also allows the opportunity to morselize and thereby reshape the dome and lower lateral cartilages into more desirable configurations.

A between-the-cartilage incision is made bilaterally. This is done with a #15 blade between the upper and lower cartilages extending to the inferior edge of the nasal bones. A swivel hook is then used to evert the nasal rim while the middle finger of the same hand presses and also everts the lower lateral cartilage. An incision is made from the inferior edge of the lower cartilage dome three-quarters of the way, laterally hugging the inferior aspect of the lower lateral cartilage. When this is completed on both sides a Foman scissors is used to separate the overlying skin from the underlying lower lateral cartilage. Care must be taken that the scissors also separates the lower lateral cartilage from the upper lateral cartilage. A single hook is then placed on the inferior aspect of the nasal dome and traction is exerted inferiorly.

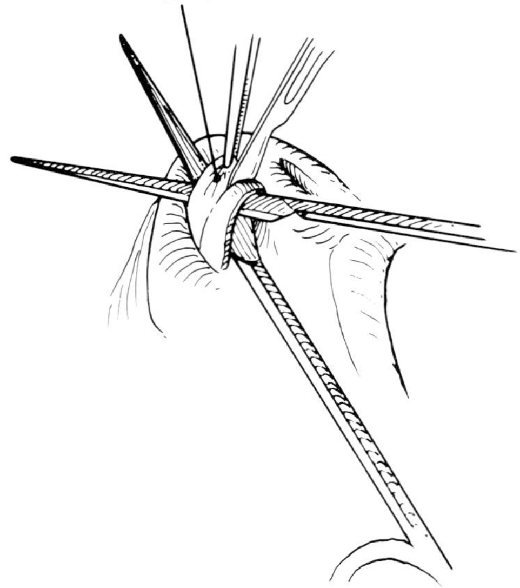

Fig. 10-1. Delivery approach to the nasal tip. (From Berman WE: Rhinoplasty, ed 2, Washington DC, 1984, American Academy of Otolaryngology-Head and Neck Surgery Foundation, Inc.)

The Foman scissors is then placed in the between-the-cartilage incision, and the scissor points are brought out of the nose between the lower lateral cartilage and the overlying skin, through the prior marginal incision. This maneuver everts the lower lateral cartilage, affording an excellent view of the lower lateral dome and the lateral and the medial crura, if the dissection was carried out in that direction. The scissors is advanced until its screw becomes the fulcrum under the dome. The handles are then spread to allow the scissors to become a self-retaining retractor while the lower cartilages are shaped. The handles of the scissors are stabilized on either side of the chin. With both lower lateral complexes in view, symmetry is obtainable (Fig. 10-1).

Excessive fibrofatty tissue is removed from the dissected side of the lower laterals, between the domes, and possibly from the medial parts of the cartilage (Fig. 10-2). When thinning or debulking the nasal tip is deemed necessary, a 5 mm strip of cartilage is left at the inferior border of the lower lateral cartilage. This will ensure an intact line postoperatively without irregularities at the nasal tip. With the single hook still in place, the lower lateral complex is everted from the nose as a chondroplastic bipedicle flap. The Foman scissors is removed after the incisions are made in the lower lateral cartilage and a blunt retractor is substituted to retract the nares. No vestibular skin is removed. The lateral extent of cartilage removal is varied 50% to 75%. Further removal may cause a collapse of the external nares. Fibrofatty tissue attached to the undersurface of the overlying skin is then removed with a Brown-Adson forceps (Fig. 10-3).

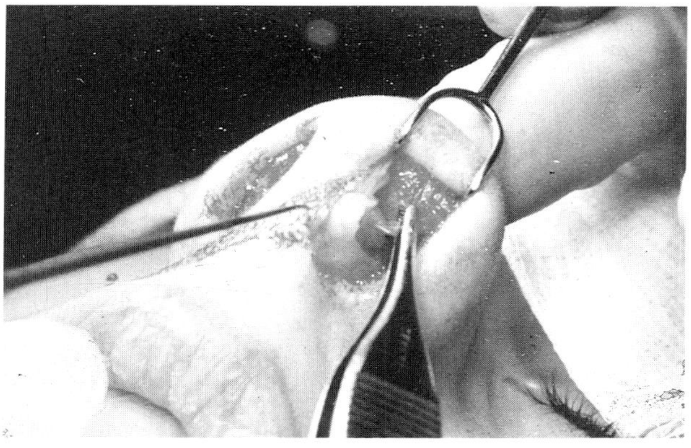

Fig. 10-2. Picking out the fibrofatty tissues from the subcutaneous areas and between the domes.

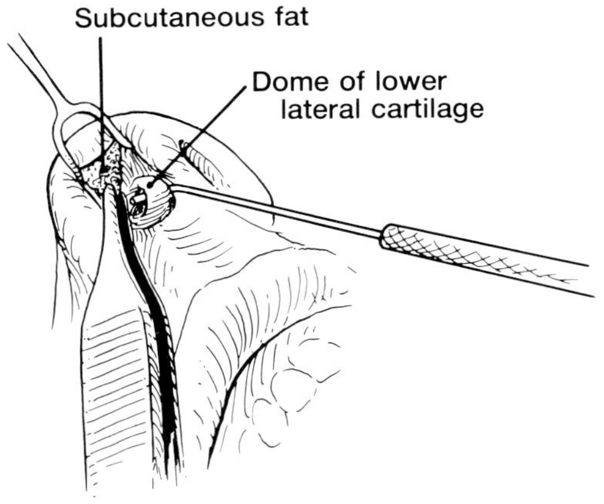

Fig. 10-3. Removal of subcutaneous and interdomal fat and fibrous tissues with a Brown-Adson forceps. (From Berman WE: Rhinoplasty, ed 2, Washington DC, 1984, American Academy of Otolaryngology-Head and Neck Surgery Foundation, Inc.)

I like a small one-sided morselizer such as the Rubin for morselization of the nasal dome and adjacent areas of the cartilage (Fig. 10-4). This allows further molding of the nasal tip and repositioning of the lower lateral cartilages. Further modifications of the lower lateral cartilages and nasal tip will be discussed subsequently under appropriate sections (Fig. 10-5).

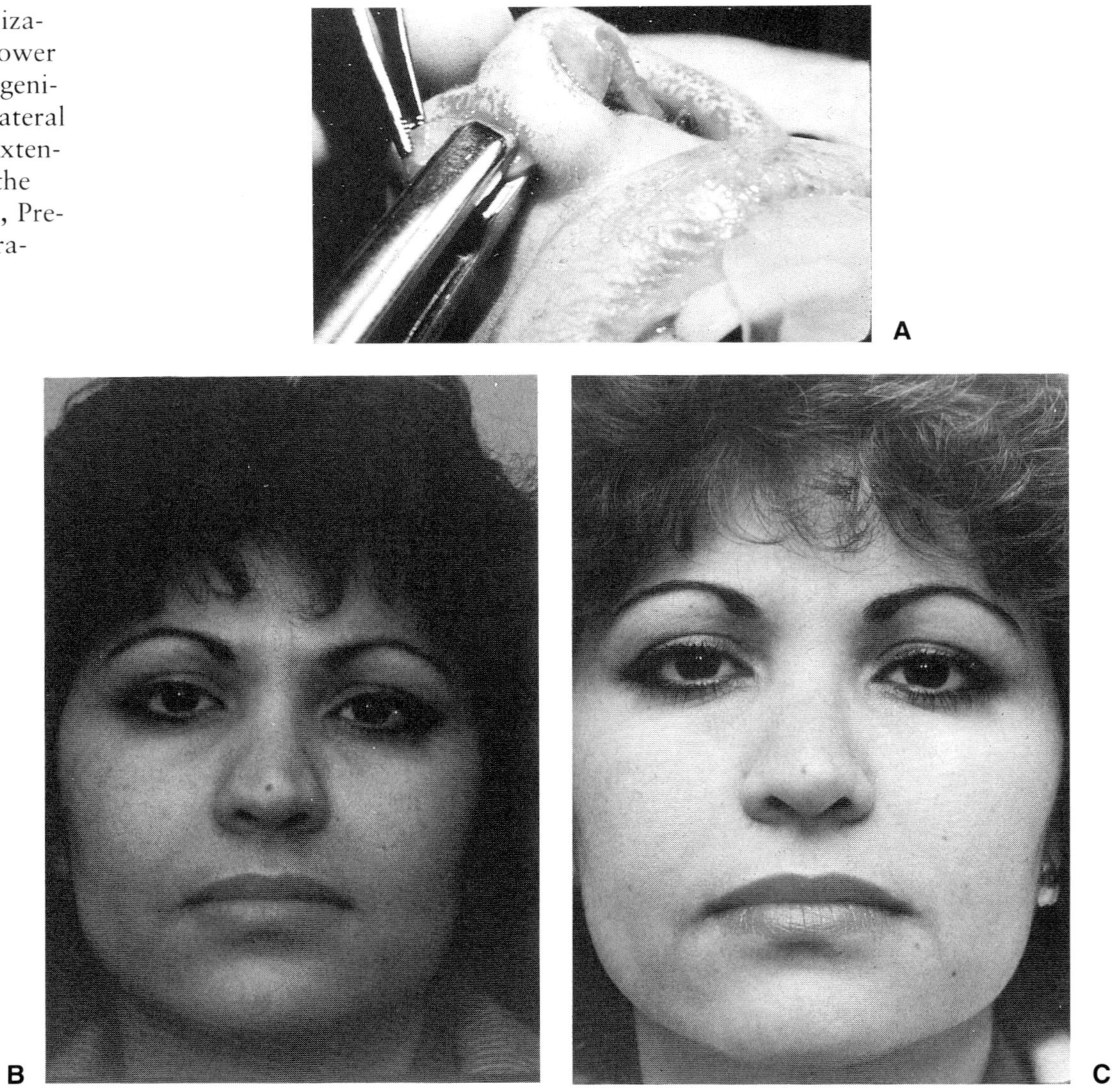

Fig. 10-4. A, Morselization of the delivered lower lateral cartilages. Congenital corrugated lower lateral cartilages treated by extensive morselization of the delivered cartilages. B, Preoperative. C, Postoperative.

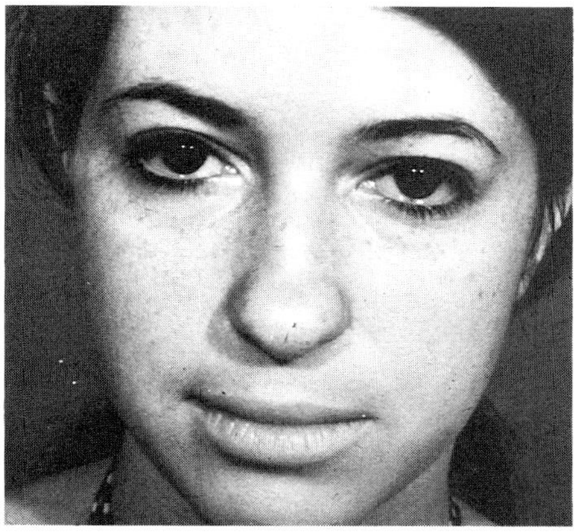

A

Fig. 10-5. Bulbous nose treated with delivery of the lower lateral cartilages, superior excision of same, morselization, removing fibrofatty tissues and a double dome suture. **A** and **B,** Preoperative C and **D,** Postoperative. (From Berman WE: Rhinoplasty, ed 2, Washington DC, 1984, American Academy of Otolaryngology-Head and Neck Surgery Foundation, Inc.)

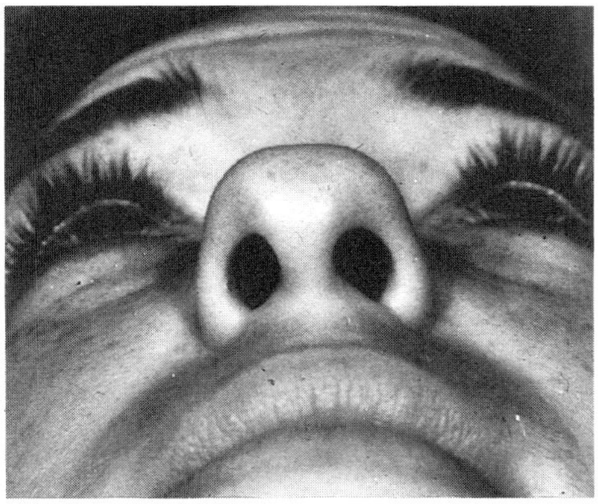

B

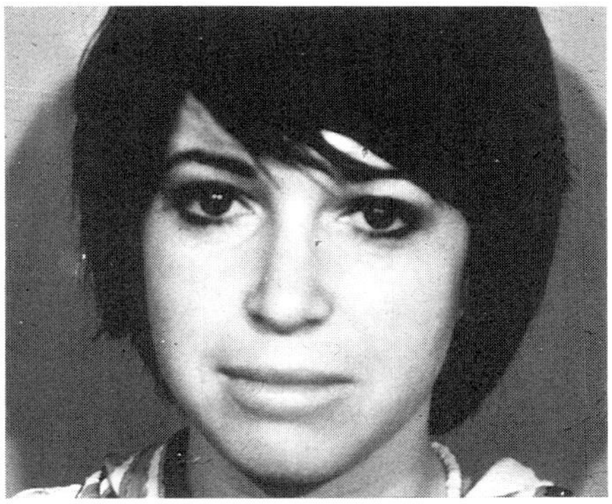

C

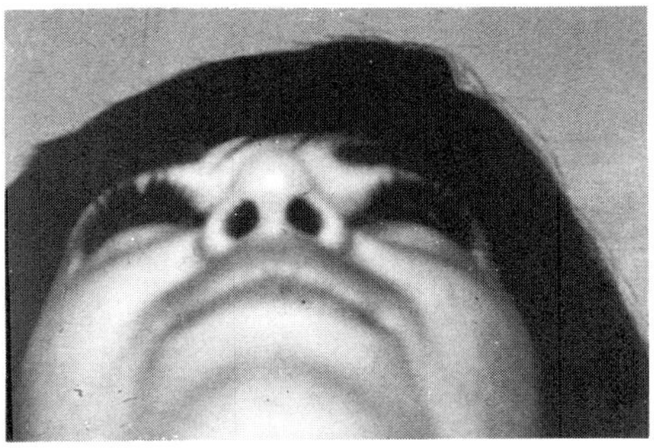

D

Tip Thinning/Cartilage Splitting (Intracartilaginous)

A common method of thinning the nasal tip without delivery is the 'split' (intracartilaginous) approach. This is merely another variant of removing the superior aspect of the lower lateral cartilage. The inferior border of the lower lateral cartilage is determined by examining the same through the vestibular membrane. An incision through the vestibular membrane is made parallel to the inferior border of the lower lateral cartilage, about 5 mm from that inferior edge. The more superior aspect of the lower lateral cartilage is then denuded of the remaining vestibular skin under the cartilage with a straight Stevens iris scissors. Next, the overlying skin is separated from the same piece of cartilage in a similar manner. With both sides of this cartilage freed, it is a simple matter to grasp and excise this cartilage and thereby thin the nasal tip (Fig. 10-6).

What are the advantages and disadvantages of this procedure? The advantages are that it is relatively simple, quick, and, unlike the delivery method, requires no between-the-cartilage incision. Its disadvantages are that it is not possible to evaluate the two sides as well as in a delivery.

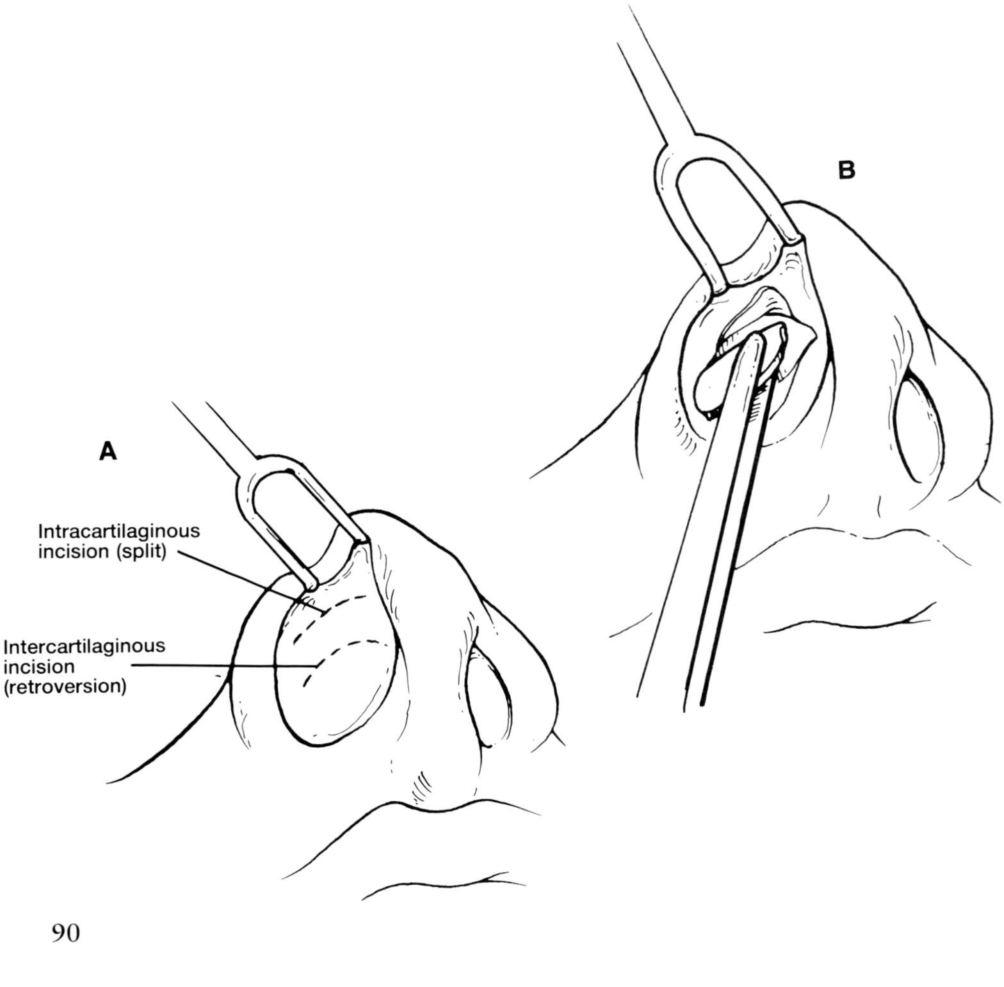

Fig. 10-6. Split (intracartilaginous) removal of lower lateral cartilage. **A**, Incisions: lower is the between-the-cartilage; upper marks the extent of cartilage to be removed. **B**, Superior lower lateral cartilage being removed.

Possible asymmetry may result and it is impossible to remove the fibrofatty tissues both over the undissected lower lateral cartilages and between the nasal domes. It is also impossible to morselize the remaining cartilages to define the nasal tip. This procedure is useful when a nasal tip is already thin before surgery and merely needs some debulking of the lateral tip.

Retrograde (Intercartilaginous)

Removal of the excessive lower lateral cartilage through the between-the-cartilage incision is a reverse technique of the split approach. The edge of the nares is everted with a double swivel hook. A straight Stevens iris scissors is used to separate the vestibular skin from the undersurface of the lower lateral cartilage to be removed and the overlying skin of this same cartilage. The freed piece of vestibular skin is also retracted and the desired amount of lower lateral cartilage is excised with a scissors.

I feel that it is best to leave the between-the-cartilage incision unsutured at all times. This promotes drainage and causes less subsequent swelling of the nasal structures.

The retrograde is particularly suited in a male traumatized nose when some debulking with little definition of the tip is desired. The pros and cons of this procedure are similar to the split tip technique, but may allow better visualization and surgical access than the split technique.

External

The external incisions are a combination of an inferior skin incision on the columella, the previously described marginal incisions, and connecting incisions along the sides of the columella. The skin over much of the nasal tip cartilage is then dissected from the underlying structures and reflected.

This technique allows an excellent view of the tip structures with direct surgical access. However, there are disadvantages: more surgical time, external scarring, and greater difficulty may result if a secondary procedure is necessary. Chapter 17, by Dr. Jack Anderson discusses external rhinoplasty in greater depth.

Procedures: Tip Rotation and Definition

The four procedures to modify nasal tip architecture each have their own benefits and risks.

Primary Rotation

The inferior border of the lower lateral cartilage (LLC) and dome are left intact. Such is the case when the LLC is delivered and a portion of its superior aspect is removed. The rotation point is the most lateral point of the LLC.

Secondary Rotation

When the nasal tip is rotated with the inferior edge of the lateral crura intact, the rotation point is from the most lateral edge of the lower lateral cartilage (complete strip). When further rotation, or shortening, is desired, a secondary point of rotation is created by excising a triangle of cartilage towards the mid area of the lower lateral cartilage (lateral crural flap) (Fig. 10-7). The apex of the removed triangle of cartilage is on the inferior aspect, while the base of the triangle is on the superior aspect of the LLC. This is an excision of cartilage completely through the width of the LLC while sparing the vestibular skin. When rotation takes place, the space at the base of the excised triangle disappears and the nasal tip is rotated in that proportion (Fig. 10-8).

In order to facilitate this surgical technique, the lower lateral cartilages are delivered through a marginal and between the cartilage incision. A small skin hook is used for traction at the dome and the cartilage is excised without removing any underlying vestibular skin. Care must be taken not to make this excision towards the dome. The triangle is removed about halfway lateral to the dome. Overlying skin is thinner near the dome and sharp edges of cartilage may be evident postoperatively.

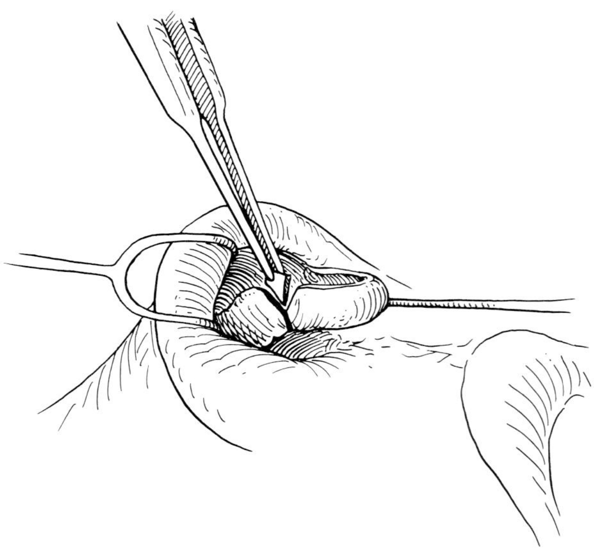

Fig. 10-7. Secondary rotation: removal of superior cartilage. (From Berman WE: Rhinoplasty, ed 2, Washington DC, 1984, American Academy of Otolaryngology-Head and Neck Surgery Foundation, Inc.)

Free Rotation

The LLC is freed from its most lateral attachments, namely the sesamoid cartilages, ligaments, and fibrous tissues. This allows the lateral aspect of the LLC to float more freely and be replaced in its new position. This is useful in the wide nasal base such as the ethnic nose.

Vertical Dome Division

The lower nasal cartilages are separated at the dome area where the LLC meets the medial crura. This often causes tip irregularities, occasionally a few years after surgery. With morselization of the dome area, removal of the underlying fibrofatty tissues and the permanent dome suture that holds the domes together, vertical dome division is not necessary (Fig. 10-9). I believe that this should hardly ever be done. The only exceptions would be in cases of gross asymmetry of the domes such as a post-cleft lip nose or where there has been severe nasal trauma.

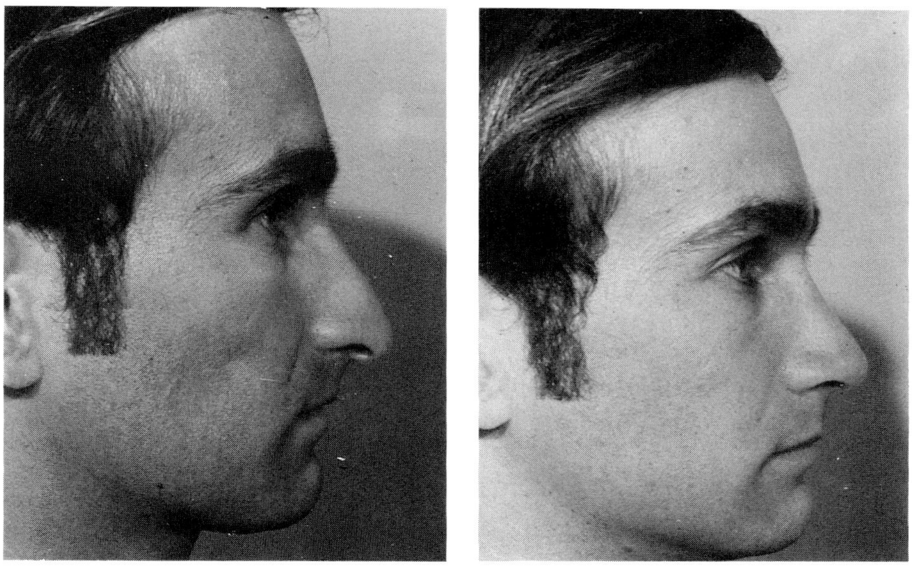

A B

Fig. 10-8. **A**, Preoperative and **B**, Postoperative photos of a secondary rotation for a long nose with a soft central segment.

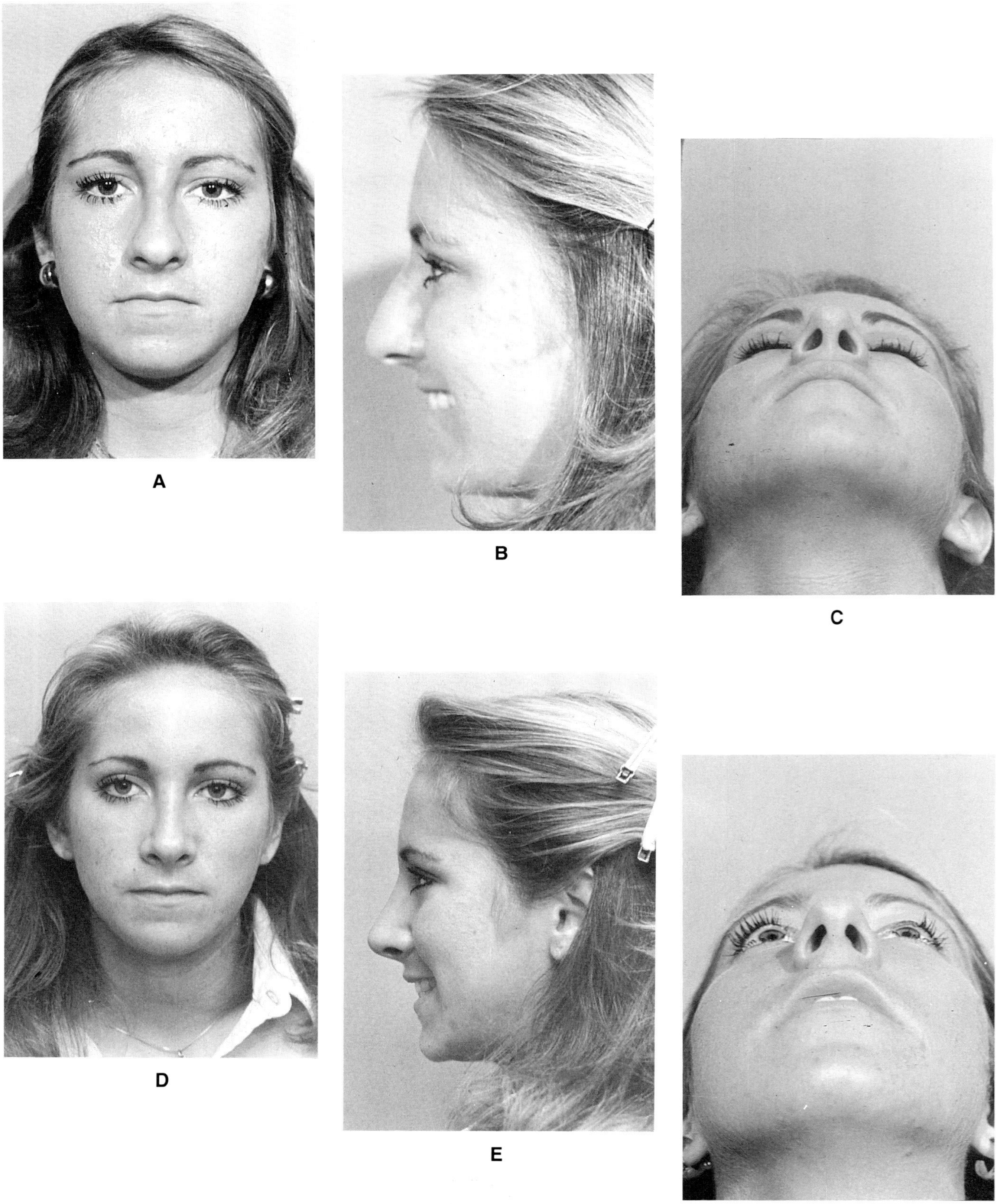

Fig. 10-9. **A-C,** Preoperative and **D-F,** Postoperative photos showing repaired vertical dome division in which a permanent non-buried double dome suture was used to hold the two nasal domes in closer apposition.

Through the years I have seen many split nasal domes. Even after several years patients say that bumps appeared on the tips of their noses. It is certainly safer to split the nasal domes when there is very thick overlying tip skin than when it is fairly thin. When these bumps (horny tip) appear postoperatively in cases when the domes were *not* split, they are caused by an insufficient border of cartilage having been left in place.

Final Evaluation and Correction of Tip Projection

After completion of the septum, turbinate, tip, and osteotomy surgery, we turn to the definitive finishing touches. These include checking for future tip support, any protrusions anterior to the anterior septum and/or upper lateral cartilages, any irregularities, and correcting these when they occur.

Checking for Future Tip Support

Mild digital pressure in a posterior direction, inferior to the nasal spine, should cause little, if any, loss of tip projection. This test should be done before any septal-columellar suturing. We must remember that local injection over the anterior nasal spine acts like a temporary implant that holds the nasal tip up during surgery. It is, therefore, imperative not to inject this area with a local anesthetic. Injections in surrounding areas will not cause this deceptive phenomenon while affording local anesthesia. If the tip is readily depressed with minimal pressure, some type of supporting mechanism is required.

Increasing Tip Projection

When the surgical literature is replete with many ways of accomplishing a result, it only means that none of them is foolproof. This is certainly true of the task of increasing nasal tip projection. Small wonder that the definitive result of a nasal surgery is often based on what could be accomplished with the nasal tip and how the corresponding parts of the nose were altered to fit the tip.

I would like to keep an aesthetically pleasing nasal tip intact whenever possible. It is preferable to raise the entire tip complex when necessary rather than to add tissue to the tip and increase tip projection in that manner. Inadvertently creating irregularities and asymmetries by cutting through the nasal domes or adding cartilage has occurred too often.

My armamentarium to increase tip projection has consisted of permanent placement sutures and cartilaginous grafts from below.

Permanent placement sutures. After an inferior septal incision has been made, a permanent #4-0 clear suture is taken from a higher point on the inferior quadrilateral cartilage to a lower point on the medial crus (Fig. 10-10). This suture is from cartilage to cartilage and is buried deep to the mucosa and the vestibular skin (Fig. 10-11). Usually a similar secondary suture is taken posteriorly to the first for added support. I have used this type of suture for more than fifteen years with good results. This type of support is adequate for a mild loss of tip projection, but not for the more severe cases.

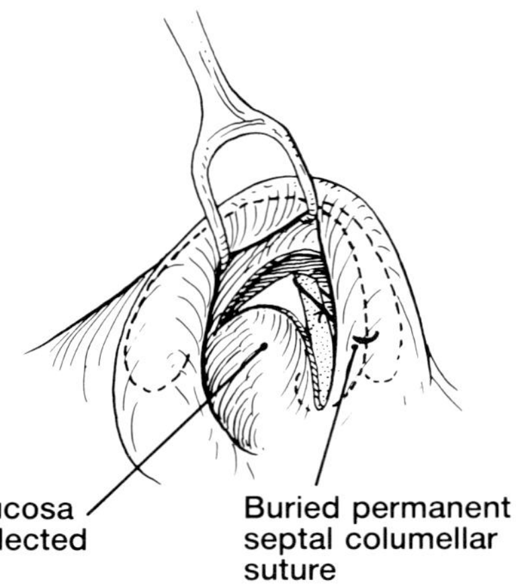

Fig. 10-10. Permanent placement suture extends from a more anterior point on the quadrilateral cartilage to a more posterior point on the medial crura. (From Berman WE: Rhinoplasty, ed 2, Washington DC, 1984, American Academy of Otolaryngology-Head and Neck Surgery Foundation, Inc.)

A
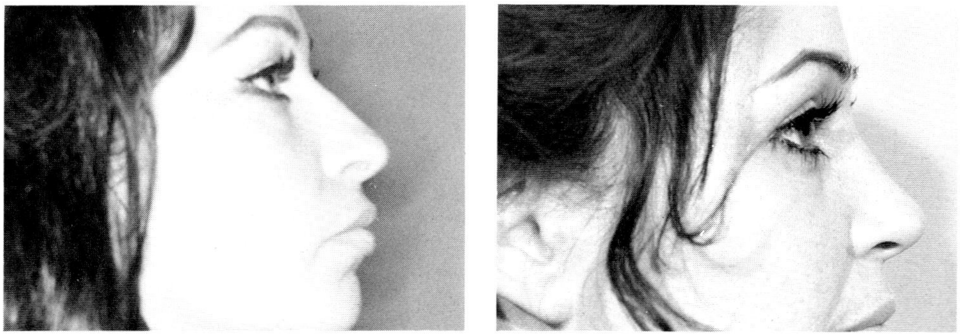
B

Fig. 10-11. **A,** Preoperative and **B,** postoperative photos showing result of using a permanent buried placement suture from a higher point on the inferior edge of the septal cartilage to a lower point on the medial crus. (From Berman WE: Rhinoplasty, ed 2, Washington DC, 1984, American Academy of Otolaryngology-Head and Neck Surgery Foundation, Inc.)

Columellar cartilaginous grafts. When the placement sutures are not sufficient, cartilage grafts that are often called *struts* are used. The bed for the graft will be inferior to the medial crura. These grafts are placed inferiorly, caudal to the medial crural cartilages. They may extend from the anterior nasal spine to the feet of the medial crura or to an area between the nasal domes. I prefer to start the graft site with an incision on the lateral side of the right medial crus to prevent any marginal postoperative scarring. A prior medial rim incision may also be used. A straight Stevens iris scissors is then used to tunnel posteriorly down to the nasal spine. This dissected pocket is inferior to the crural cartilages. The cartilage graft is fashioned to the desired size, both in height and breadth, and is placed through this incision along the previously created tunnel down to the nasal spine (Fig. 10-12). Care must be taken that the cartilaginous graft, the strut, is not too long. Especially, in thin skin nasal tips, the anterior edge of the graft may be visible. This can be nullified by placing the anterior edge of the graft between the nasal domes or by shortening the length of the cartilaginous strut. When the medial

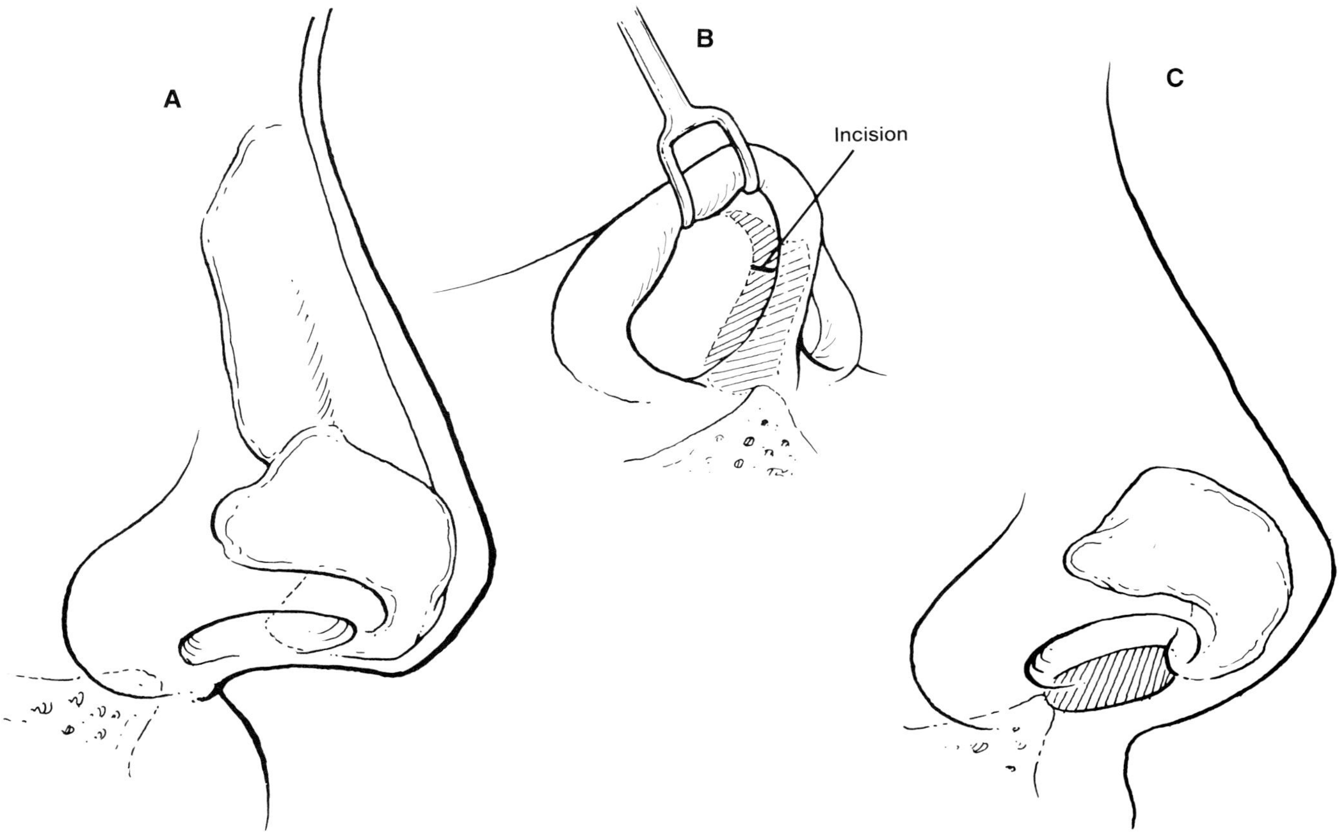

Fig. 10-12. Placement of columnellar grafts. **A,** Before placement. **B,** Hidden vestibular skin incision with a Stevens iris scissors forms a pocket to place the grafts. **C,** Graft in place.

crura are too close to the nasal spine, a cartilage graft placed between the spine and the feet of the crura will raise the medial crural complex. This loss of projection may be developmental or caused by an inferior septal transfixion incision. This supporting graft is sutured in place.

The sutures to hold the graft in place are long-lasting dissolvables such as Vicryl. Horizontal mattress sutures are used. These encompass the inferior border of the quadrilateral cartilage, the graft, and often the mucosal flap from the septal surgery. Both the placement sutures and the cartilaginous grafts may be used together when warranted.

The clinical determination of whether to use a graft and how much to use is made with a Brown-Adson forceps. The forceps moves the medial crura until the desired effect is obtained. Measurements are taken and the graft is sculpted to size.

For many years I have preferred to use megarad cartilage from a bank. This necropsy rib cartilage receives between 2 and 3 million rads for sterilization. Various studies have shown that they hold up as well as autogenous grafts. My reasoning has been that this rib cartilage is thicker, is usually straighter, and is readily obtainable from a bottle. These grafts have less of a tendency to curl and no greater incidence of absorption than autogenous tissues.[1] The rib grafts are obtainable from various commercial laboratories throughout the country.

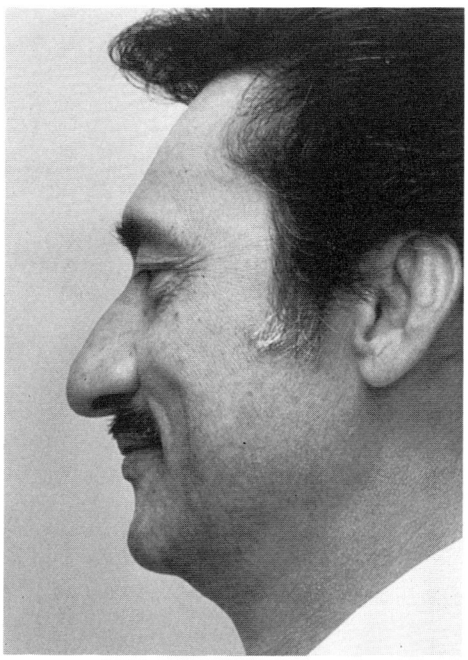

A

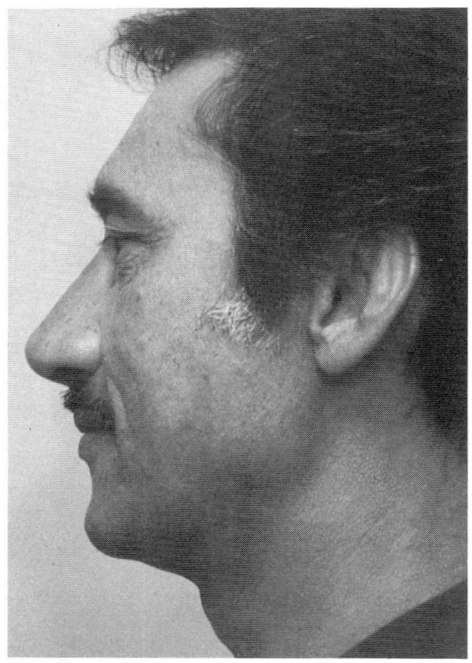

B

Fig. 10-13. **A**, Preoperative and **B**, Postoperative photos showing result of using inferior septal graft of megarad bank rib cartilage to increase tip projection.

In many cases where this type of reconstruction is mandatory, the septum is worthless for graft material, either from prior surgeries or trauma. Auricular cartilage seldom has sufficient strength. An autogenous rib is more difficult both for the patient and the surgeon.

In a sense these are onlay grafts that are placed inferiorly or posteriorly to the medial crura. They serve a dual purpose of also providing support for tip projection (Fig. 10-13).

When the nasal tip meets our aesthetic criteria but needs projection, I would rather use the existing nasal tip and project it to a better height (Fig. 10-14). Onlay grafts over the nasal domes often get absorbed and show irregularities with the passage of time.

Given adequate nasal domes that are merely at too posterior a level, increasing the projection of the entire tip complex is preferable to adding tissue on top of the domes. This technique will prevent the slipping of the grafts and the broadening of the nasal tip.

When there is columellar retraction, and thereby loss of crural support, the nasal tip may lose projection. A shorter graft of cartilage is substituted in much the same manner as the longer grafts that are needed for greater tip projection (Fig. 10-15). This type of cartilaginous graft often serves the dual function of aiding the posterior columellar retraction while raising tip projection.

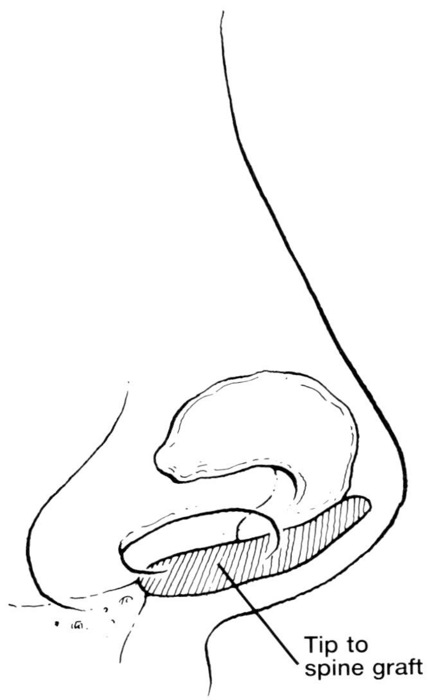

Fig. 10-14. Inferior (caudal) graft to increase tip projection from the nasal spine to the tip.

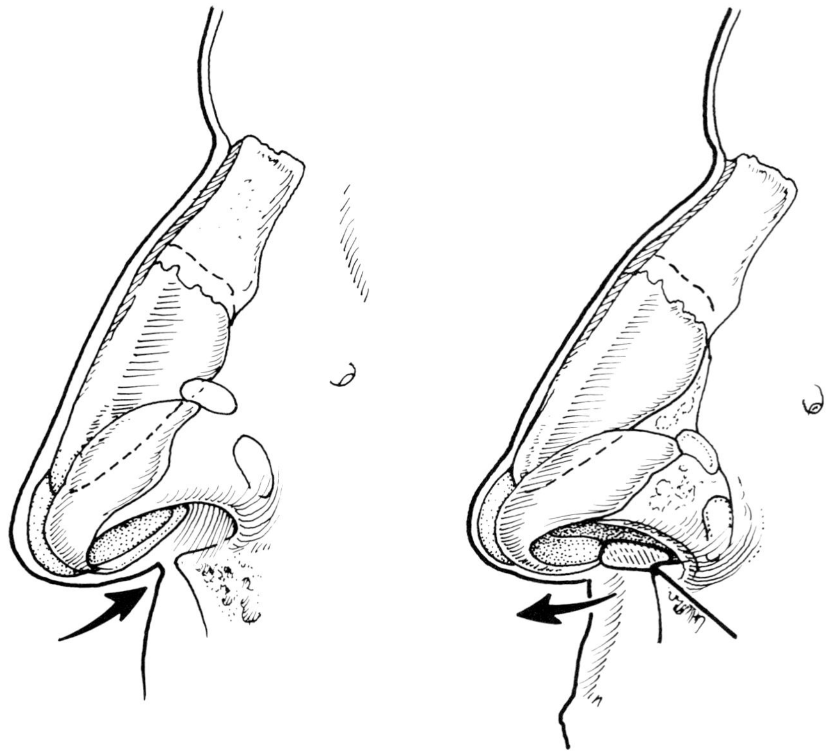

Fig. 10-15. Cartilage graft between the nasal spine and the feet of the medial crura. This treats loss of tip projection and mild columellar retraction.

Composite grafts. When columellar retraction is severe, requiring epithelium and cartilage, a composite graft from the auricle (composed of epithelium attached to cartilage) is indicated to replace both skin and cartilage deficits. It will also increase tip projection. This type of autogenous grafts is discussed further in the section on secondary surgeries in Chapter 21.

Decreasing Tip Projection

When the tip projects excessively from the face of the maxilla, we must lower this projection while maintaining smooth nasal domes without widening the base of the nares (Fig. 10-16). The following steps help to achieve this end (Fig. 10-17):
(1) Extensive delivery of the lower lateral domes and medial crural cartilages.
(2) Removal of a cartilaginous segment of the medial crura posterior to the nasal domes. The length of the removed cartilage equals the amount of desired decreased tip projection. The underlying mucosa is left intact.
(3) The remaining lower lateral dome and medial crural cartilages are thoroughly morselized.
(4) The morselized cartilage complex is rotated and advanced medially. Part of the former lower lateral becomes the dome and the former dome becomes part of the medial crus. This technique lowers the domes without broadening the nasal base and maintains smooth nasal domes (Fig. 10-18).

A 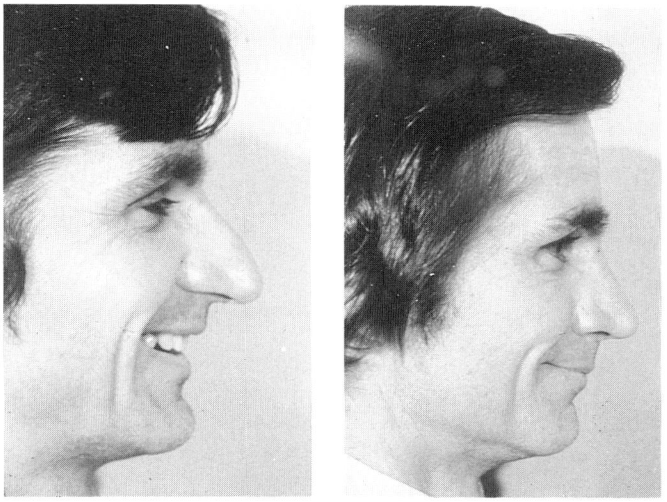 B

Fig. 10-16. Overly projected male nasal tip. **A,** Preoperative. **B,** Postoperative.

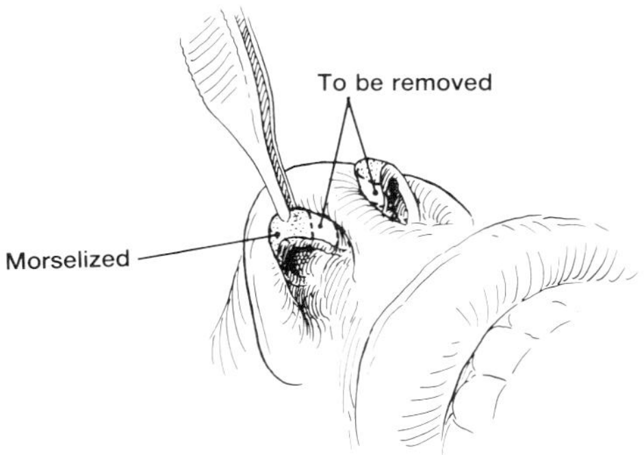

Fig. 10-17. Decreasing tip projection: removal of medial crural cartilage, morselizing dome, and lower lateral cartilage and rotating former dome into new medial crus and lateral cartilage into the new dome. (From Berman WE: Rhinoplasty, ed 2, Washington DC, 1984, American Academy of Otolaryngology-Head and Neck Surgery Foundation, Inc.)

A 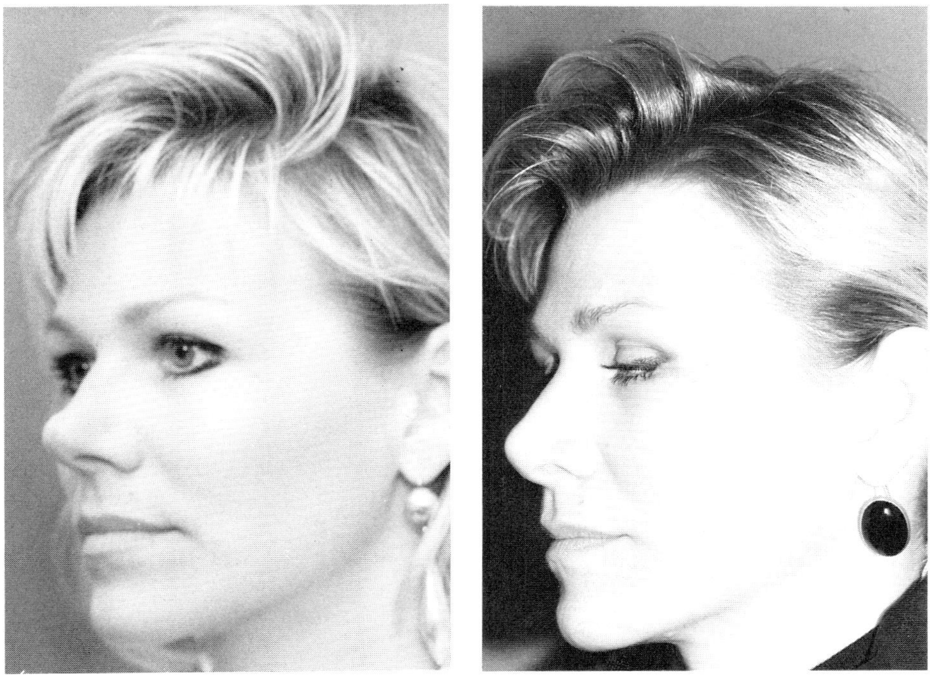 B

Fig. 10-18. An overly projected and wide nasal tip. **A,** Preoperative. **B,** Postoperative.

REFERENCES

1. Ersek RA and Delerm AG: Processed irradiated bovine cartilage for nasal reconstruction, Ann Plast Surg 29:540, 1988.

11

Tip-Columella-Lip Aesthetic Surgery

Richard C. Webster, Nabil S. Fuleihan, Usama S. Hamdan, Richard C. Smith

Achieving aesthetically acceptable relationships between the nasal tip, the infratip lobule, the columella, the columellar-labial junction, and the upper lip remains one of the most important and challenging tasks for the surgeon performing rhinoplasty. The presence of multiple structures involved in the anatomical definition of this small area requires meticulous analysis of the variables that result in deformity in order to plan the best treatment modalities. Within reasonable ranges, predictable changes may be made easily in this entire area; the goal is to select the best combination of surgical alterations or displacements of the complex for a given patient.

Let us describe the tip-lip or tip-columella-lip complex as the tissues running from the most anteriorly projecting parts of the lobule of the nasal tip (the tip defining points) to the free border of the central upper lip, these tissues being capable of gliding on the fixed central skeleton consisting of the septal cartilage, anterior nasal spine, and premaxilla. In the unoperated nose, these tissues may be moved forward and upward or backward and downward on the skeletal structures because their attachments are relatively loose or elastic.

Anatomical and Aesthetic Considerations

Orientation is important in the descriptions that we shall give. All terms used apply to a patient sitting or standing and looking forward. We use the term *superior* to mean toward the top of the head; the term *retrodisplacement* means toward the back of the head.

Space does not allow a detailed description of the anatomy of the tip-lip complex, but a presentation of some pertinent structural relationships is necessary for understanding the goals, dynamics, and results of the surgical procedures modifying the complex itself.

The infratip lobule is that part of the nasal tip extending forward and superiorly from the junctions of the lateral margins of the nostrils with the anterior columella to the most anteriorly projecting portion of the tip.

The columella consists of two medial crura, with intervening areolar or fibrous tissue, covered by thin skin. Anteriorly these crura flare to a greater or lesser extent in providing the framework for the width of the tip. Posteriorly the curved ends of the medial crura flare to override the caudal edge of the quadrilateral cartilage of the septum.

The angle formed where the columella meets the central upper lip is the columellar-labial angle; its position is determined partially by the caudal border of the septum and the nasal spine and the anterior surface of the premaxilla. The soft tissues contributing to the formation of this angle are skin, muscle (mainly depressor septi nasi), and some fat and fibrous tissue. Not uncommonly the junction of the columella with the central upper lip visually occurs somewhere along a concave curvature rather than having a clear-cut demarcation (such as a crease or a groove). In the unoperated nose, the skeletal area behind the junction is the premaxillary portion of the skull. Extending forward from the upper part of the premaxilla is the anterior nasal spine, which lies behind and at a higher level than the columellar-labial junction. In rare cases, the most anterior portion of this spine may extend forward to sit above the junction itself. Much more commonly the junction of the anterior nasal spine with the caudal or inferior margin of the septal cartilage is situated above and behind the columellar-labial junction. The caudal margin of the septal cartilage is usually the fixed skeletal element found immediately superior to the columellar-labial junction.

The columellar-labial junction is not necessarily a precise anatomical entity; rather, it is a visual and/or mental interpretation of where the observer believes that the columella ends and the central or philtral portion of the lip begins. When a groove or crease exists, the junction is defined; when a concave curve is present, the exact junction is somewhat subject to interpretation.[3]

The central part of the upper lip consists of two philtral crests with a depression or dimple between them. This is called the philtral dimple or groove. For the most part, the lateral profile of the central upper lip is relatively vertical, but it may run obliquely downward and may be relatively straight or may have a series of curves before it gets to the vermilion border. If, just above the vermilion border the curvature is concave with its lower end protruding forward, this appearance frequently is described as a labial "pout." Generally, below the Cupid's bow (at the junction of the vermilion with the white skin of the central upper lip) sits a vermilion-covered part of the lip that is vertically wider or at least protrudes lower than the portions located just laterally. This bulge is the median labial tubercle. The lower border of the median labial tubercle is the free border of the central upper lip. In some cases, this free border, at rest with the lips slightly parted, may cover or hide the incisal edges of the central maxillary teeth. In others, 2 to 4 mm of the anterior surfaces of the teeth may show; and, in still others, the free border may sit so high that part of the gum is exposed or seen. Rarely is a smile attractive if it reveals an appreciable amount of gum. When the free border hides the maxillary incisal edges, the patient has a "swollen" or "lippy" look, which is also unattractive. If the central upper lip is so short in the vertical dimension that it results in a toothy or, worse, a gummy appearance, then the patient may have a functional difficulty with closing the lips or with achieving a so-called "lip seal."[4]

We do not intend to go into a detailed discussion of aesthetics or into a presentation of supposed "ideal" ratios between lengths of upper lips and lengths of columellas and lengths of noses or projections of noses. Obviously, these "ideals" vary depending upon the aesthetic sensibilities of various cosmetic surgeons. Instead, we shall use terms like *excessive nasal projection* (meaning that, in our opinion, the tip of the nose is too far forward from the vertical profile of the upper lip) or *short upper lip* (meaning that, in our opinion, the central upper lip is too short relative to the length of the columella and infratip lobule, or that, when at rest or when smiling, the patient shows too much tooth or gum). We shall try to indicate here selected techniques that are of value in solving problems of malposition, or of too much or too little length of the components of this tip-lip aesthetic complex. Our comments on the varied techniques described will be based on what *we* consider to be too long, too short, or malpositioned.

We shall not try to tell other cosmetic surgeons what an ideal feminine or masculine columellar-labial angle is. Instead, in this goal-oriented chapter, we shall merely describe the angulation as being "too acute" or "too obtuse" in our aesthetic judgment. We also are not advocates of any hard and fast rules about how many millimeters of columella in the vertical dimension should show inferior to the alar margins because so many variations are possible. Instead, we will talk here about *retraction,* which means too little columellar show for our taste, and *excessive columellar show,* meaning too much. A study of many models' noses, female and male, will demonstrate that 4 to 5 mm or more of columella may show at the columellar-labial junction.

There are three other factors that we consider important in aesthetic or cosmetic diagnosis. The first is the extent of obliquity of the profiles of the white skin of the upper lip and the columella-infratip lobule entity. Too vertical an infratip lobule profile gives a blunted or too-short nasal appearance. The same is true of the profile of the columella. If the profile of the central upper lip slopes posteriorly too much as the eye observing it travels upward from the vermilion border to the columellar-labial junction, an uncouth, somewhat ape-like appearance is produced. Too much of a slope in the opposite direction produces a web-like or ferret-like appearance. The second factor is the relative lengths of the infratip lobule and of the columella. If the infratip lobule is too long, not only may the tip project too much, but postsurgically the nose may have a abnormal appearance; if it is too short, a blunted or infantile appearance may be produced. The third factor has to do with aging. A dependent nasal tip or too acute a columellar-labial angle gives the effect of aging. A squared-off, central upper lip that is excessively long vertically, particularly when observed in combination with too little show of vermilion makes the lip and the patient look older. By "squared off" here, we mean a somewhat tightly drawn upper lip with no pout.

There is still another factor that must be considered in tip-lip aesthetic complex surgery. This is what happens to the upper and central portions of the central upper lip when the patient laughs or smiles. Of course, the nasal tip tends to retrodisplace and to rotate inferiorly during smiling. However, in some patients, when the lower part of the central upper lip moves superiorly, a horizontal groove may appear in it. The compressed part of the lip just above this groove curves outward. This seems to be because of the mobile lower portions moving against the relatively fixed and immobile portions above, the latter being held in place by the premaxilla, anterior spine, and caudal septal skeletal structures. When the convexity and groove are present before surgery, moving more tissue or bulk into this area by sliding maneuvers or by grafts or implants may make this bulge more apparent and may even, in some cases, produce it where it did not show before surgery.

In summary, aesthetic diagnosis must take into consideration the following variables: (1) tip projection, (2) tip level, (3) supratip slope, (4) supratip profile length, (5) infratip lobule slope, (6) infratip lobule length, (7) infratip region-columella angulation, (8) columellar length, (9) columellar curvature, (10) columellar-labial angulation, (11) columellar-labial junction position, (12) central upper lip slope, (13) central upper lip length, (14) central upper lip prominence, (15) central upper lip white skin-vermilion relationships and, (16) central upper lip free border position at rest and when smiling and laughing. Moreover, (17) width factors, and (18) the profile of the anterior cheeks must be considered. One of the most important factors limiting alterations of these relationships is (19) the total length of skin from the nasal tip to the free border of the upper lip. Without production of external scarlines, it is almost impossible to achieve significant changes of this length.

Surgical Techniques that Alter the Complex

A mechanistic but practical way of thinking about the manifold approaches to tip-lip complex surgery is to classify the modalities into six divisions: (1) subtraction of subdermal or skeletal tissue from the columellar-labial junction region, (2) augmentation of the columellar-labial area by implants or grafts, (3) sliding the complex forward and upward or downward and backward on fixed skeletal structures, (4) repositioning of fixed skeletal structures, (5) additions to, and (6) subtractions from lengths of skin between tip and free border of the upper lip.[4] Limitations of space will not allow a detailed description of all of these approaches in this text. Repositioning of fixed skeletal structures implies orthodontic, orthognathic, or maxillofacial surgery beyond the scope of many surgeons who confine their practices to cosmetic surgery alone. Changing the length of skin between the nasal tip and the free border of

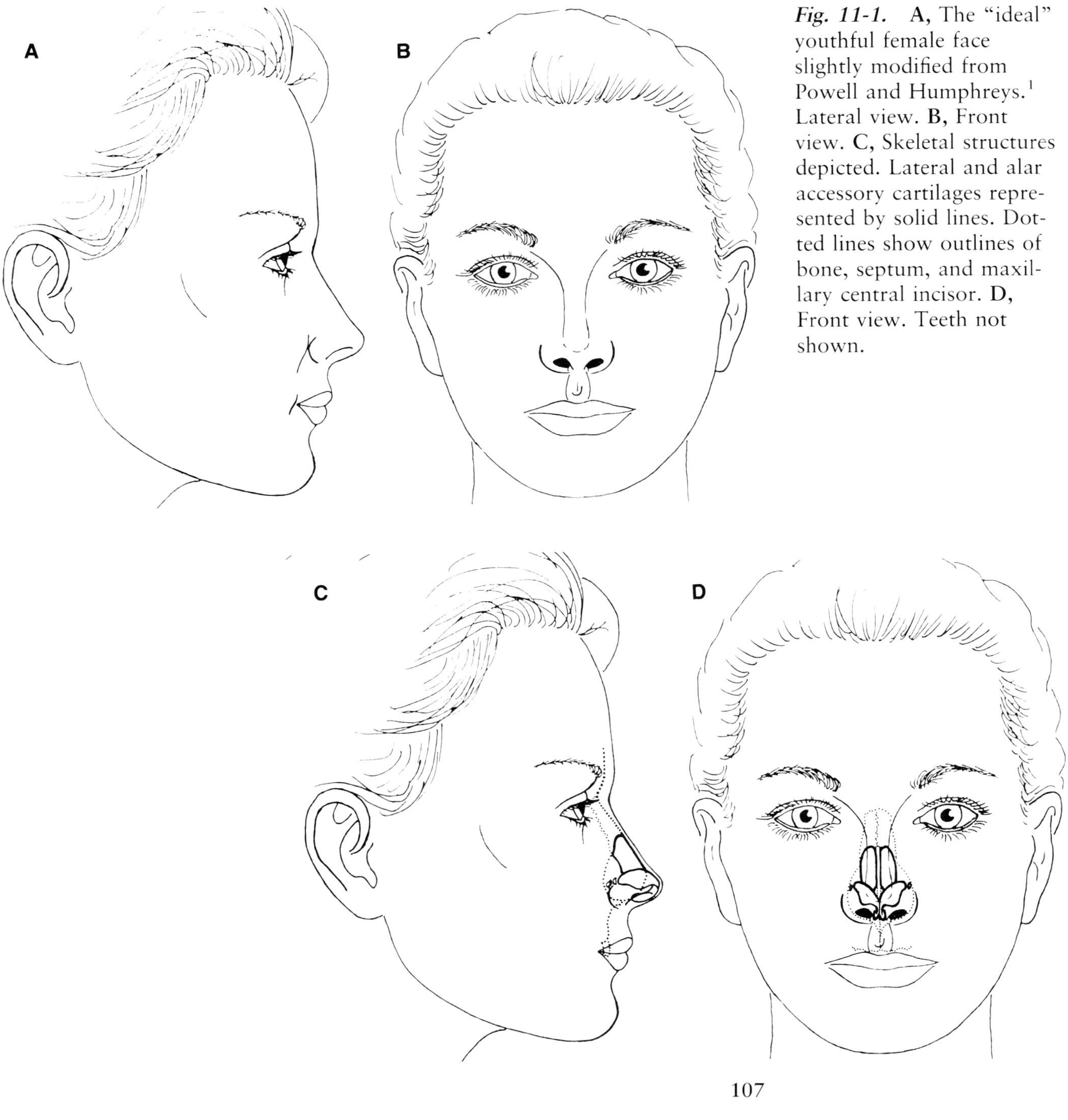

Fig. 11-1. **A,** The "ideal" youthful female face slightly modified from Powell and Humphreys.[1] Lateral view. **B,** Front view. **C,** Skeletal structures depicted. Lateral and alar accessory cartilages represented by solid lines. Dotted lines show outlines of bone, septum, and maxillary central incisor. **D,** Front view. Teeth not shown.

the lip dictates external scarring, something assiduously avoided by many in cosmetic surgery. Therefore, these techniques for altering the complex will not be described here. Instead, we shall confine ourselves in this chapter to the first three subjects listed.

Many of the diagrams showing the deformities and surgical changes made in the following three sections depict a female face modified slightly (see Fig. 11-1) from that used in the excellent monograph of Powell and Humphreys.[1]

Fig. 11-2. A, "Ideal" view of face modified by moving columellar-labial junction 4 mm lower (in life-size proportion) than in Fig. 11-1, **A. B,** Underlying skeletal structures shown by line of dashes. Removal of stippled parts of anterior nasal spine and caudal septal cartilage will allow an upward displacement or correction of the position of the columellar-labial junction to that of the profile shown in Fig. 11-1, **A. C,** Earlier surgery elsewhere. Note compression of upper lip and extent of "show" of columellar-labial region inferior to alar margin. **D,** Resection of portions of anterior nasal spine and septal cartilage, as shown in Fig. 11-2, **B,** allowed superior displacement of columellar-labial junction and less compression of upper lip downward against the lower lip. One year following revision.

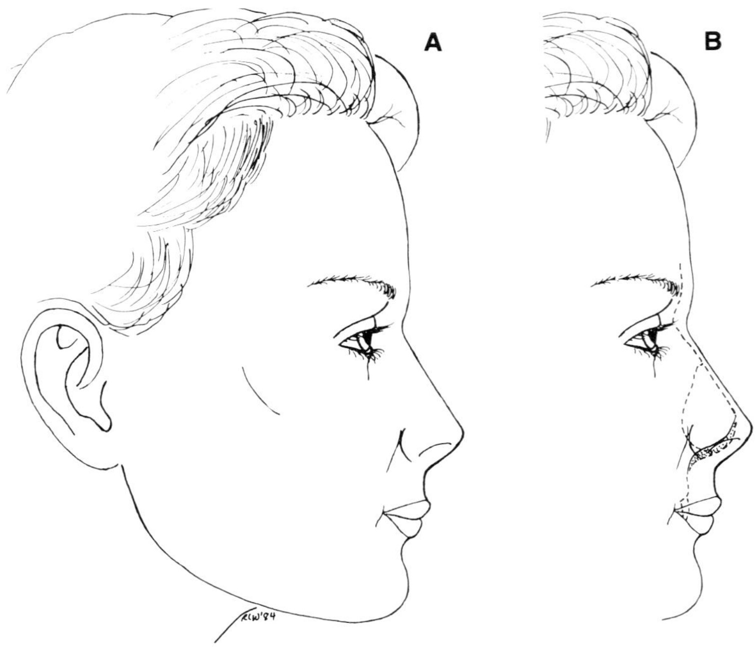

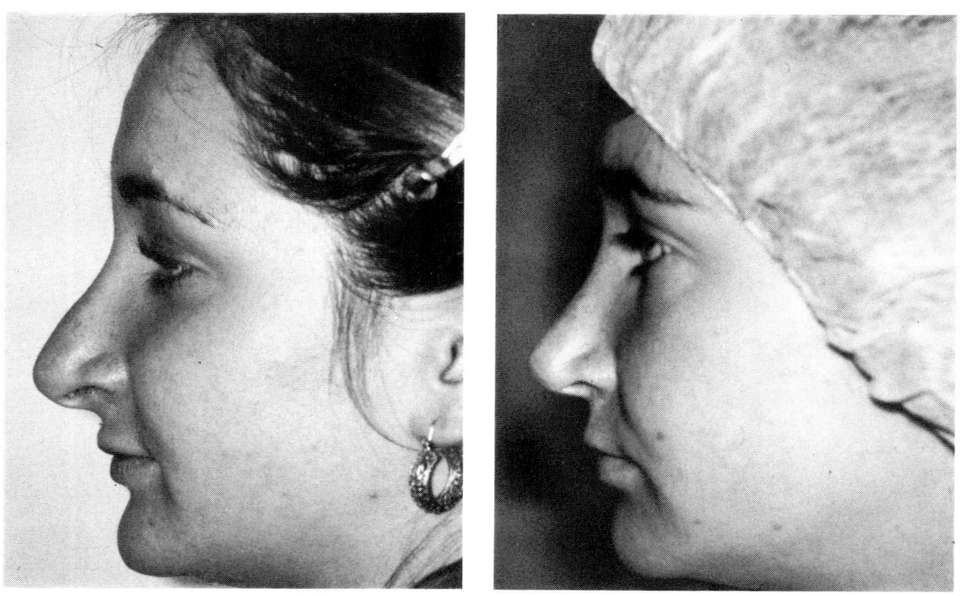

C

D

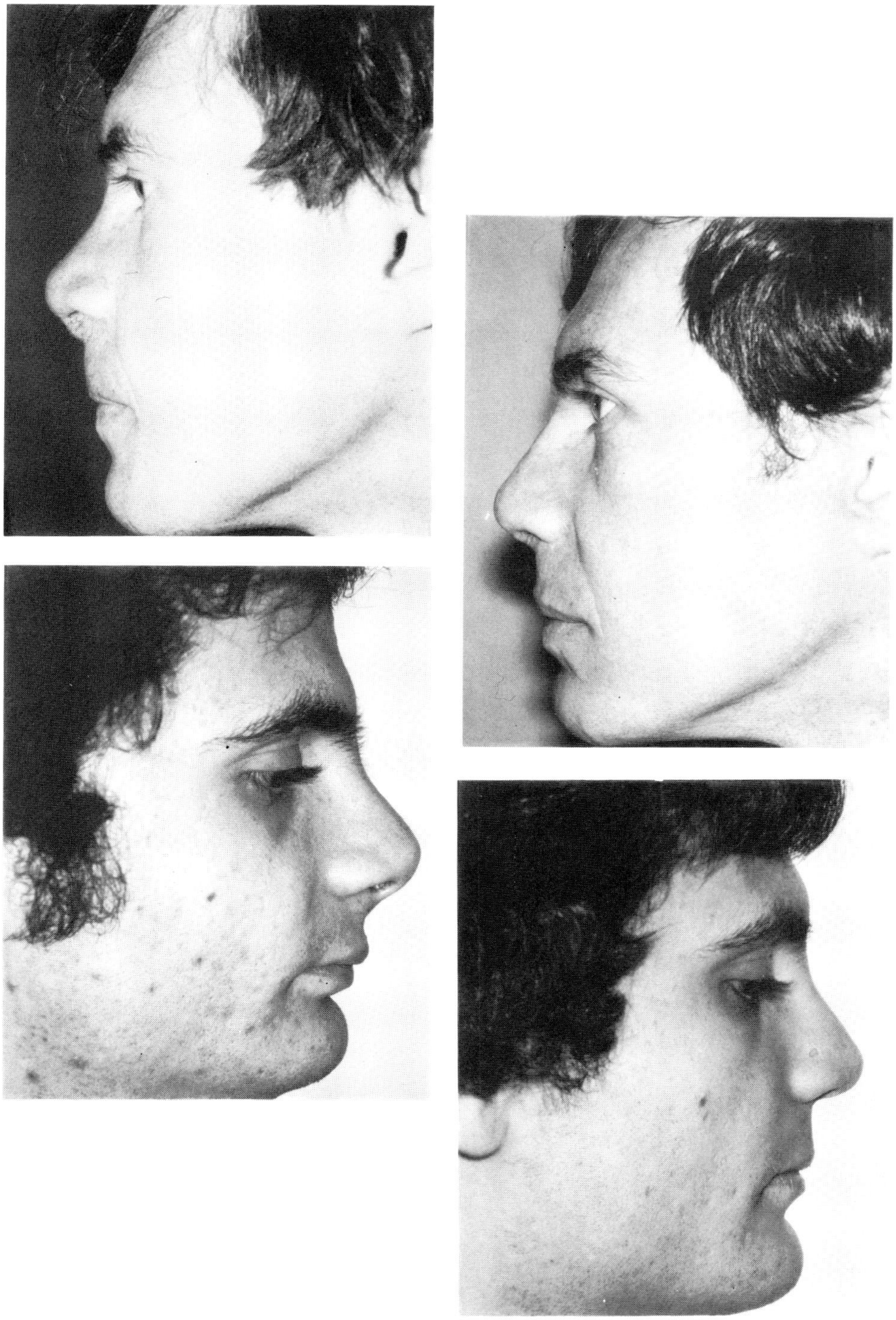

A

B

C

D

Fig. 11-3. A, Several operations elsewhere previously. B, Observe profile of columella and improved position of columellar-labial junction after resections of portions of spine and septum. Result over one year following revision. C, Another male needing similar revision. Note upper lip hanging over lower lip. D, One year after correction. Just a little too much was resected giving central upper lip a long vertical look and a slight superior retraction of the columellar-labial junction.

Fig. 11-4. **A,** If columellar-labial junction sits 4 mm (life-size) anterior to position shown in "ideal" (Fig. 11-1, **A**), and if columella and infratip lobule length are the same as those shown in Fig. 11-1, **A,** then the profile would be as shown. **B,** Resection of stippled parts of septum, spine, and premaxillary region will allow retrodisplacement of the involved landmarks to more "ideal" positions. **C,** Skeletal structures behind columellar-labial junction position the junction too far forward. Slight resection above the junction and greater resection behind it will allow improvement. Over-resection of spine and septum above junction will allow superior displacement of central upper lip, the free border of which is already satisfactorily positioned relative to the lower lip. Proper resection, mainly from behind the junction, will allow the white skin portion of the upper lip to look longer vertically. **D,** Profile improvements five months postoperatively. **E,** This patient has an upper lip already drooping slightly over the lower lip. Also, the vertical length of the white skin of the upper lip already is long enough. Therefore, excision mainly behind the columellar-labial junction and slightly above it will allow appropriate retrodisplacement of columellar-labial junction and tip without adding to the overhang just mentioned. However, more must be resected superiorly than in Fig. 11-4, **C,** if excessive downward thrust of central upper lip is to be avoided. **F,** Three years after surgery.

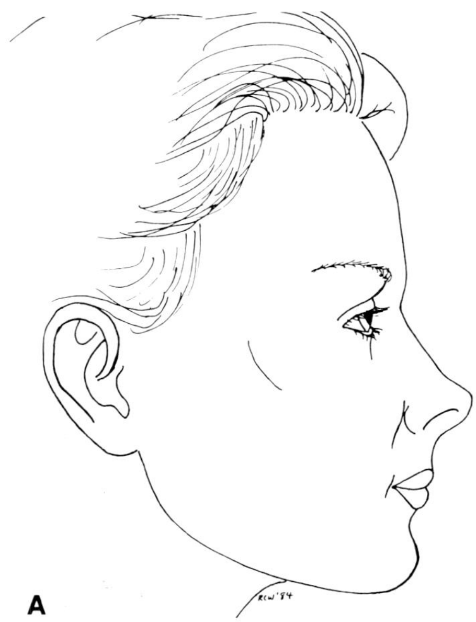

A

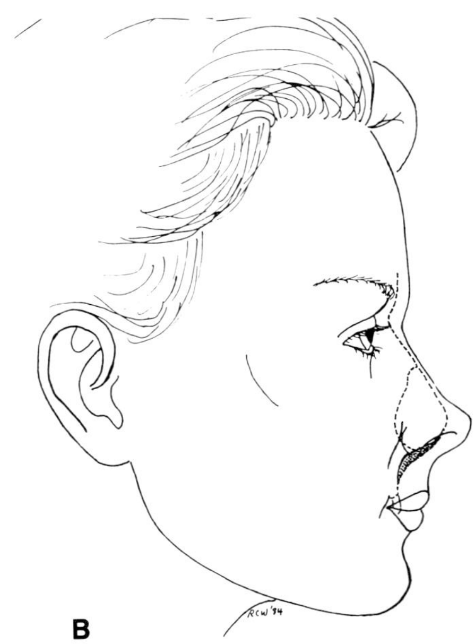

B

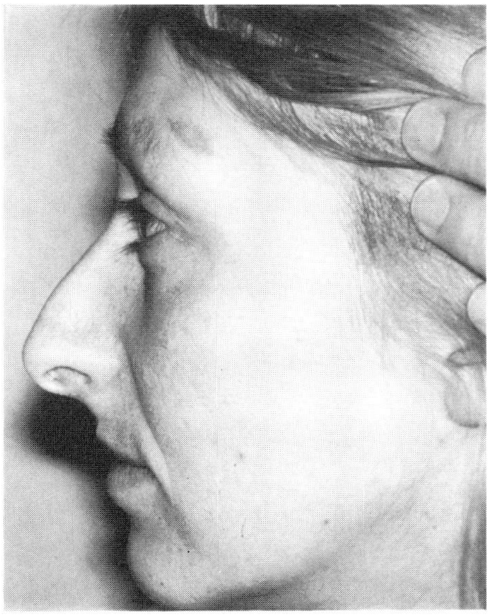

C

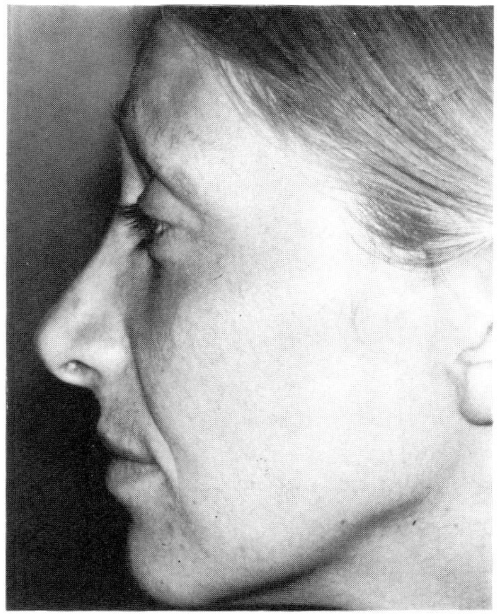

D

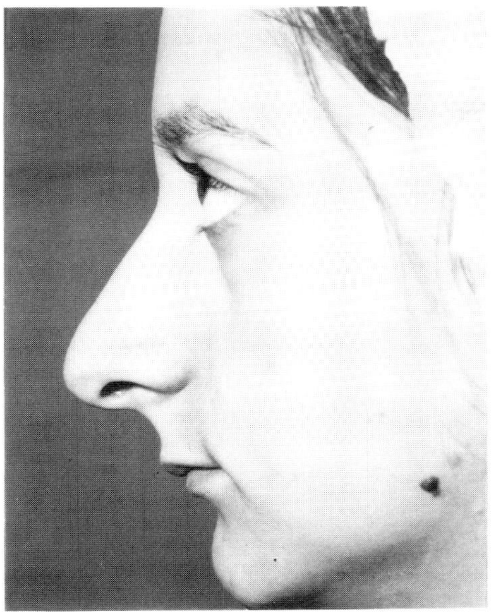

E

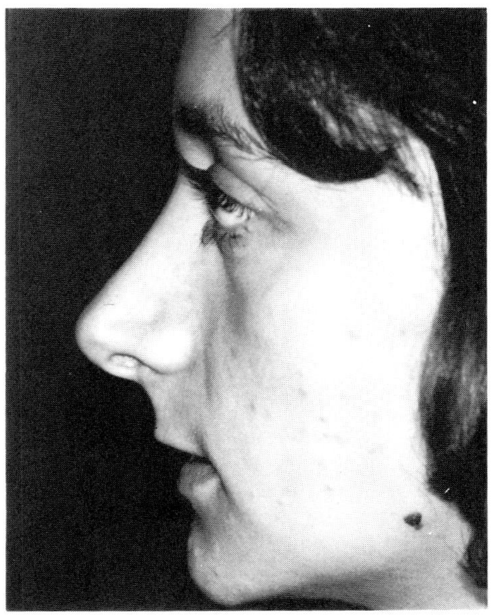

F

Fig. 11-5. **A**, Upper lip already long. Tip slightly projecting. Chin needs augmentation. **B**, Five months after retrodisplacement of columellar-labial junction and tip, mainly by skeletal resection behind junction and very slight resection above it. **C**, Excessive anterior positioning of columellar-labial junction and protrusion of upper portion of central upper lip combined with projecting nasal tip. **D**, Too much skeletal resection superiorly rather than posterior to the columellar-labial junction caused new columellar-labial junction position to be too high and emphasized excessive vertical length of central upper lip. **E**, Before surgery. **F**, Fourteen months after surgery. Observe that much of what was positioned between the alar lobules in **E** and what some would call posterior columella is now clearly central upper lip. Now look back at **C**. Arrow shows where true columellar-labial junction is.

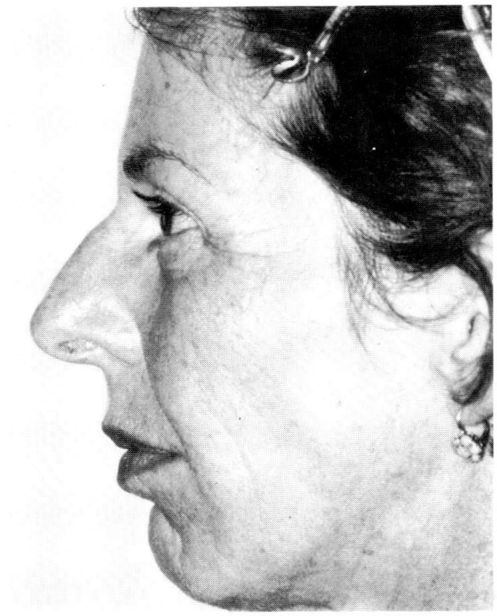
A

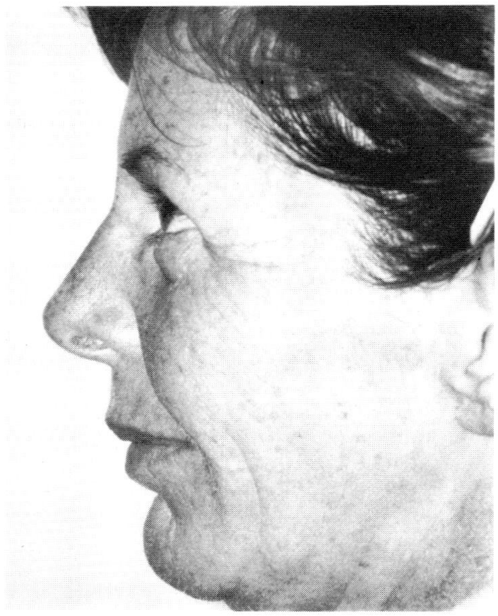
B

C
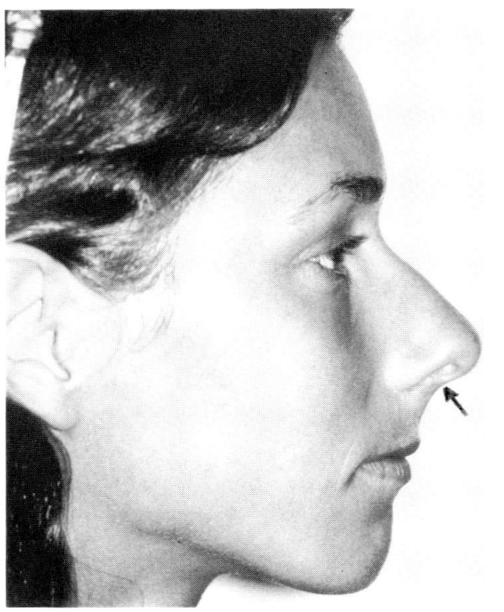

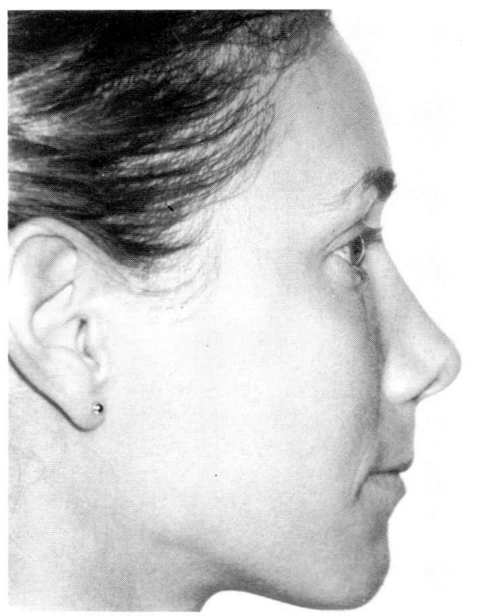
D

Subtraction of Subdermal or Skeletal Tissue

Subtraction or removal of soft tissue and/or parts of skeletal elements is used where the goal is to move the columellar-labial junction upward and/or posteriorly when the free border of the upper lip does not need to be moved inferiorly.[3,2,5] Resection of soft tissue, bone, or cartilage (caudal part of the septum) above and behind the columellar-labial junction tends to produce a superior or superior and posterior displacement of the junction, retrodisplacement of the columella and tip, and superior displacement of the central upper lip (Figs. 11-1–5, **B**). The columellar-labial angle becomes more acute. Too generous an excision may produce deformities such as too acute a columellar-labial angle with a plunging tip, a retracted columella, and/or a posteriorly sloping upper lip (ape-like) or a lip that appears too long and block-like (Figs. 11-5, **C-F**).

Access for these subtractions may be obtained easily through postero-inferior extension of the typical columellar-septal transfixion incision, columella-splitting incisions,[6] or small intraoral incisions near the central superior labial sulcus.[7] High or cartilaginous septal transfixion incisions and open rhinoplasty incisions may be extended to provide access to this area above and behind the columellar-labial junction when these approaches are used for the other septo-rhinoplastic work as well.[2]

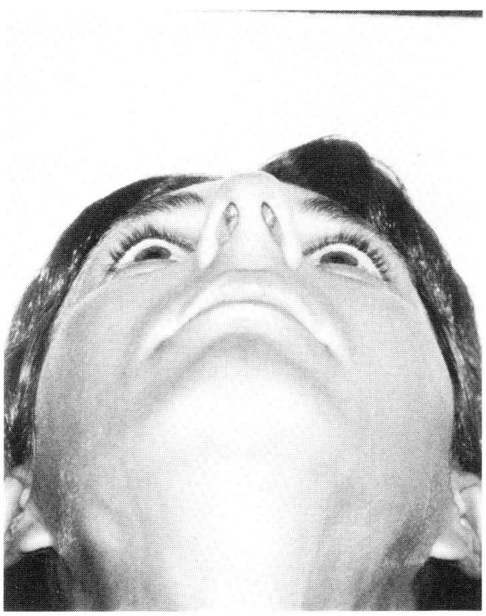

E

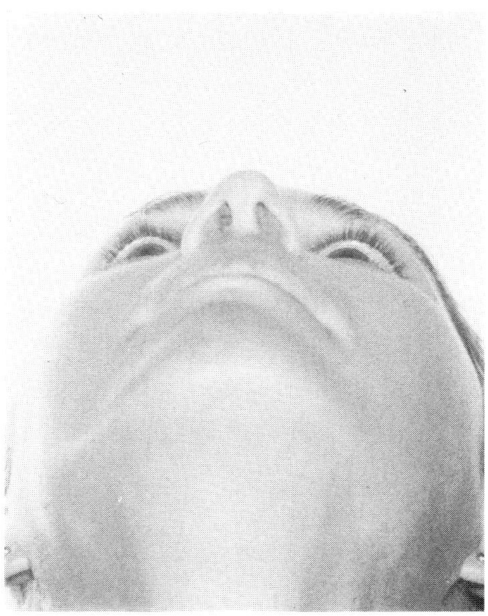

F

Augmentation of Columellar-Labial Area by Implants or Grafts

The goals of augmentation may vary from increasing the columellar-labial angle with no appreciable change in position of the nasal tip or free border of the central upper lip to significant inferior and/or anterior repositioning of the columellar-labial junction and marked displacements of the tip in a forward direction and the labial free border in a downward direction.[3,2,5] Sliding or gliding maneuvers may be used to "pile up" or augment the soft tissue just above and behind the columellar-labial junction, but these will be described in the next section. Grafts and/or implants are used when augmentation is needed and no tip retrodisplacement or elevation of the central upper lip is desired (Figs. 11-6 to 11-22).

To date, the most valuable and predictably successful grafts are those from the patient himself. Depending upon their purpose and availability, grafts may be of fascia, bone, cartilage, or other tissues. For the most part, we prefer the use of septal cartilage. When it is not available, septal bone, nasal cartilage and bone, conchal cartilage, or other tissues may be used. To augment grafts of the patient's own tissues, we occasionally use implant materials buried deeply, with the patient's tissue grafts placed more superficially. If lining tissue is required, local flaps or composite grafts may be used. We generally use one or two types, a thin linear graft or one or several nonlinear plumping grafts; selection of the type is dictated by the goal.

Pockets for reception of grafts or implants should be carefully planned to confine the augmenting material precisely where it is wanted to give the desired thrusts. A pocket made 2 mm larger than it needs to be can allow at least 2 mm of displacement of the augmenting material into an area where it is not needed or where it may produce an asymmetry or an undesirable obliquity or slope, excessive width, or an unwanted bulge.

The surgical approach for pocket preparation behind and/or above the columellar-labial junction may be a retrograde one from a septal transfixion incision, an incision close to the margin of the columella and nostril sill on one or both sides, an incision splitting one medial crus near its posterior end, an incision at the junction of the columella with the philtral region, an approach from one or both nostril sill resection sites or one or both (Weir) alar lobule resection sites, a columella-splitting incision, or from an intraoral incision. For the larger or longer grafts, we generally prefer intraoral incisions or columella-splitting incisions. When implant materials other than the patient's own tissues are going to be used to build flattened cheeks, retropositioned alar lobules, and the lateral superior portions of the upper lip forward, ordinarily we have preferred columella-splitting incisions that allow access to all of these areas and that place the epithelial surface of the closed wound far away from the artificial material, the patient's own tissues being used close to the external incision line. Also, we prefer columella-splitting incisions when grafts are to be inserted along the dorsum or in the radix or glabellar regions.

The remarks just made in regard to pocket size and selection of incision site do not apply when we use open rhinoplastic approaches with incisions made at the junction of the columella with the lip or some-

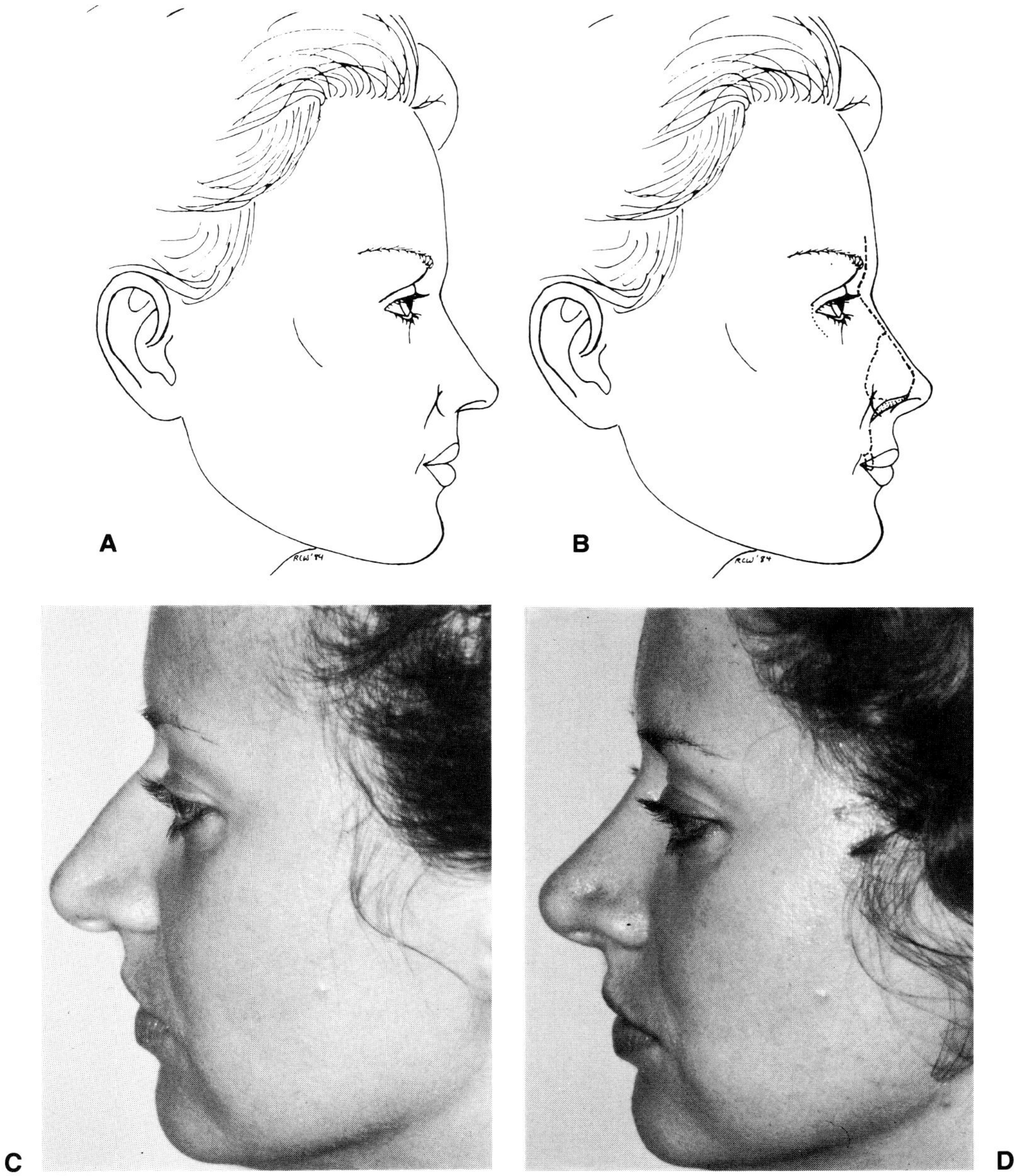

Fig. 11-6. **A,** Columellar-labial junction is depicted here 3½ mm (life-size) above its "ideal" position shown in Fig. 11-1, **A.** The retraction is obvious. **B,** The stippled portion shows a graft or implant used to correct this deformity. Plumping or filling material also can be used in the same location for the correction. **C,** Superior retraction of columellar-labial junction. **D,** Plumping grafts of diced septal cartilage inserted above the junction. One year after surgery.

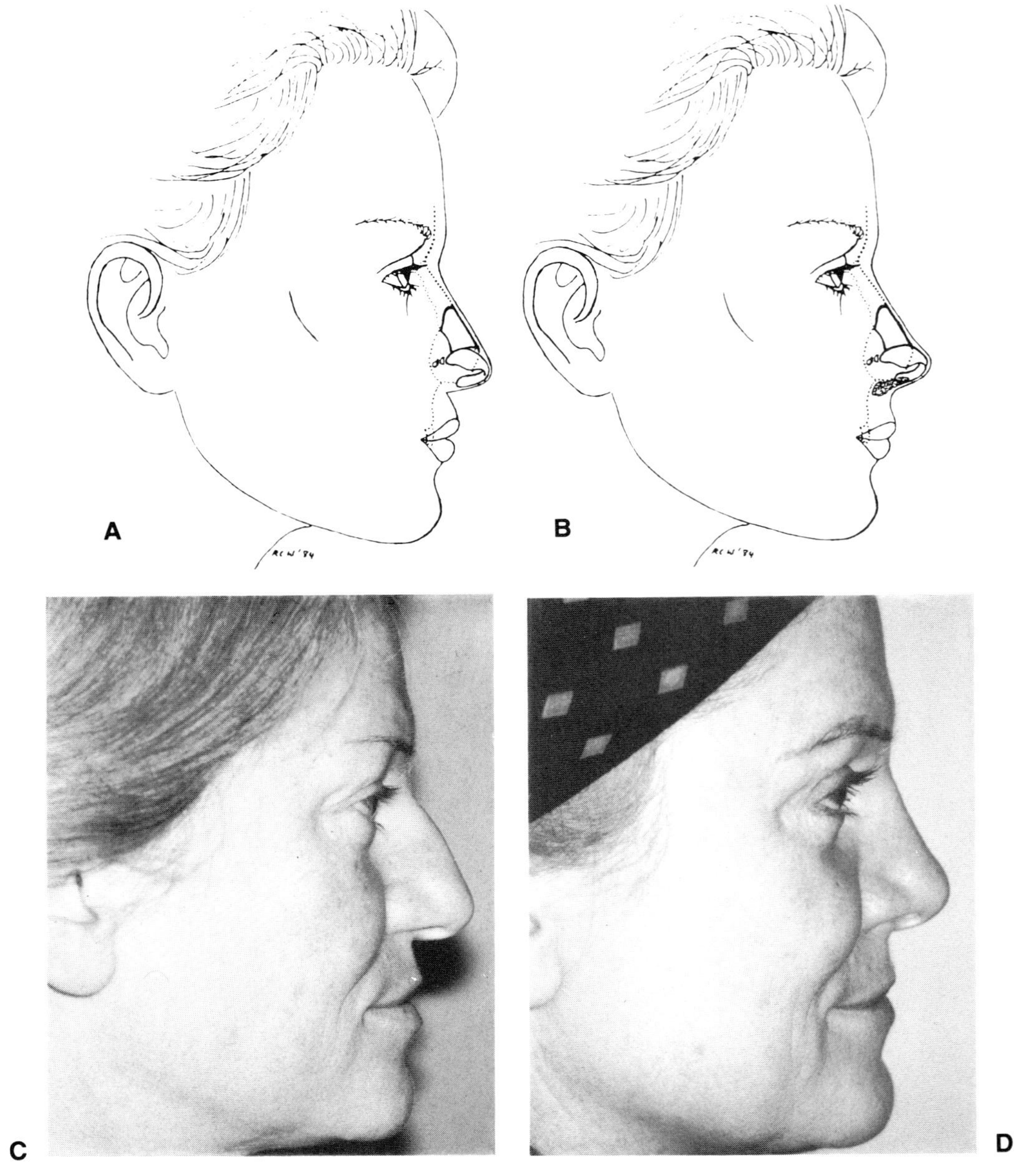

Fig. 11-7. A, Nasal tip and columellar-labial junction retrodisplaced. Unattractive, ape-like posterior sloping of upper lip. B, Plumping material pushing medial crura and tip forward and columellar-labial junction forward and slightly downward. Upper lip contacting lower in more normal relationship. C, Similar findings shown in profile of patient. D, Plumping cartilage grafts placed in carefully prepared pocket behind the medial crura, columellar-labial junction, and central upper lip. Pocket should be limited in size, shape, and position to achieve desired effect with minimal amount of augmenting material and with little chance of displacement of material.

where along the columella anterior to the columellar-labial junction. With open rhinoplasty, where grafts can be sutured in place, pocket size and shape along the dorsum or in the lateral walls do not have to be precise, but the pockets prepared in the columellar-labial region should be tailored to precise position and proportion.

Text continued on p. 130.

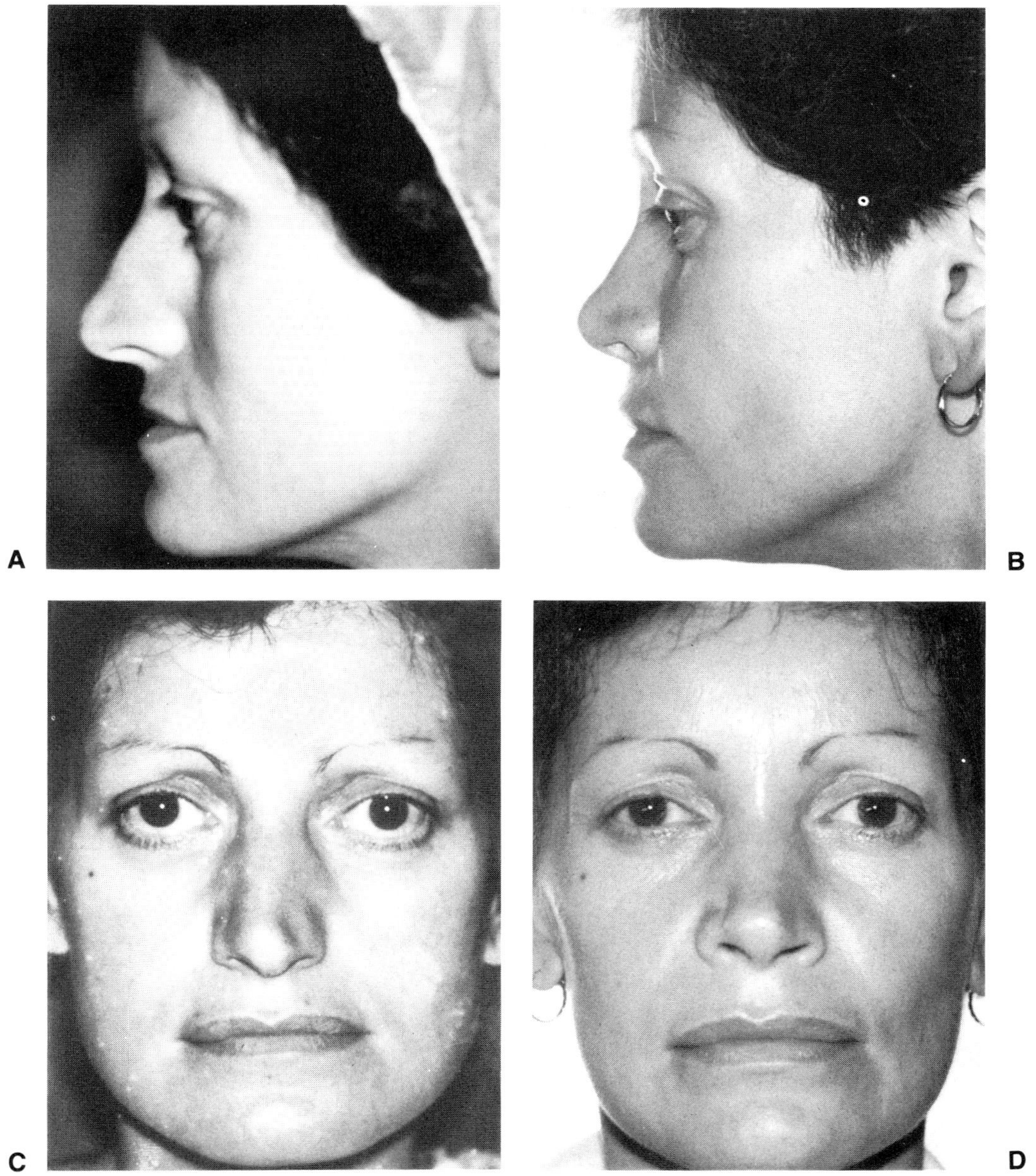

Fig. 11-8. **A**, Cheeks flattened. Columellar-labial junction and central upper lip retrodisplaced. **B**, Three years after plumping material used behind retrodisplaced soft tissues. **C**, Front view. **D**, Silicone rubber, bone, and plumping grafts of septal cartilage used to advance alar lobules, sunken cheeks, upper lip, and columellar-labial junction. Three years postoperative.

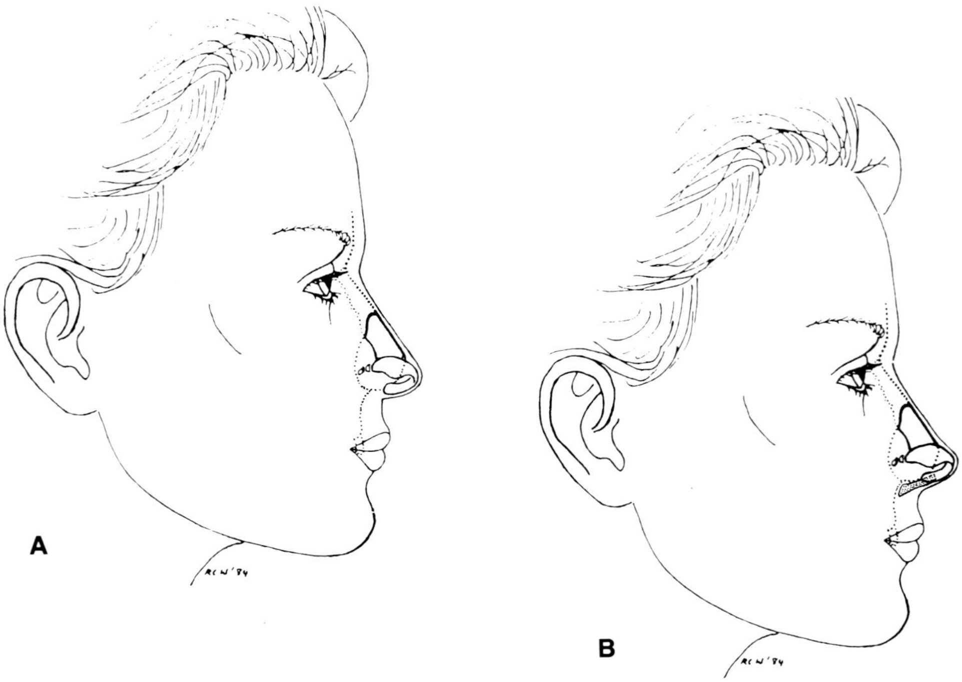

Fig. 11-9. **A,** Nasal tip and columellar-labial junction retropositioned. Length of central upper lip is adequate without superior displacement of free border of upper lip. Here, a forward thrust is needed to push medial crura of adequate strength forward, thus projecting the retrodisplaced tip and pulling columellar-labial junction forward. Plumping grafts sufficient to produce the desired forward thrust would push the already long enough central upper lip too far inferiorly. Therefore, a carefully carved linear graft limited in its vertical measurement is the indicated choice. **B,** Stippling shows the carved graft. It is inserted in a confined pocket running back almost to the premaxilla, but not quite to periosteum or bone and running forward to fibrous tissue connecting one medial crus to the other. If pocket extends to bone or periosteum, graft posteriorly tends to slip out of its central and elevated position. If pocket extends too far forward, graft must be longer than needed in patients with strong medial crura. **C,** Columellar-labial junction retrodisplaced. Nasal tip inferiorly rotated and retrodisplaced. Upper lip obviously long enough and posteriorly sloping. Medial crura do not bend or bow downward when pushed forward preoperatively from behind. Earlier rhinoplasty performed in 1963. **D,** Septal cartilage graft limited in vertical dimension is pushing medial crura and tip forward. Two months postoperative. Observe that distance between the columellar-labial junction and the cheek profile has increased as the thrust of the graft drags the columellar-labial junction forward. Contrast this finding with Figs. 8 A and 8 B where plumping material was used to push the cheeks, alar lobules, and columellar-labial junction forward. **E,** Before revision. **F,** Eight months after revision.

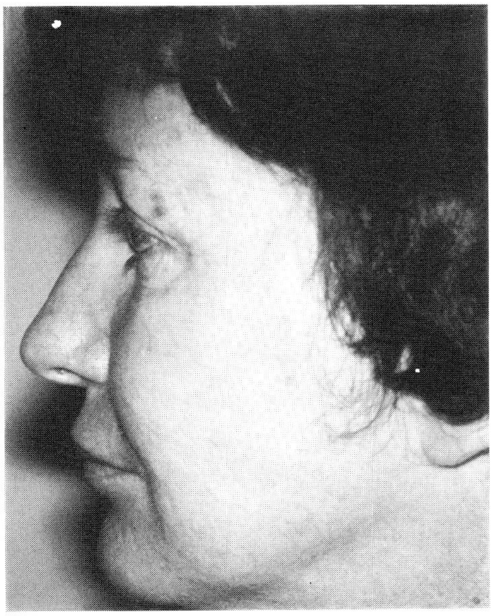

C

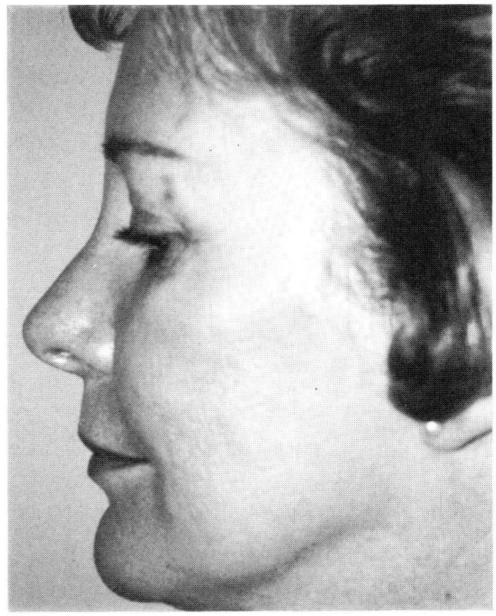

D

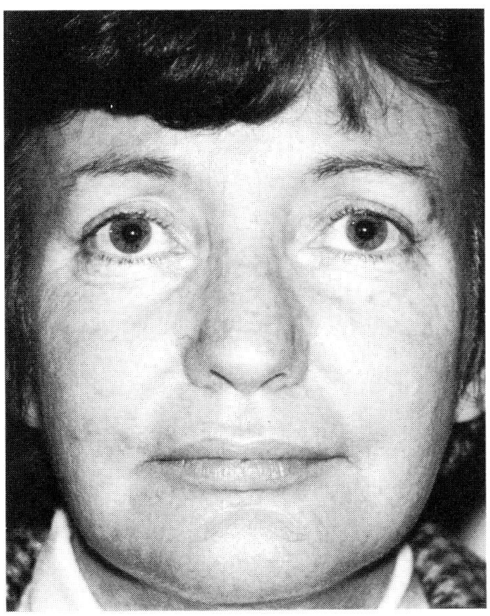

E

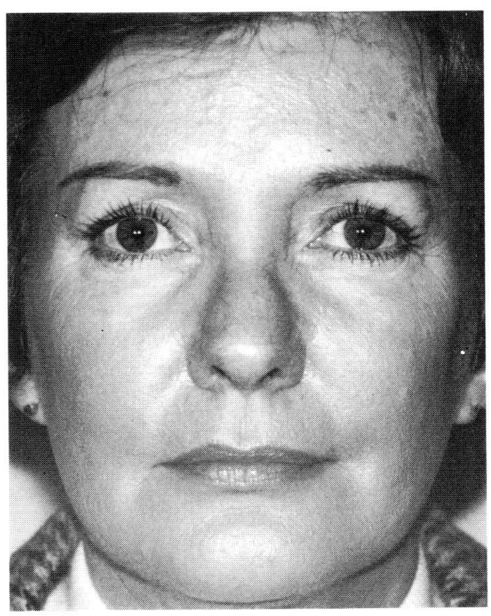

F

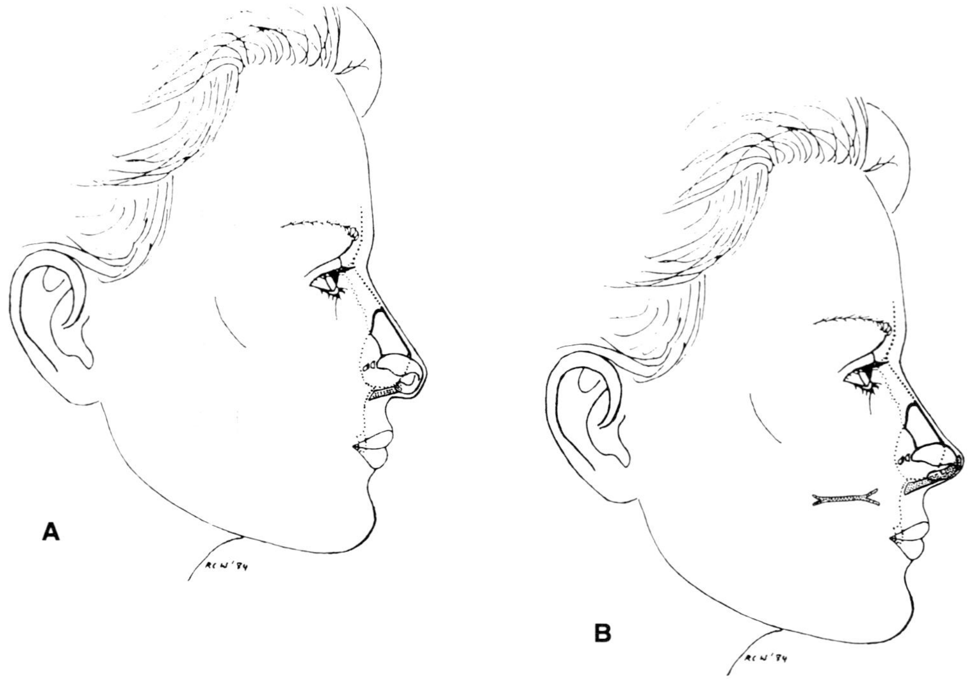

Fig. 11-10. **A,** Shown here is an upper lip already long enough vertically, a somewhat retrodisplaced columellar-labial junction. The stippled graft, in this case pushing forward on fibrous tissue connecting the two medial crura, is bending these downward. They are not strong enough to remain straight and to effectively transmit the forward thrust to the tip. Therefore, a longer graft going between the medial crura directly to the tip is needed to produce the tip definition and required projection. **B,** The stippled graft here shown is long enough to reach the tip. A view of the superior edge of this graft is shown overlying the right cheek. It is split at each end. At the anterior end, the split is designed to provide two forward thrusting portions imitating the medial crura that will be bypassed. At times, it is wise to place small pieces of cartilage between the split ends anteriorly to keep them appropriately apart; occasionally, a carved triangular piece of cartilage is sutured between them to provide required strength and separation. **C,** Revisional advancement of tip and columellar-labial junction required. **D,** Long graft inserted through columella splitting incision.[6] Six months postoperative. **E,** Before revision. **F,** Observe apparent lengthening of columella and change in nostril shape and inclination after the revision.

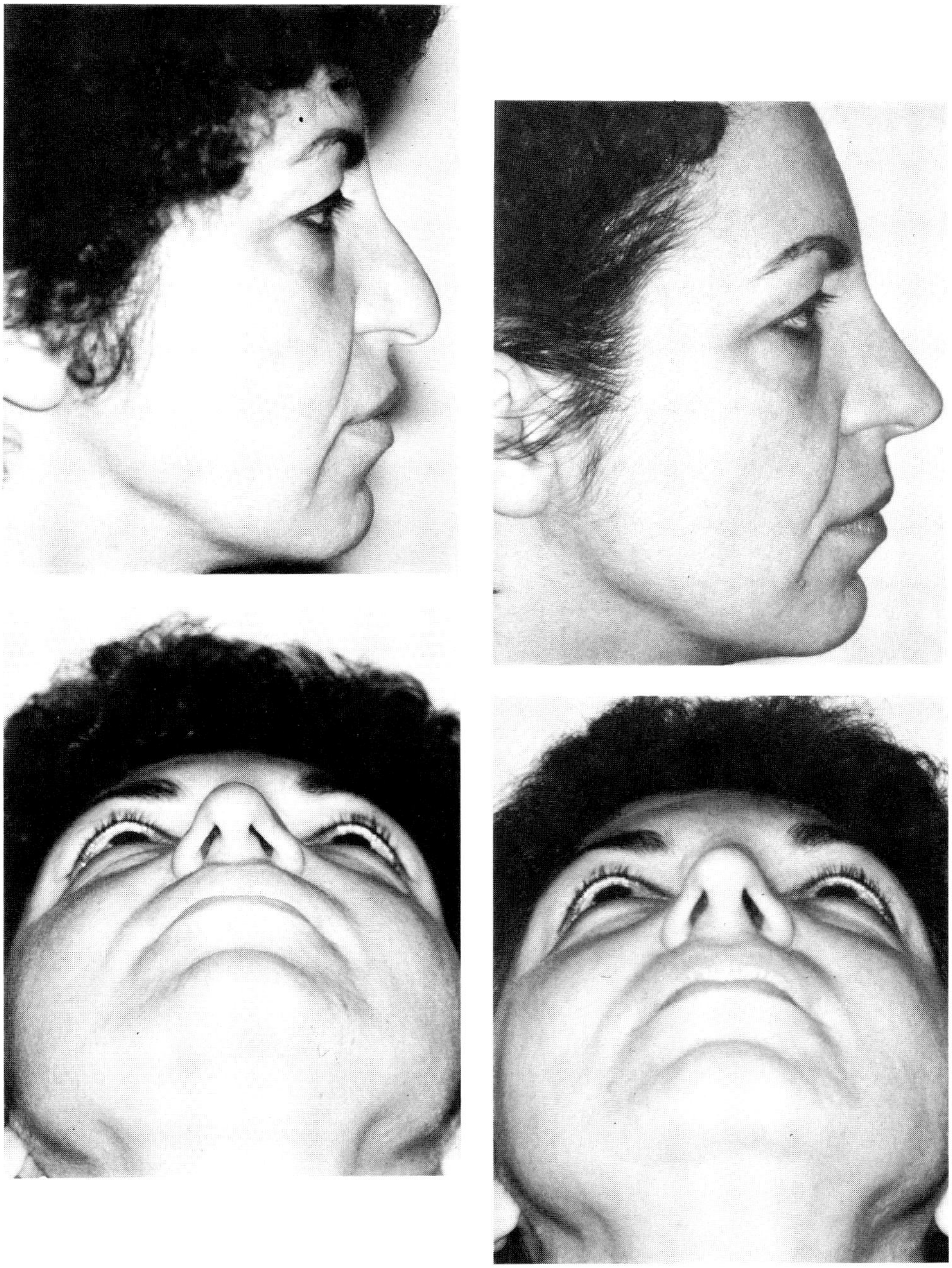

C D E F

A 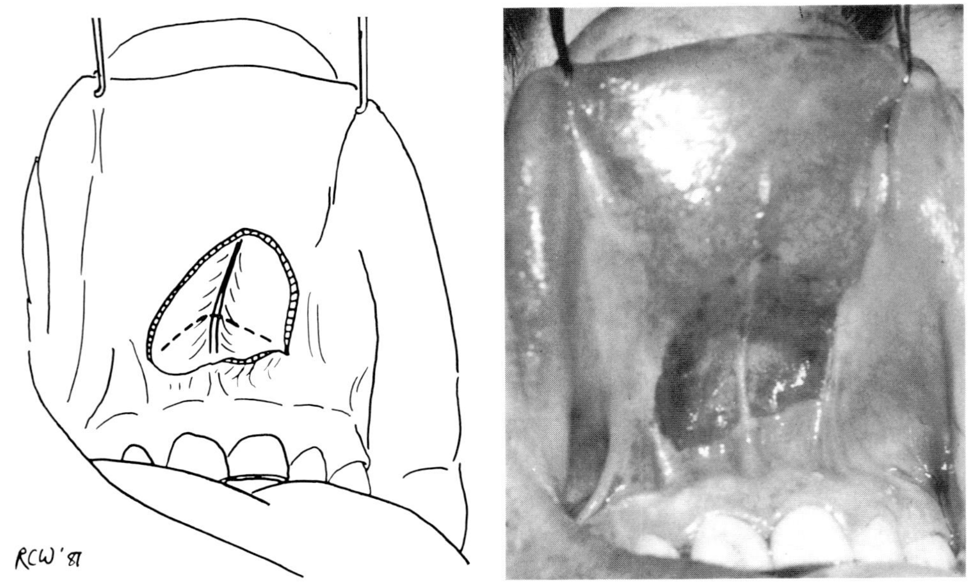 B

Fig. 11-11. **A,** Hooks everting upper lip so that its posterior surface can be seen. U-shaped or V-shaped incision through mucous membrane shown by cross-hatching. It begins approximately 5 mm on lip side of superior labial sulcus. Line of dashes shows incision across the submucosal tissues of the midline frenulum. **B,** Operative photograph from which **A** was made.

A 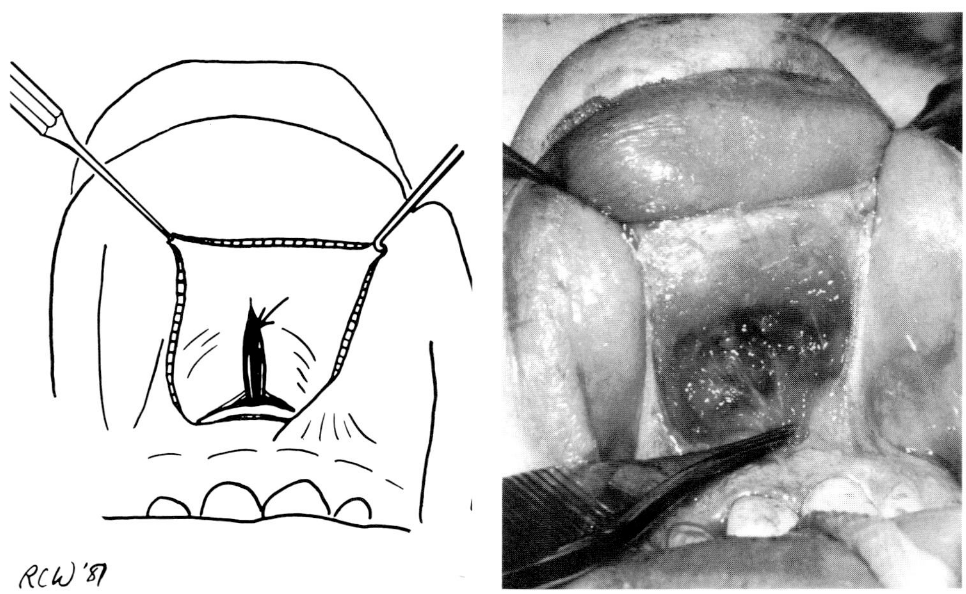 B

Fig. 11-12. **A,** Arrow points to area where frenulum has been split vertically. The incision made across the frenulum shown in Fig. 11-11 is only made to a depth of 1 or 2 mm, thus allowing the flap of mucous membrane to retract toward its base about 5 mm from the labial sulcus. The deeper splitting of the frenulum region in the vertical dimension allows access to the area close to the anterior nasal spine. **B,** Operative photograph.

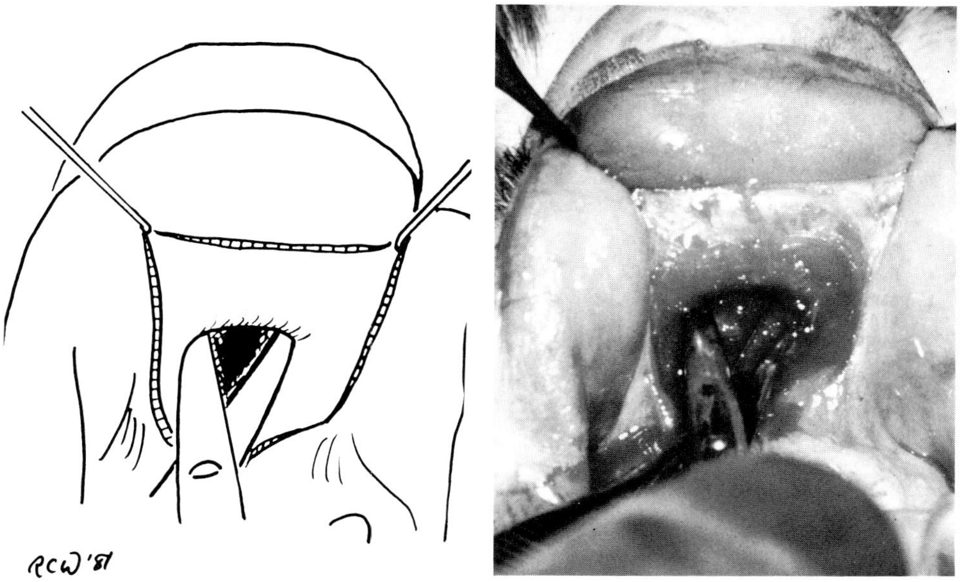

Fig. 11-13. Blunt-ended scissors now being gently spread to separate musculature on either side of midline.

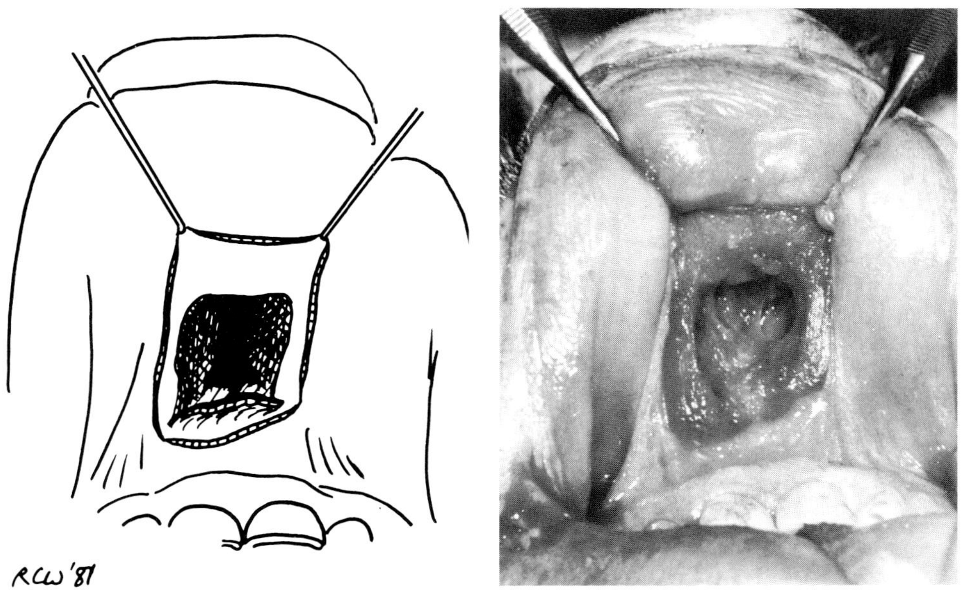

Fig. 11-14. Pocket going almost to anterior nasal spine. Caudal margin of septal cartilage is depicted in black.

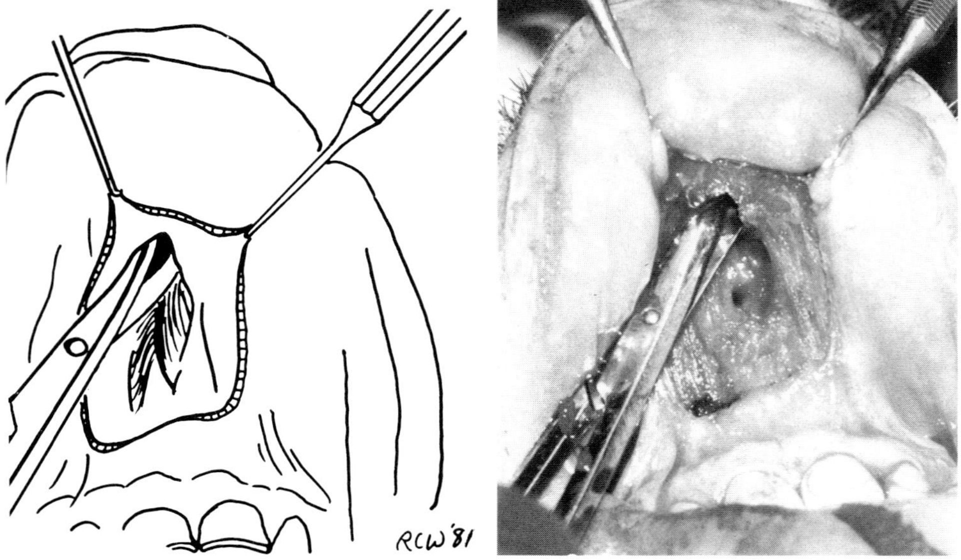

Fig. 11-15. Curved blunt-ended scissors pushed toward columella and gently opened to spread posterior portions of medial crura apart. Closing scissors and pushing forward on the fibrous tissues connecting the medial crura allow the operator to determine whether a graft similarly thrusting forward will produce the desired tip projection and rotation with or without bending or bowing the medial crura anterior to the forward thrusting object.

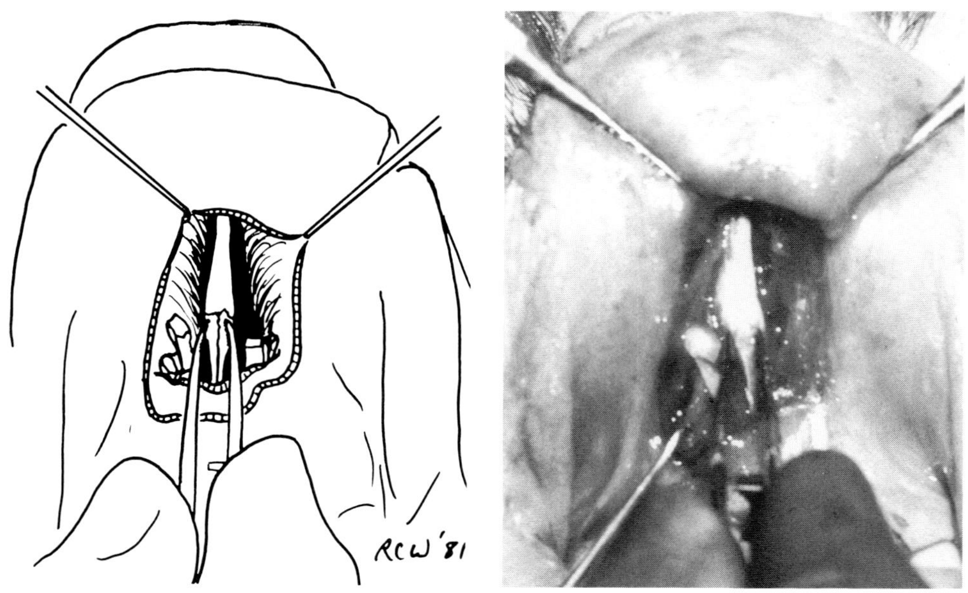

Fig. 11-16. A graft long enough to produce the desired effect is being inserted. On either side of it, small grafts or pieces of implant material may be inserted to help keep the long graft centered and/or to produce more augmenting effect lateral to the midline.

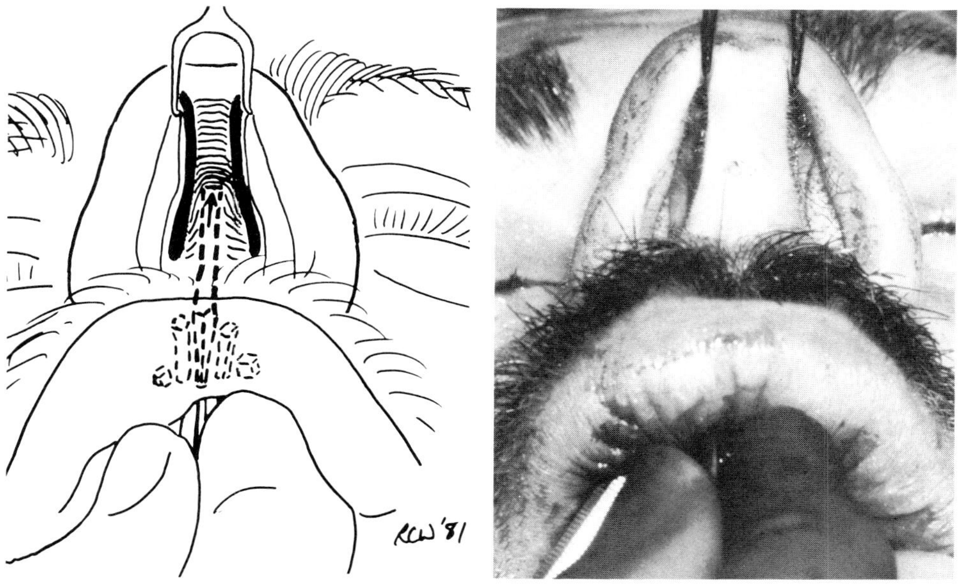

Fig. 11-17. Dashed lines show graft with stabilizing smaller grafts on either side. Forward end of graft is inserted between posterior portions of medial crura, shown in black. The fine lines running between the medial crura depict unsevered fibrous tissues connecting the medial crura, this fibrous tissue and the medial crura being pushed forward by the graft. Double hook is holding tip forward in slightly over-corrected position of projection. Slight over-correction should be provided. Excessive over-projection can be handled by incising the fibrous tissue a little farther forward or by shortening the graft.

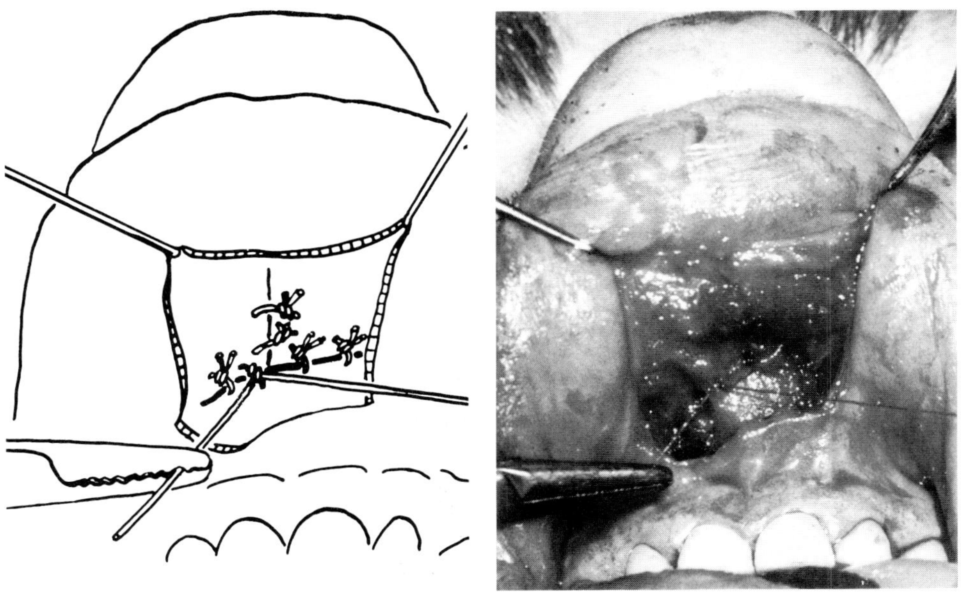

Fig. 11-18. Deeper closure with fine catgut. Mucous membrane closure will be provided next with same material.

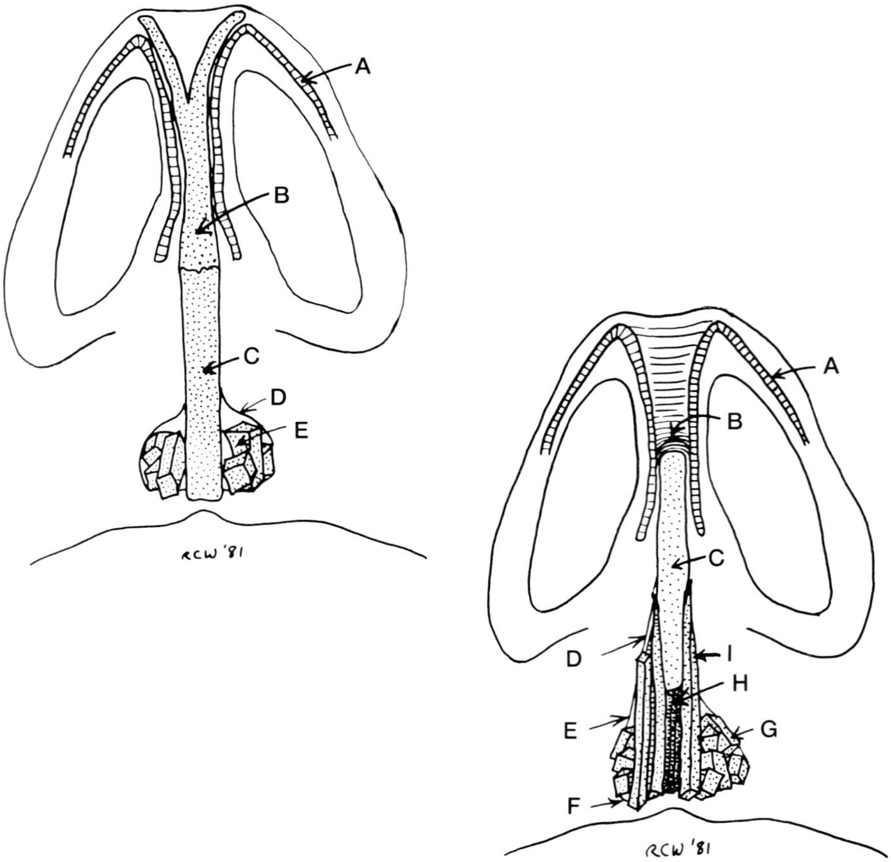

Fig. 11-19. (left) Long graft and smaller grafts on either side are stippled. **A**, Tip cartilages are shown cross-hatched. **B**, Cartilaginous portion of long graft split at anterior end. **C**, Bony part of long septal graft. **D**, Pocket edge. **E**, Small pieces of cartilage, bone, and/or implant material. Note that long graft shown from below runs back almost to premaxilla in midline, but not quite. Anterior split ends are bypassing medial crura and are providing the tip defining points and the tip projection. (right) Here, the longest graft **C** is pushing anteriorly on fibrous tissue connecting the medial crura at **B**. The tip defining points here are provided by the tip cartilages themselves, and the anterior projection and rotation is produced by the tip cartilages, which are being thrust forward by graft **C** as it pushes on the fibrous tissue at **B**. When the longest graft available will not reach back to the posterior end of the pocket close to the premaxilla, how may the operator effectively lengthen the graft? The way that we do it is to keep the pocket small, pull the anterior nostrils with the double hook up and forward until they are in a position of over-correction, push the long graft **C** forward against the fibrous tissue connecting the medial crura, and then fill the pocket behind the larger graft with smaller pieces and then with slivers, as shown. **D**, **E**, and **F** show the edges of the pocket. **G** depicts stabilizing grafts or implants. **H** shows grafts behind the larger implant **C**, and **I** shows stabilizing and splinting sliver grafts wedged in to fill the confined pocket and to prevent retrodisplacement of the large graft.

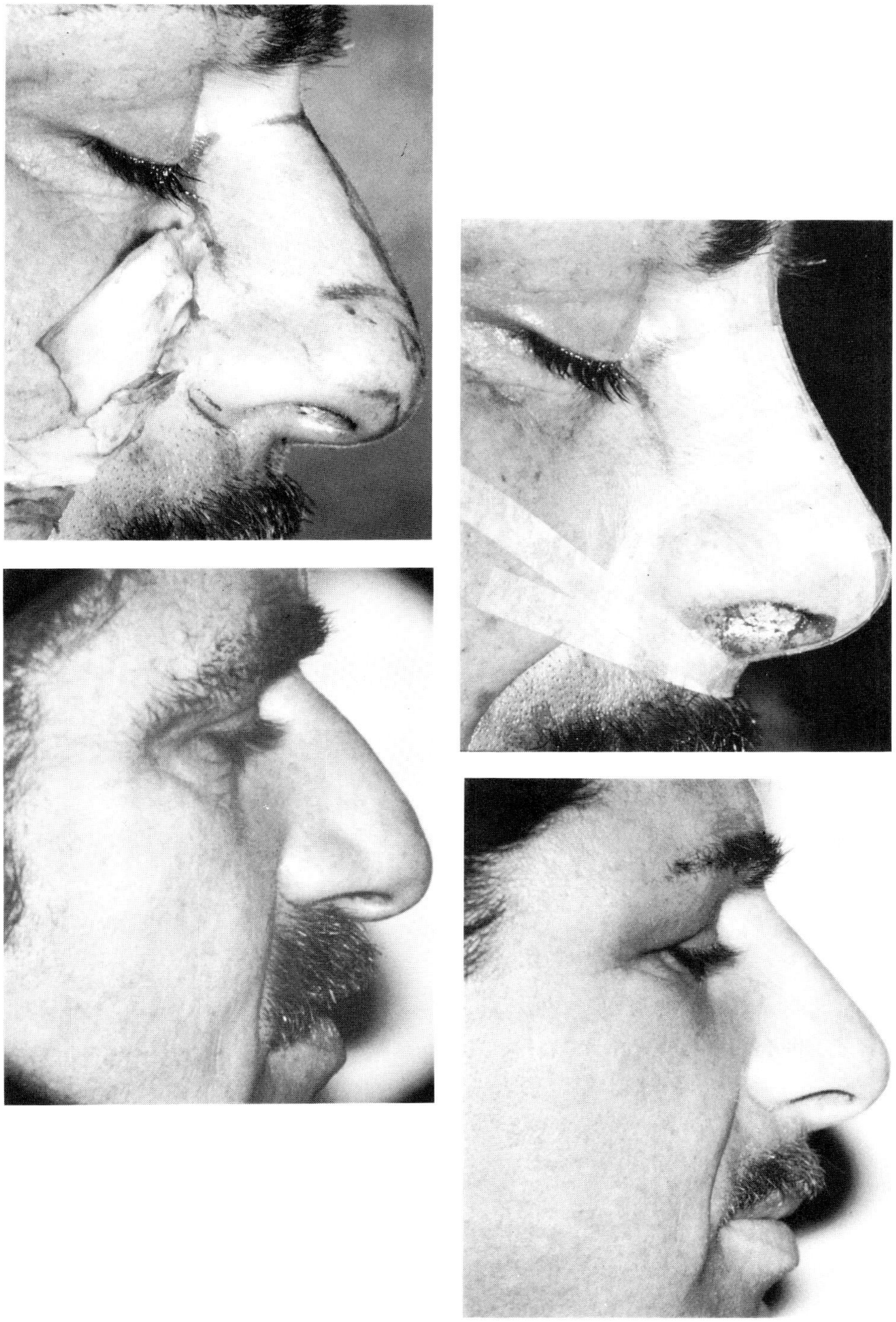

A B C D

Fig. 11-20. The patient whose operative photographs have just been shown. **A**, Septal bone and cartilage are sitting on the patient's right cheek. Note the downward inclination and retrodisplacement of the tip. **B**, Tip rotated upward and advanced forward with intraoral insertion of the grafts as just shown. Note paper tape dressing. Essentially no work has been done on the bony dorsum. **C**, Preoperative. **D**, One week postoperative. Only slight rasping performed on bony dorsum.

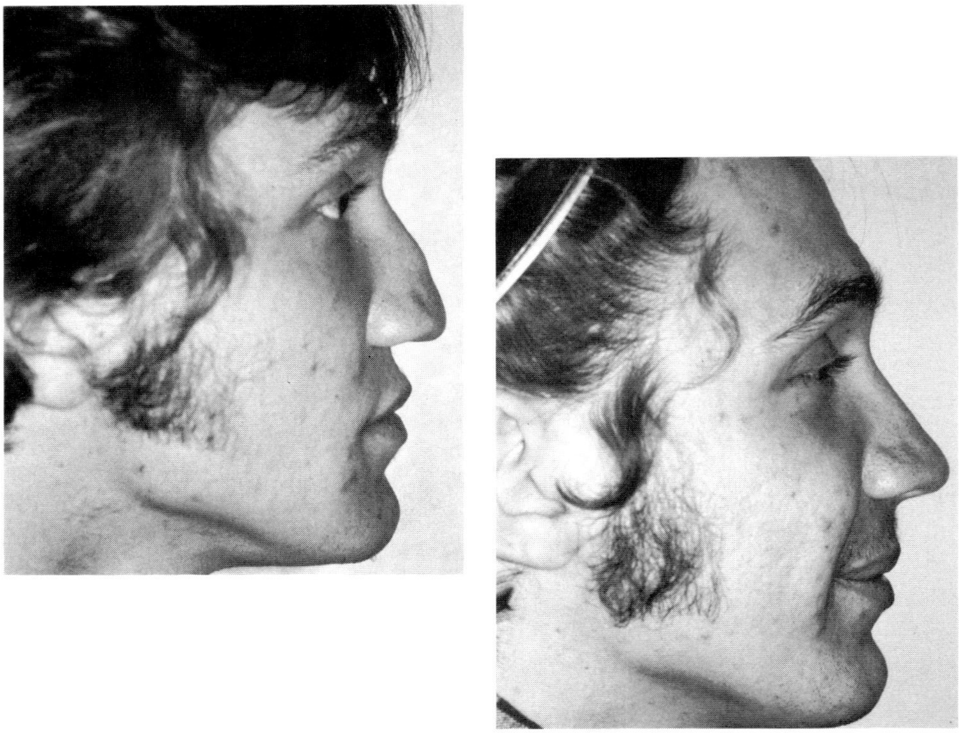

A
B

Fig. 11-21. **A,** Observe flattening of cheek, posterior and superior retraction of columella, and retrodisplacement of tip and upper portion of upper lip. The posterior sloping of upper lip is readily apparent. **B,** Grafts and implants inserted through columella-splitting incision into pockets behind alar cheek junctions and columellar-labial junctions. The grafts ran from the premaxillary region through the columella into the tip. Very little surgery was needed on this patient's dorsum.

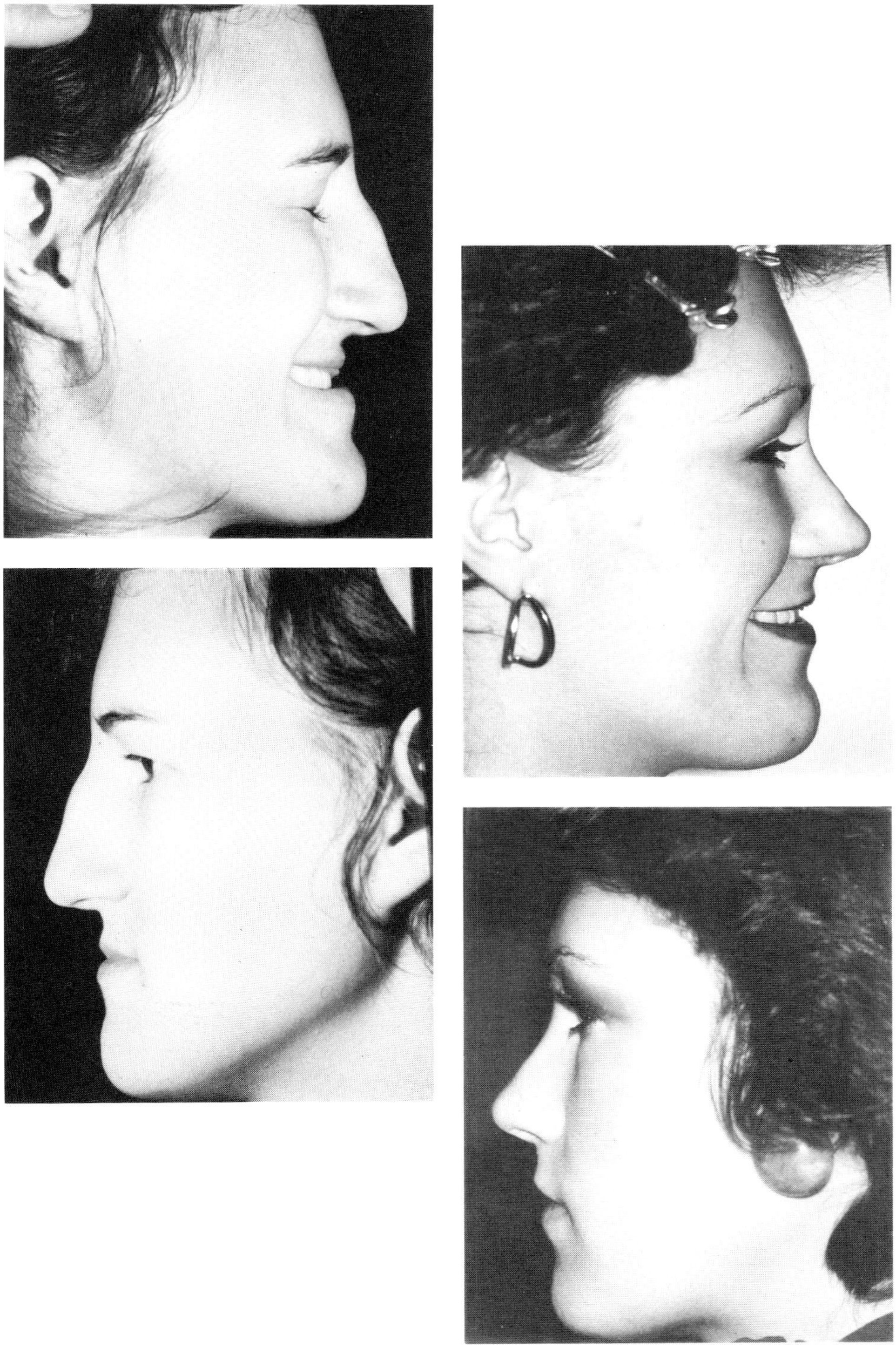

A B C D

Fig. 11-22. A, Nasal deformity, maxillary retrusion and mandibular prognathism. B, Over four years after septal grafts (cartilage and bone) to central maxillary areas and to columella. Long graft ran to tip. Columella-splitting incision used. C, Before surgery. D, Almost three years postoperative. Compare preoperative and postoperative relationships between columellar-labial junction and upper lip to the lower lip.

Sliding the Tip-Lip Complex Forward and Upward or Downward and Backward on Fixed Skeletal Structures

We have already mentioned the fact that the tip-columella-lip complex is made up of tissues running from the most anteriorly projecting parts of the nasal tip to the free border of the central upper lip. The cosmetic surgeon has but to grasp his own columella between his index finger and thumb and slide it forward or backward as far as it will go in order to observe the profound changes taking place in the positions of the supratip and tip regions, the columella and columellar-labial junction, and the positions of the vermilion border and free border of the central upper lip. Prior to surgery more than 4 mm of anterior or posterior displacement of the columella can be produced easily, these displacements taking place with the tissues of the complex still attached to fixed skeletal structures. If a membranous or cartilaginous (high) septal transfixion incision is made running from the tip back to the junction of the anterior nasal spine with the premaxillary portion of the upper jaw, even more extremes of displacement can take place. Any cosmetic surgeon should be able to produce significant changes in the positions of the parts of this complex because technically they are very easy to make. The transfixion incision and the separation of the soft tissues from the fixed tissues is one of the simplest maneuvers in all of rhinoplastic surgery.

Again, space limitations will not permit a full description of all of the variations on the theme of tip-lip complex sliding surgery, but we shall use cases to explain most of the important aspects. Generally, adequate transfixion incisions and separation of the sliding tissues from the fixed skeletal structures (septum, anterior nasal spine, and premaxilla) accompanied by the appropriate work to the tip cartilages and dorsum will allow posterior and downward sliding of the components. Mere suturing of the retrodisplaced columella to the septum above with one or two catgut stitches will provide permanent retropositioning and inferior displacement of the columellar-labial junction and central upper lip. There is practically no tendency in the healing phase for the complex to return to its former position (Figs. 11-23 to 11-28). Going the opposite way, however, is more of a problem. Either permanent sutures must be used, or grafts or implants must be added to the gliding surgery to provide permanent forward thrusting (Figs. 11-29–11-31), or skeletal structures must be locked and sutured into one of several arrangements of carpenter-like joints (Figs. 11-32 and 11-33), the fourth of the six divisions listed earlier.

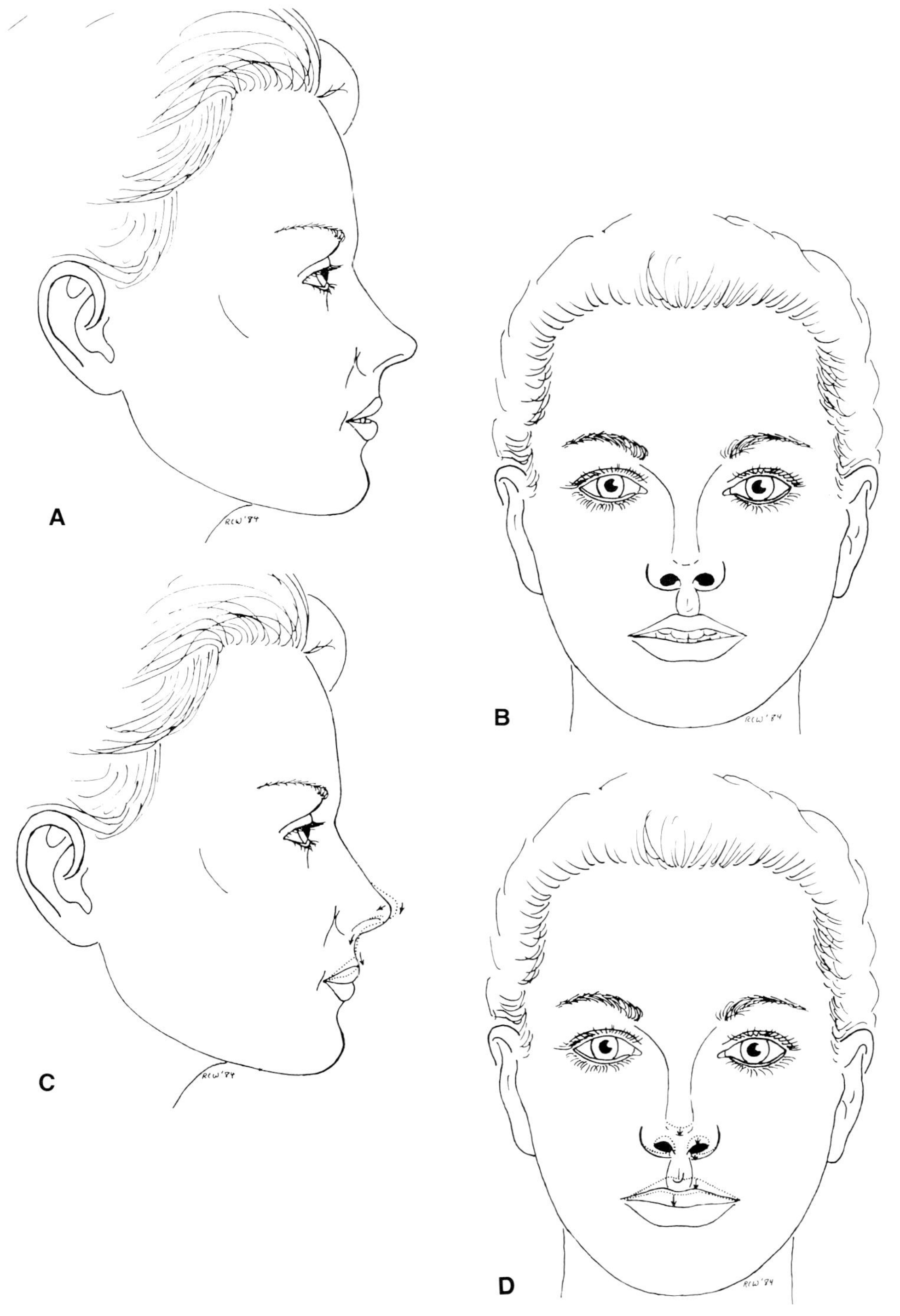

Fig. 11-23. **A,** Projecting tip with anteriorly positioned columellar-labial junction, slight superior retraction of columella, upper lip tethered superiorly. Its free border at rest does not adequately cover maxillary incisor teeth. Lip seal difficult. **B,** Front view. **C,** Dotted lines show preoperative positions. Continuous lines show changes after sliding the tip-lip complex postero-inferiorly on the fixed skeleton. Arrows depict directions of movement or displacement with this surgery. **D,** Front view after surgery.

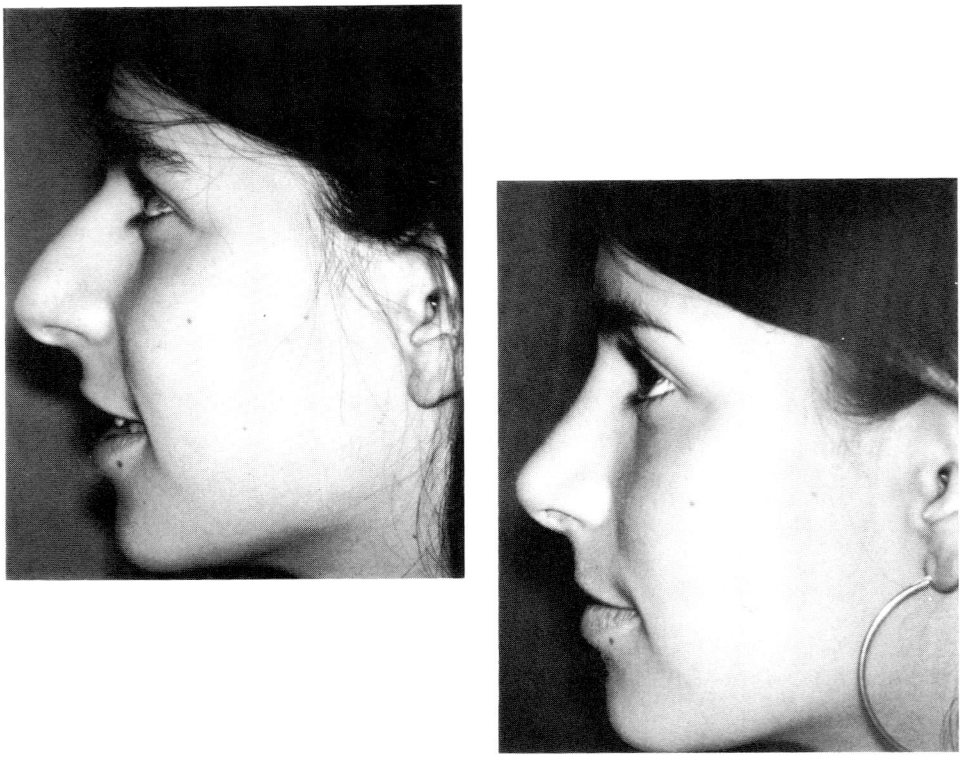

A B

Sliding maneuvers may be used in combination with many other rhinoplastic or cheiloplastic techniques; the selection of modalities depends on the combination of defects or deformities being improved. A very common combination of deformities seen is a projecting nasal tip with what seems to be a short upper lip, the free border of which sits so high that maxillary teeth or, at times, even the maxillary gum is exposed and lip seal may be difficult. Here, an almost ideal correction of two significant deformities can be achieved by appropriate resection of tissues making up the prominent dorsal profile combined with retrodisplacement of the tip and columella and inferior displacement of the columellar-labial junction and central upper lip (see Figs. 11-23 to 11-28).

Text continued on p. 140.

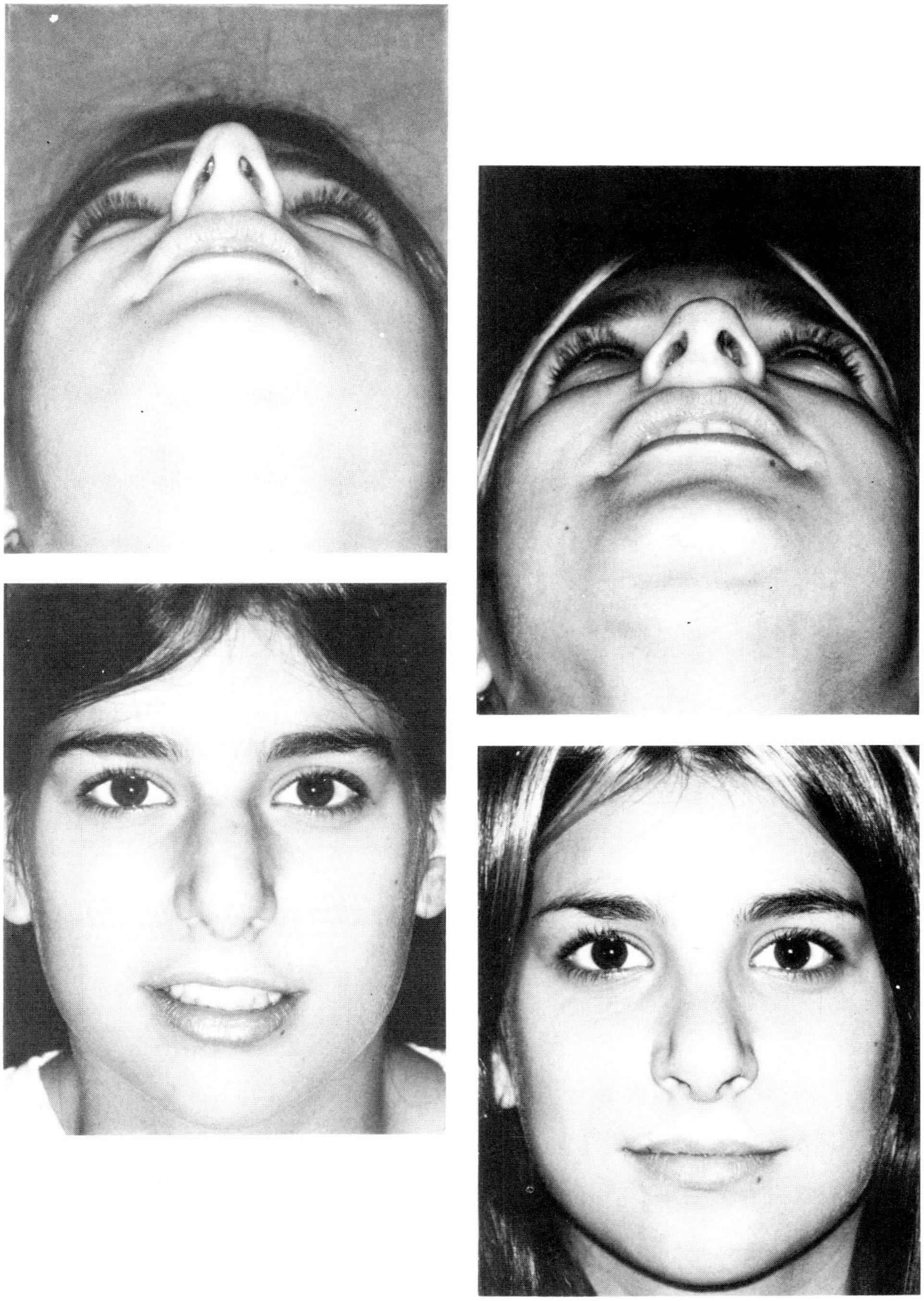

C

D

E

F

Fig. 11-24. **A**, Superiorly situated central upper lip with projecting tip **B**, six months postoperatively. **C**, Note what seems to be great width of posterior columella. **D**, Observe that what seemed to be columella has now become part of philtral portion of the lip. Eleven months after surgery. **E**, Preoperative. **F**, Eleven months postoperatively. Easy lip seal. Nostril base only slightly wider than before surgery.

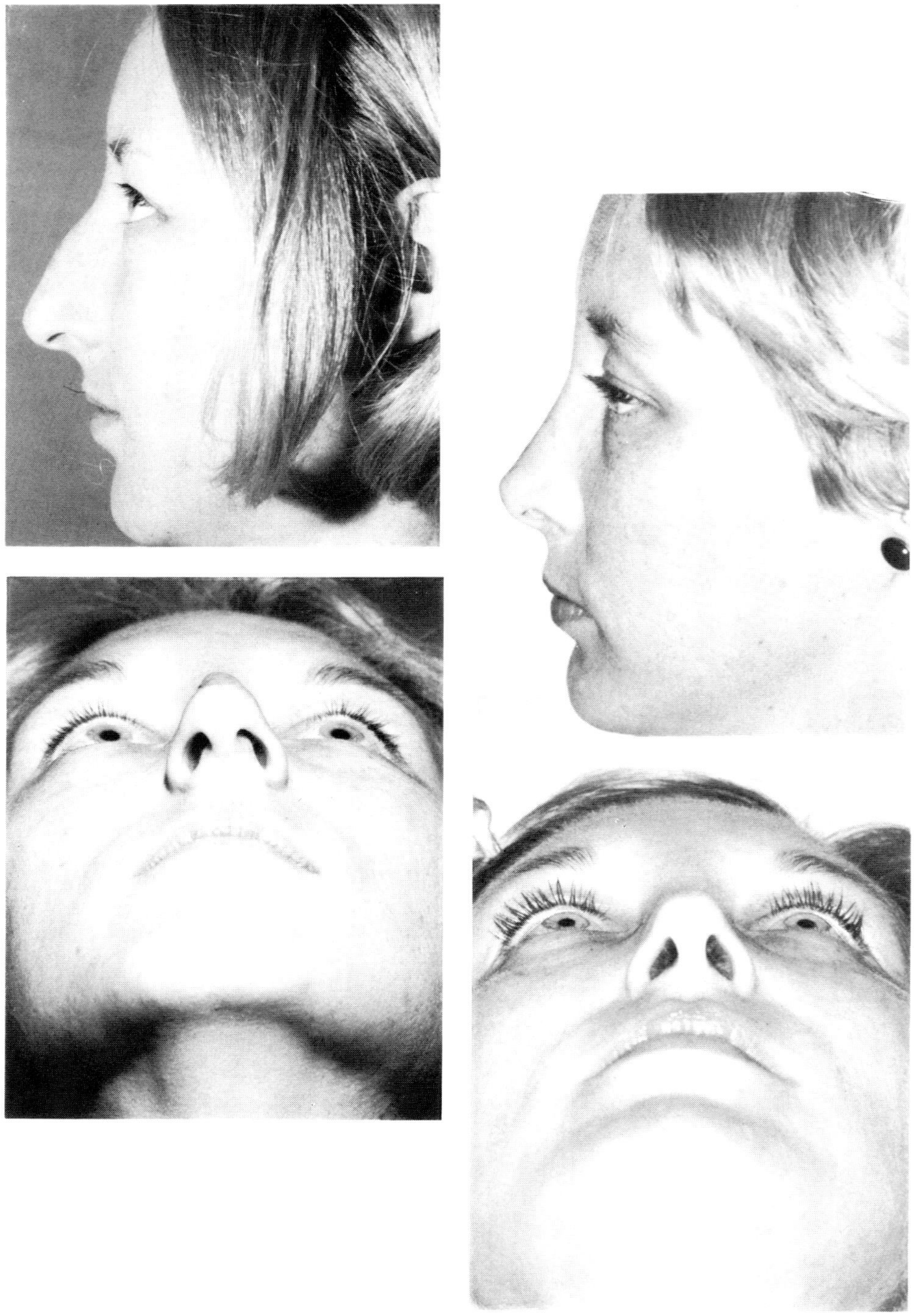

Fig. 11-25. **A,** Projecting tip and what might be considered a short upper lip. **B,** Six years after surgery. **C,** Observe position of medial crural foot plates before surgery and what seems to be a very wide columella between the alar lobules. **D,** Six years postoperatively. What seemed to be posterior columella before surgery now obviously has become part of philtral region of lip. Very little widening of alar base apparent.

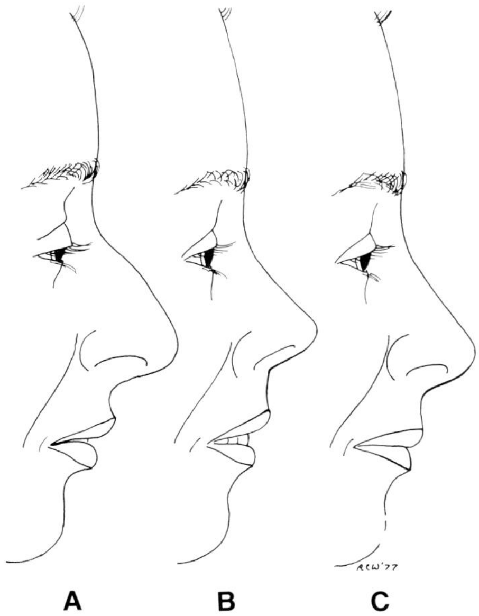

Fig. 11-26. **A,** Tracings of female patient with central upper lip that "rides high" and a projecting nasal tip. Alar lobule has high or superiorly positioned junction with lip. "Columella show" already excessive. Anterior nasal spine resection frequently performed under this latter circumstance. **B,** A likely profile after anterior nasal spine and caudal septal cartilage resection. The columellar-labial junction would be situated higher than before surgery. Central upper lip would tend to look long in relation to nasal length. Free border of upper lip would be pulled even more superiorly than in the preoperative condition, a mistake. **C,** After tip-lip gliding retrodisplacement without spine and septal cartilage resection. "Columella show" accepted in order to provide tip retrodisplacement and better positioning of central upper lip.

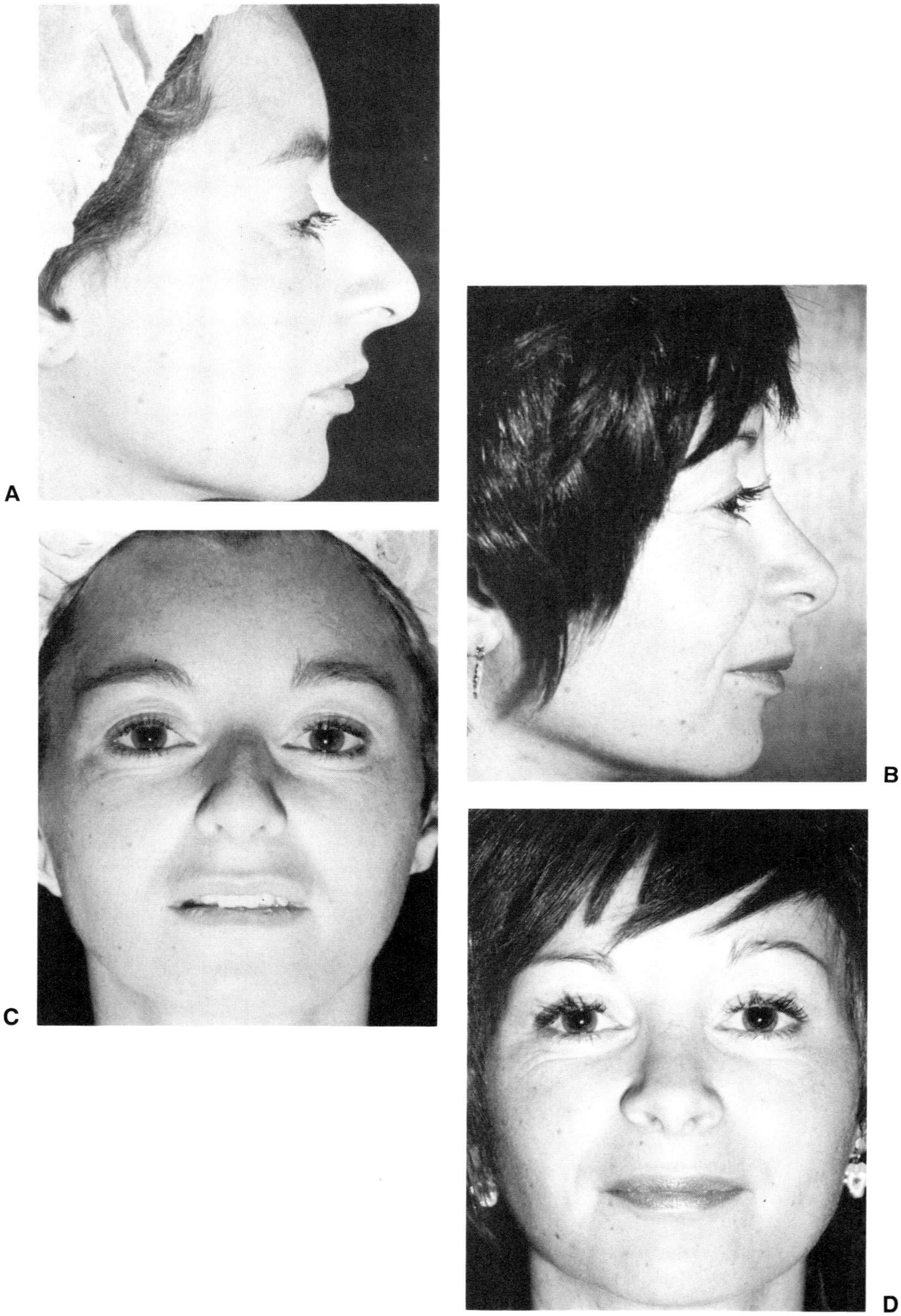

Fig. 11-27. **A,** Preoperative profile from which tracing (Fig. 26, A) was made. **B,** Postoperative profile. Tracing shown in Fig. 26, C made from this photograph. Four years after surgery. **C,** Observe "carrying" position of upper lip preoperatively. **D,** Postoperative. Has easy lip seal.

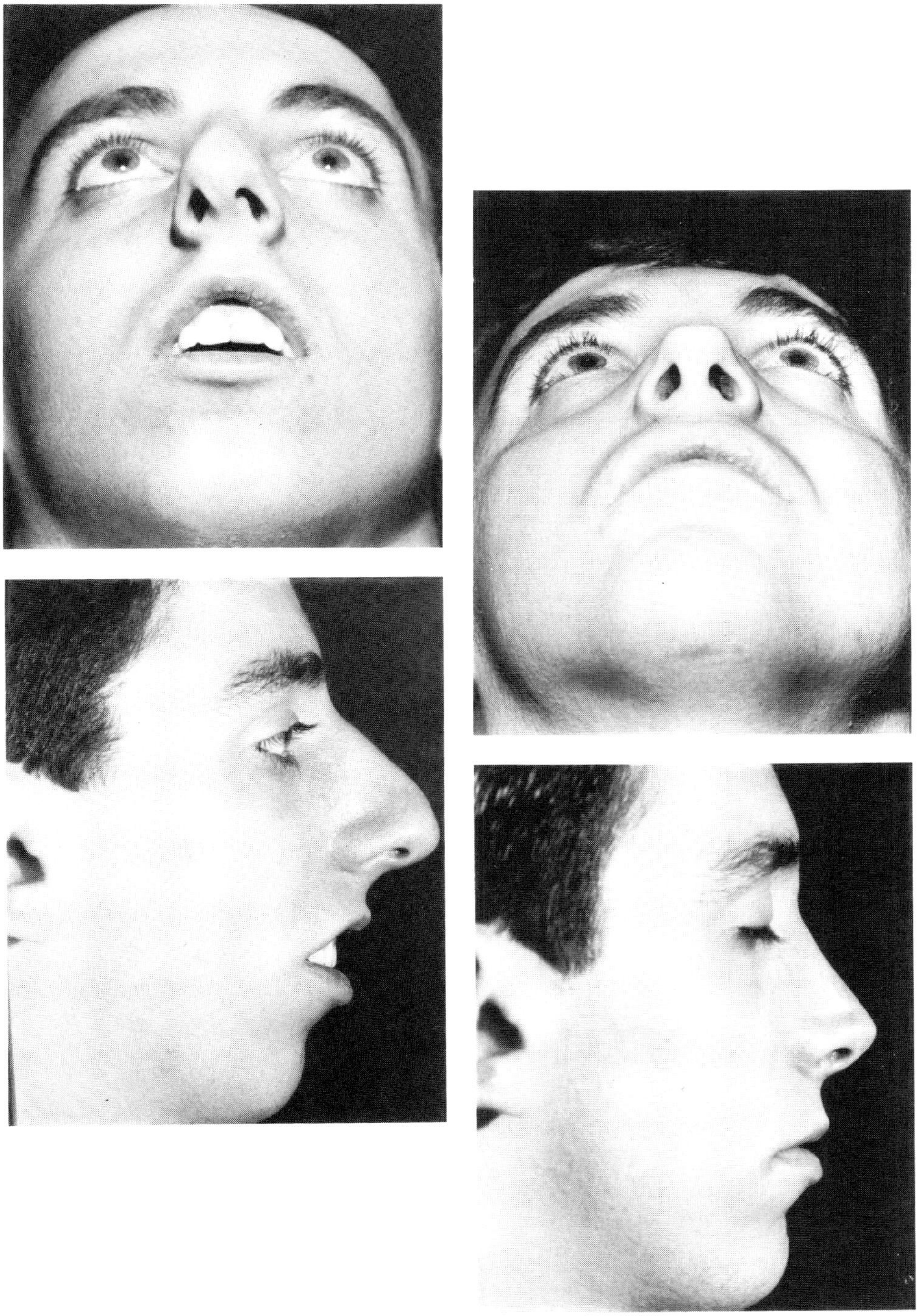

A B C D

Fig. 11-28. **A,** Note positions of tip, columella, and upper lip before surgery. In particular, observe exposed teeth and gum and positions of medial crura. **B,** Three years after surgery. Today we would use a different technique to avoid "boxy" tip. Compare lip seal and positions of medial crura with preoperative condition. **C,** What seems to be a difficult combination of problems (tip projection and extreme shortness of upper lip) easily and conveniently treated with retrodisplacing tip-lip complex sliding surgery. **D,** Chin augmentation, of course, performed as well. One year after surgery.

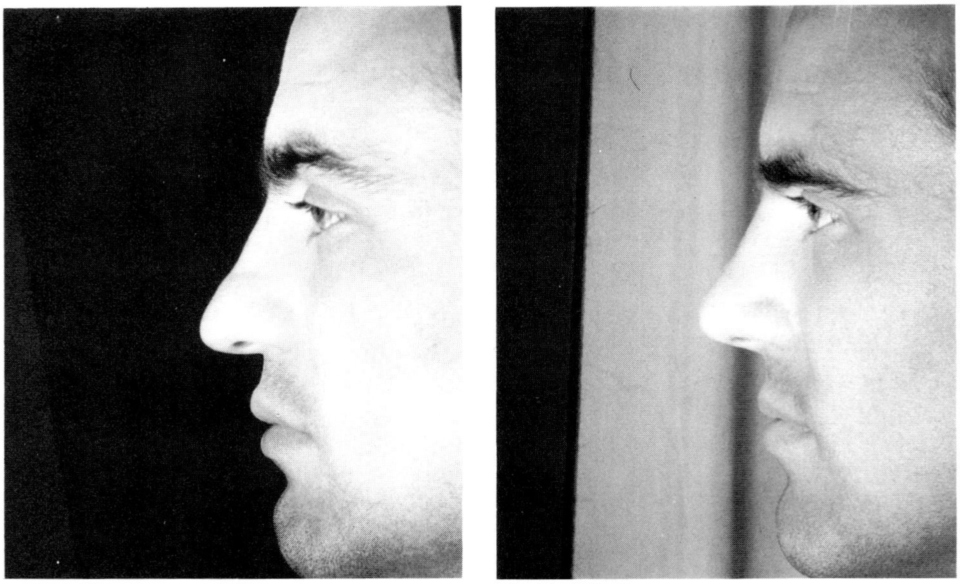

A B

Fig. 11-29. A, Anterior gliding combined with grafting, as discussed under augmentation of columellar-labial area, will be carried out. See also Fig. 11-6 to 11-22. B, Seven months postoperatively.

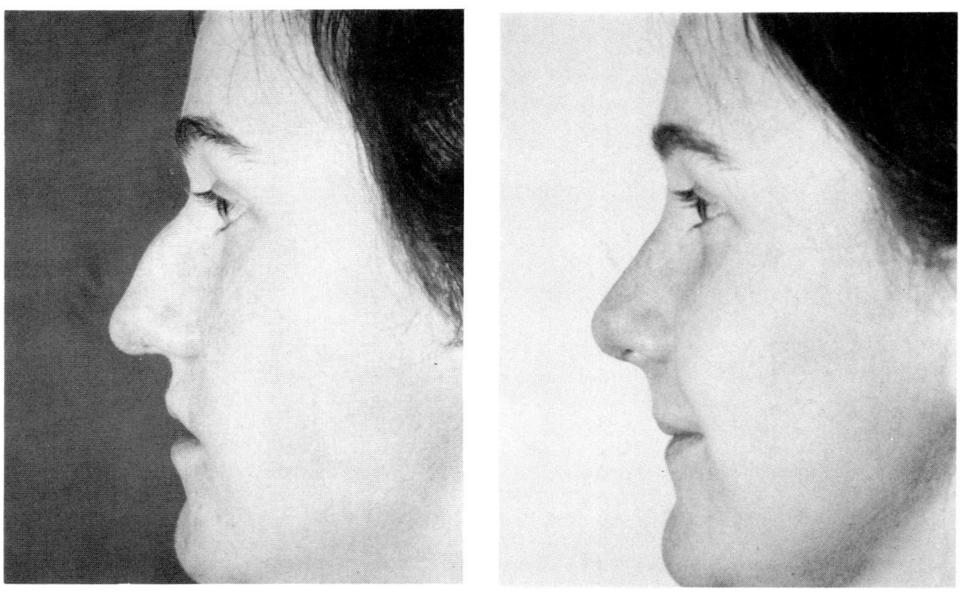

A B

Fig. 11-30. A, Retrodisplaced tip, upper part of central upper lip, columellar-labial junction, alar lobules, and anterior cheeks. B, Augmentation with grafts to or behind areas just listed, combined with anterior gliding. Columellar-labial junction antero-inferiorly positioned when compared with preoperative condition. Short-term result.

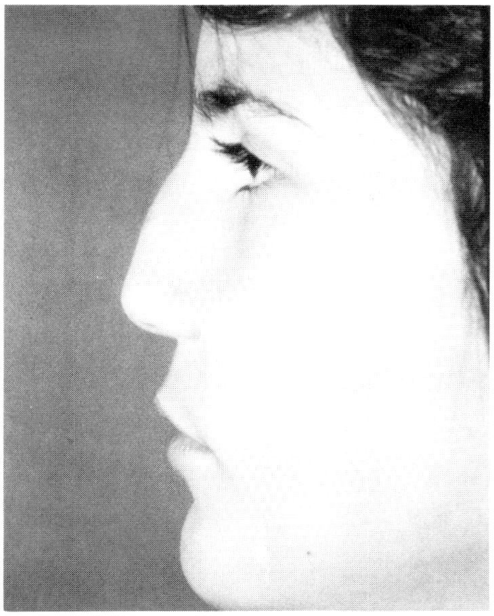

A

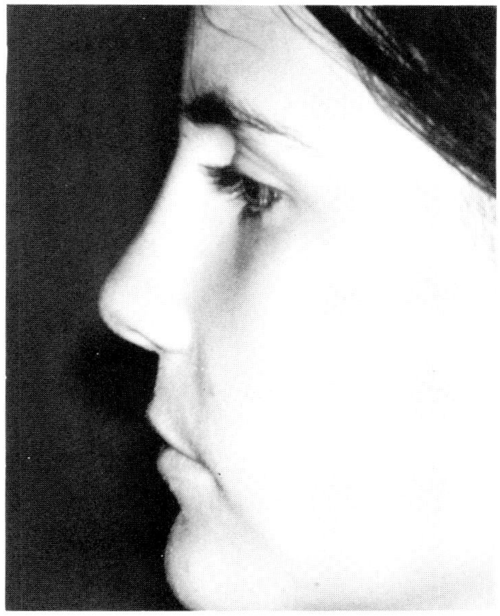

B

Fig. 11-31. **A,** Post traumatic deformities. Posteriorly sloping upper lip. Retrodisplacement of tip and columellar-labial junction. Lip obviously long enough. **B,** Anterior gliding (supplemented with grafts behind the now anteriorly placed structures) moved the tip far enough forward so that very little profile trimming of dorsum was needed.

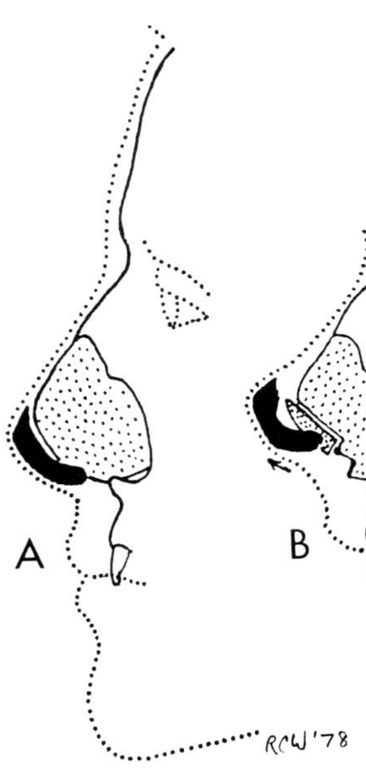

Fig. 11-32. **A,** Dotted lines show soft tissue profiles. Stippled portion shows septal cartilage. Solid black section shows medial crus, postero-superior part of which overrides and is attached to septal cartilage. **B,** If vertical septal shortening is to be performed, high septal transfixion incision may be made back to a site close to the anterior nasal spine. The septal cartilage "strut" inferior to septal transfixion incision (with medial crura still attached) may be separated from septal cartilage above and behind by a right-angled incision near the anterior spine. A rectangular defect stepped forward of the right angle incision just described may be provided to allow the desired septal shortening. Into the rectangular defect the "strut" may be placed and sutured. So much forward thrust can be placed on the still attached medial crura that they may bend excessively. Strong medial crura, of course, transmit forward thrust better. This technique is occasionally used for forward and upward gliding and fixation when the tip is retrodisplaced and dependent and the septum is too long vertically. Grafts placed near anterior spine help in fixation and maintenance of the correction.

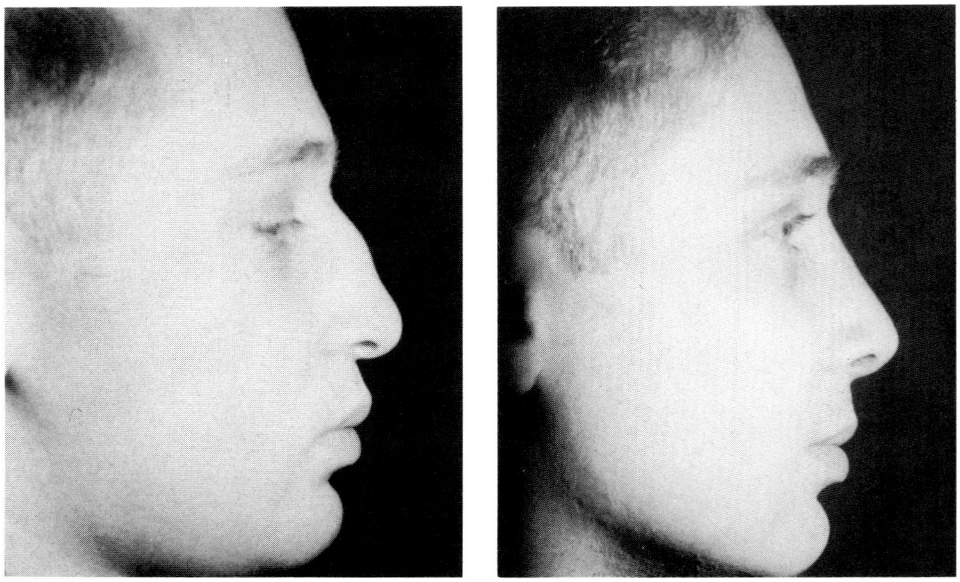

A B

Fig. 11-33. **A,** Condition just described. **B,** After septal "orthopedic" or "carpentry" surgery combined with anterior gliding (as shown in Fig. 11-32).

However, if the nasal tip shows the same excessive projection just described, but the central upper lip is longer and adequately covers the teeth and gum, the same posterior sliding of the columella and inferior displacement of the columellar-labial junction and central upper lip would position the free border of the central upper lip down so far that the edges of the teeth would be hidden and the patient would have a deformed or "lippy" smile. Moreover, there often would be far too much "columellar show." The same basic tip-lip aesthetic complex surgery (namely, the gliding maneuver) may be performed, but room must be made for the tissues sliding into the area just below the anterior spine and caudal septum. This space can be provided by appropriate resection, under these conditions, of caudal septal cartilage and bone of the anterior nasal spine (Figs. 11-34 and 11-35).

In the patient with excessive tip projection, too long a columella, and excessive vertical length of the white skin of the upper lip, sliding of parts of the complex may have to be combined with excision of some of the skin of the columella and/or upper lip to provide the best cosmetic compromise possible (this would involve the sixth of the six divisions listed earlier).

Another frequently seen combination is a retrodisplaced tip with retraction of the columellar-labial junction superiorly and posteriorly. Here, as described in the section on augmentation, grafts or implants may be needed to provide the thrusts necessary to allow the anterior parts of the columella and tip to glide forward and upward (see Figs. 11-29 to 11-31). Occasionally we see a retrodisplaced tip that is also po-

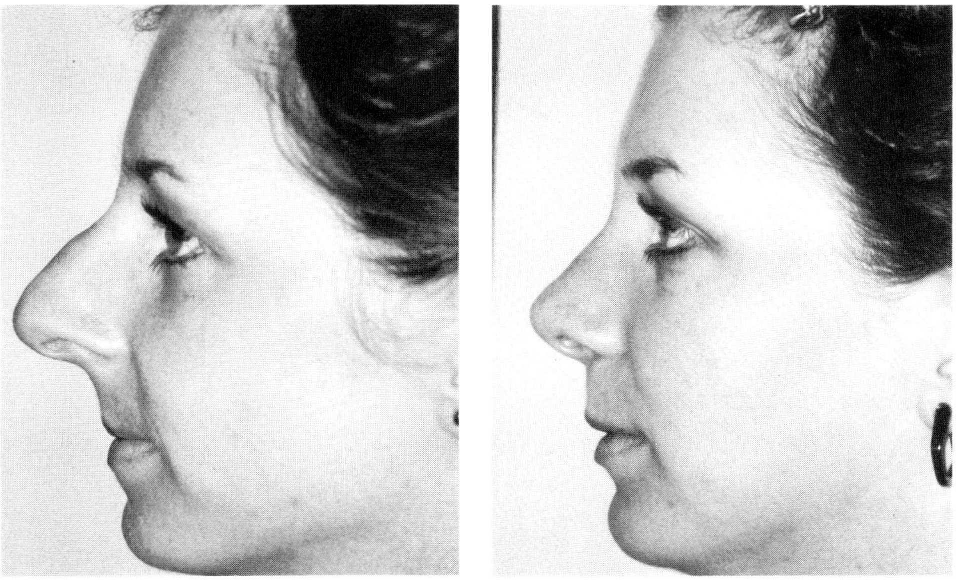

Fig. 11-34. **A,** Projecting tip and anterior positioning of columellar-labial junction, central upper lip long, lip seal adequate. **B,** If anterior spine and caudal septal cartilage had not been resected at all, free border of upper lip would be situated too far inferiorly. Therefore, postero-inferior gliding is combined here with appropriate resection (see also Figs. 11-1 to 11-5).

sitioned too far inferiorly (dependent tip) with excessive vertical length of the anterior part of the septum. This combination allows vertical shortening of the septum to take place at the same time that the lower border of the septal cartilage anteriorly is detached and moved forward and then locked into its new upper and anterior position with fixed septal cartilage just above and behind the piece just moved forward and upward (see Figs. 11-32 and 11-33). The medial crura are left attached to this piece of caudal septal cartilage and, under these circumstances, they are slid forward and upward and the tip is moved superior to and forward of its former location.

We have found it enormously helpful to be able to play with these many factors in order to select what may be the very best combination in truly complex diagnostic problems. However, one must be aware of the possibilities and take the time to break the appearance of the patient into the many factors involved in order that appropriate and sophisticated diagnoses are made. Added to usual rhinoplastic thinking, we must always keep in mind that two paradoxical concepts are involved in gliding maneuvers of the tip-lip aesthetic complex when it is retrodisplaced.

We know that resection of the anterosuperior portions of the lateral crura will allow thinning in the upper tip region. This narrowing resection leaves an intact strip of lateral crus running from the dome to the

Fig. 11-35. **A**, Excessive tip projection, marked anterior position of columellar-labial junction, lip long enough, but drawn or tethered antero-superiorly somewhat. The patient is not edentulous and has had carcinoma of left nasal tip removed, with skin graft closure earlier. **B**, Three and a half years after subtraction or resection of bone and cartilage just above and behind columellar-labial junction combined with postero-inferior sliding of tip-lip complex. **C**, Before rhinoplasty. Note long axis of nostril, positions of medial crura, and what seems to be a very wide posterior columella. **D**, Observe change in columella and nostril shape and length. Here change in slope of nostrils, with this extent of tip retrodisplacement, has led to some widening of alar base. **E**, Before rhinoplasty and flap repair of skin grafted tip. **F**, One year after tip-lip surgery and local flap repair of nasal tip.

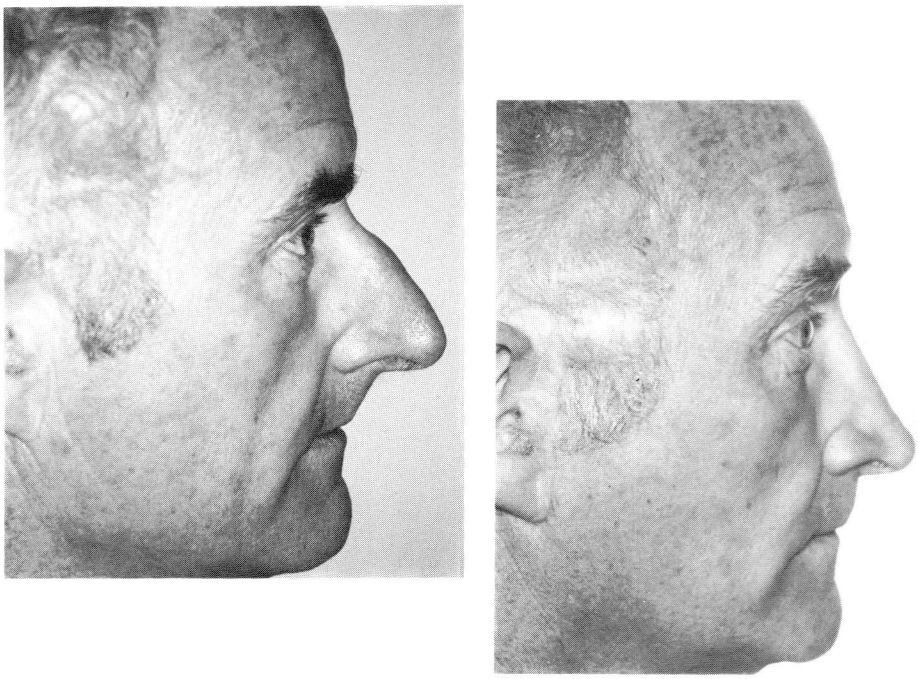

A

B

posterosuperior attachments of the lateral crus to the upper lateral cartilage and to relatively fixed fibrous tissues near the pyriform aperture. This basic tip technique, called the intact or complete strip technique, tends to prevent retrodisplacement or inferior or superior rotation of the tip, as long as the medial crural attachments to the caudal septal cartilage are intact. Every observation that we have made over the years indicates that Anderson's "tripod" concept is correct. If the middle leg (the conjoined medial crura) of the tripod is shortened or retrodisplaced and the two lateral legs are left intact with their attachments to relatively fixed structures also left intact, then retrodisplacement of the columella and tip should produce inferior rotation of the tip. However, when we slide the tip and columella back in the typical tip-lip complex

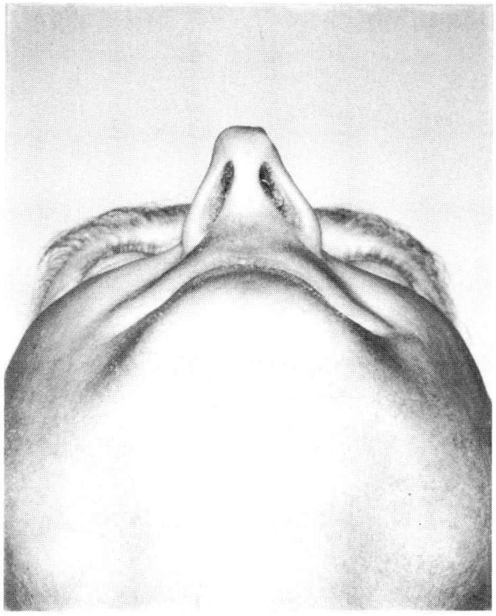
C

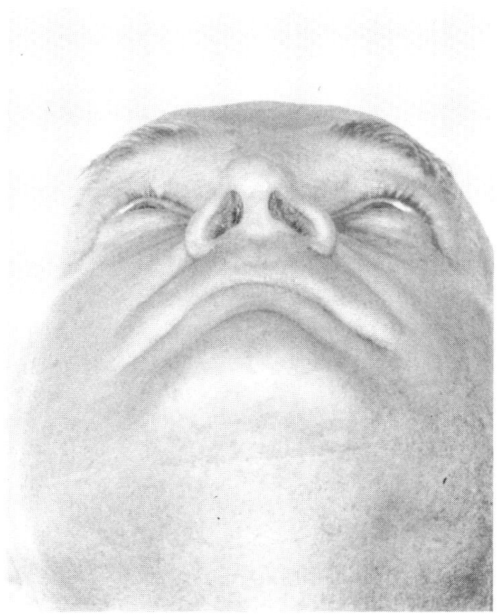
D

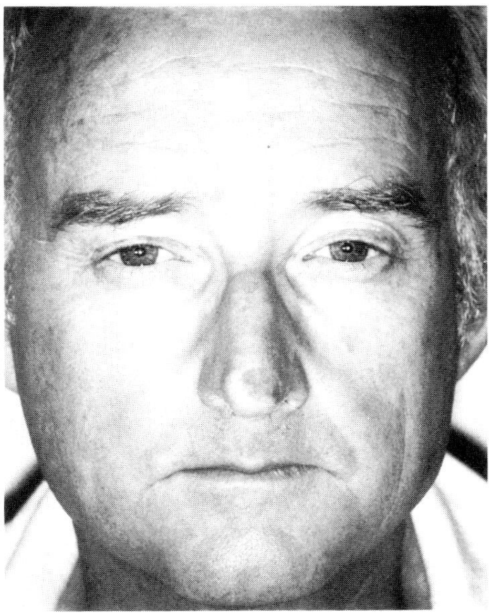
E

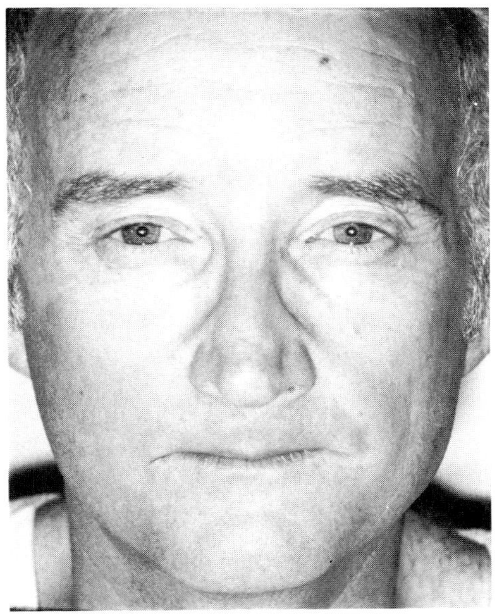
F

maneuver, both front and side views seem to show that there has been superior tip rotation. The nose usually looks vertically shorter. How can this be? What actually has happened is that, as the tip does rotate inferiorly, say by 2 mm, the columellar-labial junction has moved inferiorly more than 2 mm. The appearance of shortening of the nose and superior rotation of the tip is based more on our perception of the slope of the columella and the degree of acuteness of the angle made up by the

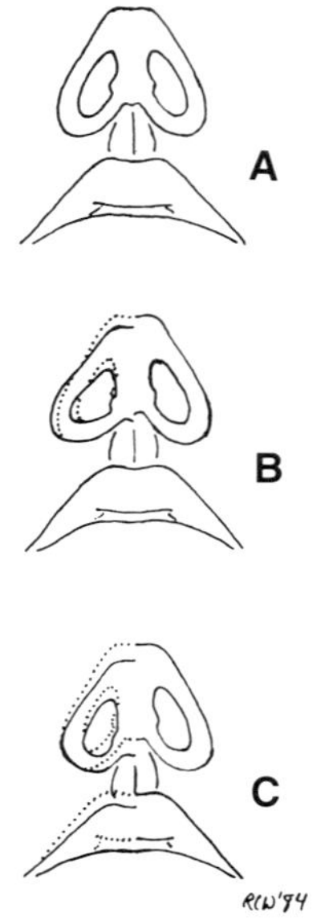

Fig. 11-36. **A,** Base view of nose and lip. Lip seal is incomplete because of forward and upward displacement of columellar-labial junction into what might be considered by some to be a wide posterior columella. Little bulges inside nostrils represent medial crural foot-plates. Tip is depicted as slightly projected. Note slope of nostril and long axis of nostril. **B,** Dotted lines show preoperative positions. Solid black lines on reader's left show retrodisplacement of nasal structures and change in the aesthetic factors just described. Here, though, tissues have not been thoroughly "freed up" or separated from skeleton in anterior nasal spine region. Tissue "piling up" in columellar-labial junction area pushes junction back a small amount and pushes alar lobules apart. Condition is somewhat similar to that noted in "tip drop" cases, where little displacement of free border of lip occurs. **C,** On reader's left, the solid lines show position after tip-lip gliding surgery has been performed. Here, instead of "piling up" between the alar lobules, the posteriorly and inferiorly displaced tissues have moved downward to give good lip seal without undue widening of alar base.

profile of the columella-infratip lobule complex and the profile of the central upper lip than it is on actual or true positioning of the tip. If the columellar-labial angle is made more obtuse and the columella has a greater vertical slope after the displacements, the appearance is that of a superiorly rotated tip (Figs. 11-36 and 11-37).

Fig. 11-37

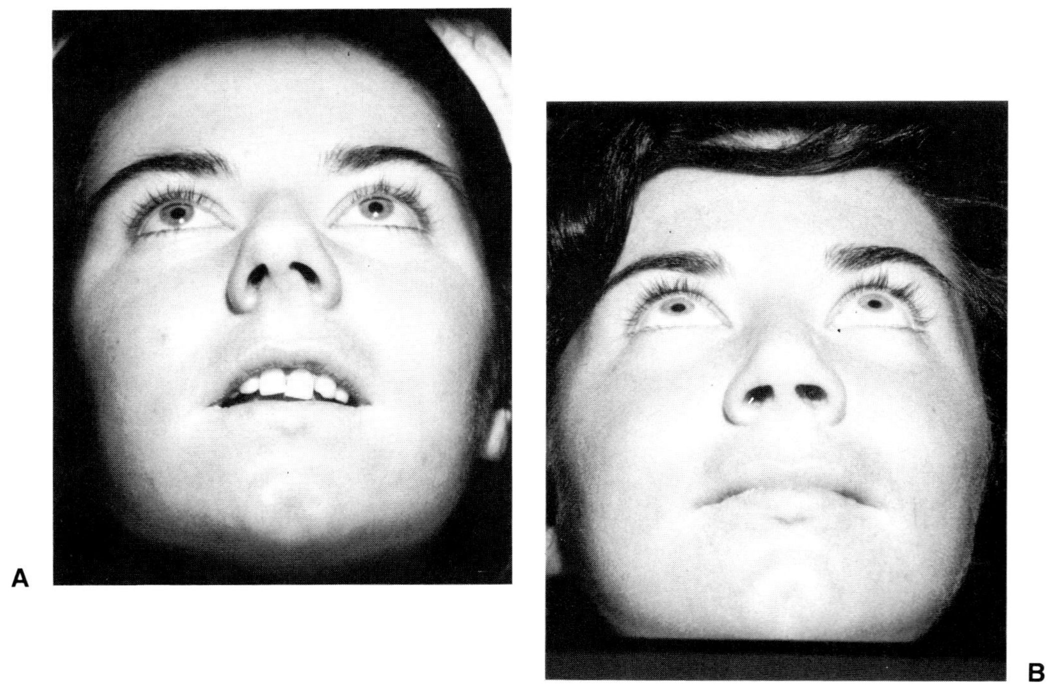

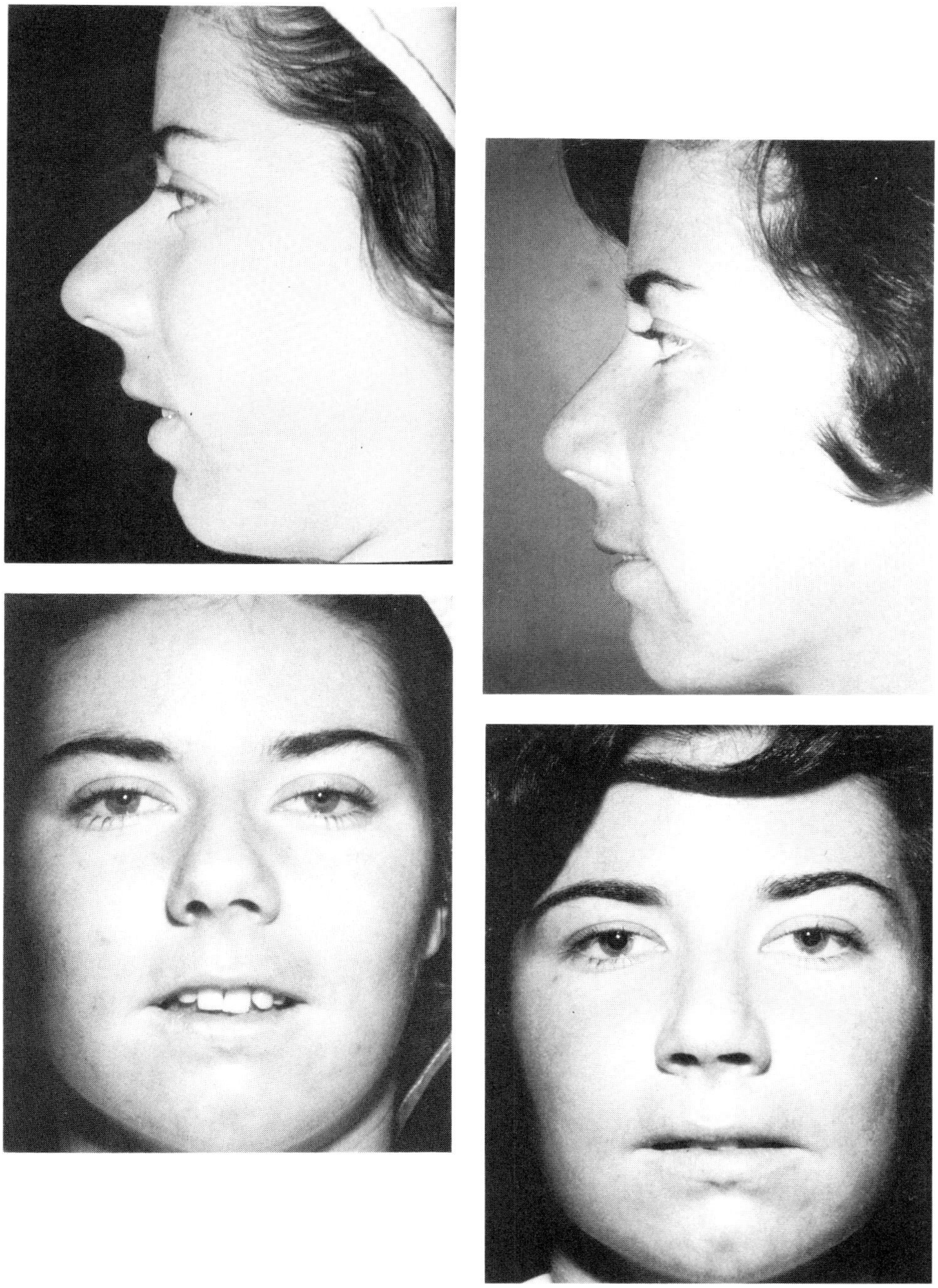

C D E F

Fig. 11-37. Patient showing changes shown in Fig. 11-36. **A,** Note obliquity of nostrils, location of medial crural foot-plates, exposure of maxillary teeth, and what seems to be a wide columella between the alar lobules and nostril sills. **B,** Observe changes after tip-lip sliding produced retro- and inferior displacement. Part of what seemed to be the columella is now obviously not the columella. There is a slight widening of alar base; lip seal is easily accomplished now. **C,** Lateral view before surgery. **D,** Note locations of tip, columellar-labial junction, and central upper lip. **E,** Difficulty with lip seal apparent before surgery. **F,** Nostril base is only slightly widened after tip-lip surgery. The lip has obviously improved.

A second paradox exists. One of the most frequent problems involved in rhinoplastic surgery in the past was so-called "tip drop." After the swelling from the local anesthesic and surgery had subsided and healing had progressed for a while, the tip was found to have dropped closer to the face or to have been retrodisplaced, leading often to supratip fullness or, if anticipated at the time of surgery, to over-resection of the dorsum in order to prevent supratip prominence or fullness. In addition, the alar base widened. Therefore, large numbers of Weir resections or nostril sill resections were performed to correct or prevent this aspect of "tip drop." In other words, most rhinoplastic surgeons know that one effect of retrodisplacement of the tip is widening of the nostril base. Why then, when we retrodisplace the tip with this sliding surgery sometimes as much as 5 mm or more, do we not see gross widening of the alar base in most cases? Obviously, as the tip moves closer to the alar base, unless it too is retrodisplaced, the slope of the external sides of the nostrils changes. With less tip projection, even if the alae have not been pushed apart somewhat, the lower part of the nose will look a little wider than it did before the surgery. However, in the usual unplanned "tip drop" the lip was not slid downward to any appreciable extent. Tissues near the columellar-labial junction tended to pile up in that area. We all know that tissues made up largely of water are virtually noncompressible. Something had to give. What we believed happened was that with fixed bone above and behind these retrodisplaced tissues, a small downward displacement did occur in the columellar-labial junction and central upper lip region, but a larger lateral and posterior shift occurred near the nostril sills and anterior nostril floor regions, thus pushing the alar lobules apart and adding to the effect of widening of the alar base. What we know happens, if the separation of the soft tissues is complete enough with the transfixion incision running almost to the nostril sills and the soft tissues separated all the way back to the premaxillary area, is that the retrodisplaced soft tissue shifts downward mainly, thus pushing the central part of the upper lip downward enough to adequately cover exposed maxillary incisors or gum. Although some widening of the alar base does occur, the main displacement of this soft tissue is downward (Fig. 11-38). Therefore, it is imperative that adequate separation be carried out. Actually, it is technically possible to pull downward on these freed tissues (by putting a hook in the central upper lip) so that the nostril sills become distorted and inferiorly displaced and the alar lobules then begin to move closer together.

Of course, it is true that the degree of columellar-labial junction "show" is greater than it was before one of these retrodisplacing maneuvers, and often the nostril base is widened slightly. Generally, the latter does not require nostril sill resection for narrowing, and, in our aesthetic judgment, the increased columella show is more than acceptable when the improvement in position of the free border of the upper lip is taken into account. Compromise is the order of the day here, and

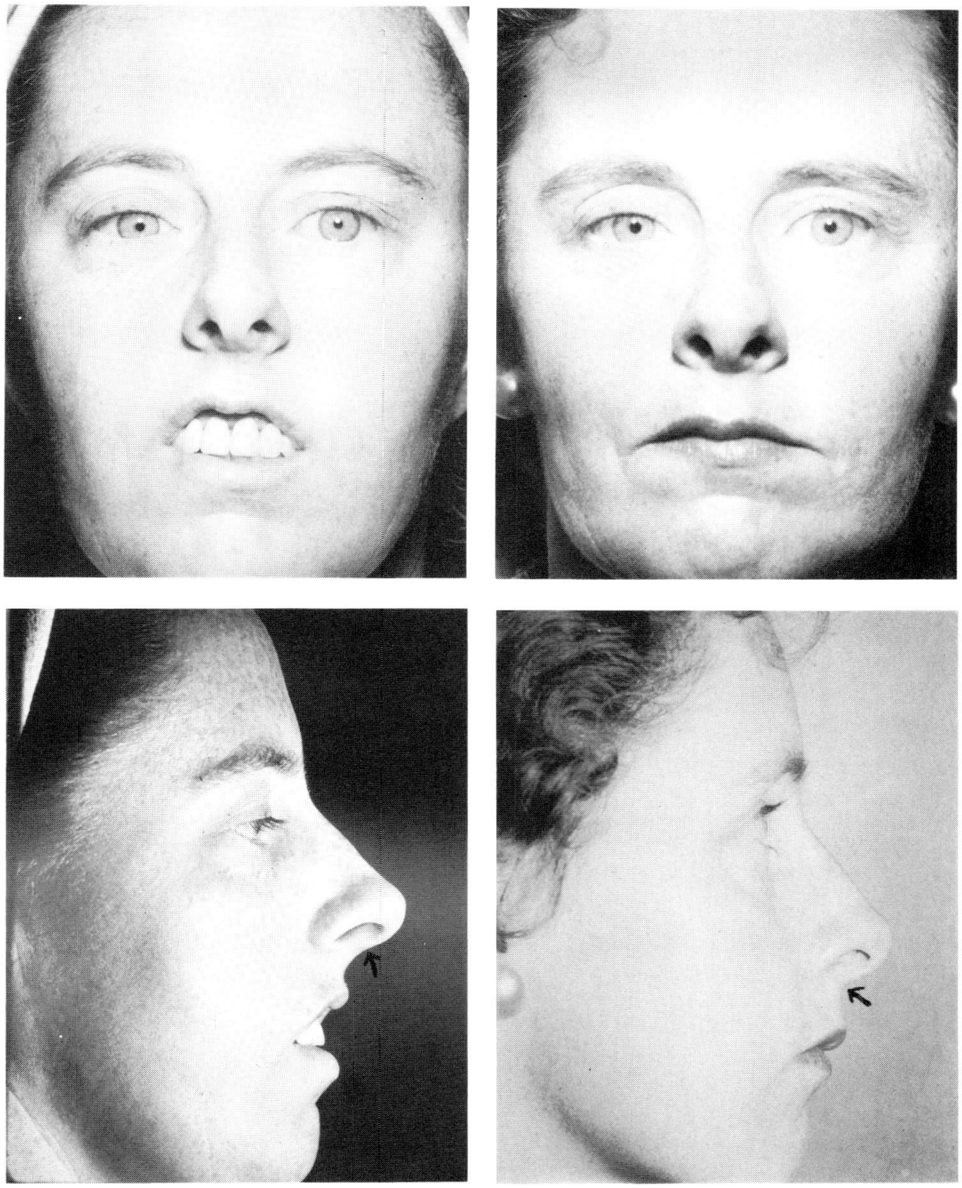

A B C D

Fig. 11-38. **A**, More extreme case with gum, as well as teeth, exposed. **B**, despite extreme postero-inferior sliding, there is very little widening of the nostril base. **C**, Note marked shortening of central upper lip. **D**, Compare carefully with preoperative profile. At first glance the tip does not seem to be rotated inferiorly, but accurate measurements would show that it is situated at a significantly lower level than it was before surgery. Because the columellar-labial junction has moved farther downward than the tip has, the inferior tip rotation actually taking place is not apparent. Note more acute arching of the alar margin taking place as nostril length in antero-posterior direction was diminished with retrodisplacement of tip. Nostril sills and columellar-labial junction moved inferiorly so that very little lateral compression to widen nostril base occurred (see **A** and **B**). Instead, gliding tissues moving postero-inferiorly carried the free border of the central upper lip downward to give appropriate lip seal. Arrows in **C** and **D** show how the real or true columellar-labial junction moved in this tip-columella-lip sliding surgery.

one must balance the advantages against the disadvantages to try to get the best total result in each case.

Summary

We have discussed in some detail but not completely three of the aspects of tip-columella-lip aesthetic complex surgery. We believe that these techniques should be known and used more widely in rhinoplastic surgery because they often allow more accurate diagnosis and treatment of the more complex cosmetic problems involving the upper lip and lower part of the nose. Their use, combined with other more standard rhinoplastic modalities, frequently allows these other modalities to be used to less than extreme degrees or extents. Results often are more predictable when several modalities can be used conservatively than when one approach has to be used to an extreme degree. Our primary message here is that the nose is not an independent structure; it is joined to the upper lip and anterior cheeks. Aesthetically, subtle and important relationships exist between all of the facial landmarks. The cosmetic surgeon would be well advised to consider these relationships in every patient. When he can improve two or all three of these facial components in one operation, he is likely to do better than when focusing all his attention on just one.

REFERENCES

1. Powell N and Humphreys B: Proportions of the aesthetic face, JD Smith (ed.), Thieme Medical Publishers Inc., 1984.
2. Webster RC: Advances in surgery of the tip. Intact rim cartilage techniques and the tip-columella-lip esthetic complex, Otolaryngol Clin North Am 8:615, 1975.
3. Webster RC, Davidson TM, and Smith RC: Importance of the columellar-labial junction in rhinoplasty, Head Neck Surg 1:423, 1979.
4. Webster RC and Smith RC: Rhinoplasty: lip improvements as adjuncts. Plastic and reconstructive surgery of the head and neck. Proceedings of the Fourth International Symposium, Los Angeles, 1984. Ward PH and Berman WE, editors, St. Louis, 1984, The CV Mosby Co.
5. Webster RC, Smith RC, and Kazda G: Columella-labial changes in solution of rhinoplasty problems, Laryngoscope 95: 629, 1985.
6. Webster RC, et al.: Columella-splitting incisions in rhinoplasty, J Otol 8:417, 1979.
7. Webster RC, et al.: Intraoral insertion of grafts to project the nasal tip, Arch Otolaryngol 108:187, 1982.

12

Mid-Nose Surgery

Walter E. Berman

The mid-nose is critical to nasal function and appearance. Its skeleton is composed of the upper lateral cartilages and cartilaginous septum. The position of these structures is dependent on each other, as well as being influenced by the nasal, ethmoid, and vomerine bones superiorly and posteriorly, and the nasal spine, and maxillary and palatine crests inferiorly.

Approach to the Mid-Nose

Separating Skin From Skeleton

To uncover the mid-nose skeleton, a sharp scissors or scalpel is inserted through the "between-the-cartilage" incision. Hugging the cartilage, the instrument is used to conservatively deglove this portion of the nose.

Junction Tunnels

Junction tunnels involve constructing submucosal tunnels at the junction of the upper lateral cartilage and the nasal septum, as opposed to simply cutting the membranes (Fig. 12-1). This area, the internal nasal valve, plays a crucial role in respiration and should be kept intact, thus avoiding the vagaries of mucosal healing and possible postoperative cicatrix. Additionally, keeping the membranes intact virtually eliminates postoperative anterior ethmoidal bleeding.

Technique

1. The perichondrium is elevated at the septal angle. This elevation is carried along the anterior or dorsal border of the septum, continuing under the periosteum of the perpendicular plate of the bony septum.
2. This same elevator is moved laterally to elevate the periosteum and perichondrium as needed. The extent will depend on how much anterior bone and cartilage will be removed. The developed mucosal envelope is intact from the "between-the-cartilage" incisions superiorly and posteriorly into the nose.

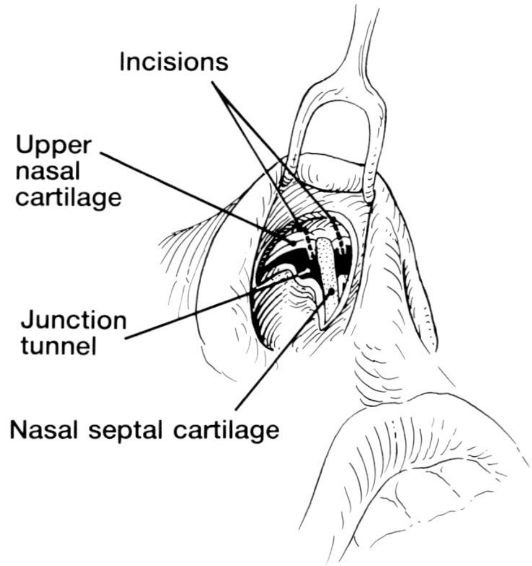

Fig. 12-1. Junction tunnel: the underlying mucosa is intact. (From Berman WE: Rhinoplasty, ed 2, Washington DC, 1984, American Academy of Otolaryngology-Head and Neck Surgery Foundation, Inc.)

3. The junction tunnels just created are then used to separate the upper lateral cartilages from the attached septum with a scalpel. The overlying skin is protected from the scalpel with a thin flat retractor such as a Converse, Alfrecht, or Neivert placed through the between-the-cartilage incisions and under the overlying skin.
4. Junction tunnels may also be accomplished from the anterior or dorsal position. After the anterior overlying skin is separated from the nasal framework, the incision is made through and between the cartilage incision. The upper cartilages are separated from the cartilaginous septum with a scalpal, sparing the underlying mucosa.

After degloving and creating juction tunnels, the upper lateral cartilages are usually separated from the septum and the septal and lateral cartilage components are operated on separately.

Septum

Lateral Deformity

Any significant lateral deviation of the anterior cartilaginous septum must, of course, be repaired. Specifically, the twisted nose often has much of its pathology in this area. As discussed in the chapter of septoplasty, stripping the septal cartilage in both cardinal directions and carrying the cuts through the anterior cartilaginous border is very helpful. In cases of severe deviation, the cartilage may have to be completely disassociated from its bony attachments and strips of cartilage may have to be removed to obtain a straight septum. Only one side of the septal perichondrium is elevated, except where thin strips are removed.

Vertical Deformity

Adjustment of the definitive height of the cartilaginous nasal hump is aesthetically dependent of the projection of the nasal tip and, to a

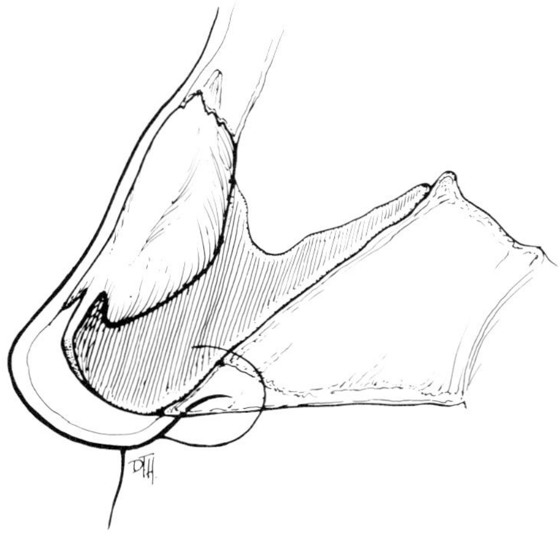

Fig. 12-2. Anatomical components of the mid-nose.

lesser degree, on the overall length of the nose, At times, the height of the anterior cartilaginous components of the nose distorts the nasal tip. A partial reduction of these component parts must be made before the final tip projection can be assessed.

A 135-degree angulated serrated scissors is used to remove an appropriate amount of anterior septal cartilage. This also creates the level at which the gouge or straight osteotome will be placed and is used to remove the more superior and anterior aspect of the nasal bones.

Excessive anterior cartilage may also be decreased with a rasp, cut with scissors, or shaved with a blade. I prefer to use scissors or a blade because rasping may leave irregularities from minute residuals. Until the lateral osteotomies have been completed, no attempt is made at this stage to definitively smooth the top of the nose.

Upper Lateral Cartilages

After completing the septal work, the upper lateral cartilages are addressed. Having been freed from the septum, they generally "seek their own level." In the case of the twisted nose, simply freeing the lateral cartilages and repairing the septum can significantly improve nasal appearance. Conservative trimming of these cartilages, however, is often necessary.

Trimming

As discussed in Chapter 14, the upper lateral cartilages are shaped like triangles with their bases laid along the septum. Trimming may be needed along their bases to lower vertical height, or along their inferior angles, which underride the lower lateral cartilages (See Color Plate VI, Chapter 2).

When addressing the upper lateral cartilages, a thin flap elevator, a

Neivert or Alfrecht, can be inserted through the between-the-cartilage incision. This readily exposes the anterior aspects of both upper lateral cartilages as well as the septum.

Only gentle retraction with the elevator may be used. Portions of the cartilage are then trimmed in conservative fashion. Strong retraction in an anterior direction may give the illusion that the severed upper lateral cartilages are higher in relation to the septum than they actually are. This false perception may cause the surgeon to remove more of the upper lateral cartilage than necessary.

After trimming the base, if any residual "scrolling" of the inferior upper lateral cartilage is evident, conservative removal of this will aid air flow. If this is not done, the internal valve may be compromised. At times, excessive "telescoping" of the upper lateral cartilage beneath the lower lateral cartilage occurs. Some of this may be removed to further protect the airway at the internal valve and to allow for nasal tip rotation when necessary.

13

Osteotomies

Walter E. Berman

An osteotomy, which is the cutting of nasal bones and naso-maxillary processes, is performed on the bony pyramid. The type and degree of the osteotomy will be as varied as the individual case. Whether the osseous changes are removal of the anterior (dorsal bones) or repositioning of the lateral nasal bones, there are two general principles to observe. First, the periosteum should be elevated and preserved when feasible because this will aid the regeneration and healing of the osseous tissues. In addition, it may hide the small irregularities in the skeletal framework, as a blanket hides wrinkles in the sheet beneath. Second, the surgical procedure should cause the least trauma possible.

Anterior Hump Removal

The anterior hump is usually composed of bony and cartilaginous components. The anterior soft tissue coverings are separated from the underlying bony and cartilaginous components. This is accomplished by a bilateral between-the-cartilage incision and elevation of the overlying skin and subcutaneous tissues. In reality, if possible, the tissues over the upper laterals are separated from the overlying tissues with a scalpel, while the tissues overlying the bone are elevated with a periosteal elevator under the periosteum. The latter is very difficult, indeed sometimes impossible, in cases of secondary surgeries or post-trauma. Junction tunnels are then developed.

We now have bony tissues devoid of coverings both anteriorly and posteriorly on top and underneath the nasal bones. The covering or periosteum is only separated from the bone to the extent that the bony tissues will be removed.

I have found that the best exposure for hump removal is after the upper lateral cartilages have been separated from the septum. Using a small anterior dorsal nasal retractor, the anterior aspects of both upper laterals and the septum are brought into an excellent view.

Septal Upper Lateral Cartilage Removal

After a 135-degree serrated scissors is used to conservatively remove the desired amount of excessive cartilaginous septum and upper lateral cartilages, a base or bed is formed for the osteotome to carry this plane more superiorly through the anterior part of the nasal bones. I normally prefer a gouge that actually removes a slightly deeper part of the perpendicular plate of the ethmoid rather than the two adjacent nasal bones. This allows for better apposition of the nasal bones (Fig. 13-1). Also the nasal gouge prevents a deviated anterior (dorsal) ethmoid plate from splaying the medialized nasal bones.

If the nasal pyramid is exceptionally broad, it is best to start with a wider flat osteotome until the radix area is approached, then switch instruments and complete with the gouge. This is necessary with the wide pyramid because the gouge is not wide enough to contact both nasal bones inferiorly. Initial trimmings of the anterior upper lateral cartilages and rasping is then carried out. I do not think it pragmatic to finish polishing these anterior borders or the nasal bones and upper cartilages until the lateral osteotomies have been completed because slight changes to the anterior aspect of the nasal bones may occur after the lateral osteotomies.

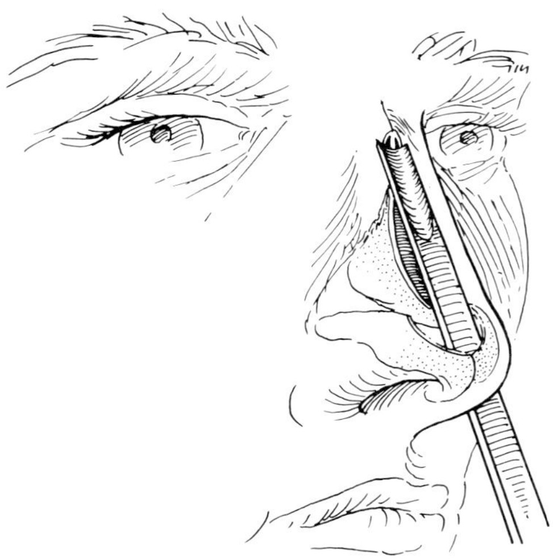

Fig. 13-1. Nasal gouge removing more perpendicular ethmoid plate than lateral nasal bones. This allows closer apposition of the nasal bones.(From Berman WE: Rhinoplasty, ed 2, Washington DC, 1984, American Academy of Otolaryngology-Head and Neck Surgery Foundation, Inc.)

Medial Osteotomies

When a significant hump is removed with osteotomes on the anterior surface of the nasal bones, medial osteotomies have in effect been performed. The nasal bones have been separated from the septum and each other.

Medial osteotomies are needed in the twisted or traumatized nose. They help control the single or multiple lateral osteotomies and the resultant transverse or back fractures. If not, the previous fracture sites may cause undesirable fracture lines when the lateral osteotome is used for infracturing. The wide flat nose that necessitates removal of bone lateral to the septum to narrow the pyramid also requires medial osteotomies. In this case, double medial osteotomies are made on each side and the intervening bone is removed with rongeurs to enable narrowing.

The previously elevated "junction tunnels" are followed by a medial osteotomy (Fig. 13-2). The flat, guarded osteotome is placed alongside the anterior septum and gently tapped with a mallet as the osteotome proceeds superiorly. If the very dense bone of the radix is encountered, the osteotome is angled slightly in a lateral direction for the last part of the cut. This is repeated on the contralateral side. The osteotome should be kept perpendicular to the nasal septum at all times.

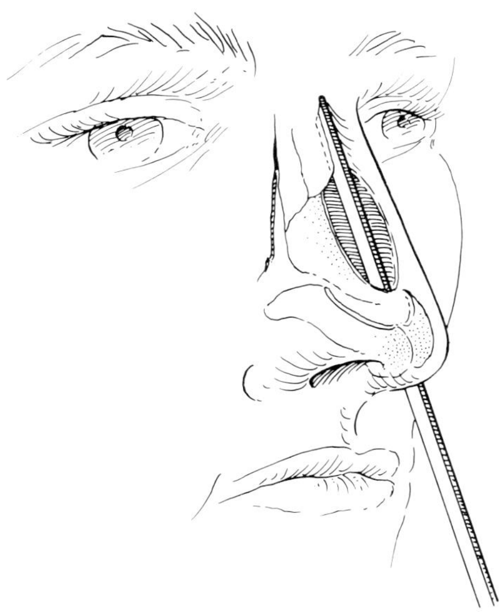

Fig. 13-2. Medial osteotomy through prior "junction tunnel." (From Berman WE: Rhinoplasty, ed 2, Washington DC, 1984, American Academy of Otolaryngology-Head and Neck Surgery Foundation, Inc.)

Lateral Osteotomies

There are many instruments available to perform these cuts in the nasal bones. It is far more important to know what needs to be accomplished than what tool to use. I personally make a small horizontal incision in the pyriform aperture and use a thin 3 to 4 mm straight guarded chisel. Cadaver dissection has shown that the formation of tunnels before using the osteotomes is not necessary. A thin guarded osteotome will readily raise the periosteum at the same time.

In the average nose, the lateral osteotomy is made on the outside of the naso-maxillary process practically on the face of the maxilla. Depending on the width of the nasal pyramid the cut is carried towards the radix. If the radix is thin, there is no need to carry this cut to the thick nasal process of the frontal bone. In fact, the cut can be made from one-third to one-half up the maxilla as indicated (Fig. 13-3). If a complete lateral osteotomy is contemplated, the cut should be gently angulated towards the anterior surface in the last quarter of the cut towards the radix (Fig. 13-4). This technique will help control the transverse fracture when the lateral cut through the nasal process of the maxillary bone is infractured (Fig. 13-5).

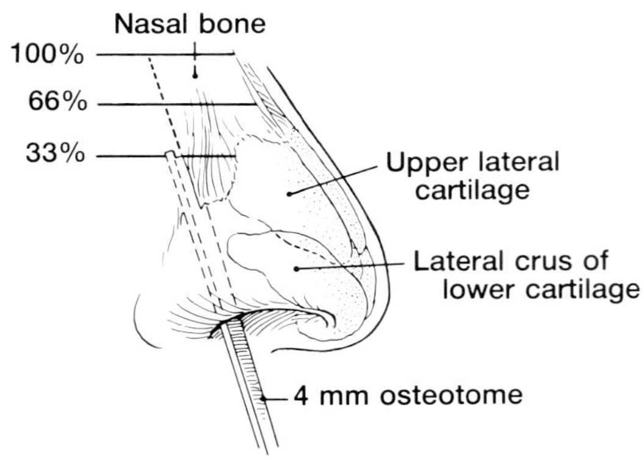

Fig. 13-3. Partial to complete osteotomies as needed. (From Berman WE: Rhinoplasty, ed 2, Washington DC, 1984, American Academy of Otolaryngology-Head and Neck Surgery Foundation, Inc.)

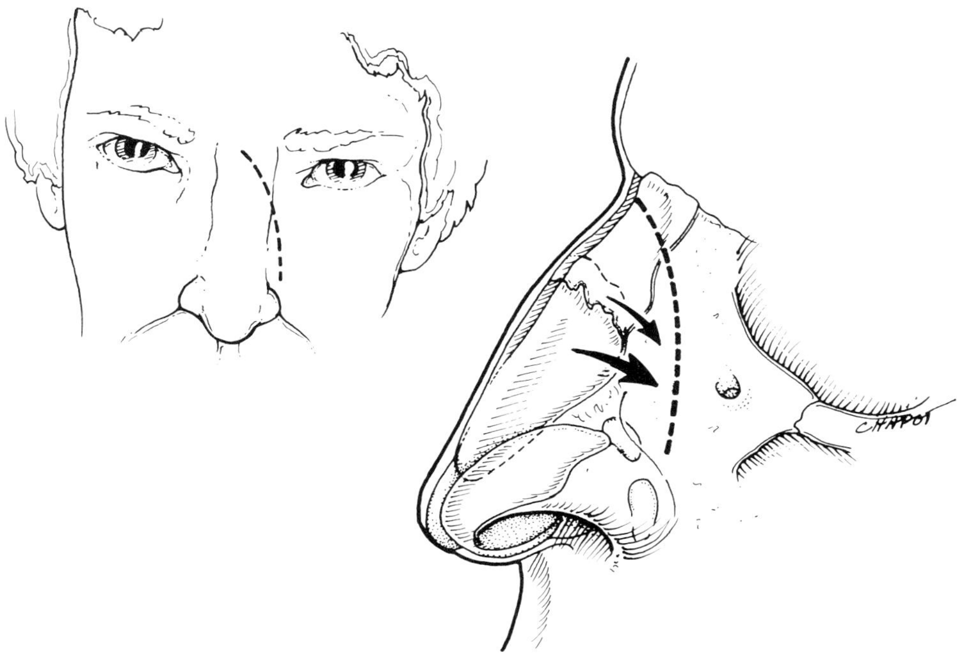

Fig. 13-4. Lateral osteotomy curving anteriorly at the radix to prevent transverse or backfracture.

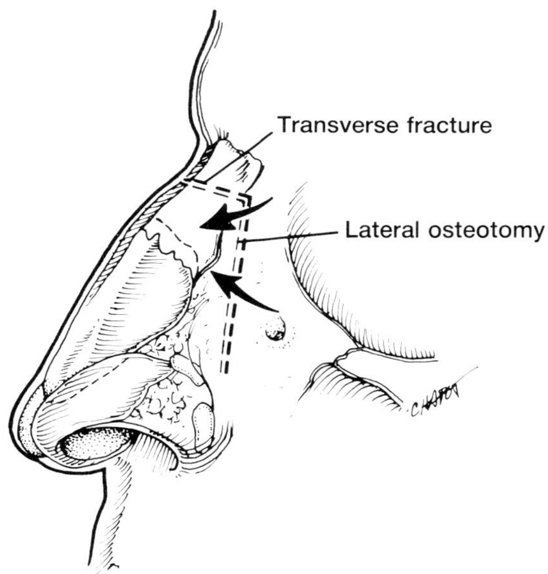

Fig. 13-5. Lateral osteotomy with infracturing causing resultant transverse or backfracture.

An even thinner straight osteotome may be used through the same pyriform aperture opening as described. This 2 mm osteotome is used with a puncture technique, postage-stamp effect (Fig. 13-6) in three or four areas along the same line as the lateral osteotome cut. The bone is then digitally infractured. Other instruments such as the U shaped Rubin lateral osteotome can be used just as effectively. The Rubin has a cutting edge on one end of the U against the bone while the other end of the U is external to the nose and is hit with a mallet. All of these instruments, including the outmoded saw, accomplish similar results. It is important to use a thin lateral osteotome so that only the bone and not the internal lining of the nose is cut.

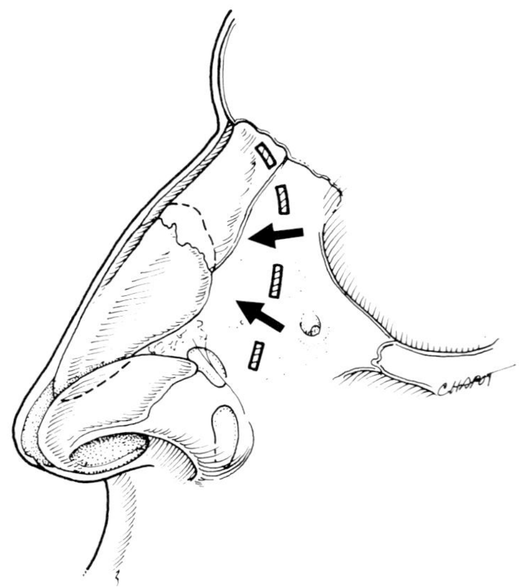

Fig. 13-6. "Postage stamp" osteotomies through the pyriform aperture, infractured with digital pressure.

When no abnormal bony hump is present and the goal is merely to thin the nasal pyramid, the suture line between the nasal bone and the nasal process of the maxillary bone is used as a hinge (Fig. 13-7). The lateral osteotomy is infractured. The above suture line "hinges" readily even though no medial osteotomy is performed. This is especially evident when the patient is under forty years of age and minimal calcification of this suture is anticipated. I have also used this technique successfully with older patients.

One straight osteotome that the surgeon carefully guides at a slight angle is all that is necessary on both sides. The angled cut of the osteotome, higher on the lateral side and lower on the medial side, allows the infractured bone to retain its new position more medially towards the nasal cavity. A thin straight osteotome can be used to curve up towards the radix very readily, instead of changing to a curved osteotome.

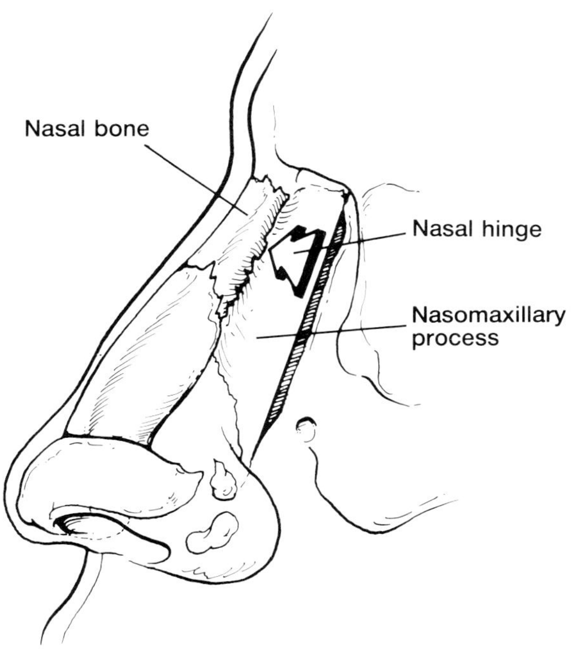

Fig. 13-7. The "hinge effect" with the nasal, naso-maxillary suture acting as the "hinge." This is useful when only the broad pyramidal base should be narrowed with a lateral osteotomy, without removing a hump.

Twisted Nasal Bones

So far the osteotomies we have discussed have been for a straightforward nasal pyramid. We must also treat the post-traumatic abnormally curved or angled framework, and patients who have developmental deformities, either congenital or secondary to growth-related trauma.

When a nasal bone twists or curves abnormally, multiple osteotomies must be used to create multiple fractures. Only by fracturing the bone where the abnormal angulations existed can we create a straighter nasal bone. When multiple osteotomies are performed, the most anterior osteotomy is carried out first; the more posterior osteotomy can then be done, and the most lateral osteotomy will be performed last. In this way the more posterior bony cuts will be made into solid bone rather than into movable structures.

I have found that two osteotomies are usually sufficient, but occasionally I have had to use three to accomplish the desired result (Fig. 13-8). A similar procedure is done on the contralateral side as indicated. In this manner, multiple compound fractures are created that allow the surgeon to mold the bony nasal framework into a straighter anatomical position.

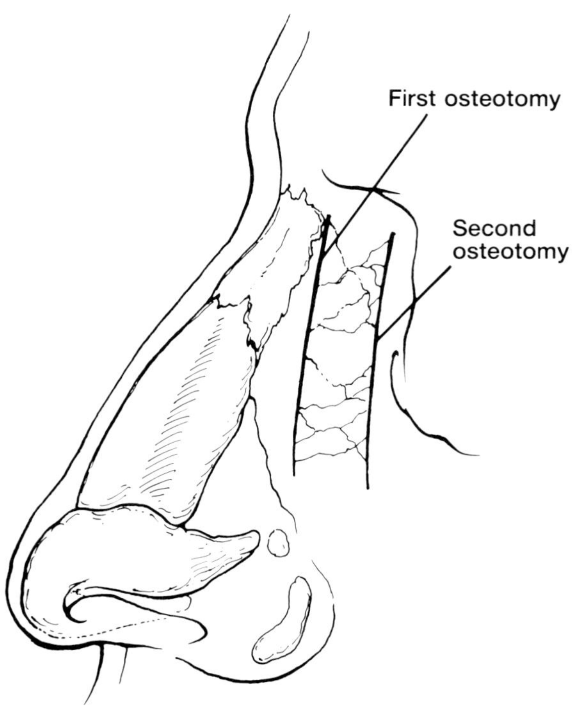

Fig. 13-8. Multiple lateral osteotomies for twisted nasal bones. The more anterior cut should be made first, two to three depending on the pathology.

The Transverse Fracture (Back Fracture)

When the lateral osteotomy is infractured, a secondary diagonal fracture from the most superior point of the cut, running inferiorly and medially often occurs. This is transverse fracture (Fig. 13-9). If the triangular piece of bone that is created is palpable, repositioning of this bony fragment must be done. The medial osteotome can be placed medial to this fragment and it can be outfractured. It can also be treated by using a 3 mm osteotome that has been passed through the pyriform incision for the lateral osteotomy. The small osteotome is then used to puncture the base of this triangular fragment and separate it from the naso-frontal process. Occasionally mere rasping of the transverse fracture edge will smooth any irregularity. Any of these techniques should succeed in lining this fragment up with the other parts of the nasal bones.

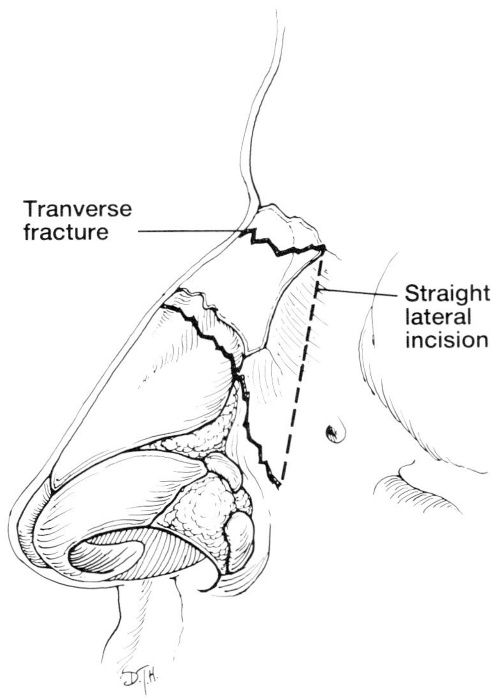

Fig. 13-9. Transverse fracture when doing an infracture after a lateral osteotomy. (From Berman WE: Rhinoplasty, ed 2, Washington DC, 1984, American Academy of Otolaryngology-Head and Neck Surgery Foundation, Inc.)

14

Shortening

Walter E. Berman

As discussed in the section on nasal dynamics, various anatomical considerations must be addressed before determining whether to shorten the nose and how to do so. Aesthetically we must assume that the length from the radix of the nasal pyramid to the nasal tip is excessive in relation to the other facial features. The firmness of the central segment must be determined. Digital pressure on the columella towards the radix will show whether the central segment is hard or soft (Fig. 14-1). Nasal shortening procedures are different in either case.

There are basically six ways of shortening the nose; some are purposeful and others are secondary to various nasal procedures.

Long Hard Central Segment Nose

In the hard central segment (see Chapter 6) shortening is done in the classical manner by removing inferior cartilage from the quadrilateral cartilage. This is performed after an inferior septal incision is done at the inferior aspect of the quadrilateral cartilage between the cartilage and the membranous septum, through both sides of the vestibular skin. When this incision is done, care must be taken to hold the feet of the medial crural cartilages inferiorly and away from the scalpel. Otherwise, the normal overlapping of the inferior end of the quadrilateral cartilage by the feet of the medial crural cartilages may cause the feet to be amputated. This will result in less nasal tip support and subsequent tip drop and/or a supratip deformity.

I like to retract the medial crural feet inferiorly with a Brown Adson forceps when this incision is performed. The actual removal of the inferior aspect of the quadrilateral cartilage is dependent on the type of deformity that exists. At times it is desirable to remove more towards the nasal tip or anterior part of the quadrilateral cartilage. This will provide for concomitant upward tip rotation. When a larger amount of the posterior aspect, which is next to the nasal spine, is removed, greater columellar retrusion is obtained. Sometimes a straight piece of cartilage is removed.

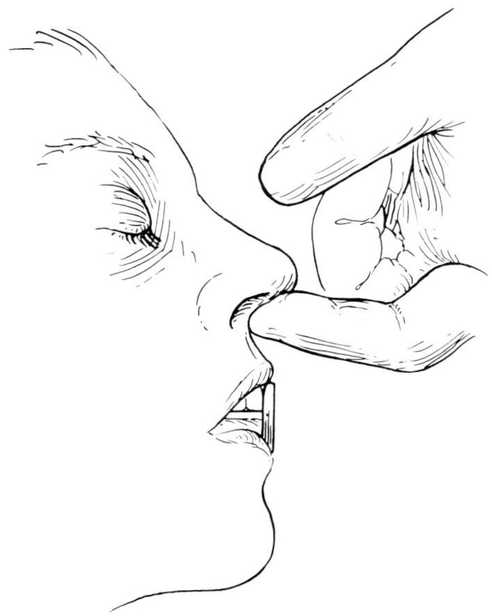

Fig. 14-1. Testing for a hard or soft central segment. (From Berman WE: Rhinoplasty, ed 2, Washington DC, 1984, American Academy of Otolaryngology-Head and Neck Surgery Foundation, Inc.)

If a complex septoplasty is part of the procedure, I certainly would advise that the septum be treated before a definitive judgment of how much inferior cartilage is to be removed is made.

Long Soft Central Segment Nose

Secondary rotation with the soft central segment nose is indicated. Removal of the inferior aspect of the quadrilateral cartilage may lead to a retracted columella. In the case of the soft central segment the overall length is determined by the lateral walls of the nose. No inferior septal incision is made; rather the lower lateral cartilages (LLC) are delivered after they are undermined and released.

The inferior aspect of the LLC is separated between the nasal dome and the most lateral extent of the LLC. This is performed when more rotation of the lateral segment of the nose is warranted. The division is placed about one third lateral to the nasal dome where the overlying skin is heavier on the LLC to prevent postoperative irregularities. The underlying mucosa is not incised. The rotation point is at the point of severance of the LLC (see Fig. 10-4).

Lower Lateral Cartilage Removal

Removal of superior lower lateral cartilage is usually done through a variety of techniques to decrease the bulk of the lower lateral cartilages. After surgery the upper and lower lateral cartilages tend to approximate each other, shortening the nose.

Removal of the Anterior Upper Lateral Cartilages

When the anterior aspect of the upper lateral cartilages is removed, the length of those cartilages is decreased. This procedure shortens the base of the triangle that comprises the upper lateral cartilages, thus shortening the nose (see Fig. 6-5).

Removal of the Inferior Border of the Upper Lateral Cartilage

Removal of the inferior border of the upper lateral cartilage will often cause the lower lateral cartilages to move superiorly, thus shortening the nose.

Excessive Septal Removal

When the quadrilateral cartilage is weakened by excessive removal of septal cartilage, retraction and shortening of the nose often ensues. We must therefore assume that there are many ways to shorten a nose.

15

Refinements

Walter E. Berman

Refinements: Conservative Removal of Anterior (Dorsal) or Inferior (Caudal) Lateral Cartilages

Beware of using too much force when using the Alfrecht or similar retractor to judge how much anterior upper lateral cartilage to remove. A heavy hand will raise the upper lateral cartilages too far above the nasal septum and cause the surgeon to mistakenly remove an excess of upper lateral cartilage. This will cause the following results.

Visible Anterior Septum

When the anterior nasal retractor is released after removing excessive anterior upper lateral cartilage, the upper lateral carilages may be more posterior than the nasal septum. This results in too thin a nose and the edges of the cartilaginous septum are visible in the midline.

Internal Valve Collapse

Especially if junction tunnels were not made, the internal valves may be in a depressed or posterior position. Numerous synechiae and interference with breathing at the valvular area may result, particularly if the mucosa had been separated in this area.

Nasal Shortening Through the Upper Laterals

There is a triangular configuration of the upper lateral cartilage. When the anterior border is resected, the nose is foreshortened by diminishing the length of the triangular base (see Fig. 6-5).

Pince-nez Effect

This also applies to the removal of the inferior border of the upper lateral cartilage when it telescopes under the lower cartilage. Therefore, no more cartilage should be removed than the amount needed to permit the upper and lower lateral cartilages to meet each other. If this dictum is not followed, a "pince-nez" effect may ensue. This was a common sequelae some years ago. The "pince-nez" collapse takes place when the external skin is directly on internal lining, without intervening cartilage. (See pince-nez in secondaries.)

Finishing Touches and Rasping

Without the aid of a retractor, I often lay a 35-degree scissors on the anterior surface of the nasal framework, under the overlying skin and through the between-the-cartilage incisions. The tip of the scissors is kept on the nasal bone. The offending bits of cartilage on the anterior surfaces of the septum and the anterior upper lateral cartilages can be safely cut away.

The final smoothing process is done with rasps. If the rasps are sharp enough, both bony and cartilaginous tissues may be removed. Even though osteotomies have been completed, with firm lateral digital support rasping can proceed. Of course, this is not the case if comminution of the bones has taken place.

The most insignificant irregularity on the surface of the nose may be the patient's focal point postoperatively. It therefore behooves us to meticulously smooth any anterior surfaces.

16

Sutures, Packs, and Dressings

Walter E. Berman

Suturing

In the majority of septo-rhinoplasties only the inferior lower lateral incisions and the septal incisions need to be sutured. The between-the-cartilage incisions are purposely left open for better drainage and less postoperative swelling. As previously mentioned, I prefer a long-acting 4-0 dissolvable suture for the septal and columellar incisions, preferably one that lasts for one to two months. A 5-0 plain suture is used to coapt only the vestibular edges of skin of the marginal incisions.

Nasal Packs

Internal splinting is usually taken care of with suturing. The same long-acting 4-o sutures are used to splint various parts of the septum with horizontal stitches as necessary. If only a minimal support system is needed, bendable straws wrapped in telfa coated with polysporin are inserted on each side of the septum and are kept in place for three to four days (Fig. 16-1). If stronger packing is desired, a hydrophylic pack with a built-in silicone tube is inserted on each side for three to four days. These packs are also coated with polysporin to aid insertion and prevent infection.

Fig. 16-1. A, Forceps holding flex straw and telfa and polysporin. B, Short end of flex straw, with telfa and polysporin on septal side, inserted into nose; permits breathing and support.

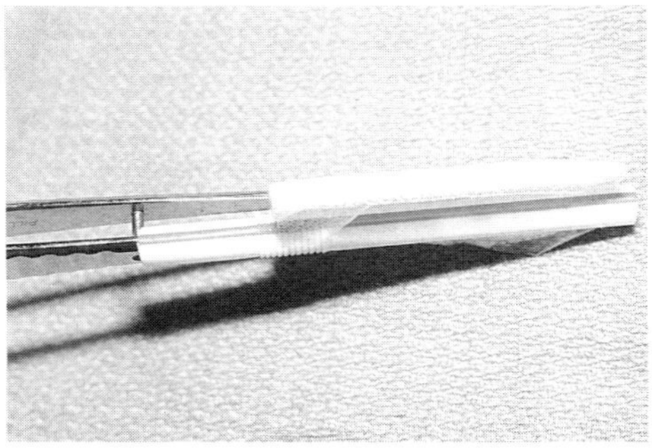

A

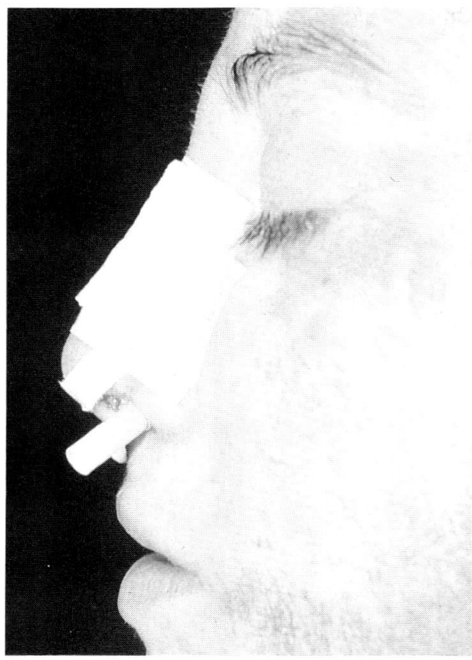

B

Dressings

Dressings are about as variable as the weather or tip techniques. Fundamentally, we need a material that will protect the skin and also bond to the splint material. Mastisol is applied to the external nose, followed by a layer of hypo-allergenic paper tape. Two layers of water-absorbent, not plastic, tape are then placed over the first layer. None extend past the lateral osteotomies. One-half-inch tape is used. Two slings of one-quarter-inch tape are placed over the inferior edge of the nasal tip, not below the nares as this could cause some retraction with swelling. A thin piece of aquaplast is then softened in hot water and placed over the tapes and held in place or quickly hardened with an ice water sponge (Fig. 16-2). Throughout the dressing the nose is milked of any serous or bloody drainage to prevent the formation of clots and any potential subcutaneous scarring later.

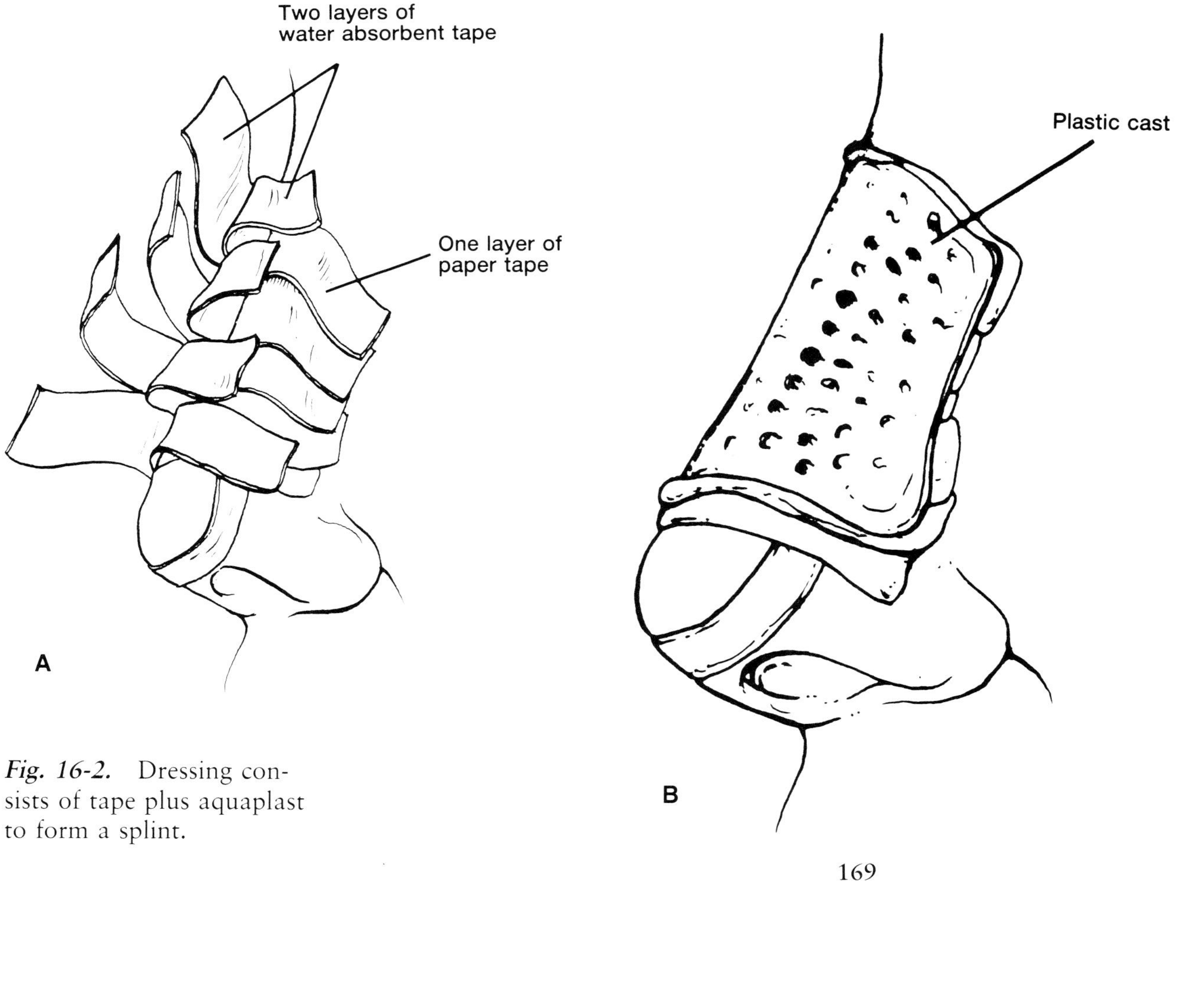

Fig. 16-2. Dressing consists of tape plus aquaplast to form a splint.

17

The External Approach to Rhinoplasty

Jack R. Anderson

For many years the use of the external approach to rhinoplasty had been on the wane because surgeons feared the scar it leaves across the columella. Lately, however, it has been learned that the once-dreaded scar can be so imperceptible that it has high patient acceptance. This has sparked a resurgence of interest in the external approach because it provides unparalleled exposure of the nasal elements, and it is generally conceded that poor exposure is a large factor in making endonasal rhinoplasty a difficult operation to learn and perform.

Actually, whichever approach is used, the basic steps of the operation remain the same: the contour and perhaps the length of the nasal dorsum is altered, the nasal pyramid is narrowed, and the lobule is remodeled. But shades of difference do exist between the two operations and the purpose of this presentation is to discuss some of these delicate distinctions.

It should be emphasized that performing rhinoplasty via the external approach does not automatically guarantee a good result; the surgeon must also master the dynamics of this fascinating operation.

Indications

Even though we have successfully performed thousands of endonasal rhinoplasties during the past 30 years, we now believe that the public would be better served if every rhinoplasty was performed via the external approach. However, this dictum does not generate universal agreement. It is embraced most enthusiastically by residents in training and by surgeons who have been struggling for years to improve the predictability of their efforts.

Many concede that the external approach might be indicated when treating twisted and/or badly traumatized noses, cleft palate noses, "fatty" noses, and for the purposes of revisional surgery; oddly enough, however, they resist using it when there is minimal deformity, which is precisely where the margin for error is smallest and when good visualization would be most advantageous.

The resistance to change that develops as one grows older has been one reason why some surgeons do not use the external approach: change is sometimes unsettling and even ego-threatening. Finally, there are those who continue to fear incising the columellar skin although they would not hesitate to incise the alar margins less than 10 mm away if the base of the nose had to be narrowed.

The Incisions

The incisions used in the external approach are depicted in Fig. 17-1. The transcolumellar incision is always located just above the flare of the feet of the medial crura. Its design, along with the underlying cartilage, eliminates the possibility of distortion caused by scar contracture. The incision is extended for a short distance over the skin covering each medial crus at its lower end, but at a more superficial level than in the columella. Next, incisions are made along the caudal margins of each lower lateral cartilage extending from beyond the body of each lateral crus to about 2 mm past the transcolumellar incisions.

The intersection of the marginal and transcolumellar incisions establishes landmarks for accurate closure of the transcolumellar incision at the end of the operation and helps to ensure a good scar.

Undermining

The soft tissues are elevated from the upper and lower lateral cartilages with a stitch scissors. The level of undermining depends on the thickness of the said tissues. Usually, it is kept as close to the cartilages as possible, but, when the tissues are thick, as in "fatty" noses, the plane is created just below the dermis, leaving the bulk of the unwanted material attached to the cartilages from whence they can be removed very easily. This method of handling the problem is definitely easier and more thorough than the endonasal approach.

As usual, the tissue elevation is extended to the pyriform margins in all directions.

Then, under direct vision, we elevate the periosteum from the medial parts of the nasal bones to permit introduction of instruments for hump removal and medial osteotomy. Admittedly, this is a controversial procedure, but we believe that the presence of even a shredded layer of periosteum helps to mask the small irregularities that sometimes follow these procedures.

The source of any bothersome bleeding that occurs during the undermining can be readily determined and easily controlled with a bipolar cautery, which is another advantage of the external approach.

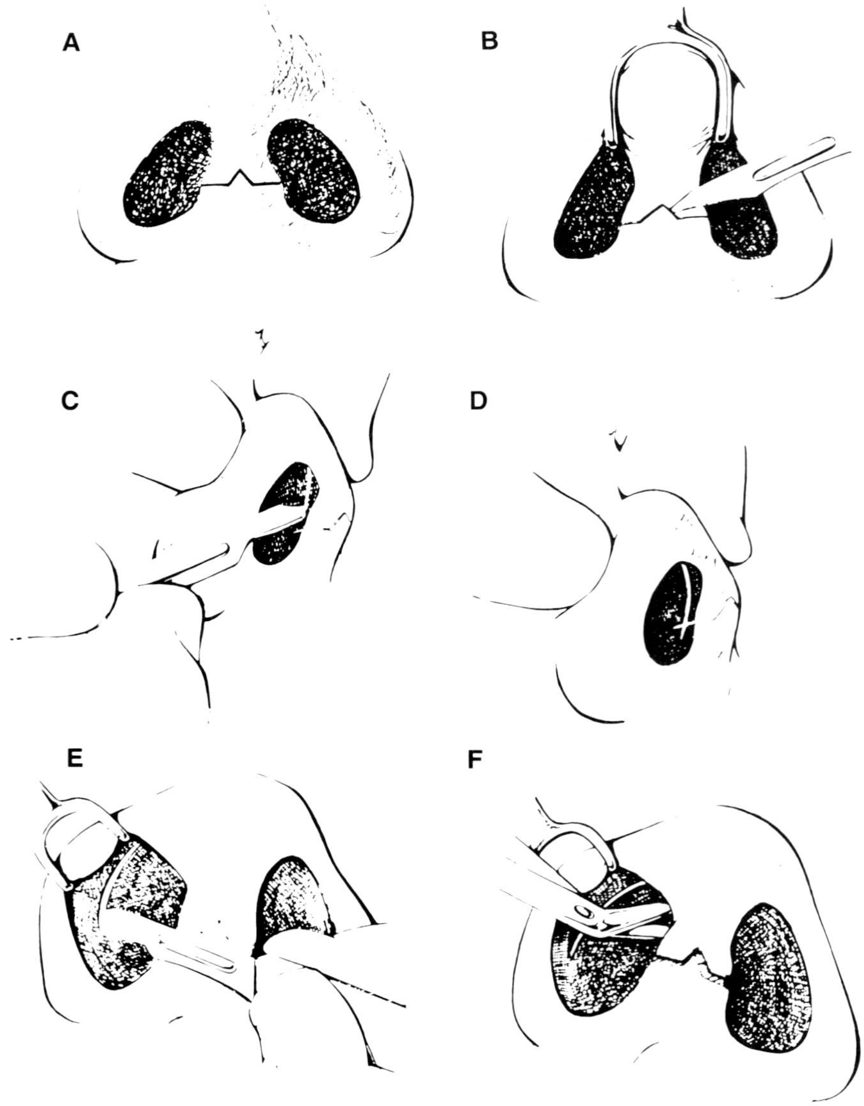

Fig. 17-1. Incisional technique. The "x" configuration created in sketch D acts as a guide for subsequent precise closure of the transcolumellar incision. (Reproduced with permission from Anderson JR and Ries W: Rhinoplasty: Emphasizing the external approach, New York, 1986, Thieme Medical Publishers Inc.)

Exposure of the Nasal Septum

Most rhinoplasties we perform require septal modification, if only to ensure adequate narrowing of the bony pyramid. The superior septal angle is exposed by dividing the so-called "ligaments" that fasten the medial ends of the lateral crura together over the caudal end of the septal dorsum. Whenever the entire caudal end of the septal cartilage and perhaps even the nasal spine area must be exposed, the ligaments joining the medial crura are similarly divided.

The upper lateral cartilages are then separated from the septal cartilage submucosally with the sharp stitch scissors, and the septal membranes are elevated bilaterally, the extent of the elevation depending on the exposure needed to carry out septal modification. The membranes will not "fall" into the nose because they remain attached to the medial ends of the lateral crura and the undersurface of the nasal bones.

The incomparable exposure obtained with the open approach facilitates septal surgery and adds a new dimension to what can be done.

Lower Lateral Cartilage Modification

Since they are completely visible, the lower lateral cartilages can be precisely modified bilaterally without incising vestibular skin or making limen vestibuli incisions.

Hump Removal

Hump removal is accomplished under direct vision with any instrument the surgeon prefers; any residual deformities are easier to correct later, rather than during endonasal rhinoplasty.

Osteotomies

Medial osteotomies are also performed under direct visualization.

Separate incisions are made along the pyriform margins at the level of the anterior ends of the inferior turbinates to permit performance of the lateral osteotomies; these are the only major steps of the operation that are not completely visible during open rhinoplasty. It is possible to perform lateral osteotomies through the lateral ends of the marginal incisions, but the practice is not recommended for fear of damaging the lateral ends of the lateral crura.

"Finishing" the Operation

After the nose is narrowed, the septal dorsum is further lowered to make the rhinion the high point of the septal profile, the caudal ends of the upper lateral cartilages are shortened, if necessary, and modification of the lower lateral cartilages is completed.

Text continued on p. 178.

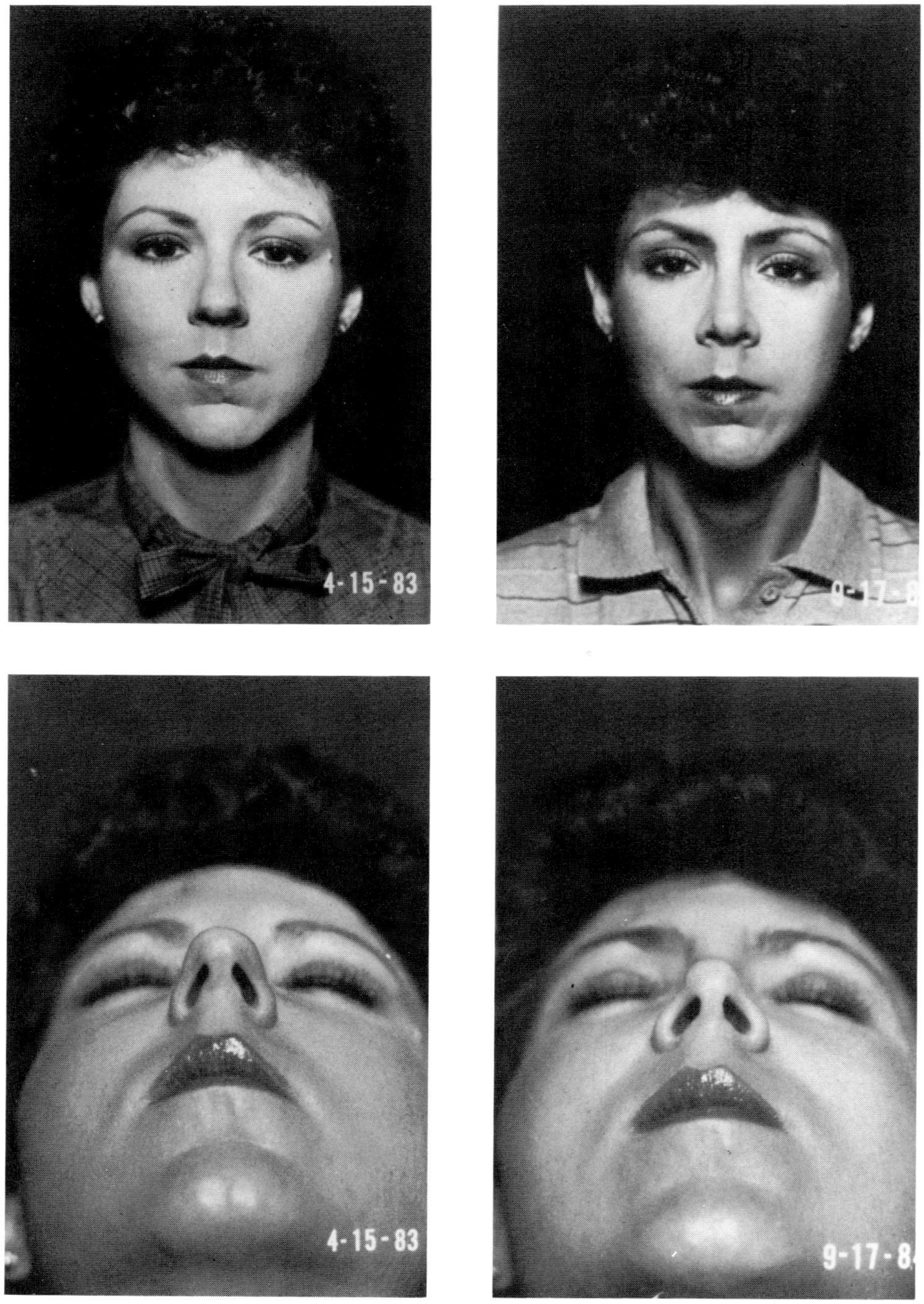

A

Fig. 17-2. Results of open rhinoplasty technique used in patient with minimal deformity. Contrary to widespread belief, the external approach is ideal for such cases because of the precision it permits. **A,** Frontal view, preoperative and postoperative. **B,** Side view, preoperative and postoperative.

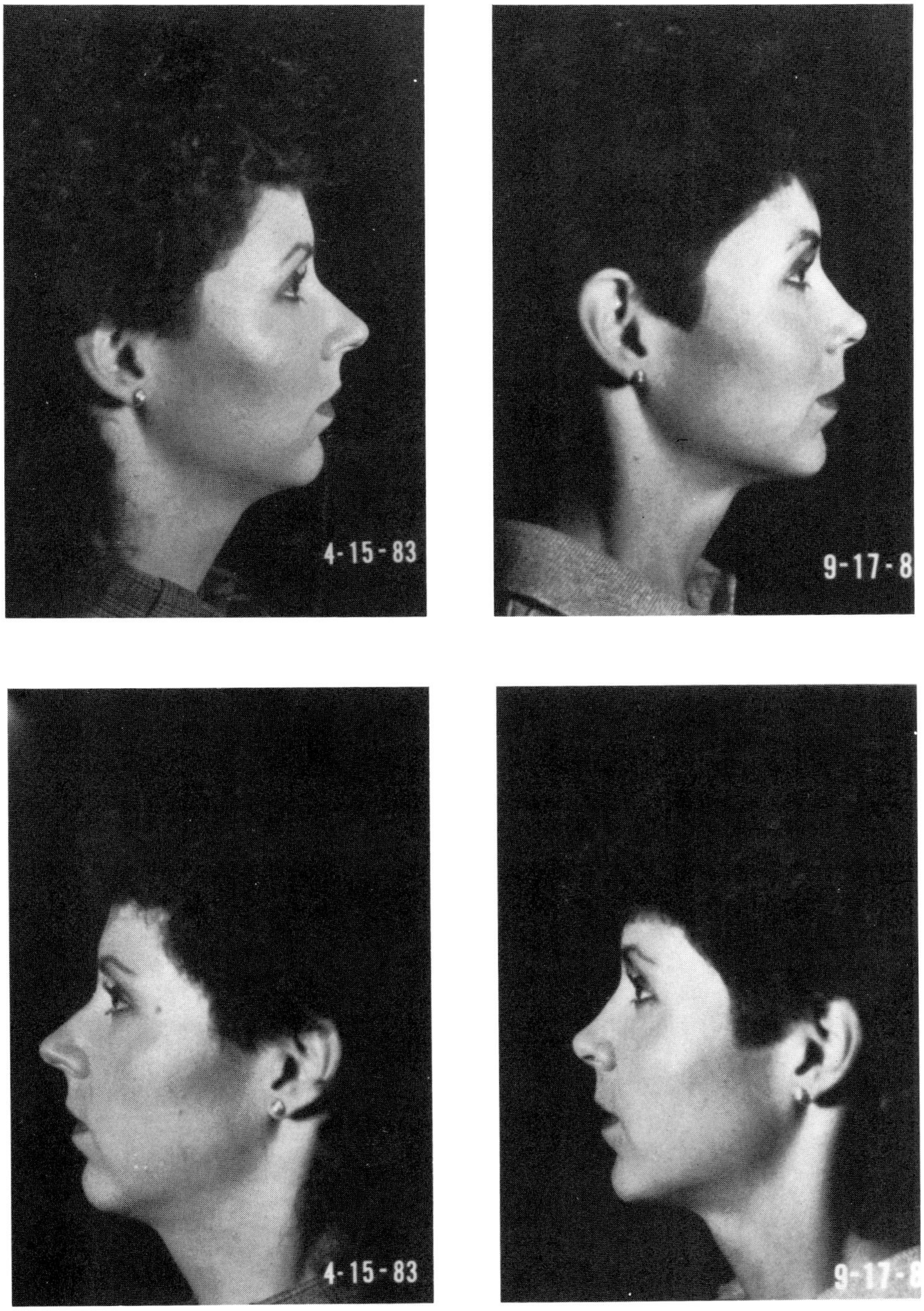

B

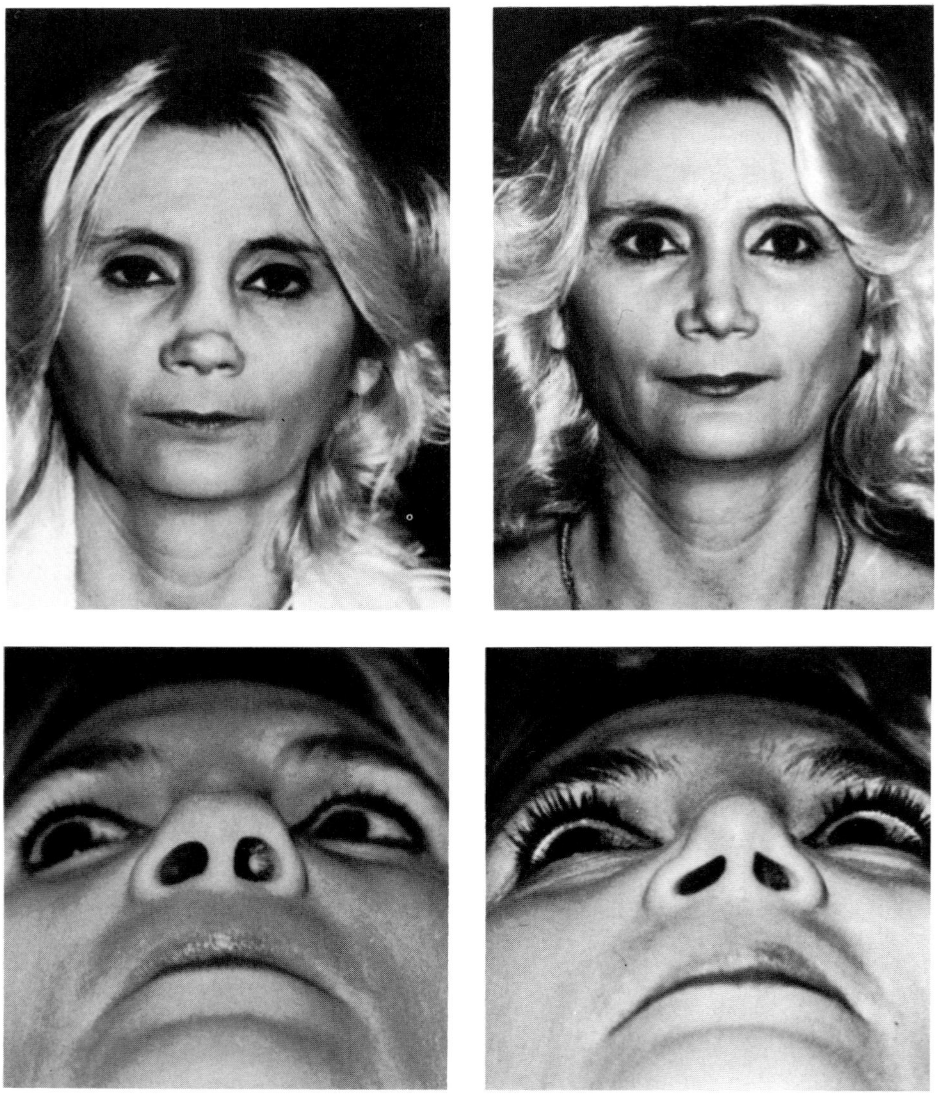

A

Fig. 17-3. Secondary rhinoplasty performed via external technique. **A,** Frontal view, preoperative and postoperative. **B,** Side view, preoperative and postoperative.

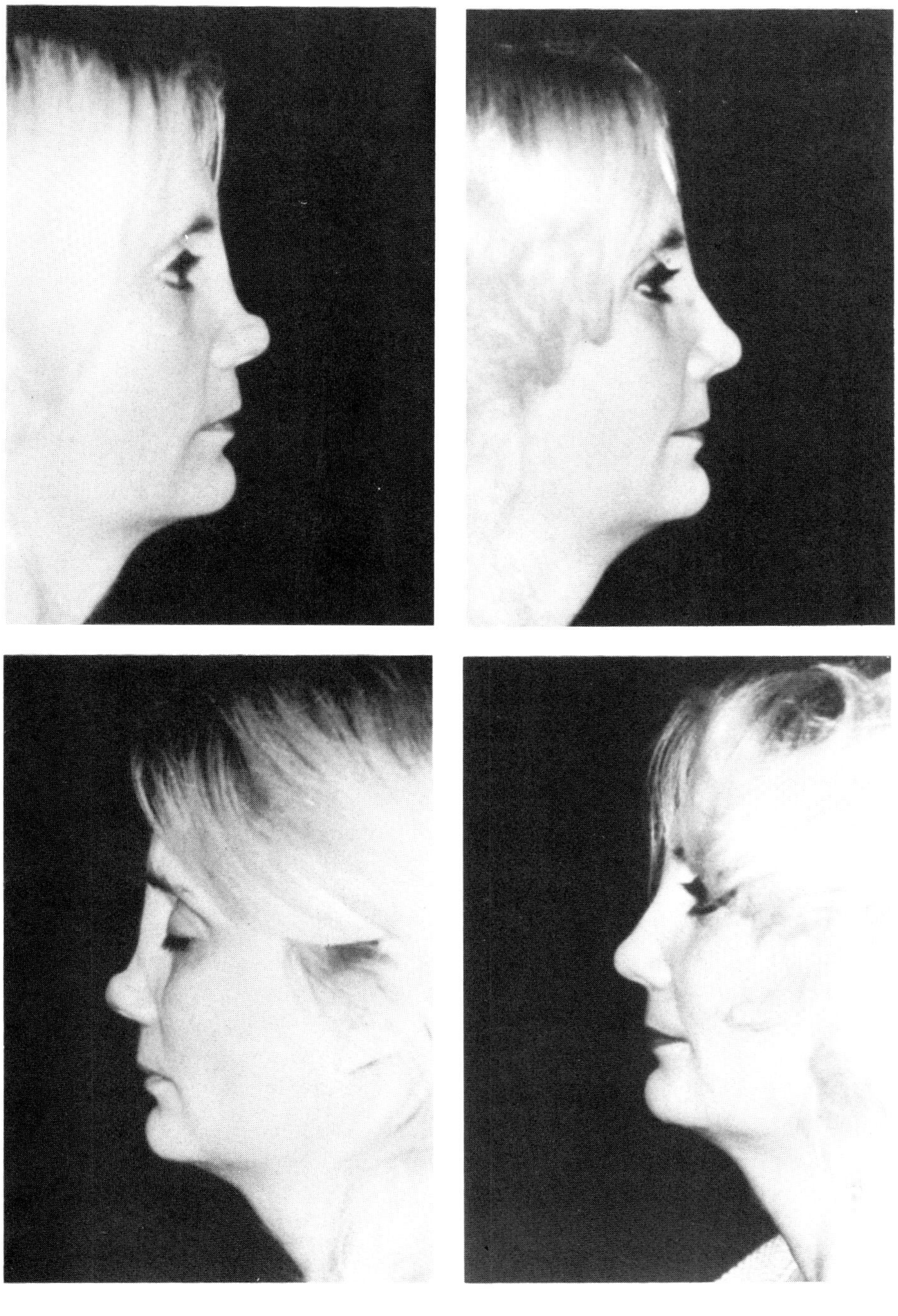

B

The septal mucosa is then elevated and sutured to the upper border of the septal cartilage; when properly placed, these sutures have two other salutary effects—they fill the dead space beneath the medial ends of the lateral crura and support those structures so they can better fill their roles as projectors of the nasal tip.

Mattress sutures are also inserted immediately behind the medial crura to stabilize those structures; in effect, they act as substitutes for the previously-divided intracrural ligaments.

Incision Closure

Single 4-0 plain catgut sutures are inserted bilaterally to close the marginal incisions; they are placed where the lateral crura veer away from the nostril margins as they proceed in a lateral direction.

Then, the apex of the transcolumellar incision is carefully sutured with 4-0 Prolene. Next, the lateral ends of the transcolumellar incision are closed, and the cruciform configuration of cuts created laterally are used as guides for suture placement. After that, the remainder of the transcolumellar incision is coapted as are the marginal incisions in the columella. Two patients who have had open rhinoplasties are depicted in Figs. 17-2 and 17-3.

Discussion

Obviously, many thousands of successful rhinoplasties have been performed endonasally. However, as Aufricht aptly said, "Rhinoplasty is an easy operation, but it is difficult to get good results," and our teaching experience has confirmed this. It takes about 8 years and numerous surgical interventions for the average surgeon to master the procedure reasonably well, mainly because the undercover nature of the operation makes it difficult to explain and to understand; the situation can be likened to trying to teach someone to play chess while his hands and the chess board are covered with a blanket.

Many surgeons will attest to the fact that using the open approach has improved their understanding of rhinoplasty and the general average of their good results. Operating time is a little longer when the open approach is used. This can be attributed to the need for special care during closure and the fact that having the nasal anatomy laid bare seems to make conscientious surgeons become even more obsessive about achieving precision and symmetry. To understand why this occurs, one need only convert an endonasal operation to an open one. Our position is that increased operating time is an acceptable trade-off for better results.

Finally, detractors of the open approach often claim that it results in more postoperative reaction than the undercover operation does; this has not been true in our experience during the past 7 years.

Part III

PROBLEMS AND COMPLICATIONS

18

The Non-Caucasian (Ethnic) Nose

Walter E. Berman

The term *ethnic nose* is really a misnomer because any of these variations can occur in Caucasian noses too. The ethnic nose is a combination of various anatomical developments. It is certainly not abnormal, but rather a genetic reflection of a particular group. It consists mainly of limited anterior and dorsal nasal projection, and extra width of both the cartilaginous and osseous parts of the nose. It is characterized by a wide nasal tip, soft or retracted columella, flared nares, and a wide nasal base. The typical ethnic nose may be a combination of any of the above. Obviously, Caucasians may also exhibit any number of these anatomical formations.

Preoperative counseling is always of paramount importance, but I feel that this is particularly essential when the nasal tip has thick, heavy skin. This is often a limiting factor in how thin a tip will evolve. As with any rhinoplastic procedure, thick nasal tip skin is most difficult to contour and is often a disappointing part of the rhinoplasty.

Systematic Approach

What can be accomplished with raising a depressed nasal tip tells the surgeon how much can be added to the anterior part of the nose if there is potential saddling. The degree of thinning that is possible with the nasal tip surgery dictates how thin to make the nasal pyramid. For instance, a thinner nasal pyramid will give the illusion of a wider nasal tip. Therefore, the guidelines for the tip surgery must be decided before appropriate measures for building up, saddling, or thinning are attempted. If not, problems of the nasal tip may increase rather than decrease.

These cases usually have a soft central segment (see Chapter 14). Therefore I would omit an inferior septal incision unless there was a hard central segment on a long nose.

Technique

On the assumption that there is no pathology of the nasal turbinates or septum, I would start with incisions between the upper and lower cartilages bilaterally. A secondary or marginal incision along the inferior borders of the edge of the lower lateral cartilages is also made. The incision along the lower edge of the lower lateral cartilage is carried medially along the inferior border of the nasal domes and often onto the medial aspect of the medial crura depending on how far medially the nasal reconstruction will extend.

The lower lateral cartilages will then be undermined or separated from the overlying skin and delivered. A thorough removal of any subcutaneous fibrofatty tissues will then be done both on the cartilaginous surfaces and the subcutaneous surfaces of the overlying skin. In a broad type of platyrrhine nose the cartilages are usually quite soft. A portion of the superior aspect would then be removed, sparing the underlying vestibular membrane. Thorough morselization of the lateral dome and medial parts of the lower cartilages would then be done with Dr. Frank Rubins one-sided small morselizer. This helps break the spring of the cartilage.

Treating the Flared Nares Without External Incisions

Delivery of the lower cartilages, removal of the superior aspect, and morselization of the cartilages all help the flaring but frequently are insufficient to accomplish the desired result. Several other procedures will help accomplish a decrease in nasal flaring.

Rotation of the Two Epithelial Covers at the Edge of the Nares

With the help of the incision along the inferior border of the lower lateral cartilage, a straight Stevens iris scissors is used to delicately separate the internal vestibular lining from the overlying external skin of the nasal nares (Fig. 18-1, A). This procedure causes a shifting of these two epithelial layers on themselves. The external nose is then gently pressed medially and the vestibular skin moves to a new relationship with the vestibular skin overlying the lower lateral cartilage. Any amount of superfluous vestibular skin overriding the lower lateral cartilage is then excised (Fig. 18-1, B and C). The opposing edges of vestibular skin are then sutured with 5-0 plain gut, which narrows the flare of the nares.

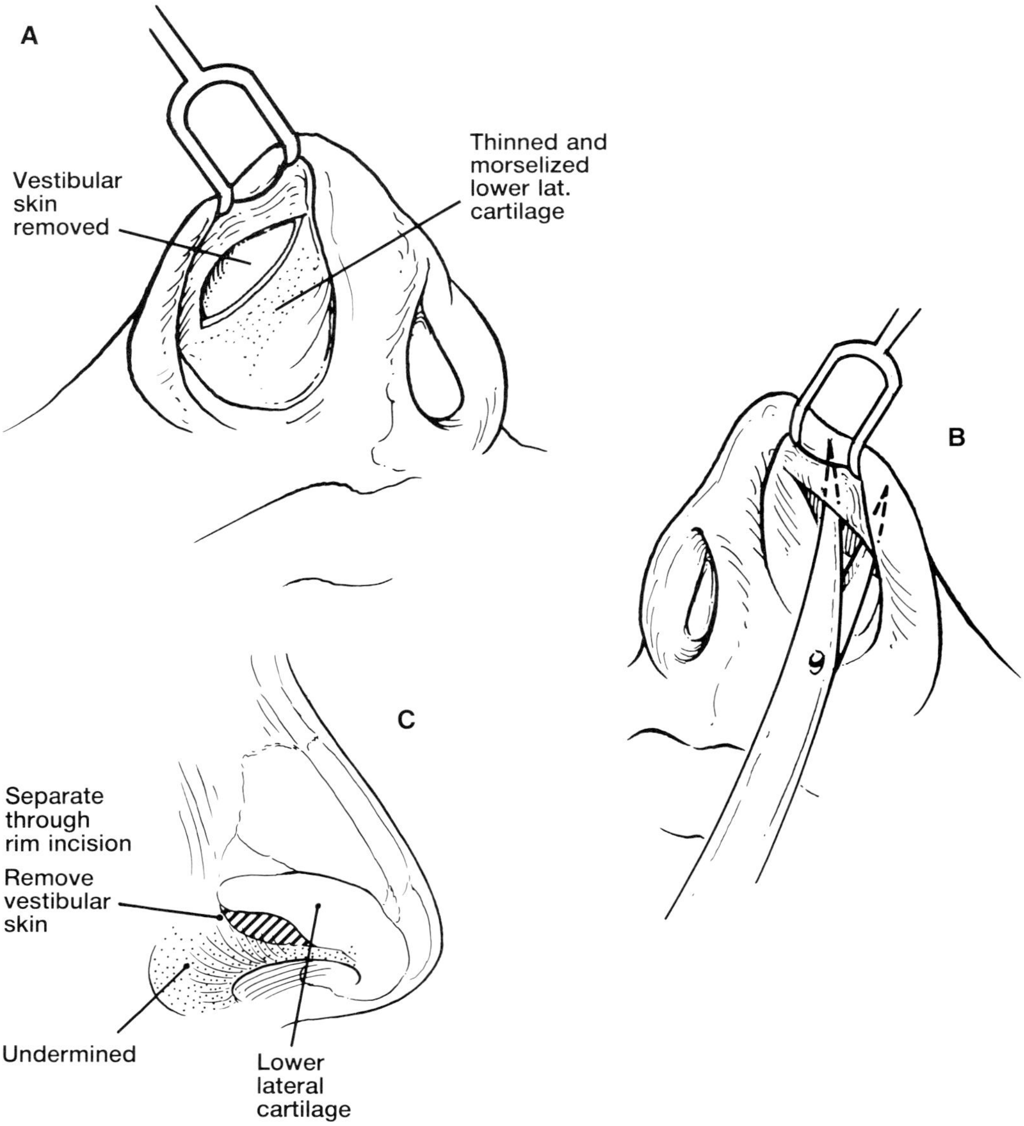

Fig. 18-1. A, An appropriate amount of dissected vestibular skin has been removed to decrease flaring of the nares. B, Separating the vestibular skin from the overlying external skin through an inferior cartilage incision. C, Undermining inferior to the lateral crura through the marginal incision.

Cinching Suture

The cinching suture is a modification of a technique that was first introduced in the 1930s by Dr. Fomon. My modification consists of using an incision on the floor of the nares (Fig. 18-2). The incision is carried internally from the 'sil' at the junction of the floor of the nares and the lateral wall of the nose. The incision is 5 to 8 mm in length and goes down to the underlying bony framework. A straight Stevens iris scissors is then placed in this internal Weir incision and dissection undermining is performed under the lateral nares and about 1.5 cm past the lateral alar groove. (Fig. 18-3). Similar undermining is also done between the two internal Weir incisions connecting them inferiorly to the nasal spine and, of course, laterally on the contralateral side of the nose (see Fig. 18-3). In effect this frees the nasal tip from the premaxilla.

I prefer using a permanent suture such as a 3-0 Mersilene on a long Keith needle. The needle is passed from an internal Weir incision through the skin in the external alar groove. The point of exit in the external groove will vary with the particular anatomy and the effect to be achieved. Exiting at a spot that is too inferior will create more bowing of the lateral nares. Usually 5 to 6 mm more superiorly in the groove will narrow the alar relationship. The placement of this suture will be obvious after a few attempts during surgery. The needle is now external to the nose and will be brought back through this external needle puncture wound into the same internal Weir incision. The needle is then guided deep under the previously dissected epithelium, emerging through the contralateral internal Weir incision. Next, a similar procedure is done on the other external lateral narial groove. The needle is then brought back to the original internal Weir incision and the suture is securely tied.

How much actual cinching is to be applied depends on the surgeon's aesthetic judgment. In the case of a wide narial base where the floor of the nares is actually bunched together from this suture, a triangular excision is done. This excision uses the original lateral nasal flood incision as the base of a triangle that has an apex in a medial direction. This is in effect an internal Weir procedure. This triangular tissue is removed with the underlying deep subcutaneous tissues. One or two 5-0 plain sutures suffice for closure.

With selected cases I have had good results when there was excessive flaring of the nares with placement of the suture anterior to the groove. A temporary depression of the external skin is noted, but it dissipates in 2 to 3 days. In more difficult cases it has been prudent to use two cinching sutures. The cinching suture prevents external scarring and the asymmetries that result from external Weir incisions. I have had a fifteen year follow-up of this procedure with good results (Fig. 18-4).

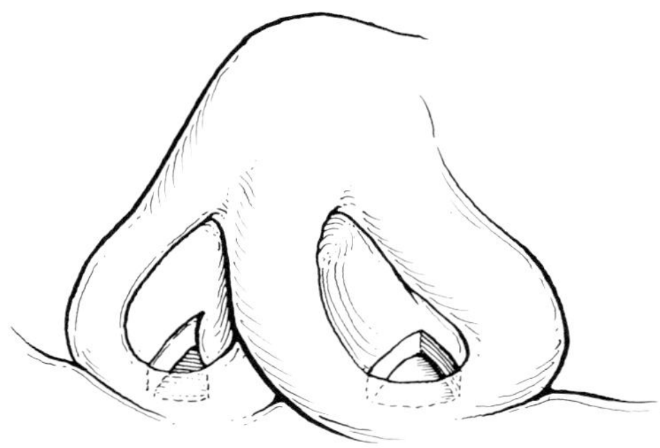

Fig. 18-2. Internal Weir incisions with removal of skin and subcutaneous tissues to narrow base of nares.

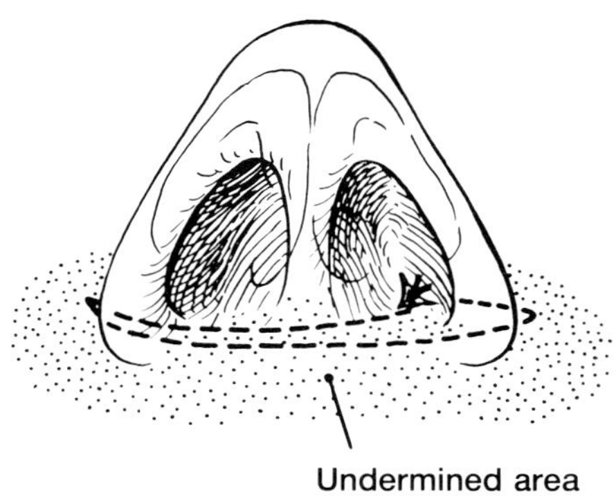

Fig. 18-3. The stippling represents the undermined area for the clinching suture to have maximum effect. (From Berman WE: Rhinoplasty, ed 2, Washington DC, 1984, American Academy of Otolaryngology-Head and Neck Surgery Foundation, Inc.)

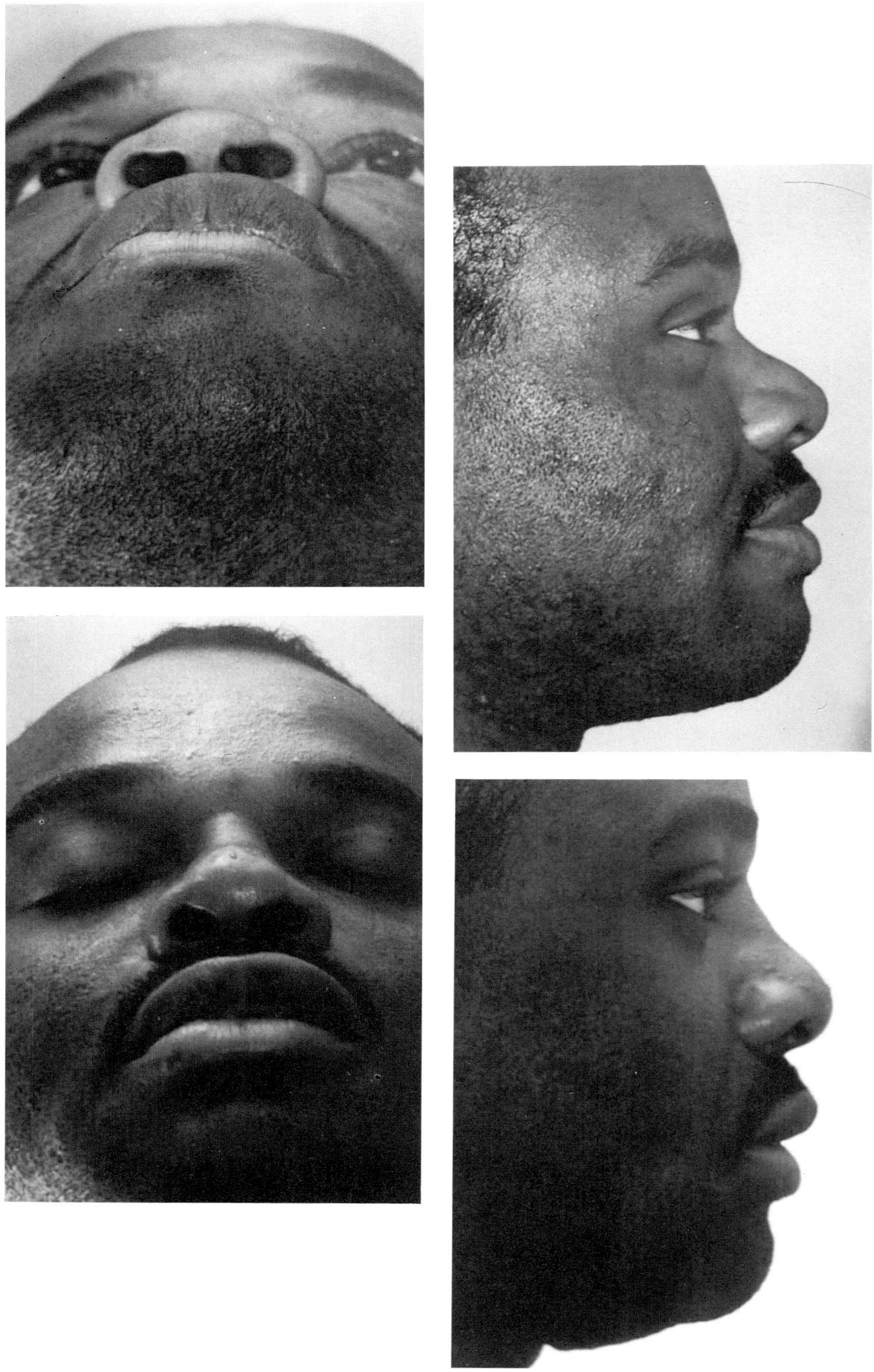

A B C D

Fig. 18-4. The platyrrhine procedure, including permanent cinching sutures, was done. Inferior septal graft to increase the tip projection and an anterior graft was also placed for the patient's saddle deformity. **A and B,** Preoperative. **C and D,** Postoperative.

The Double Dome Suture

After the lower lateral cartilages have been delivered, the superior aspect excised, morselization completed, and excessive fibrofatty tissues removed, I like to perform a very simple test: namely, placing a Brown-Adson forceps under the nasal tip and seeing if gentle pressure to oppose the medial crura will narrow the nasal tip. If so, the same forceps is held securely in as anterior position as possible while a horizontal mattress suture is placed through the vestibular skin and the most anterior aspects of the medial crura (Fig. 18-5, A). This permanent suture passes through both vestibular linings and forms a complete circle, bringing the two nasal domes into closer apposition (Fig. 18-5, B). Although the knot is exposed in the cul-de-sac of the nose, I do not recall this causing any problems. When examined years later, it seems that epithelialization had taken place over this extrusion. It is also in a difficult place for the patient to touch. It is imperative that the Brown-Adson forceps not be moved during this suturing procedure. This ensures a symmetrical constriction.

Increasing Tip Projection

When the nasal profile is depressed, either tip and/or cartilage and bony framework, the degree of surgical tip projection must be determined first. This limiting factor will then determine how much anterior projection should be achieved. This is detailed further in the tip projection chapter.

Permanent placement sutures or columellar grafts to increase tip projection is detailed in the tip projection chapter. Saddle deformity is also detailed further in the nasal grafts chapter.

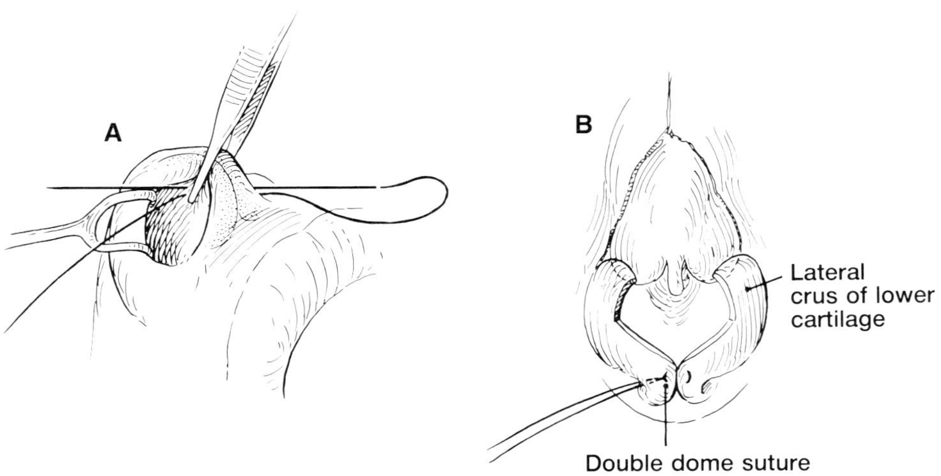

Fig. 18-5. Double dome suture. **A,** 4-0 permanent suture above Brown-Adson forceps. Tied extramucosally below the nasal domes. **B,** Opposing nasal domes sutured together. (From Berman WE: Rhinoplasty, ed 2, Washington DC, 1984, American Academy of Otolaryngology-Head and Neck Surgery Foundation, Inc.)

19

The Aging Nose

Walter E. Berman

The aging nose may be the result of a combination of factors. Although our culture expects the face, neck, and nasal tissues to relax with time, less and less relaxation is becoming acceptable and desirable. With the aging nose, it is important to realize that the patient often wants only a reversal of aging changes and not the "new" nose desired by younger patients. Picking up the fallen nasal tip is an example of this.

Tip Drop

Tissue Relaxation

The ligaments of the nose and dermal elastic tissue relax over time. The slow process of ligament stretching between the upper and lower cartilages, and between the medial crura and the septum cause the nose to elongate and the tip to drop (Fig. 19-1). As the dermal elastic tissue relaxes through maturity, further tip support is lost.

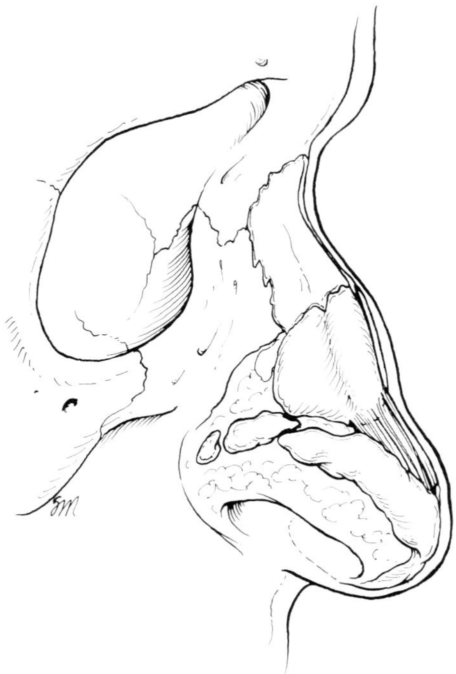

Fig. 19-1. Relaxation of nasal tissues causing tip drop. The upper and lower cartilages have separated from each other with age.

Repair

Repair of these problems consists of recreating the anatomical relationship that previously existed. Resuturing the separated upper and lower lateral cartilages with permanent sutures is of great help. The dropped tip may also be picked up with permanent sutures or columellar strut type grafts (Fig. 19-2). These techniques are fully described in the section on tip projection.

Fig. 19-2. An inferior columellar strut of mega-rad rib bank cartilage was used to replace the elevation of the tip that had dropped because of sagging tissues through the years. **A**, Preoperative. **B**, Postoperative.

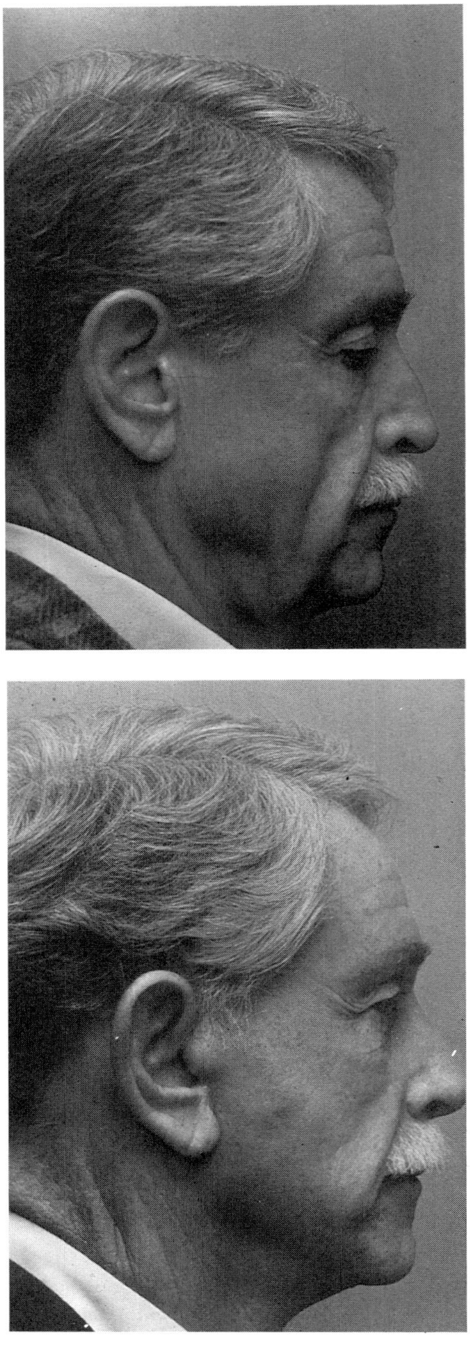

A

B

Tip Thickening

Hormonal

A non-desirable nasal tip change that occurs with time is tip thickening. This is commonly noted with hormonal changes such as menopause or pregnancy. The nasal tip thickening is probably caused by subcutaneous, soft tissue hypertrophy. I believe this is the most evident with the soft tissues between the nasal domes. Appropriate removal of these hypertrophied tissues through tip delivery methods works very well. Various modalities of treatment are described in the section on tip thinning.

Glandular Hypertrophy

Although sometimes seen in women, glandular hypertrophy is more common in men. It may range from minimal to extreme—such as an advanced rhinophyma. Minimal problems can be treated with skin drying lotions, and more advanced problems can be treated with epithelial shaving and dermabrasion.

20

Pollybeak Deformity

Walter E. Berman

The etiology of the so-called "pollybeak deformity" is quite variable. Pollybeak deformities may be caused by preoperative, intraoperative, or postoperative factors.

Preoperative

Preoperatively, false tip support may be caused by injecting a bolus of local anesthetic into the nasal spine region. This will abnormally pick up the nasal tip, which will drop postoperatively.

Intraoperative

During surgery, taking either too little or too much framework may lead to the formation of a pollybeak. The most obvious pollybeak may be caused by leaving an excess of anterior septal or upper lateral cartilage (Fig. 20-1, A). Failure to trim lower lateral cartilage when it is very wide just lateral to the dome can also directly contribute to a high dorsum anterior in the supertip area.

The very act of making an inferior septal incision, or transfixation, may cause a loss of tip support by separating the ligaments between the medial crura and the septum (Fig. 20-1, B). Various techniques of increasing tip projection will be discussed in the appropriate section.

Fig. 20-1. **A,** Excessive anterior septal cartilage left in place. **B,** Apparent pollybeak secondary to tip drop following cutting of ligaments with an inferior septal incision.

Continued.

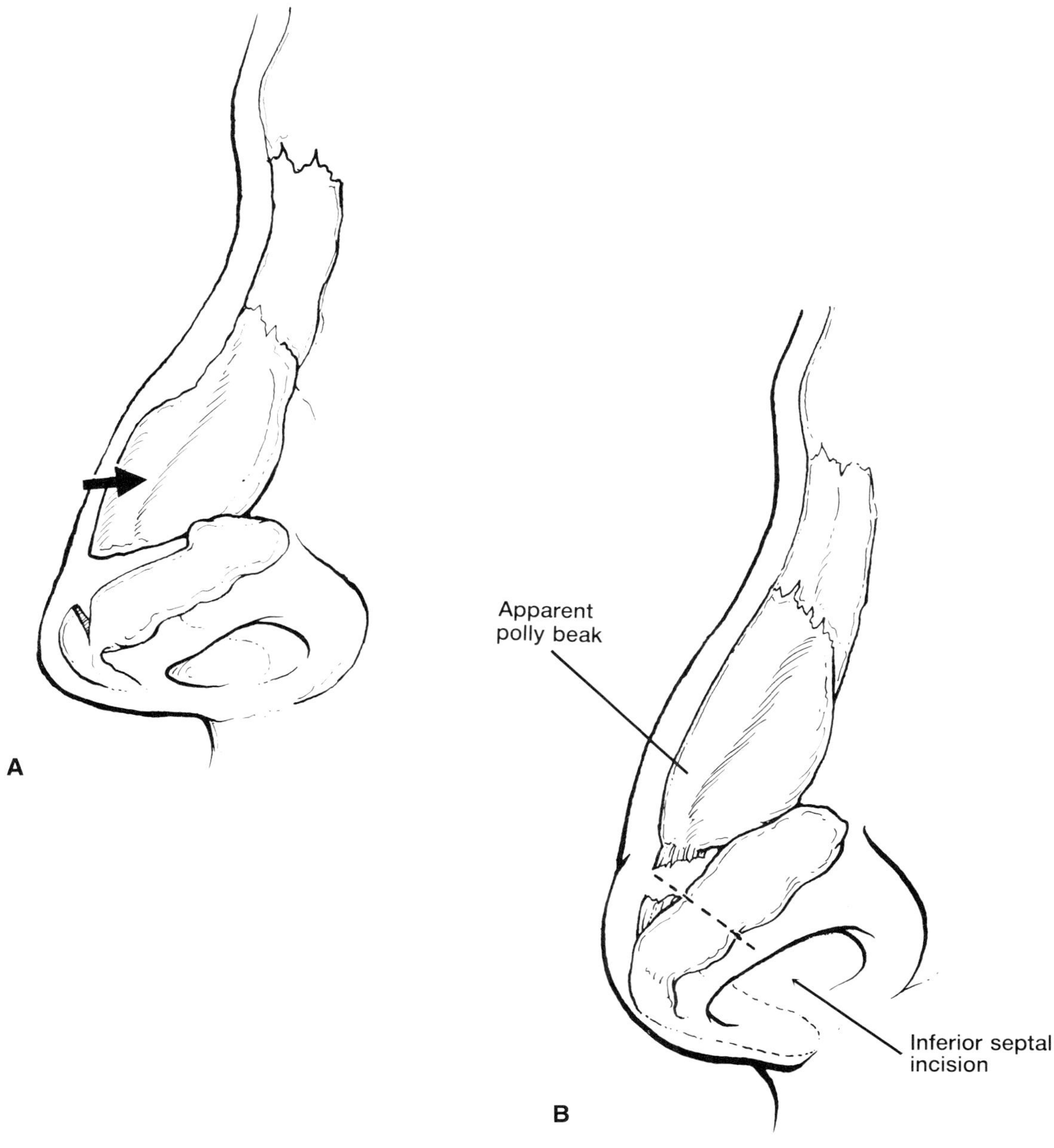

There is also an apparent pollybeak deformity caused by decreasing the height of the nasal pyramid, or osseous framework, too much. If the height is excessive, it will give the illusion that the cartilaginous septum was left too high. A graft to raise the height of the bony pyramid can correct this apparent defect.

Failure to remove fibrofatty tissue subcutaneously in the supratip area will cause a pollybeak. When there is very thick overlying skin, additional removal of the anterior nasal septum and upper lateral cartilages as a compensatory mechanism is mandatory (Fig. 20-1, C).

Fig 20-1, cont'd. C, Fibrofatty layer should be removed. Compensatory removal of anterior cartilage with thick skin. D, Postoperative splint must be firm and not allow fluid collection in the supratip area.

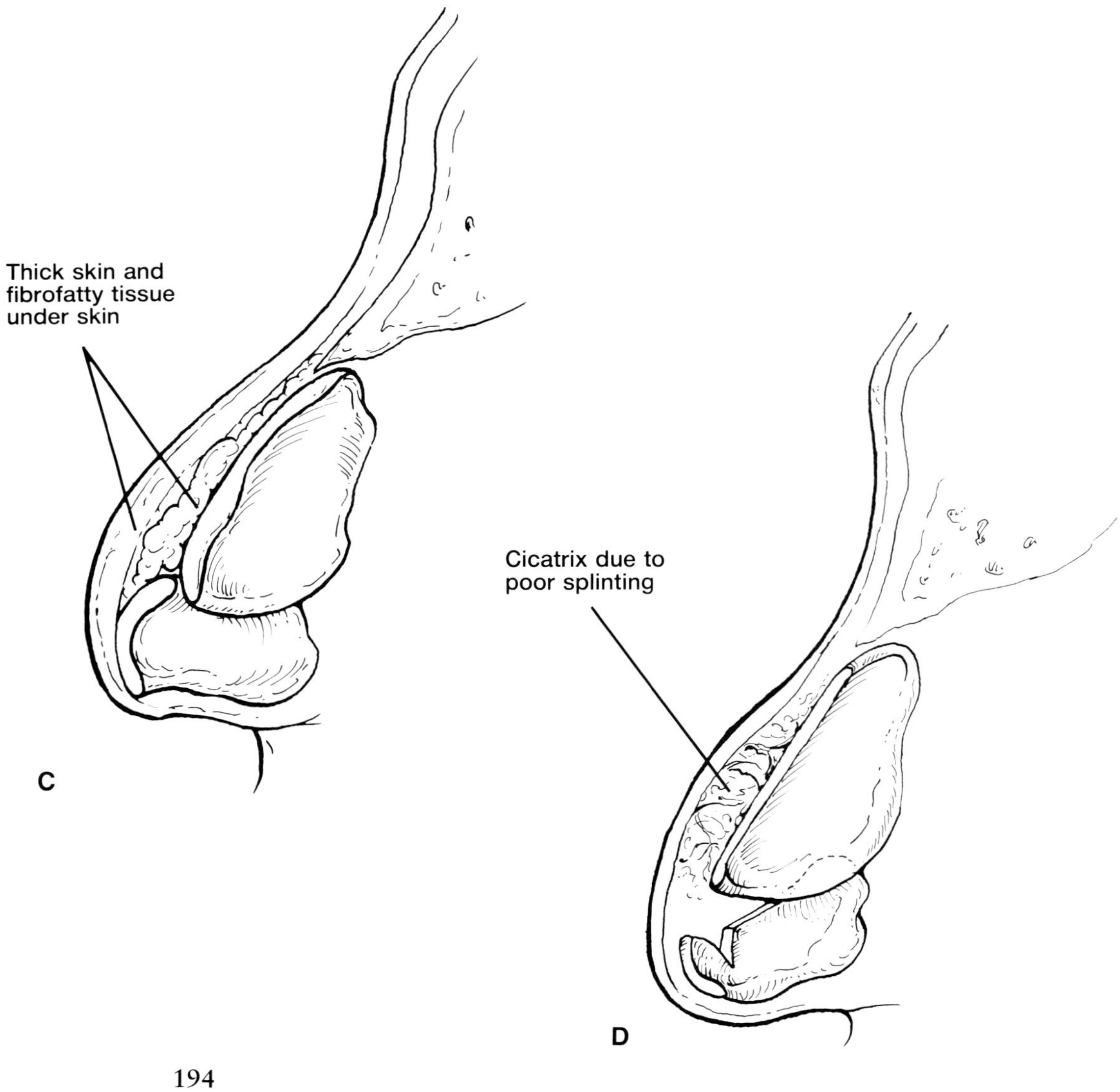

Postoperative

Postoperatively, the pollybeak deformity may be caused by poor splinting that allowed fluid to accumulate between the skin and the underlying cartilaginous framework (Fig. 20-1, D). If the fluid organizes and forms a cicatrix, thickening can result.

When administered in the early healing phases, steroids often have a beneficial effect on this thickened region. I start with about 1/4 cc or 25 mg per cc of triamcinolone diacetate injected through the skin just beneath the obvious swelling. If there is no response in two weeks, I switch to a higher dose, 40 mg per cc. When three injections have little effect, more surgical reduction of those tissues is indicated when sufficient healing transpires, usually in six to twelve months (Fig. 20-2). As we all know, excessive use of steroids may cause tissue atrophy.

The more insidious type of postoperative pollybeak is caused by tip drop from gradual support loss. This may become noticeable when the holding sutures dissolve, postoperative scar contraction occurs, or with the gradual loss of tip support with time.

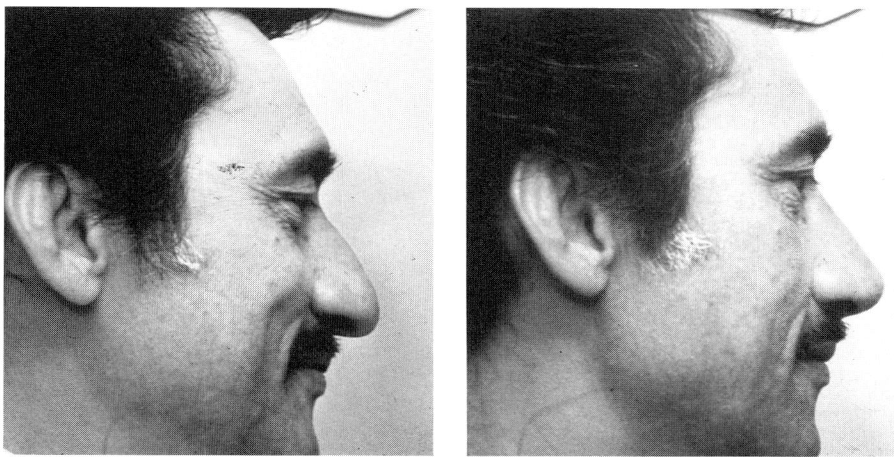

A B

Fig. 20-2. **A**, Preoperative. **B**, Postoperative photographs of a congenital pollybeak deformity.

21

Secondary Surgeries

Walter E. Berman

Secondary nasal surgery includes many factors that are akin to nasal trauma; many aspects of healed nasal trauma are found in the operated nose. Before treatment can be planned, a thorough diagnosis of the problems must be made. In particular, two key points must be decided:

(1) Are parts of the nasal framework deficient or excessive, and is further skeletal modification in order? This includes the nasal bones, upper and lower cartilages and components of the nasal septum, and

(2) Is there a loss of epithelial lining and/or cicatricial contractions that must also be addressed?

Only after a thorough chronicling of the physical problems can the reconstructive plans be considered.

Reduction Rhinoplasty

Steps of a Secondary Rhinoplasty

Many of the steps involved in a secondary nasal surgery are no different from the steps in a primary rhinoplasty.

Anterior Septum and/or Nasal Bone Height

When there is excessive anterior bone, cartilage, or scar tissue, I prefer approaching through a between-the-cartilage incision as in a primary surgery. Extra care must be taken to preserve the overlying skin, as this tissue may be atrophic. Careful evaluation of this overlying skin while dissecting the underlying framework is necessary. Sharp scissor dissection may be better than an elevator over the nasal bones. Removal of the underlying cartilaginous and bony framework is done in the same manner as a primary procedure.

Anterior Upper Lateral Cartilages

If the area of the upper lateral cartilage is satisfactorily narrow and straight, there is no reason to separate the upper lateral cartilages from the septum.

Turbinates

Turbinate hypertrophy can certainly recur, especially in the allergic patient. Therapy is the same as before. Turbinate septal adhesions are lysed with a cutting coagulating current, and any displacement of the septum or inferior turbinate contributing to, or because of, the adhesion must also be corrected or the adhesion will most probably recur (Fig. 21-1).

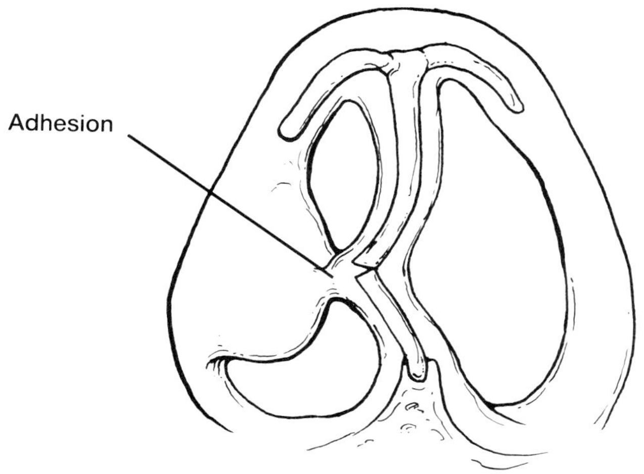

Fig. 21-1. Septal repair and separation of raw surfaces after surgery.

Tissue Replacement

When excessive tissues, mainly lining tissues, have been removed, I try to incorporate mature scar tissues into the flap. Further contraction of mature scar tissue is thus unlikely and the area that must be covered by new epithelium or full thickness grafts is also decreased.

Internal Nasal Valve

Collapse of the internal nasal valve is a particularly disturbing problem to the patient (Fig. 21-2, A). To repair this, the proximal end of the advancement flap is based on the undersurface of the upper lateral cartilage epithelium. The distal end is taken from the septal covering and rotated laterally. If the scar is quite thick, it must be thinned so that the newly placed epithelial flap will be in a more anterior position. This technique raises the depressed internal valve to improve nasal respiration (Fig. 21-2, B). It does leave a denuded epithelial surface on the septum, which quickly epithelializes. I would not recommend denuding both sides of the septal epithelium at the same surgery because of possible septal perforation (Figs. 21-3 and 21-4).

An annular cicatrix causing collapse of the internal nasal valve is most often the culmination of various nasal incisions being performed too close or in continuation of each other, resulting in a circumferential scar contraction. The annular ring of scar tissue is very restrictive to nasal respiration. Rather than a series of 'Z' plasties, as suggested by some authors, I have found it best to use a combination of the above advancement flap and a full thickness post-auricular skin graft. A few 5-0 plain sutures are placed and a sponge type of packing is inserted over the graft for a few days.

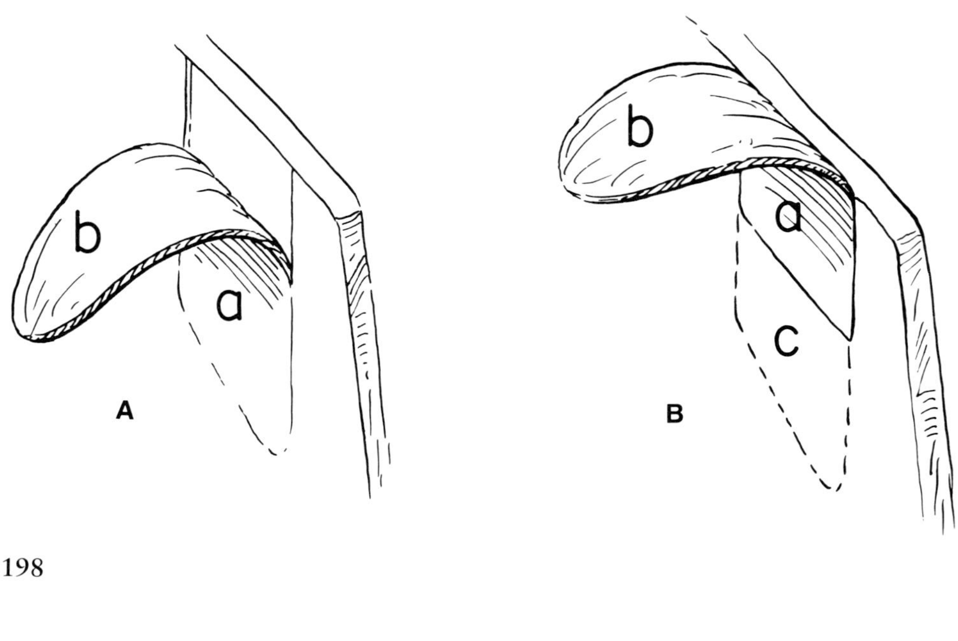

Fig. 21-2. Collapse and repair of internal nasal valve. **A,** Depressed internal valve from upper lateral cartilage to the nasal septum. **B,** The *a* mucosa is advanced to a higher point on the septum to raise the internal valve; *c* is de-epithelialized septum that re-epithelializes. (From Berman WE: Rhinoplasty, ed 2, Washington DC, 1984, American Academy of Otolaryngology-Head and Neck Surgery Foundation, Inc.)

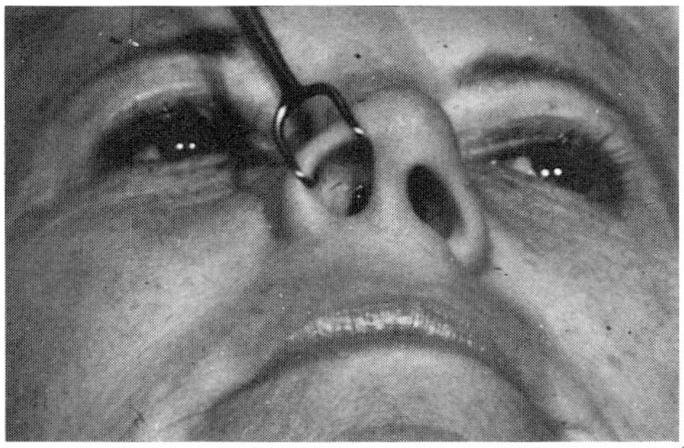

A

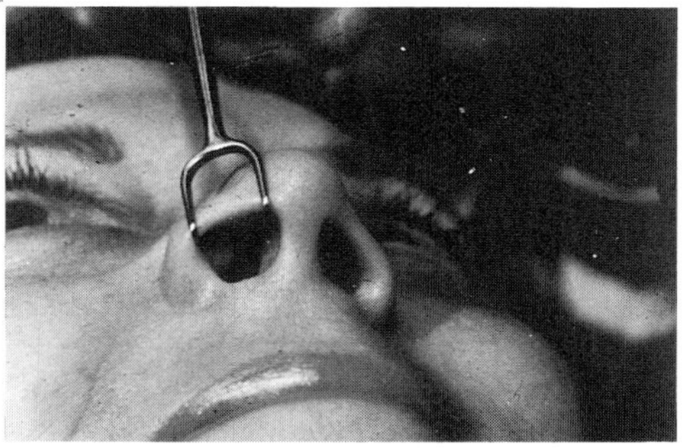

B

Fig. 21-3. An internal valve cicatrix following severance of the mucosa at the internal valve and removal of excessive soft tissues treated with an advancement flap. **A**, Preoperative. **B**, Postoperative.

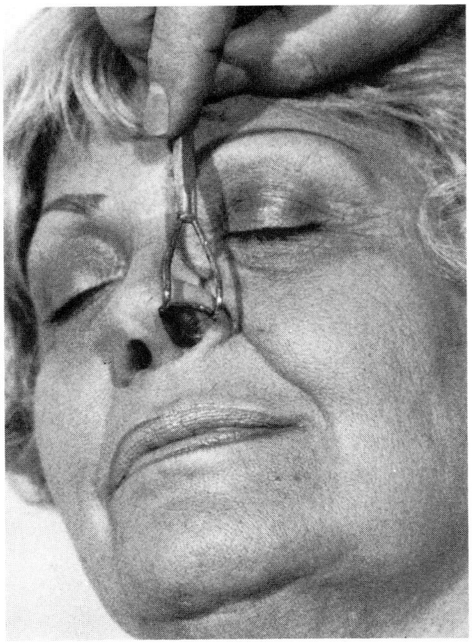

A

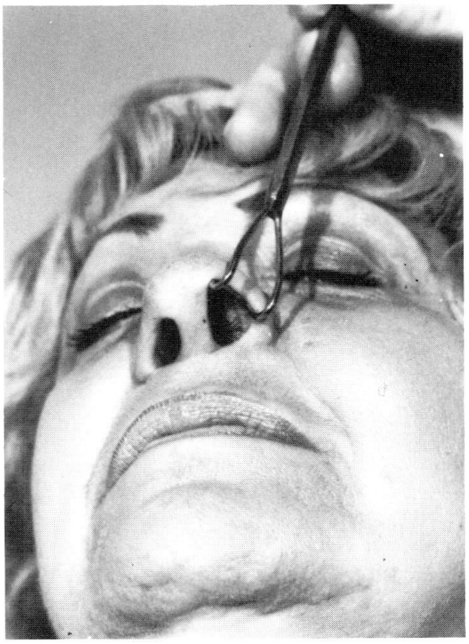

B

Fig. 21-4. Cicatrix at the internal valve following incision through the valve and membrane. Repaired with advancement flap from septum to undersurface of upper lateral cartilage. **A**, Preoperative. **B**, Postoperative.

Columellar Retraction

When a little "columellar show" is desired, a simple columellar retraction is readily treated with a cartilage graft. I like an incision above or anterior to the graft placement. A straight Stevens iris scissors is placed through this incision, which is on the lateral side of the columella. The scissors is then used to dissect a pocket and the cartilage is positioned inferior to the columella. The source of the cartilage may be autogenous from the septum, post-auricular, or irradiated bank cartilage; all work well in this area. A through-and-through columellar 4-0 Vicryl suture is then placed around or even through the graft to hold its position. If the retraction is severe, it should be treated in the same manner as for lengthening the central segment of the nose. When a nose is overly shortened, either centrally or laterally, composite grafts are most useful.

Lengthening the Nose

Short central segment. In the case of the overly shortened central segment, excessive septal surgery is the most common culprit. To repair this, an incision is made along the inferior edge of the cartilaginous septum. Two sutures are placed through the columella, superior to the medical crura. One suture is placed anteriorly (high) and one posteriorly (low). Each is held with a small clamp. Inferior traction of the columella will allow measurement of the created defect behind the columella. This measured amount of preferred inferior displacement will then be filled in with a composite graft from the medial aspect of the auricle (Fig. 21-5). Relatively large composite grafts may be taken to lengthen a nose up to two centimeters. If increased tip projection is desirable, the height of

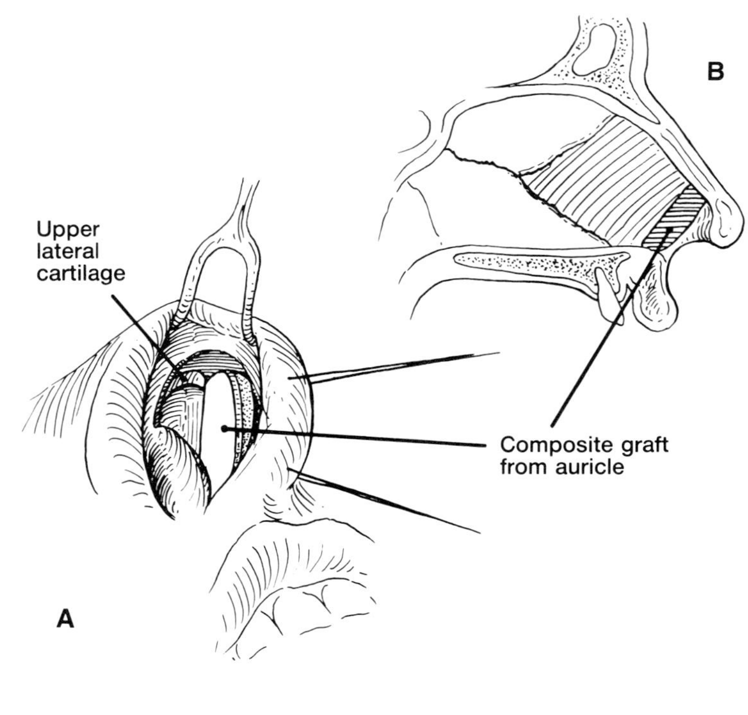

Fig. 21-5. Repair of overly shortened central segment using a composite graft. **A,** Post-auricular composite graft of skin and cartilage being placed between the septum and columella. **B,** Composite graft in place. (From Berman WE: Rhinoplasty, ed 2, Washington DC, 1984, American Academy of Otolaryngology-Head and Neck Surgery Foundation, Inc.)

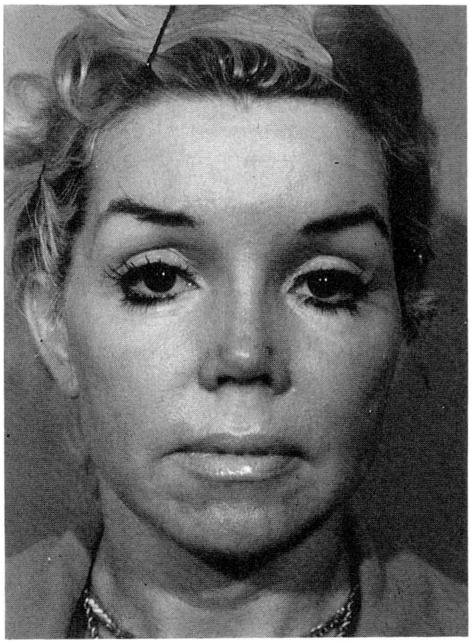

A

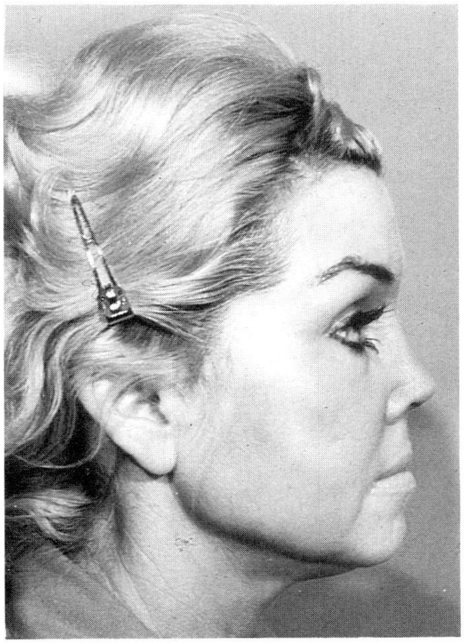

B

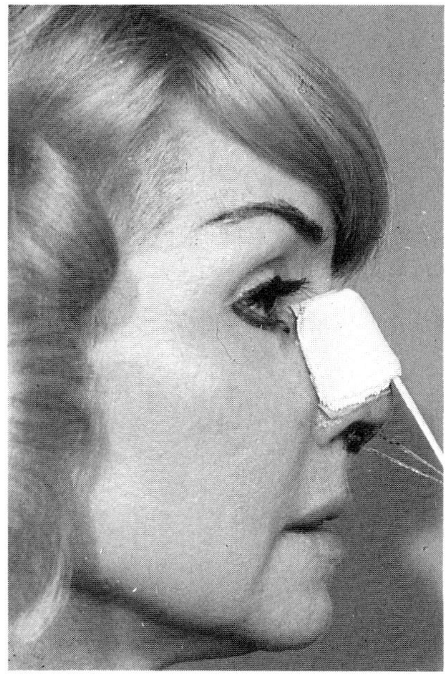

C

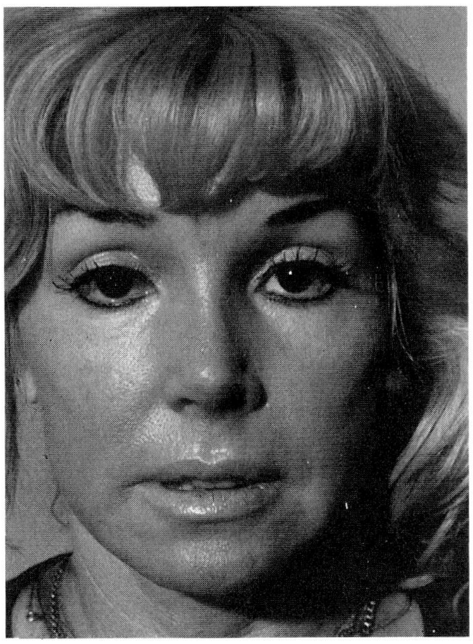

D

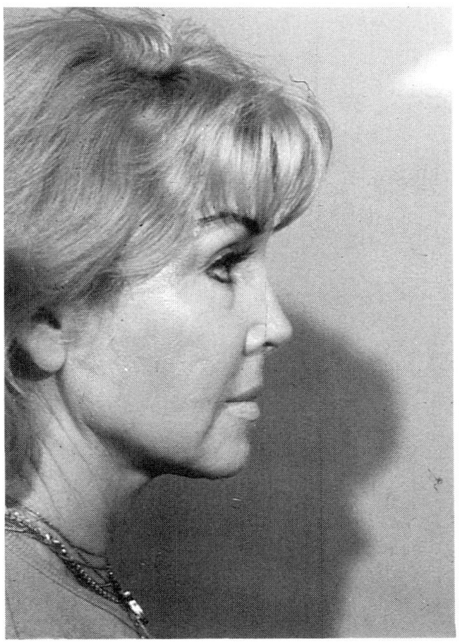

E

Fig. 21-6. Excessive septal surgery resulting in a retracted columella and foreshortened nose, **A** and **B**, Preoperative, treated with a composite post-auricular autogenous graft to the central segment placed between the columella and the medial crus. **C**, The dressing shows my traction device of permanent sutures through the columella to a point inferior to the columella which is left in place for one week. **D** and **E**, Postoperative photos.

the graft may be used to take this into allowance. Four 5-0 plain sutures are placed at the edges of the graft and our regular packs (e.g., straws and telfa) are inserted. Topical antibiotics are used on the packs. They have a straw in the center of the pack for respiration. The packs should be left in place for a week.

An external dressing of tape is applied. Two layers of casting material with a 1.5 cm wide piece of a tongue depressor held in between is then applied over the tape. The tongue depressor extends in front of the nose for 2.5 cm. The first two sutures that were placed through the anterior and posterior areas of the columella are then used as traction sutures and tied to the notched distal end of the piece of wood for the same week (Figs. 21-6 and 21-7).

A 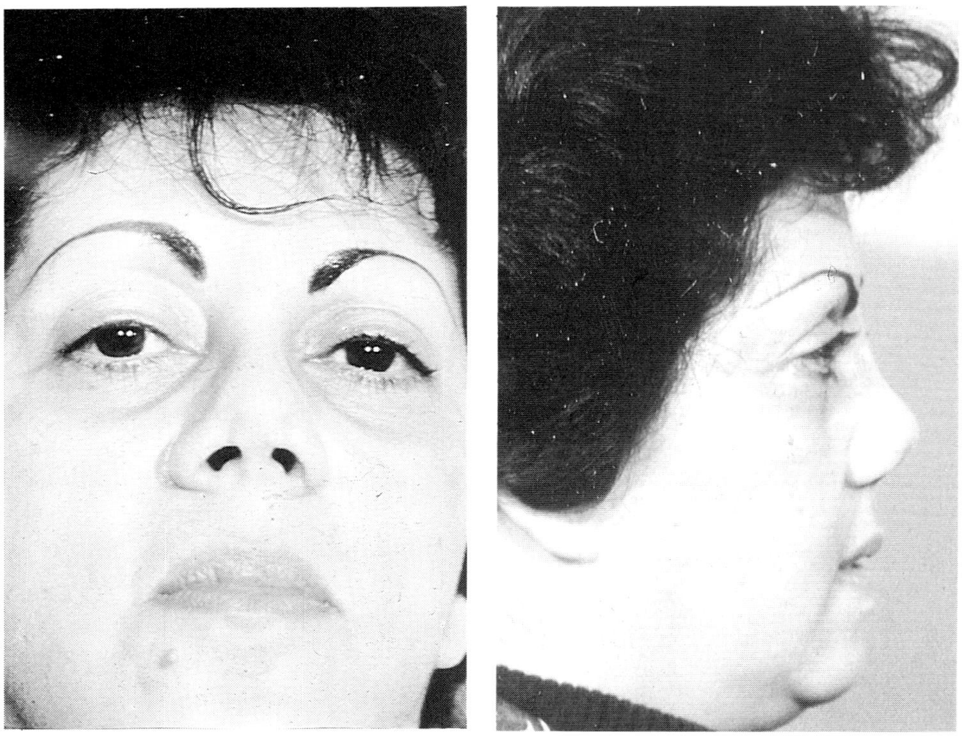 B

Fig. 21-7. Central retraction and anterior (dorsal) collapse following a septal rhinoplasty. Gross removal of inferior cartilagenous septum. Post-auricular composite graft as replacement tissue. **A** and **B**, Preoperative after the original surgery. **C** and **D**, Postoperative after the reconstructive surgery. Preoperative and postoperative views of an overzealous septoplasty with subsequent anterior (dorsal) and inferior (caudal) collapse, corrected with an anterior rib graft and a central post-auricular composite graft. **E**, Photograph taken seven days after original surgery. The swelling is causing transient support before septal and framework collapse.

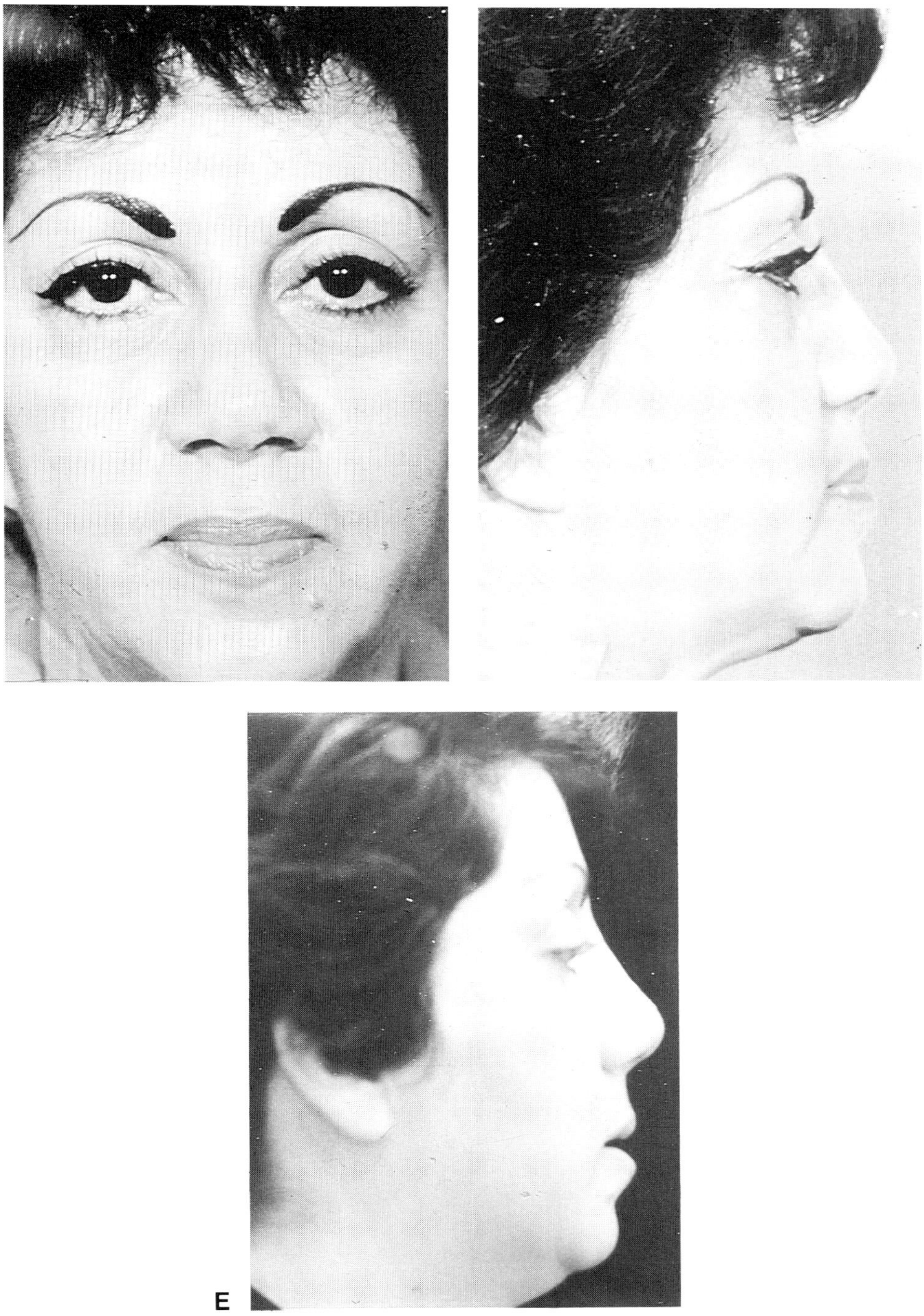

C D E

Short lateral segment. When there is lateral shortening or retracted lateral nares (Fig. 21-8, A), often referred to as the "mad dog"appearance, a similar procedure is performed. The incision is made between the upper and lower lateral cartilage only through the lining. Dissection beneath the overlying skin is done in both directions. Traction sutures are also applied through the lower lateral marginal incision, and the measurement composite graft is taken from the post-auricular region (Fig. 21-8, B). Usually both sides can have the donor grafts from the one ear. These are placed internally and likewise sutured. Traction is applied with a fashioned tongue depressor as previously noted. I have found that traction for seven full days greatly decreases or even eliminates the graft retraction (Figs. 21-9 and 21-10).

Since both the composite type grafts, either for central or lateral shortening, have at least a peripheral circumferential blood supply, the percentage of take is excellent. Whenever possible, I also try and create a septal covering flap for the side of the composite graft that is not epithelialized. This, of course, is not the case in the lateral shortening, only in the central shortening.

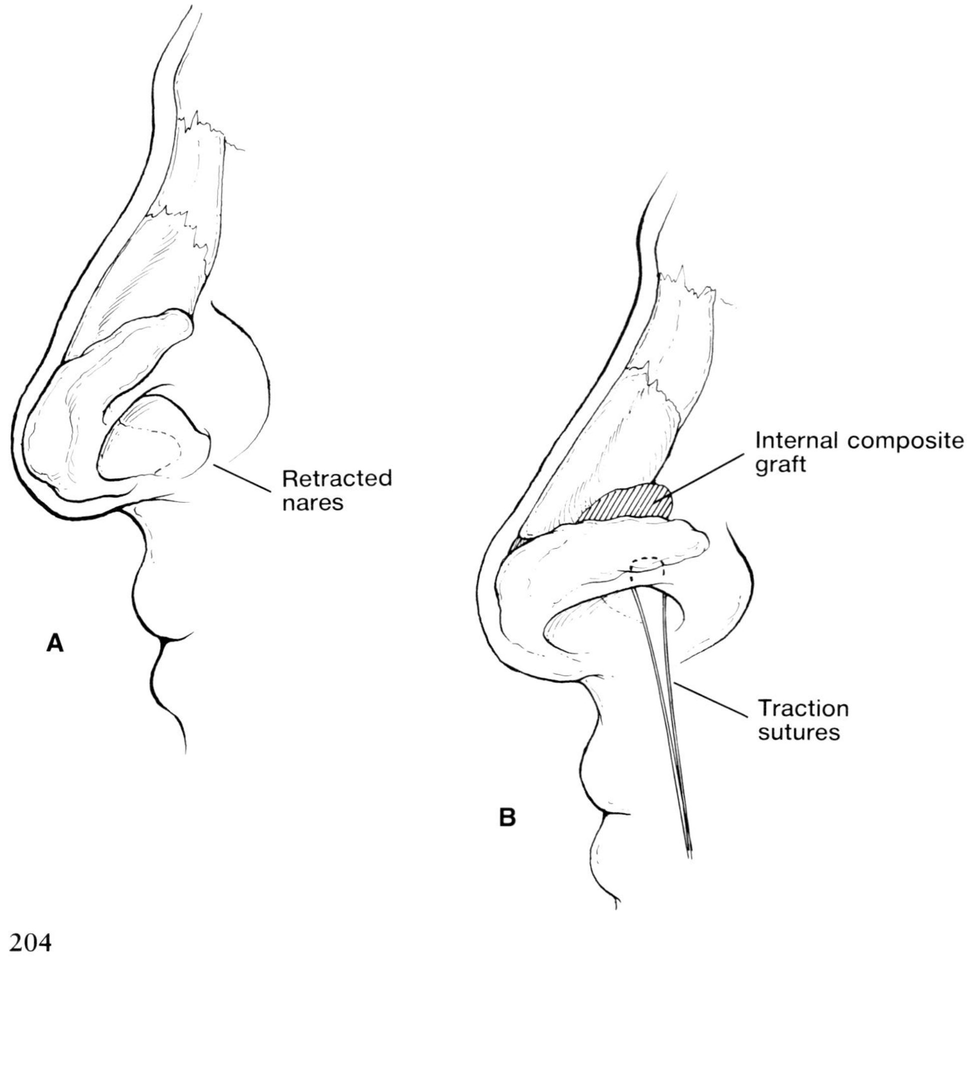

Fig. 21-8. Lateral shortening or retracted lateral nares. **A,** Snarl or "mad dog" appearance. **B,** Repair with post-auricular composite graft with epithelium as lining.

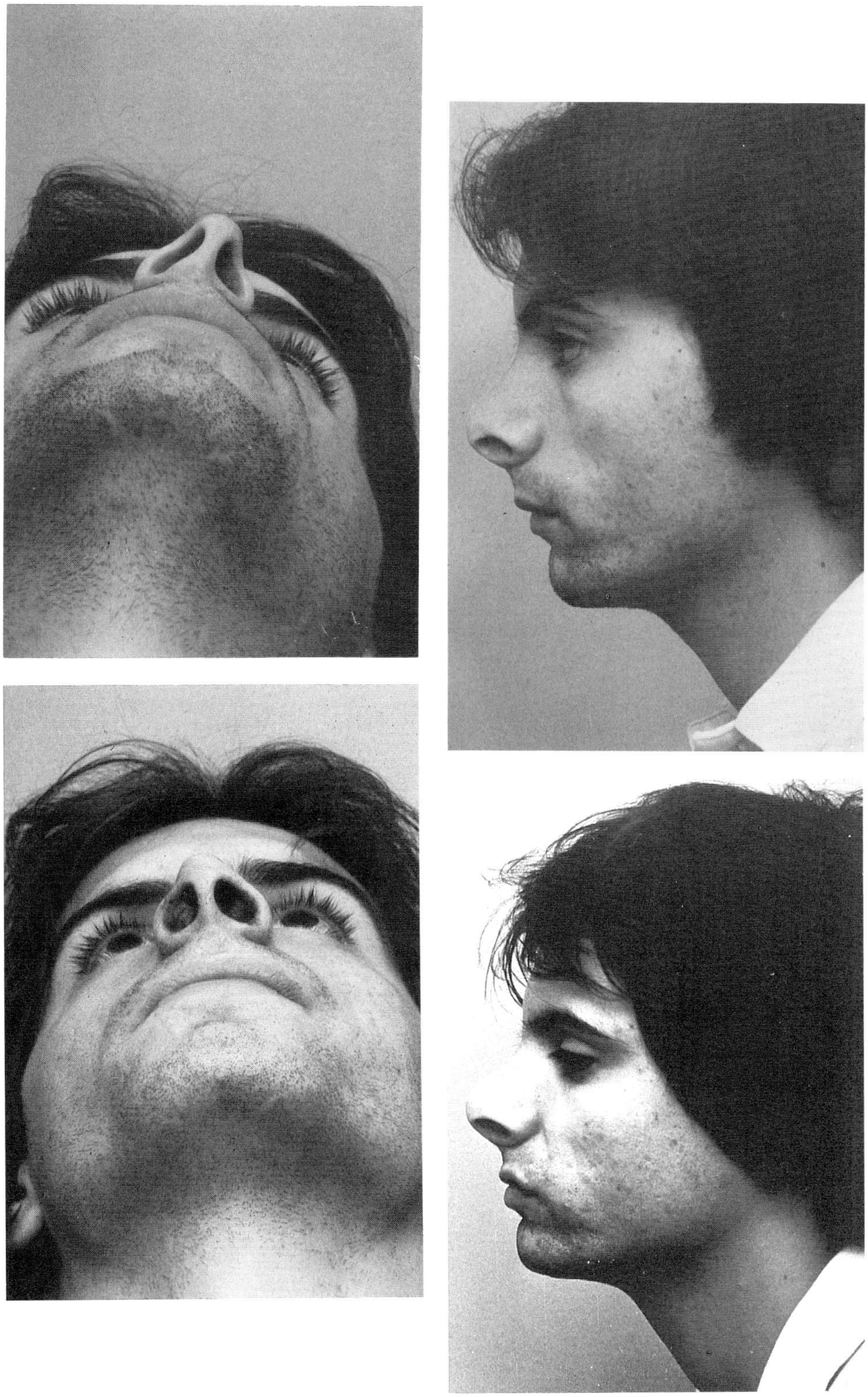

A B C D

Fig. 21-9. A lateral retraction secondary to over-zealous surgery. **A** and **B**, Preoperative. Treated with a post-auricular composite graft placed internally with external traction for one week. **C** and **D**, Postoperative.

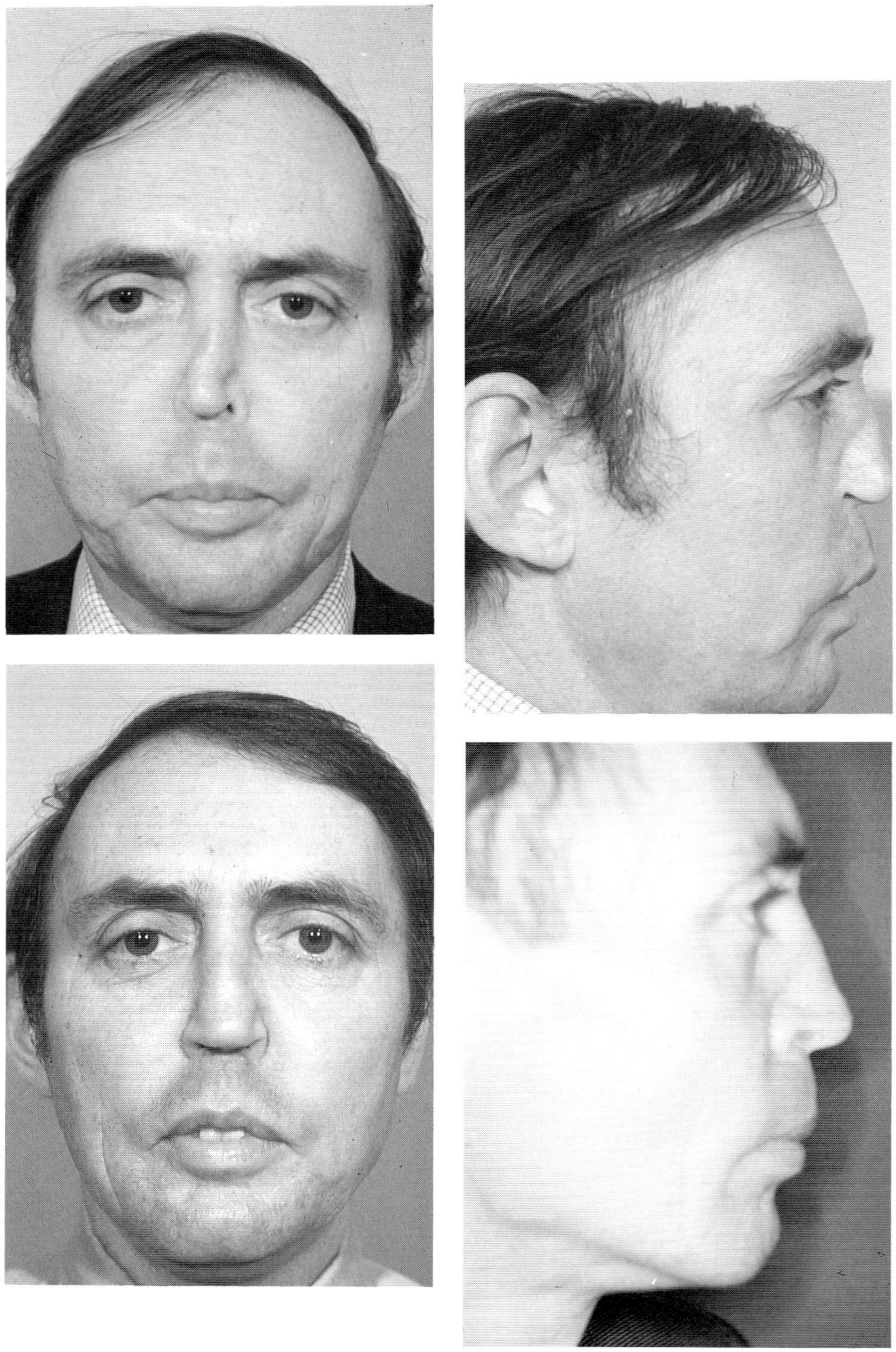

Fig. 21-10. Both cartilage and soft tissue loss at the junction of the upper laterals and lower lateral cartilages. **A** and **B**, Preoperative; a post-auricular composite graft was placed internally after undermining had restored the other tissues to a more normal relationship. **C** and **D**, Postoperative. (From Berman WE: Rhinoplasty, ed 2, Washington DC, 1984, American Academy of Otolaryngology-Head and Neck Surgery Foundation, Inc.)

Nasal Pyramid

Displacement

The possibility for problems developing with the bony pyramid are numerous. The simplest problems to solve are the displacements. Medial and lateral osteotomies are sufficient when both of the nasal bones are relatively straight; repositioning is all that is required. When one or both of the nasal bones are actually curved onto themselves with an abnormal configuration, double lateral osteotomies are needed. The first lateral osteotomy is made along the nasomaxillary-nasal bone suture line. The second is performed more laterally at the usual site of the lateral osteotomy. These double osteotomies tend to comminute the bone, allowing it to straighten (see Chapter 13). Slight irregularities of the nasal bones are often eradicated with simple rasping.

Irregularities

The "blanket" approach has been very useful, whether the irregularities are depressions or the simpler excrescences (hills and valleys). The so-called blanket is a layer of autogenous fascia—for example, temporalis (Fig. 21-11). This fascia is placed through the cartilage incision into the previously dissected space created between the underlying cartilaginous and/or bony framework and the overlying skin. The maneuver of releasing this graft, shown to me by Richard Webster, is beautiful. A forceps places the implant in its desired position. The arms of the forceps are then spread with a small hemostat, allowing the forceps to be removed without disturbing the graft layer.

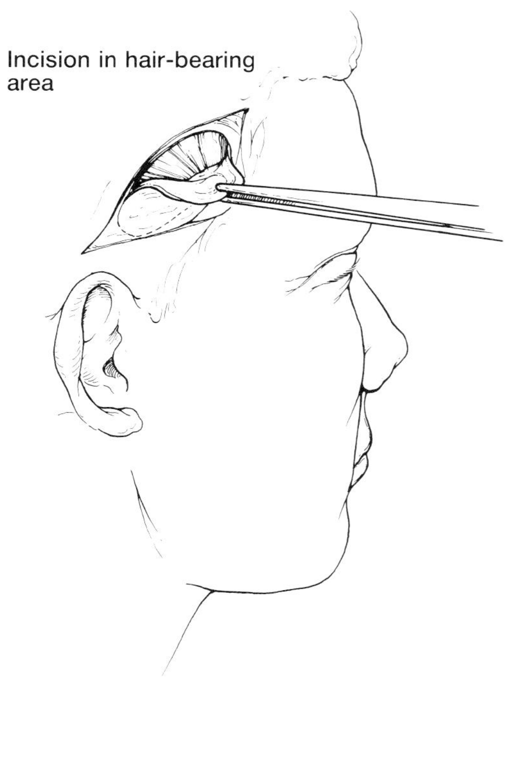

Fig. 21-11. Removing temporalis fascia through hair-bearing area of donor site.

Too narrow a bony pyramid may also be treated with a blanket. This superficial therapy is only practical when there is an adequate airway. If the airway is decreased, I prefer using cartilage wedges between the freed bones to keep the bones and the attached upper laterals apart. A fascial blanket can still be used to cover any irregularities.

Saddling (Anterior Deficiency)

Saddling of the bony dorsum and cartilaginous dorsum is treated in a similar fashion. Again, overly zealous septal surgery is the most common reason for this complication. The entry incision should be at least 1 cm distal to the point of the graft. Usually the between-the-cartilage incision is sufficient, but at times a split (intracartilaginous) or even a marginal lower cartilage incision is necessary to achieve the proper distance from the graft. Ideally, the dissected pocket should just be large enough to accept the graft but not too large to allow movement. The base of the pocket should be smooth and flat to prevent rocking of the graft at a later time. The graft itself should not have any sharp edges that may show through the skin. In thin-skinned individuals it is best to deliberately taper the edges of the graft (Figs. 21-11 and 21-12).

Autogenous cartilage from the septum or auricle is suitable for relatively small saddles. If larger, I prefer rib cartilage (Fig. 21-13). For over fifteen years, I have been using megarad bank cartilage. These rib grafts receive two million rads, which is adequate sterilization. In the hundreds that I have done, there is no more rejection or resorption of these grafts than of autogenous cartilaginous grafts (Fig. 21-14). Recently, I have also been impressed with demineralized rib grafts. The soft nature of this graft provides for malleability and lends itself very well to contouring.

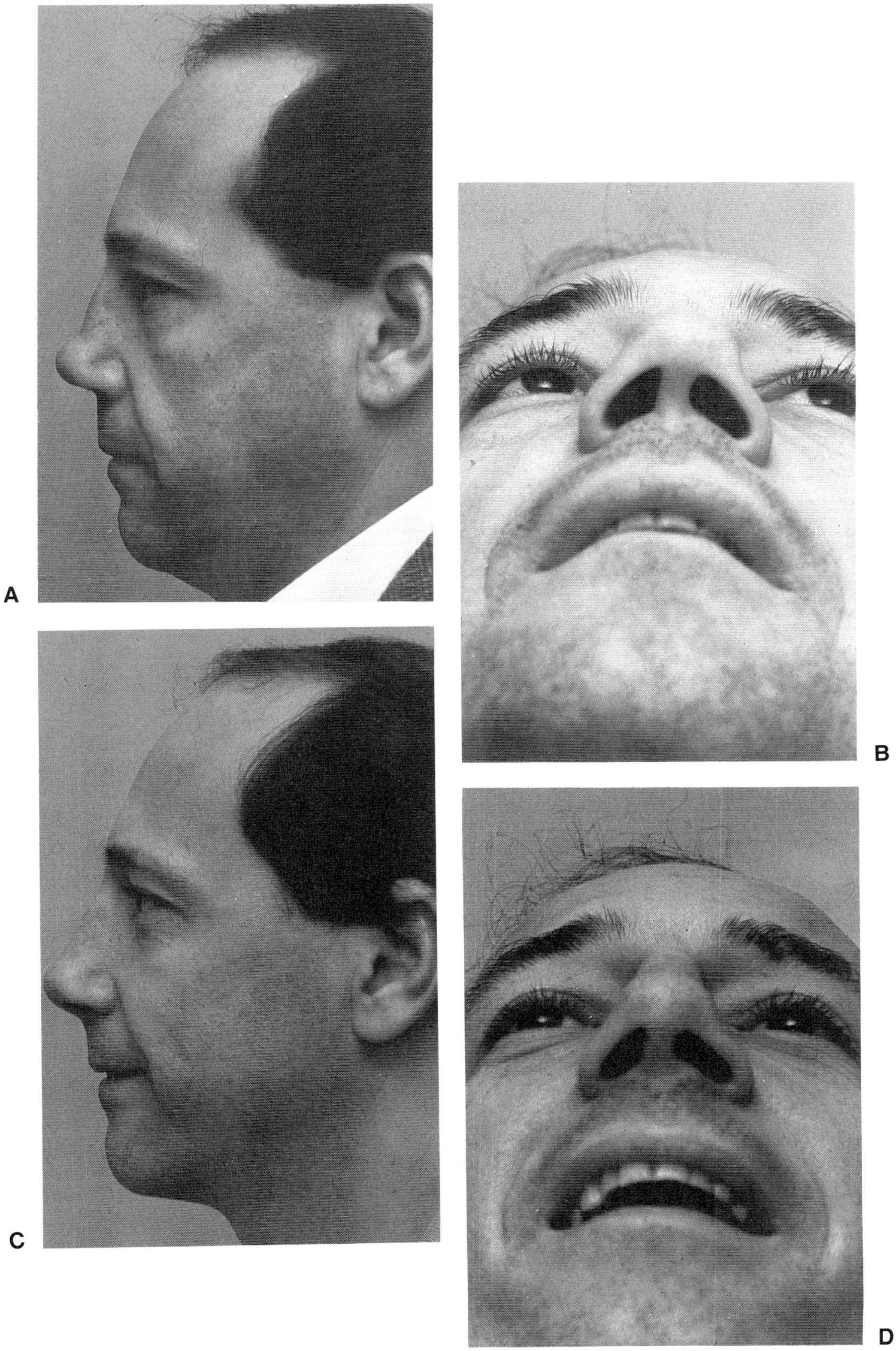

Fig. 21-12. A saddle and retracted nasal deformity. A and B, Preoperative. C and D, Postoperative.

If the case permits some motion to the graft after placement, I have used a circumferential suture around the graft and tied on a bolster overlying the skin for two days. I have not seen any long-term complications from the use of this suture.

I personally dislike the 'L' shaped grafts used by some to repair the saddle deformity. I would rather have an anterior (dorsal) and a columellar graft that are not attached to each other. This allows a more normal movement of the nose with less chance of disturbing the anterior graft when the inferior graft is contiguous with it.

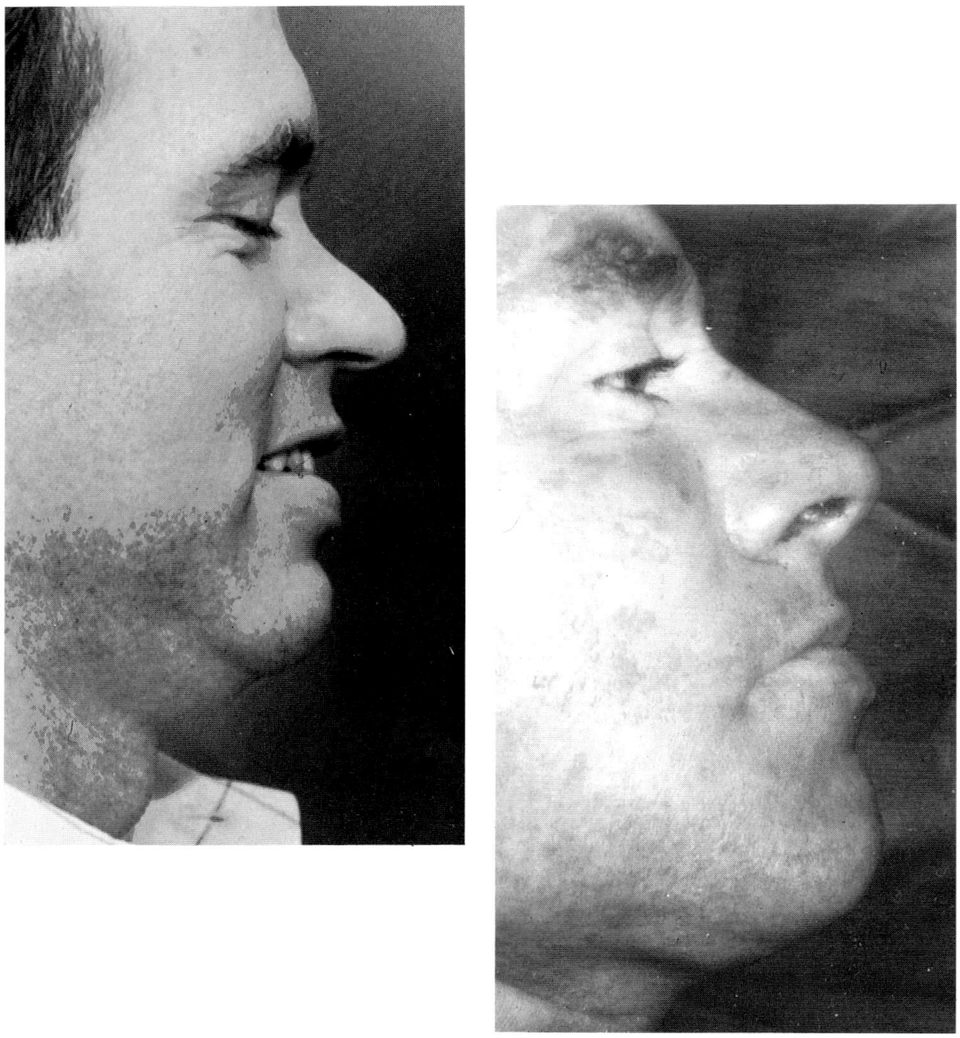

A

B

Fig. 21-13. Post-traumatic saddle deformity and loss of columellar support. **A,** Preoperative, treated with bank cartilage grafts. **B,** Postoperative.

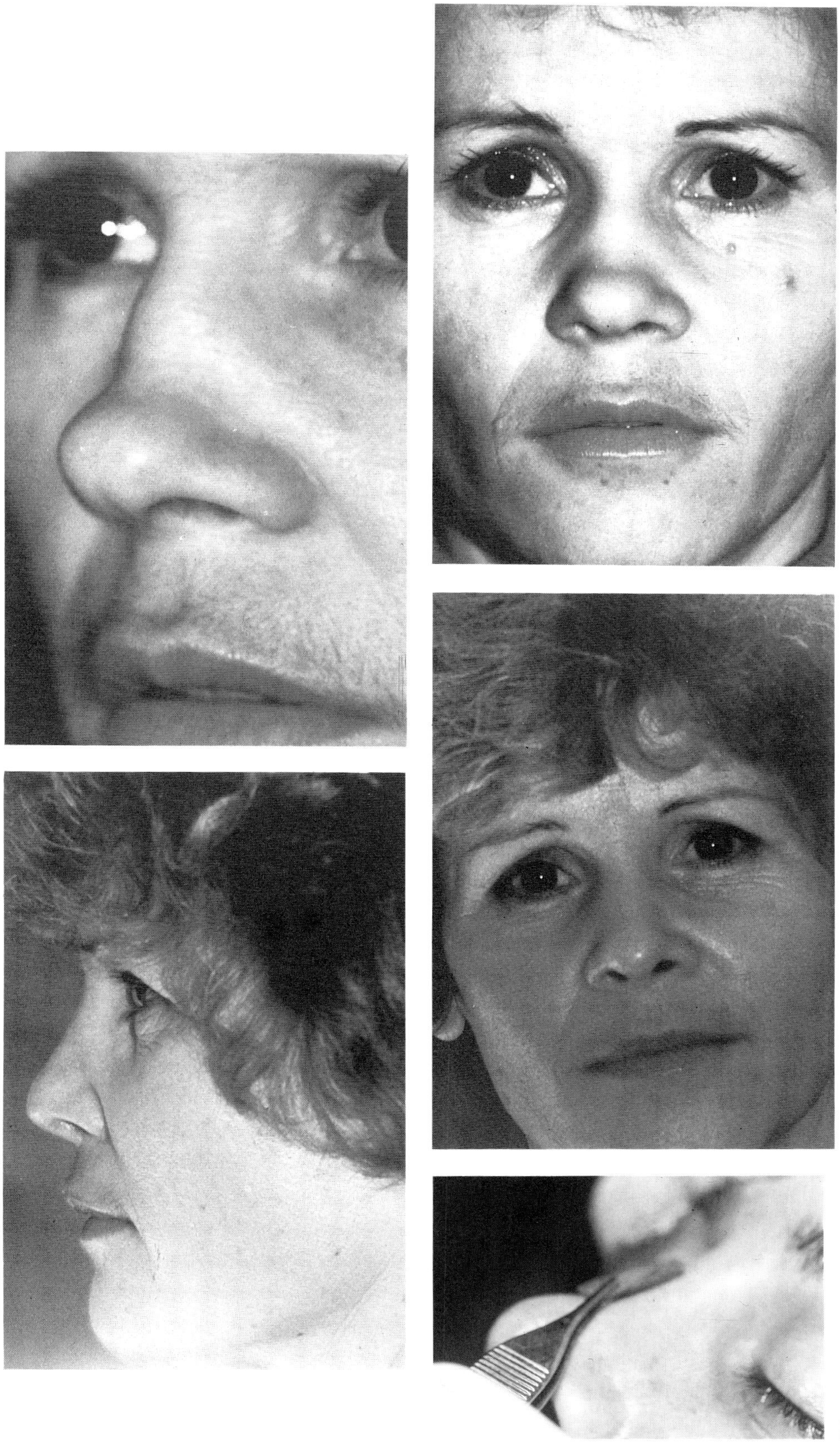

A B C D E

Fig. 21-14. **A** and **B**, Preoperative. **C** and **D**, Postoperative photographs. **E**, A surgical photograph of the graft. Megarad bank rib cartilage was used for the saddle deformity.

Secondary Nasal Tip Deformities

Secondary nasal tip problems are probably the most common cause for complaints in the postsurgical nose. Irregularities, asymmetries, and loss of tip support are the most cited problems.

In any postoperative tip problem, I prefer a delivery technique. In this way tip deformities may be directly visualized. It is of paramount importance to realize that, as Dr. Louis Fiet said in a personal communication, "It doesn't matter what you take out, it's what you leave in." This is especially true of nasal tip surgery.

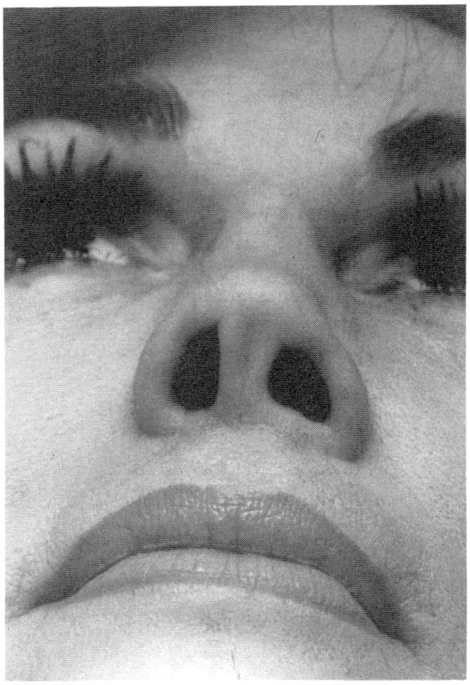

A

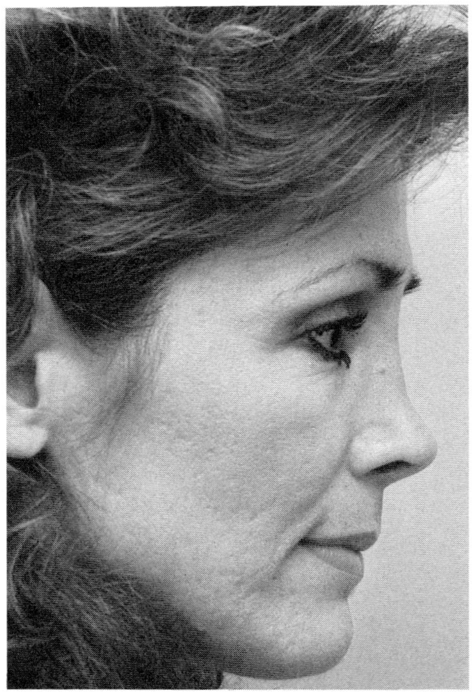

B

Fig. 21-15. A and B, Preoperative. C and D, Postoperative photographs following various surgical procedures. E, Grafts of megarad bank cartilage were placed anteriorly as depicted, and inferiorly for support. Revision of the nasal tip was also done.

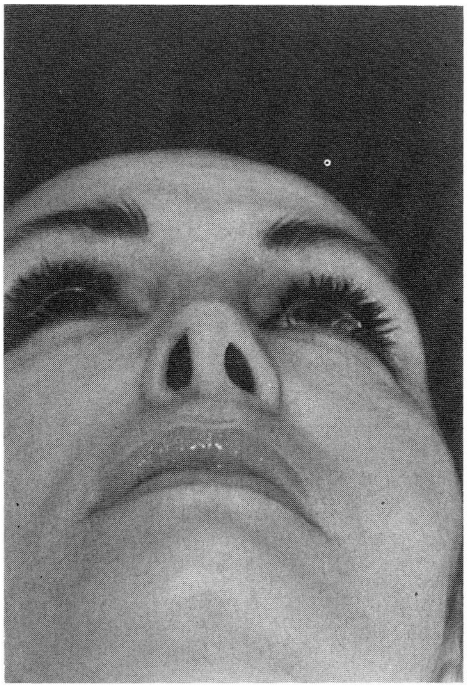

C

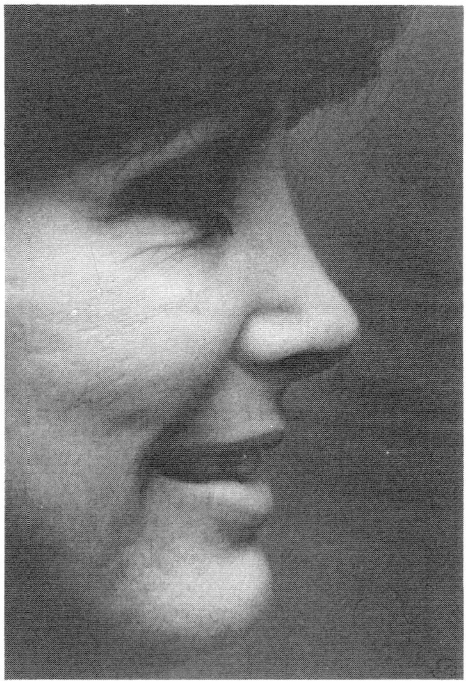

D

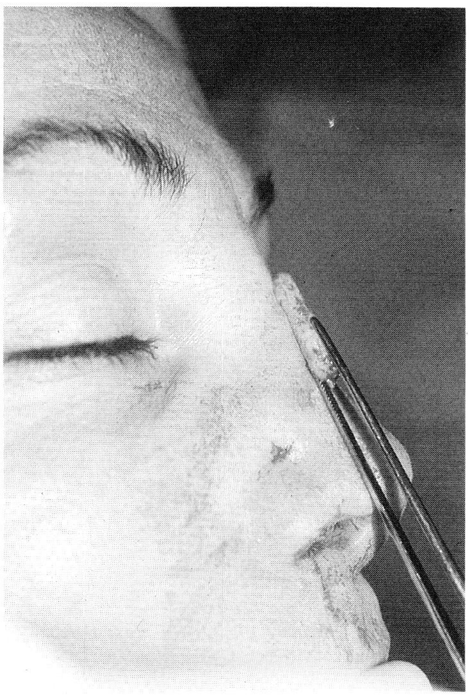

E

Asymmetries

If the domes have been severed, as in a Goldman type of procedure, and there are sharp edges, a one-sided thin morselizer like Dr. Frank Rubins' may be an excellent remedy. If using this does not eliminate the irregularities when the nasal domes are replaced under the skin, further trimming may be necessary. Any small excrescences should be conservatively cut away. Both sides should be equal in width. Interestingly, scar tissue may fill in some cartilaginous deficiencies. If the scar tissue has not filled in the deficiencies of a split nasal cartilaginous dome, cartilage grafts may be sutured in place (Figs. 21-16 to 21-19).

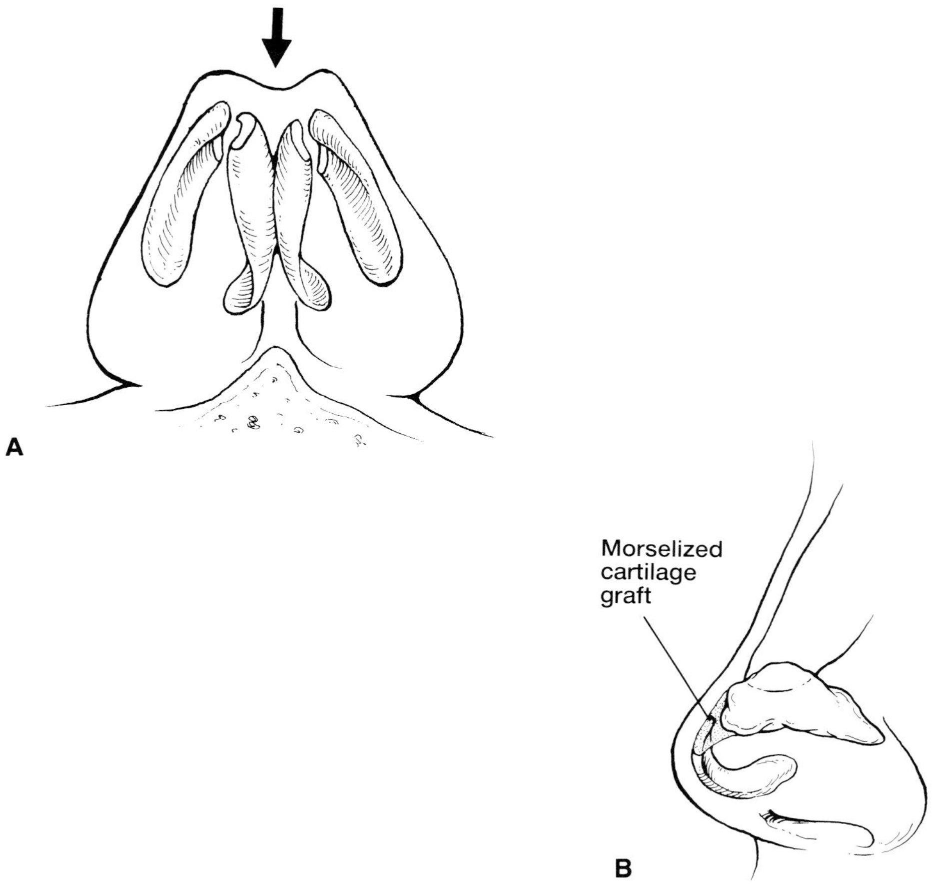

Fig. 21-16. Tip asymmetry. **A,** Split nasal dome producing irregularity following rhinoplasty. **B,** Repair of irregular tip with morselization and/or cartilage grafts.

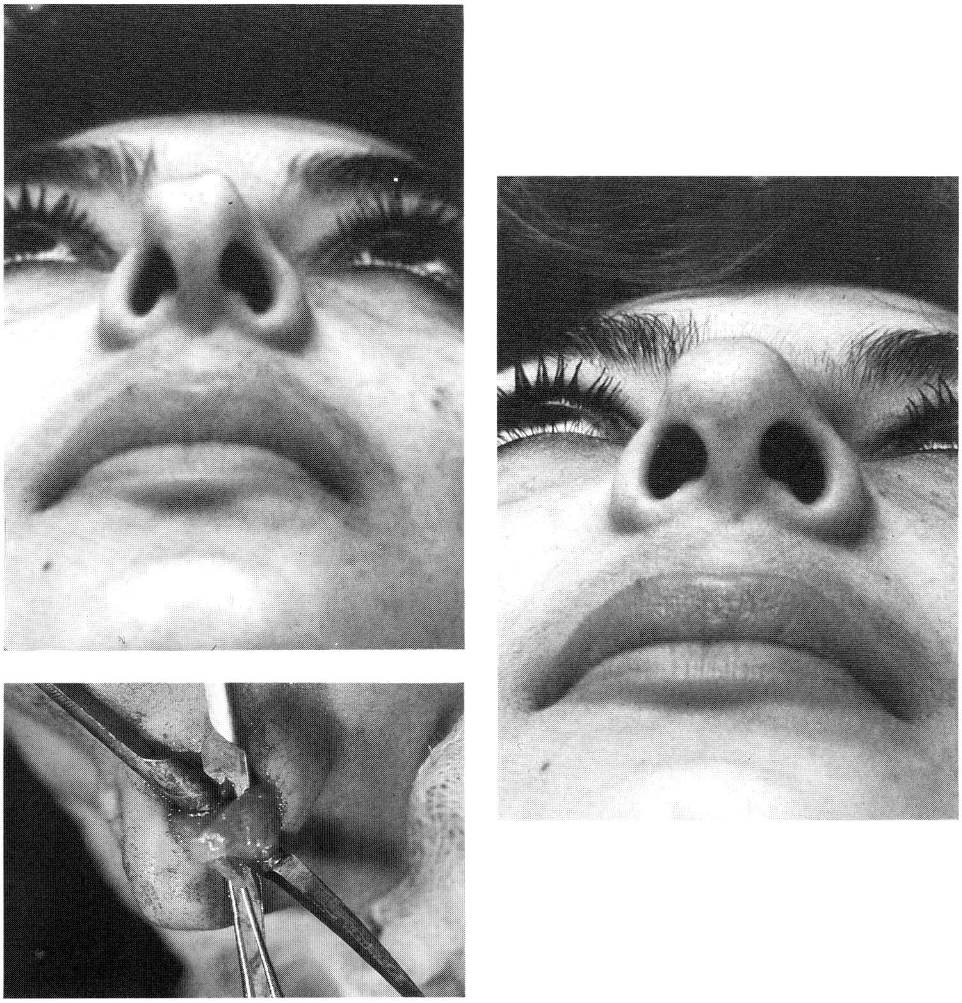

A

B

C

Fig. 21-17. **A,** Preoperative. **B,** Postoperative. **C,** A surgical photograph showing the nasal tip pathology. The nasal domes had been separated and the remaining cartilage was irregular. Treatment consisted of a delivery technique, thorough morselization of the area, and trimming as necessary.

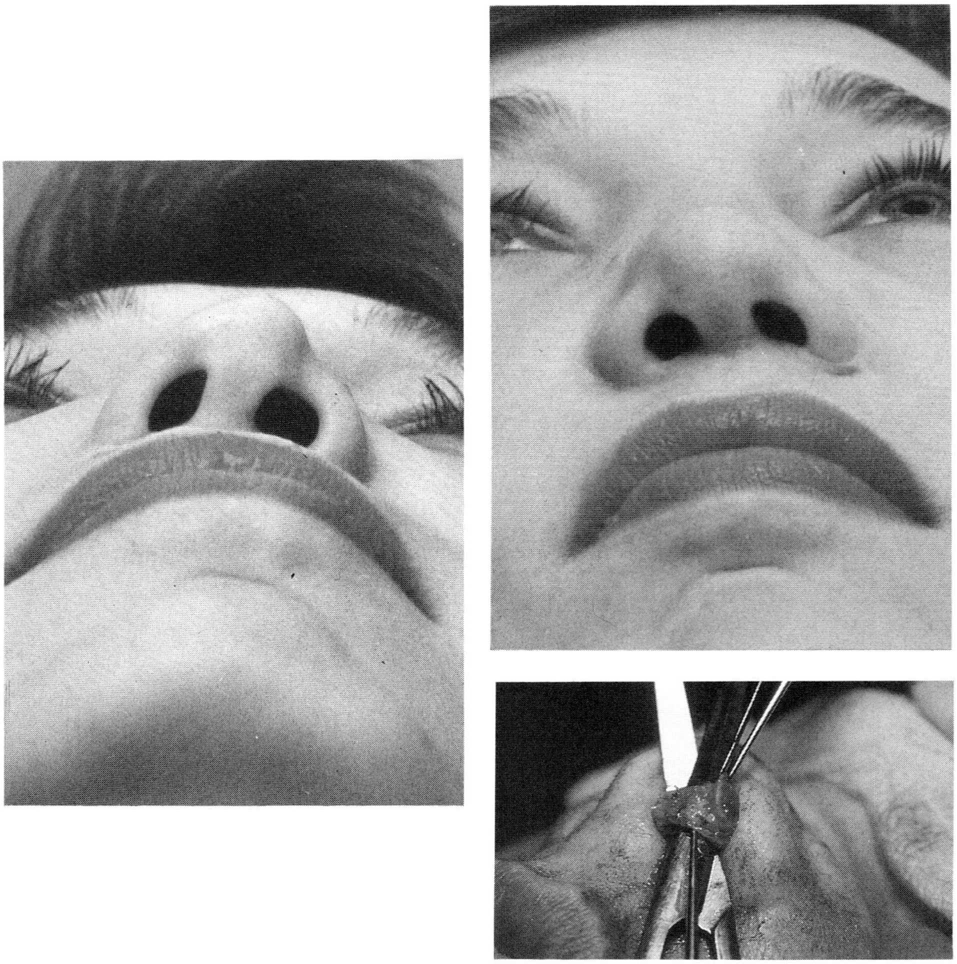

A

B

C

Fig. 21-18. **A,** Preoperative. **B,** Postoperative. **C,** A surgical photograph showing the nasal tip pathology. More lateral deformity required further undermining and repositioning of the lateral cartilages.

Dropped Tip

If the tip is depressed, columellar cartilaginous grafts from the nasal spine to the tip may be needed. I prefer smoothing out the nasal tips at their domes and raising the medial crura to the desired height rather than forming a new nasal tip with a cartilaginous graft. In my hands it produces a more natural appearance and a thinner nasal tip (see section on tip projection).

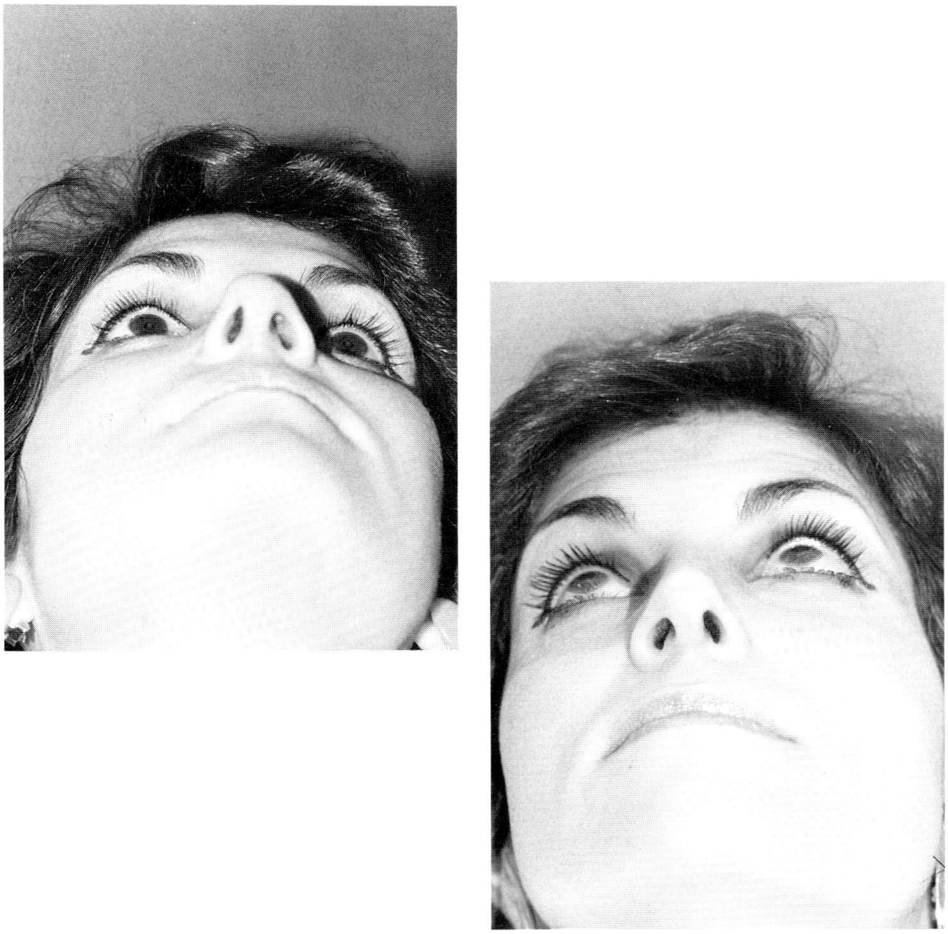

A B

Fig. 21-19. Tip asymmetry following severance of the dome. **A,** Preoperative. Treated with delivery technique and no morselization. **B,** Postoperative.

Pinched-Tip Deformity

The so-called "pince-nez" effect on an operated nose is caused by excessive removal of lower lateral cartilage and the inferior telescoping part of the upper lateral cartilage. This causes the nasal tip to have a pinched appearance. This is often associated with an overly projected thin tip. When the latter is the case, merely delivering the nasal domes and adjacent cartilages, morselization, and dropping the projection by removal of a cartilaginous section of medial crura usually cures the condition (Fig. 21-20). This procedure may fill in the pinch deformity with the excess skin and soft tissue borrowed from the tip.

In the more difficult repair, a marginal incision inferior to the lower lateral cartilage in the area of the collapse is made and the weakened area dissected. This separates the overlying skin from the chondrocutaneous flap. One or two layers of a permanent suture mesh, fascia, or thin cartilage is inserted much like a stiffening baton on a sail. This stiffens the overlying skin, providing support (Fig. 21-21).

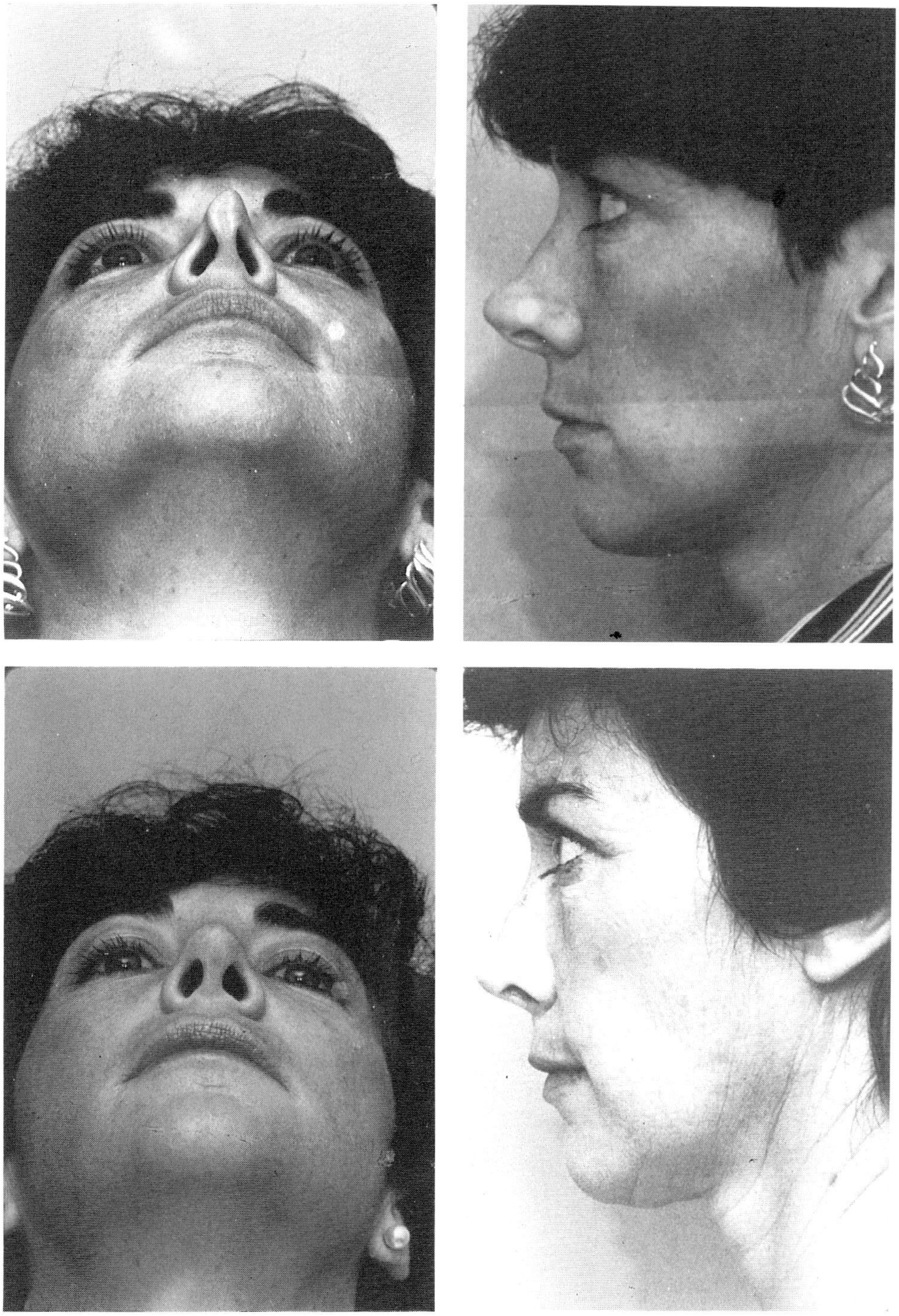

A B C D

Fig. 21-20. Excessive removal of lateral tip support while leaving too much projection. A and B, Preoperative. The tip projection was decreased, the cartilages morselized and repositioned. C and D, Postoperative.

Fig. 21-21. Excessive cartilaginous support removal with a tip collapse. **A** and **B**, Preoperative. Megarad bank cartilage used as a graft. **C** and **D**, Postoperative. (From Berman WE: Rhinoplasty, ed 2, Washington DC, 1984, American Academy of Otolaryngology-Head and Neck Surgery Foundation, Inc.)

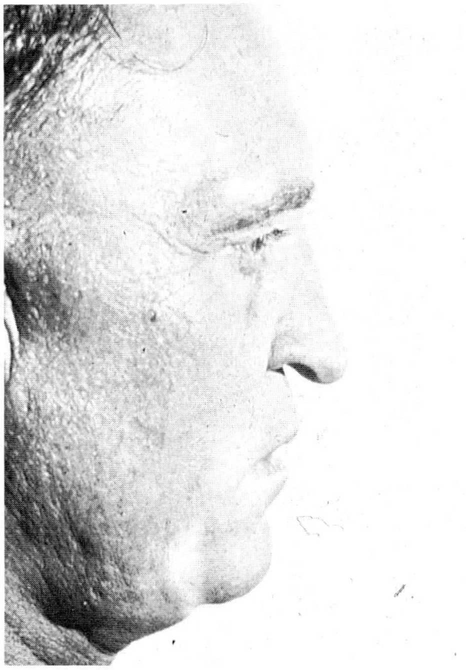

A

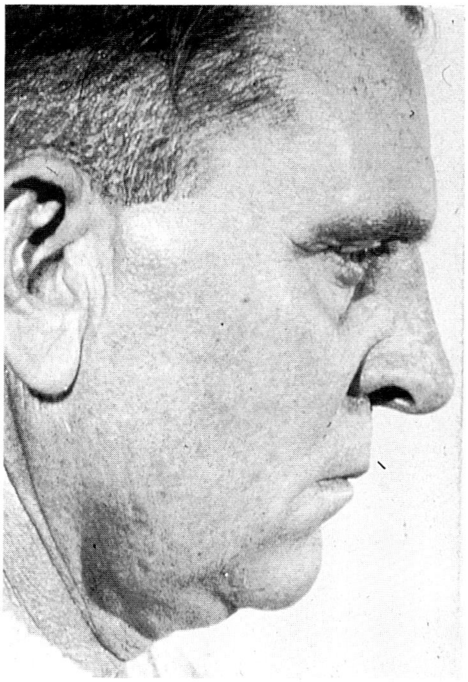

C

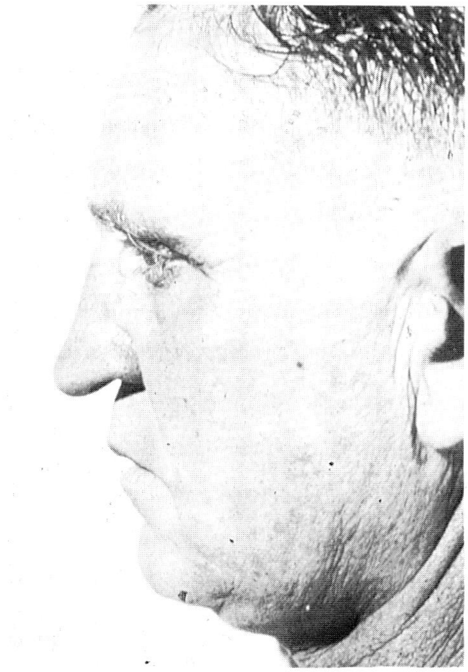

B

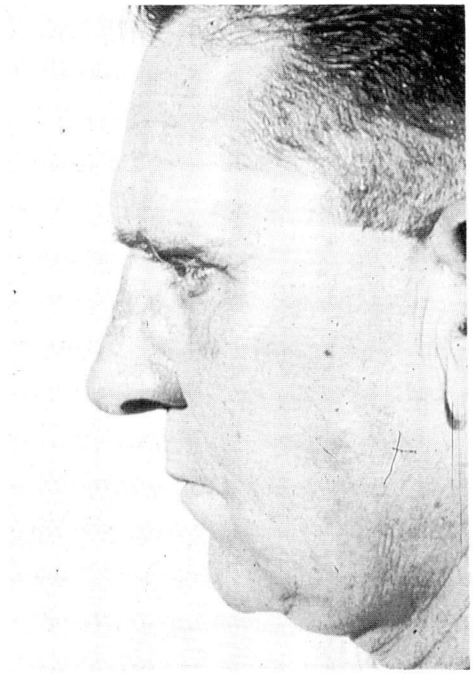

D

22

Secondary Rhinoplasty

Rodolphe Meyer, with the collaboration of Dominique M. Rheims and Louis O. Boileau

Everyone must bow to destiny. This dictum applies to every plastic surgeon, even the best, who by performing rhinoplasties will certainly be the purveyor of a certain number of cases that require a secondary rhinoplasty. If we begin by eliminating those cases arising as a result of trauma and those presenting after a surgical oncologic resection, we are left with two main groups whose indications for surgical intervention stem from either remodeling defects caused by aggressive or timid surgery, or secondary problems caused by excessive fibrosis and scarring. Only a precise topographic preoperative evaluation of such cases can guarantee a good functional and aesthetic result. We propose to study the various methods available to correct the many nasal deformities that may occur, realizing that these deformities are often interrelated and often require complex surgical techniques that call upon the experience of the surgeon.

Supratip Deformities

The so-called *pollybeak* is a frequent complication, always arising from a direct or indirect surgical error in the region of the weak triangle. Eight principal causes can be listed:
—insufficient reduction of the dorsal border of the septum
—insufficient reduction of the dorsal border of the upper lateral cartilages
—insufficient trimming of the mucoperichondrial lining
—excessive excision of the intranasal lining
—excessive resection of the alar domes
—a shortened columella left uncorrected
—under-evaluation of skin thickness
—a malpositioned nasal graft
Each of these requires specific treatment.

Insufficient reduction of the dorsal septal border must be corrected by resecting a cartilaginous wedge as per Lipsett's description, thus creating a notch in the supratip region. It is more important to ensure the presence of this depression when performing a secondary rhinoplasty as opposed to a primary rhinoplasty. A postoperative dressing left securely applied for at least 10 days maintains this depression. Patients presenting for primary rhinoplasty who have an aquiline nose with a short columella have an increased risk of developing some supratip convexity. To prevent or correct such a bird's beak deformity, one should augment the projection of the tip. In addition to performing the Lipsett depression, one should place a trapezoid or triangular graft in a meticulously dissected pocket that is separate from the supratip pocket from which fibrous tissue has been removed (Figs. 22-1 to 22-3). These onlay grafts were advocated by Eitner[4] and several other surgeons, the last being Meyer,[2] Sheen,[15] and Peck.[11]

Insufficient upper lateral cartilage reduction simply demands repeating the dissection of this area, with an additional excision of the deforming cartilaginous bands on both sides, after proper visualization of the cartilages. Sometimes insufficient elevation and trimming of the mucoperichondrial lining in the region of the lateroseptal angle results in a pollybeak deformity. Proper secondary treatment consists of reducing this mucoperichondrial "hernia" through an extramucosal dissection. This extramucosal access as advocated by Eitner,[4] Meyer,[2] Anderson,[1] Robin,[14] Pollet,[12] and Jost[5] has proved to be of prime importance in rhinoplasty and particularly in revision procedures. The lack of intranasal lining is more difficult to correct. A composite cutaneocartilaginous graft is often necessary after resection of the fibrous tissue.

As for the correction of an overly excessive resection of the alar cartilages, the secondary correction entails placing cartilage grafts in the appropriate area and holding them in place with trans-alar mattress sutures. The supratip appears unduly prominent in these cases because of the collapse of the alar cartilages, therefore it is really a pseudo-supratip deformity.

Fig. 22-1. To correct the polly beak deformity, the supratip pocket is emptied and the tip-lobule is filled with cartilage onlay to accentuate the double angle.

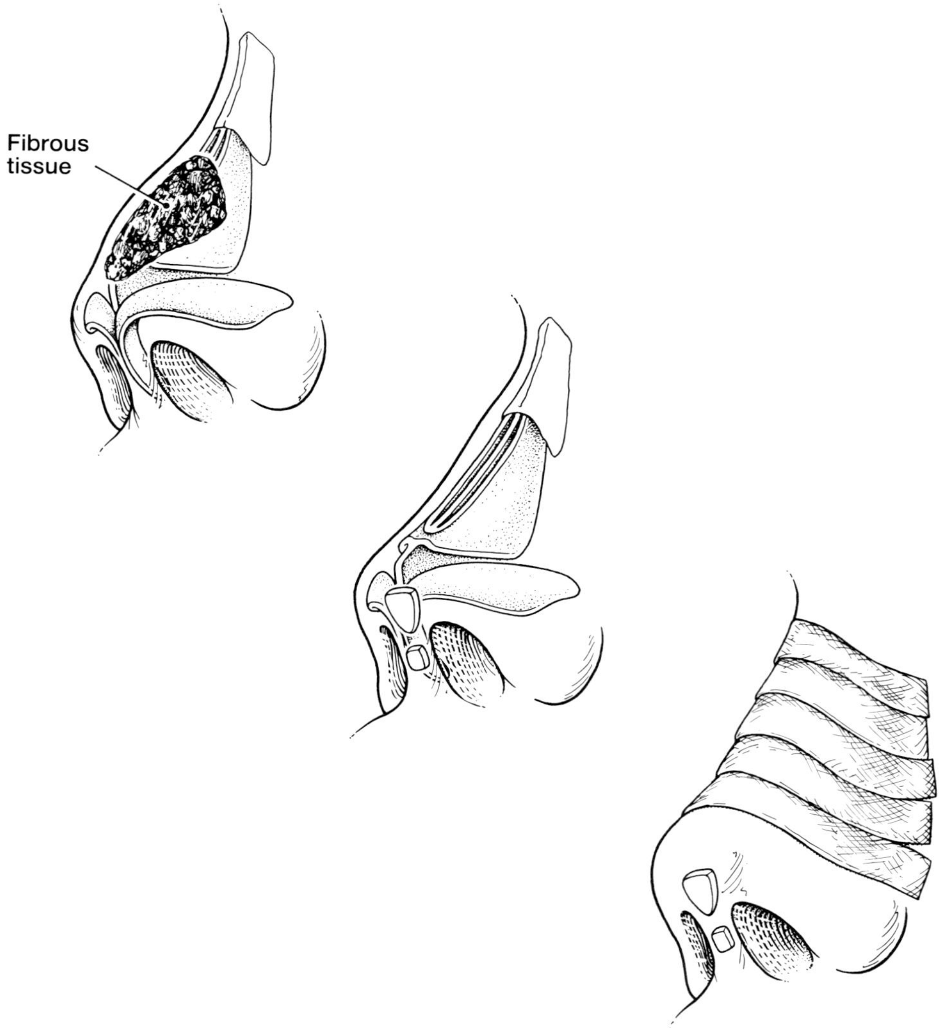

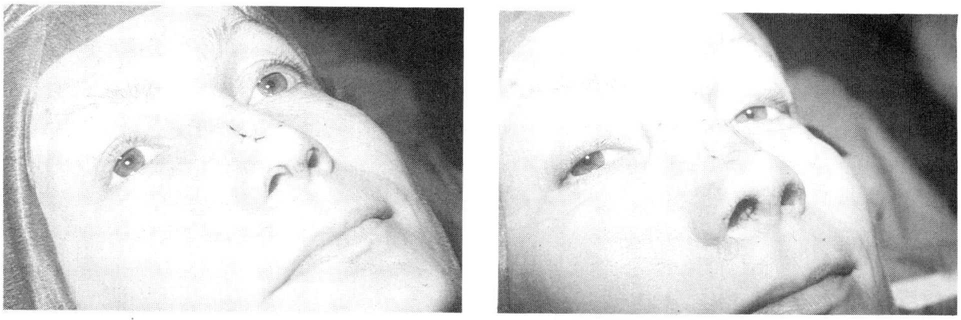

A B

Fig. 22-2. Patient with supratip convexity **A**, Before and **B**, After septal cartilage resection according to Lipsett, removal of fibrous tissue in the supratip area, and placement of a cartilaginous onlay in a tip-lobular pocket. The alar borders are reduced by marginal resections.

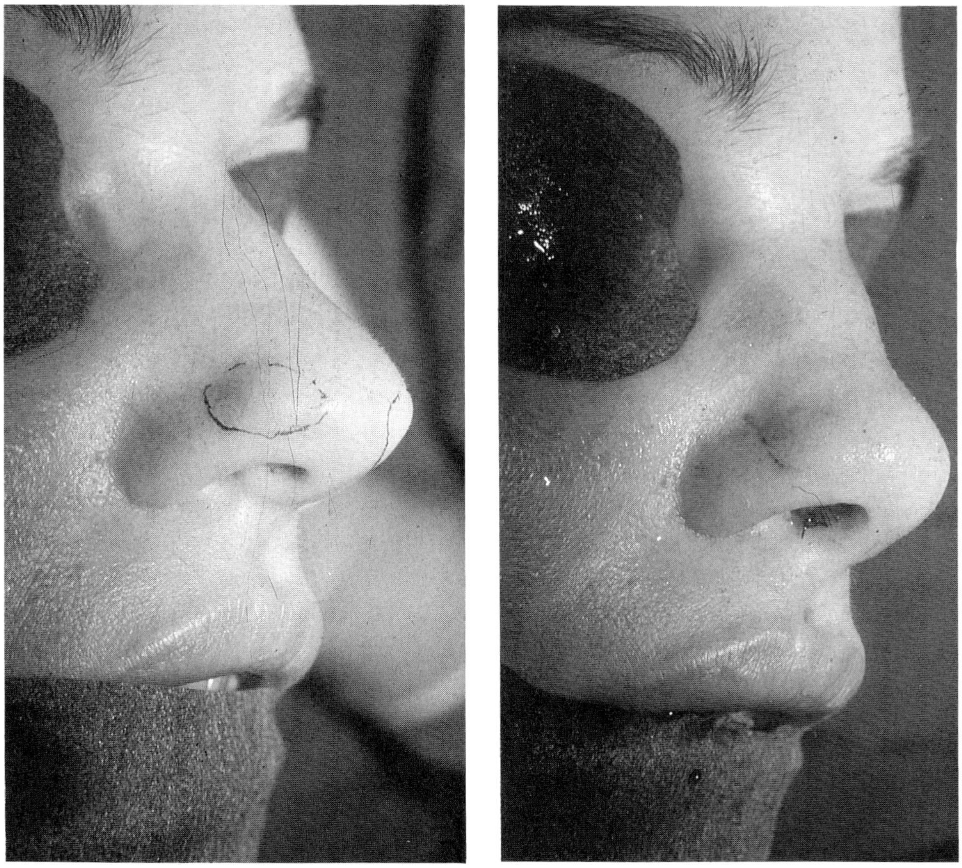

A B

Fig. 22-3. **A**, A nose seen preoperatively prior to tip-plasty and thinning of unusually thick skin in the region of the supratip. **B**, Postoperative appearance.

Excessively thick skin is often the cause of the polly beak deformity. If this is the case, one must cautiously thin the skin so as to remove the deforming fibrous and fatty tissue, but not to such a degree as to risk necrosis or furrow formation (Fig. 22-4).

Lastly, a dislodged dorsal graft is an obvious cause of the polly beak deformity. Correction demands removal of the graft, followed by its proper replacement with additional cartilaginous sculpturing if necessary.

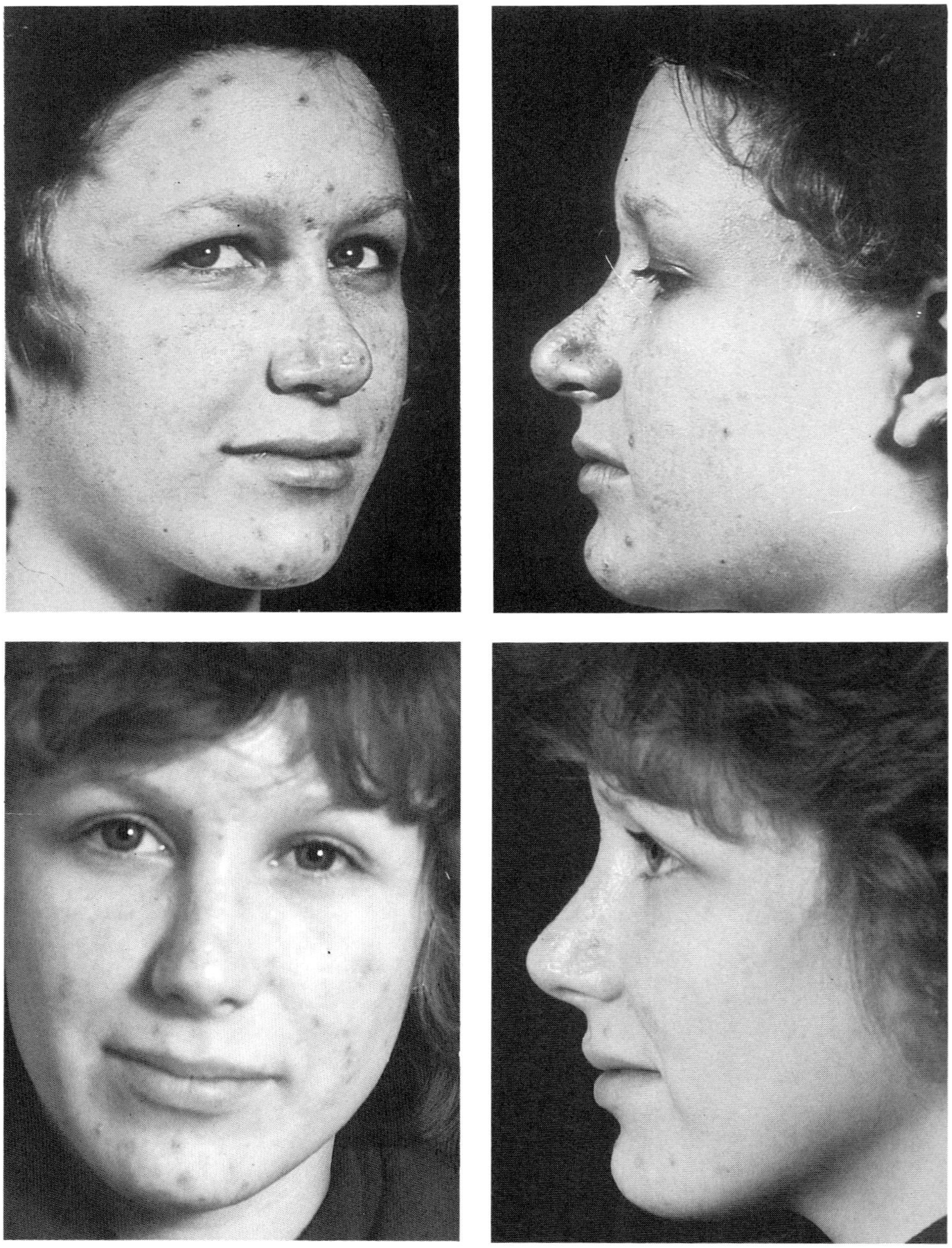

Fig. 22-4. Young female with thick acne skin before and after tip reduction with partial dome resection using the luxation technique. A plaster splint was left applied for two weeks.

Deformities of the Nasal Tip and Alae

Residual deformities of the nasal tip and nostrils are generally caused by faults in the sculpturing of the alar cartilages. In revision procedures, the recognized dissection techniques of primary rhinoplasties are used. The chief principle to be followed in these cases is to preserve the area of the soft triangle when combining an intercartilaginous incision with the infracartilaginous or transcartilaginous incisions.

Either one of the latter two incisions is chosen depending upon one's desire to expose the alar cartilage by a luxation (Fig. 22-5) or half retrograde approach or by an eversion or retrograde method when using only the intercartilaginous incision. In the more complex cases of reshaping nasal tip asymmetry, it is often preferable to carry out an external rhinoplasty using a Rethi[13] transcolumellar incision as this allows for easy access and excellent visualization of the alar dome area. There are eight types of secondary deformities of the nasal tip, which we classify as follows:

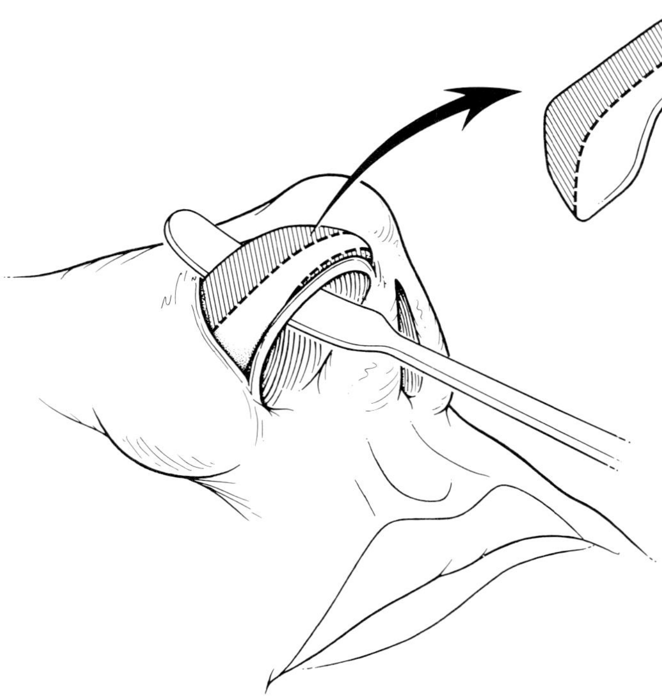

Fig. 22-5. Luxation technique. The bipedicle flap found between the intercartilaginous and the infracartilaginous incisions is delivered and rests on an elevator. The amount of cartilage that is usually resected is marked by crosshatches.

The Bifid and Broad Tip

The *bifid and broad tip* can be caused by an already present uncorrected bifidity that is only exaggerated after a primary rhinoplasty with its subsequent fibrosis, or may result after an excessive alar dome resection with subsequent scarring. To correct this deformity, all the fibrous tissue present between the two domes tending to splay these structures must be excised, followed by mattress suture placement that unites the two medial crura, thereby narrowing the tip. Scoring the cartilage may also be beneficial. If the tip still remains excessively broad, a small segment of cartilage may be resected from the dome medially (Figs. 22-6 and 22-7) and one or more cartilage grafts inserted to augment the projection and refine the tip (Fig. 22-8).

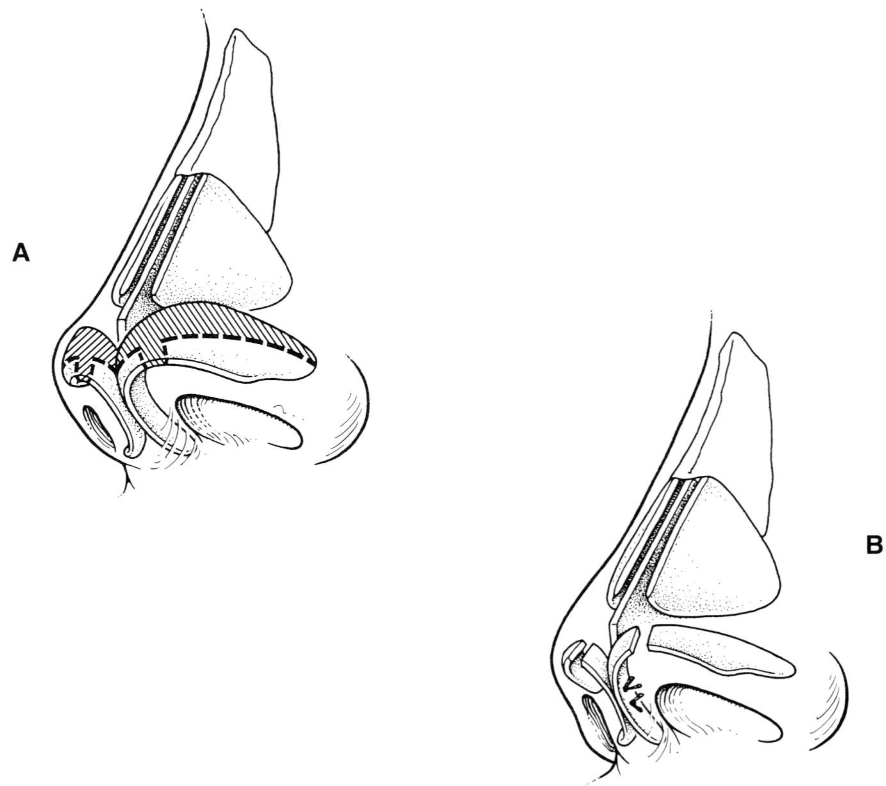

Fig. 22-6. For treating the broad tip the lateral crura may be sectioned at the dome and after resection of a segment at the dome (**A** and **B**) the medial crura are brought together with mattress sutures.

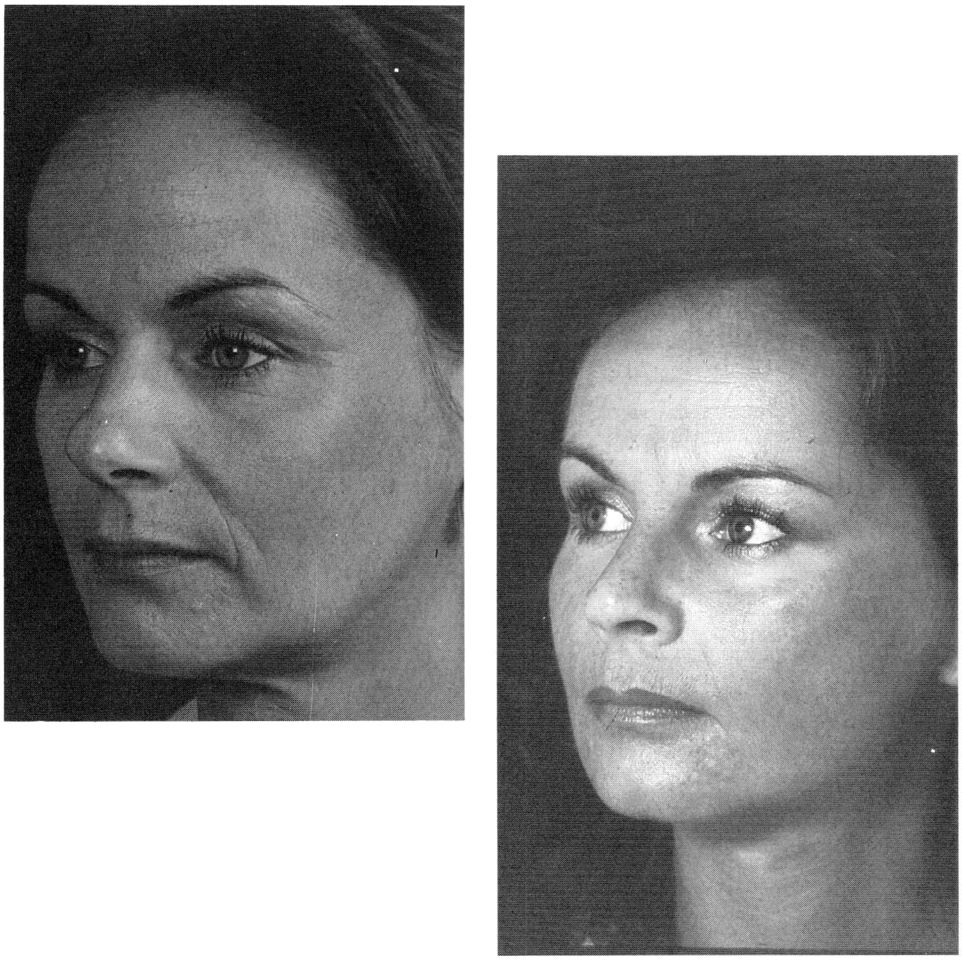

Fig. 22-7. Example of a broad nose with bifidity corrected with dome reduction seen before and after surgery.

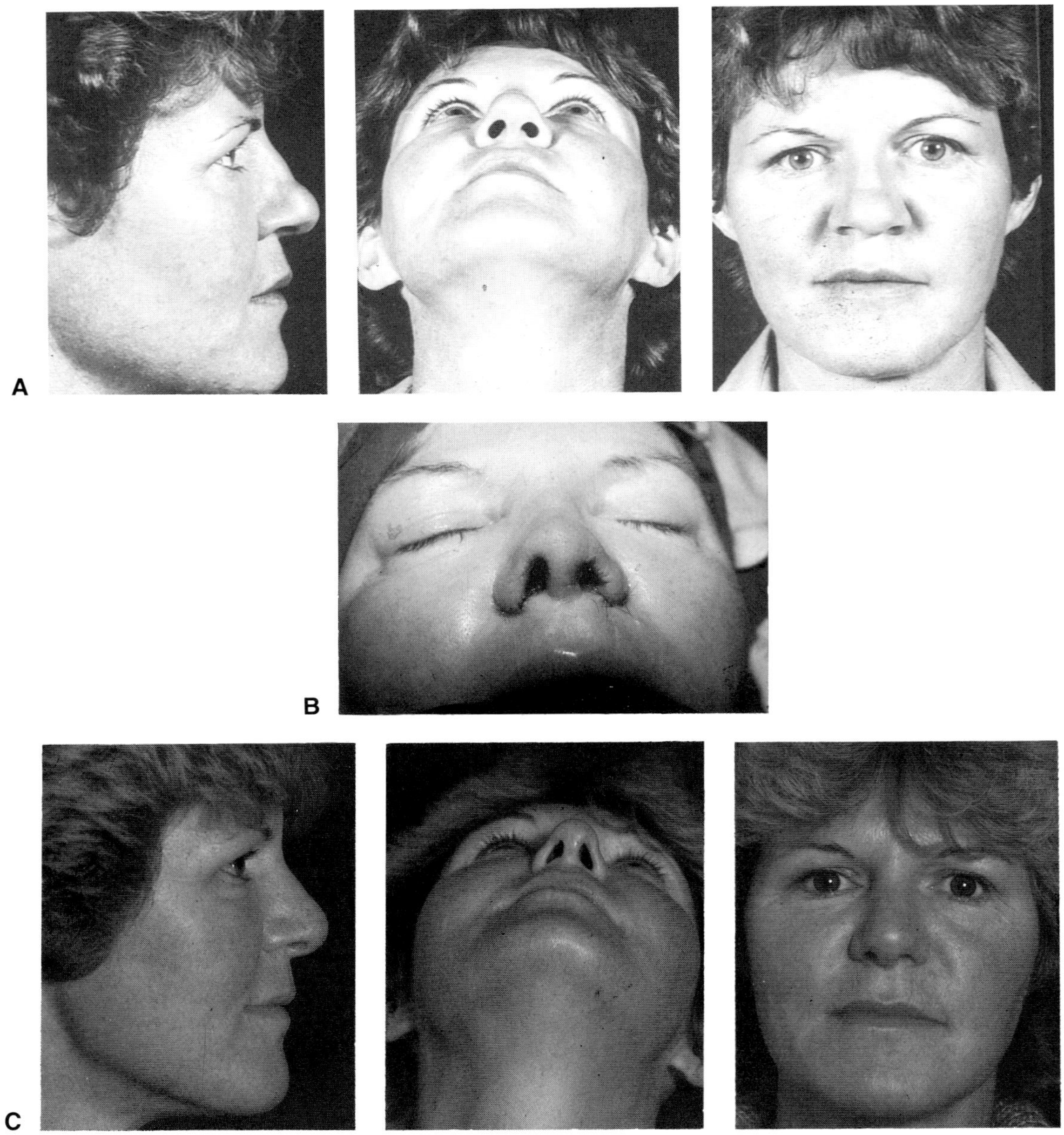

Fig. 22-8. **A,** Example of a broad, thick lobule. **B** Immediate postoperative appearance after tip-plasty with equilateral lower lateral cartilage reductions thinning of the skin, and marginal resections. **C,** Appearance 1 year postoperatively.

The Pinched Nose

The *pinched nose* is produced by an excessive resection of the lateral component of the lower lateral cartilages at the dome producing not only unpleasant aesthetic results but also functional embarrasment of normal nasal airflow. The continuity of the alar arch must be restored using cartilage grafts, held in place with mattress sutures. In cases presenting with concomitant alar retraction secondary to scar formation, the use of a composite graft from the ear may be indicated (Fig. 22-9).

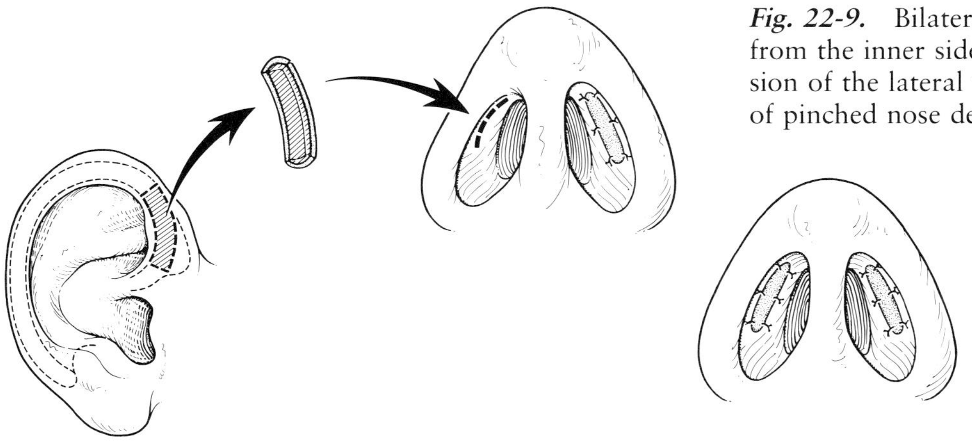

Fig. 22-9. Bilateral use of composite grafts from the inner side of the crus helicis for expansion of the lateral vestibular wall in severe cases of pinched nose deformity.

The Collapsed Ala

The *collapsed ala* stems from the same etiology as above, only in this case the entire alar cartilage is affected, narrowing the angle of the valve. It can be associated with collapse of the upper lateral cartilages increasing the valve deformity. Previously cited stiffening procedures with cartilage grafts are required to correct the flaccidity present (Fig. 22-10).

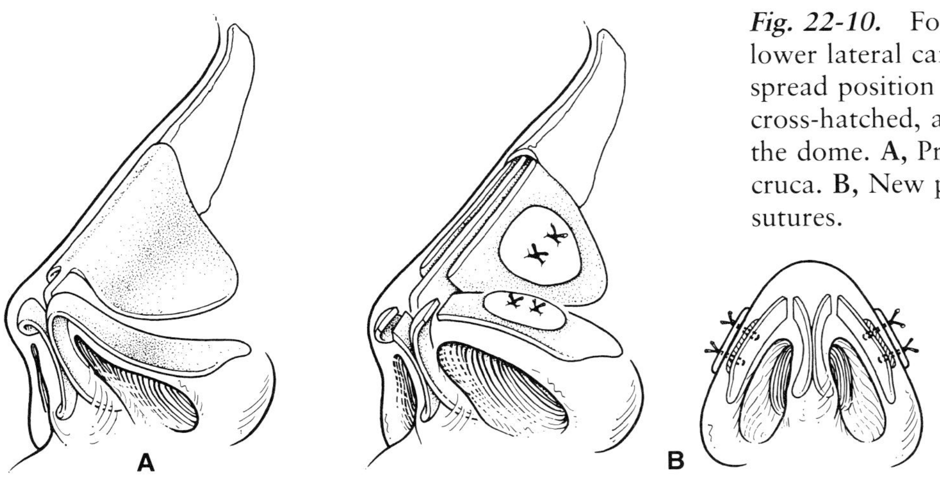

Fig. 22-10. For correction of collapsing ala the lower lateral cartilages are also fixed in a new spread position after being reduced, scored or cross-hatched, and if necessary cut vertically at the dome. **A,** Preoperative position of the lateral cruca. **B,** New position with trans alar mattress sutures.

The Retracted Alar Margin

The *retracted alar margin* is caused by a loss of tissue, usually of cartilage and vestibular lining. Treatment consists of placing a cartilage graft to fill the retraction pocket, followed by a local advancement of vestibular lining for coverage, or, if necessary, the addition of a skin graft. This local lining flap is elevated by placing an incision in the vestibule, parallel to the alar margin; the lining is then advanced and held in place together with the cartilage graft by means of one or two mattress sutures[7] (Figs. 22-11 and 22-12).

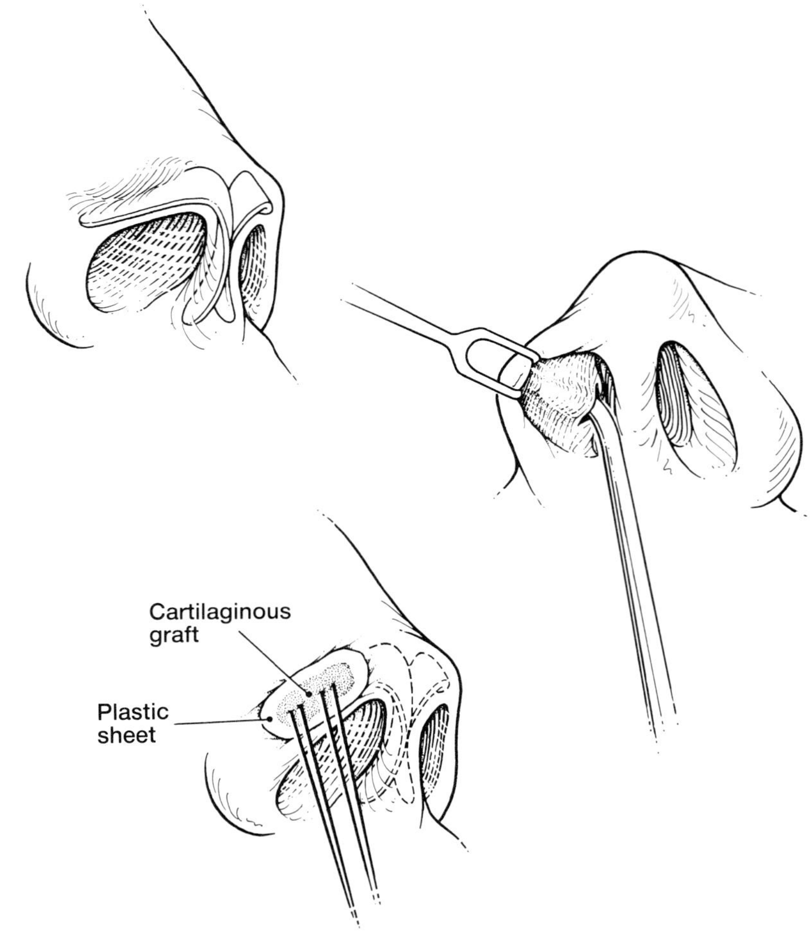

Fig. 22-11. For alar retraction one may lower the nostril border by dissecting a marginal pocket via an intercartilaginous incision, and then insert a cartilage graft, held in place with a trans alar matress suture taped to the upper lip.

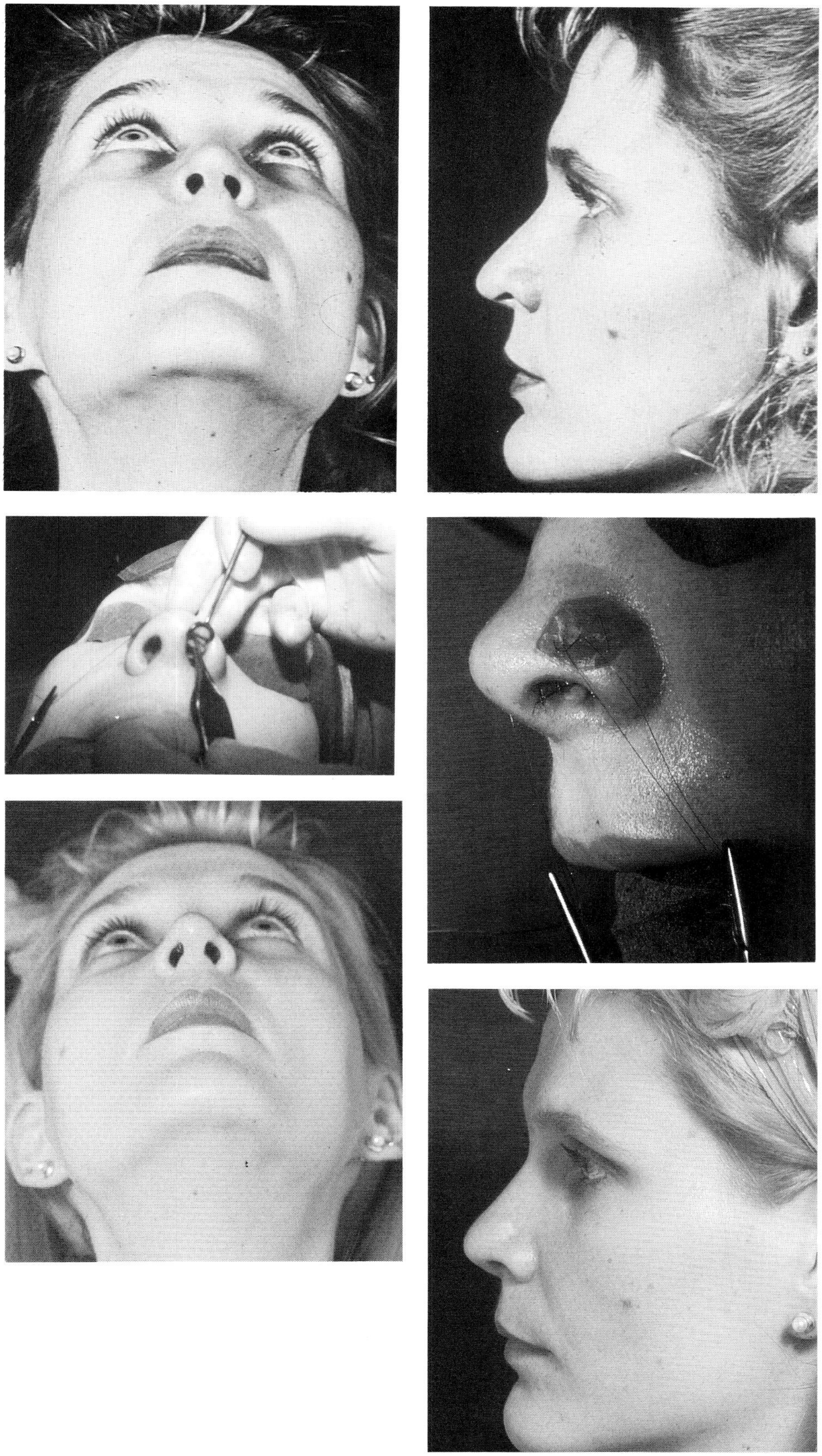

Fig. 22-12. **A,** Middle-aged female with retracted alar margins after primary rhinoplasty. **B,** Cartilage graft being inserted, and **C,** fixed in place with a mattress suture tied over a plastic sheet. **D** and **E,** Postoperative views showing the corrected alar retraction.

The Sagging Nasal Tip

The *sagging nasal tip* is also the consequence of a lack of cartilaginous support. Treatment consists of elevating and bracing the tip by means of a columellar cartilage strut combined with tip augmentation provided by a properly placed lobular onlay cartilage graft (Figs. 22-13 to 22-16).

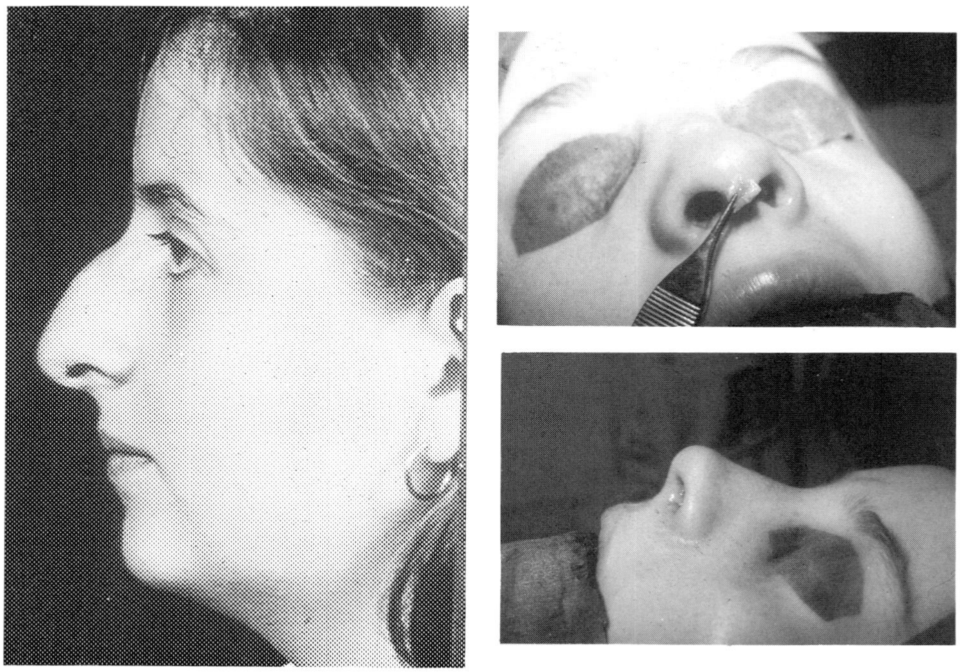
A B C

Fig. 22-13. **A,** A young girl with sagging nasal tip accompanied by a prominent dorsal hump. **B,** The cartilage graft to be placed in the lobule is shown. **C,** Postoperative appearance on lateral view with a restored double angle of the tip columella profile.

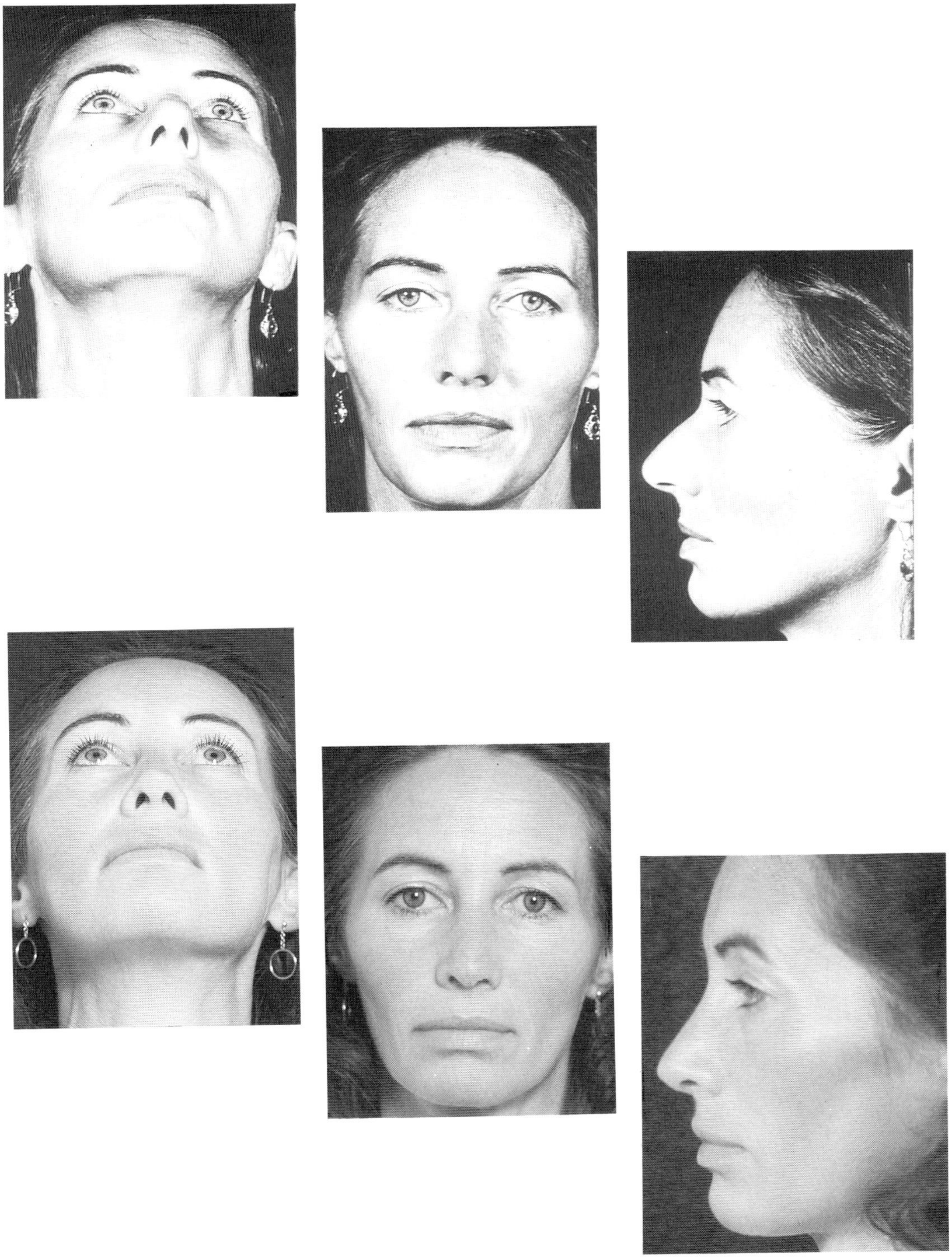

Fig. 22-14. In this young lady the double angle of the tip columella profile has been achieved with the appropriate placement of cartilage onlay grafts.

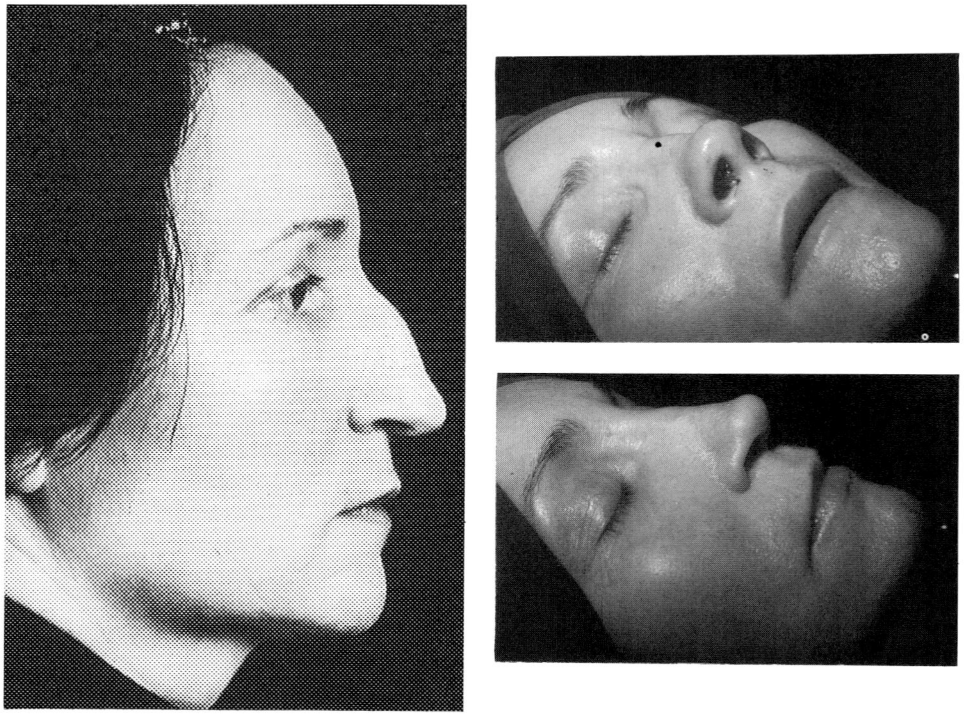

A B C

Fig. 22-15. **A,** This is an example of exaggerated tip sagging associated with a dorsal hump. **B** and **C,** Postoperative result after alar cartilage remodeling and cartilage graft insertion restoring tip projection.

Fig. 22-16. This diagrams what has been done in Fig. 22-15. The tip sagging was corrected by tip-plasty, which consisted of lower lateral cartilage remodelling and scoring, as well as the addition of a rolled ear cartilage graft to gain additional columellar support and tip projection.

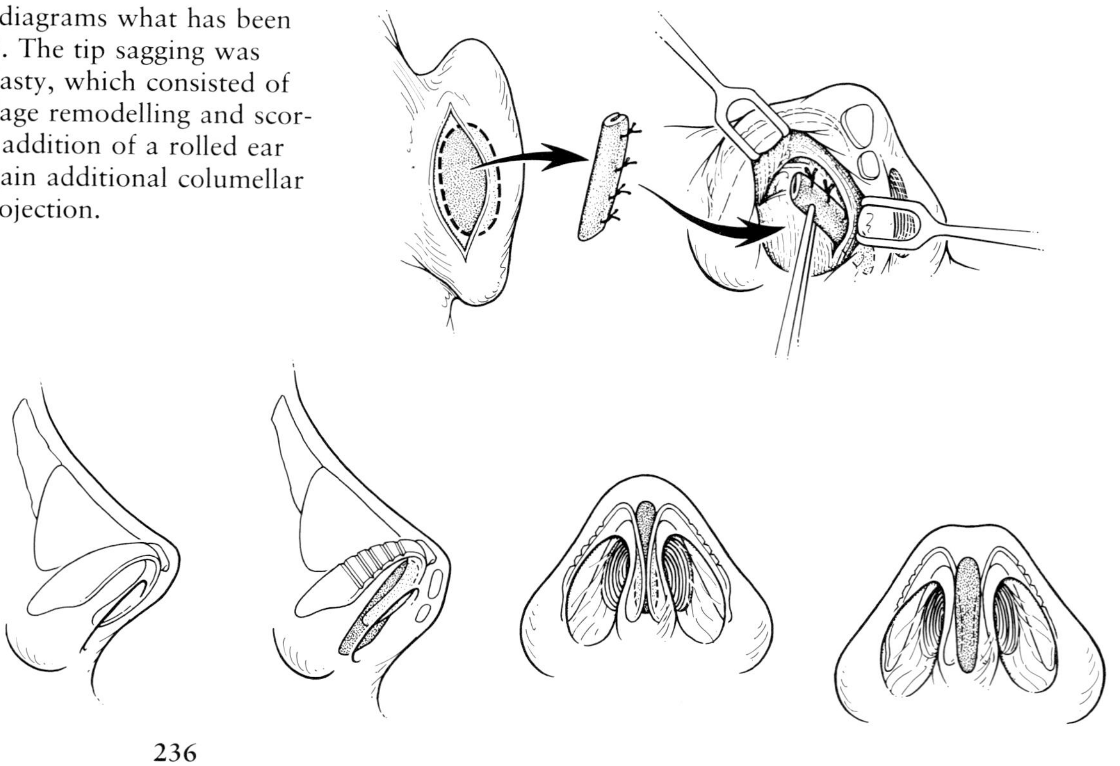

The Hanging Ala

Contrary to the preceding deformities, the *hanging ala* is caused by a tissue excess left after an imperfect nasal reduction, rather than by a deficiency of alar support. This excess tissue tongue hangs from the nostril border much like the wing of a bird. A marginal resection is the solution to this problem. This consists of removing the redundant alar border and restoring the more attractive symmetrical and harmonious curve. The resection margin is marked with a 15 scalpel blade and carried out carefully with a pair of curved sharp scissors. We meticulously close the reduced new open margin with 6-0 non-absorbable over-and-over sutures. Depending on the case, these marginal resections may be combined with thinning of the ala through the same incision and with alar base resections (Fig. 22-17 and 22-18).

The Pinocchio Nose

The *pinocchio nose* is caused by an excessive resection of the nasal dorsum with insufficient alar reduction resulting in the over-projection of the nasal tip. In the course of the secondary rhinoplasty one must adequately deliver the alar cartilages to provide the proper exposure for what at first seems to be an exceptionally timid resection of the alar domes. Any excess vestibular skin and a Lipsett flap must also be excised if required. Alar base resections may also prove beneficial. Even a horizontal skin strip resection at the columellar base may be indicated.

The Narrow Tip

The *narrow tip* can result from the preceding operation if the entire dome is excised. Treatment entails placing an oval or triangular cartilage graft composed of a columellar strut with a shell-shaped ear conchal graft sutured on top in the nasal lobule. If the loss of cartilage is severe, such an umbrella graft if indicated. In easier cases the shell graft suffices.

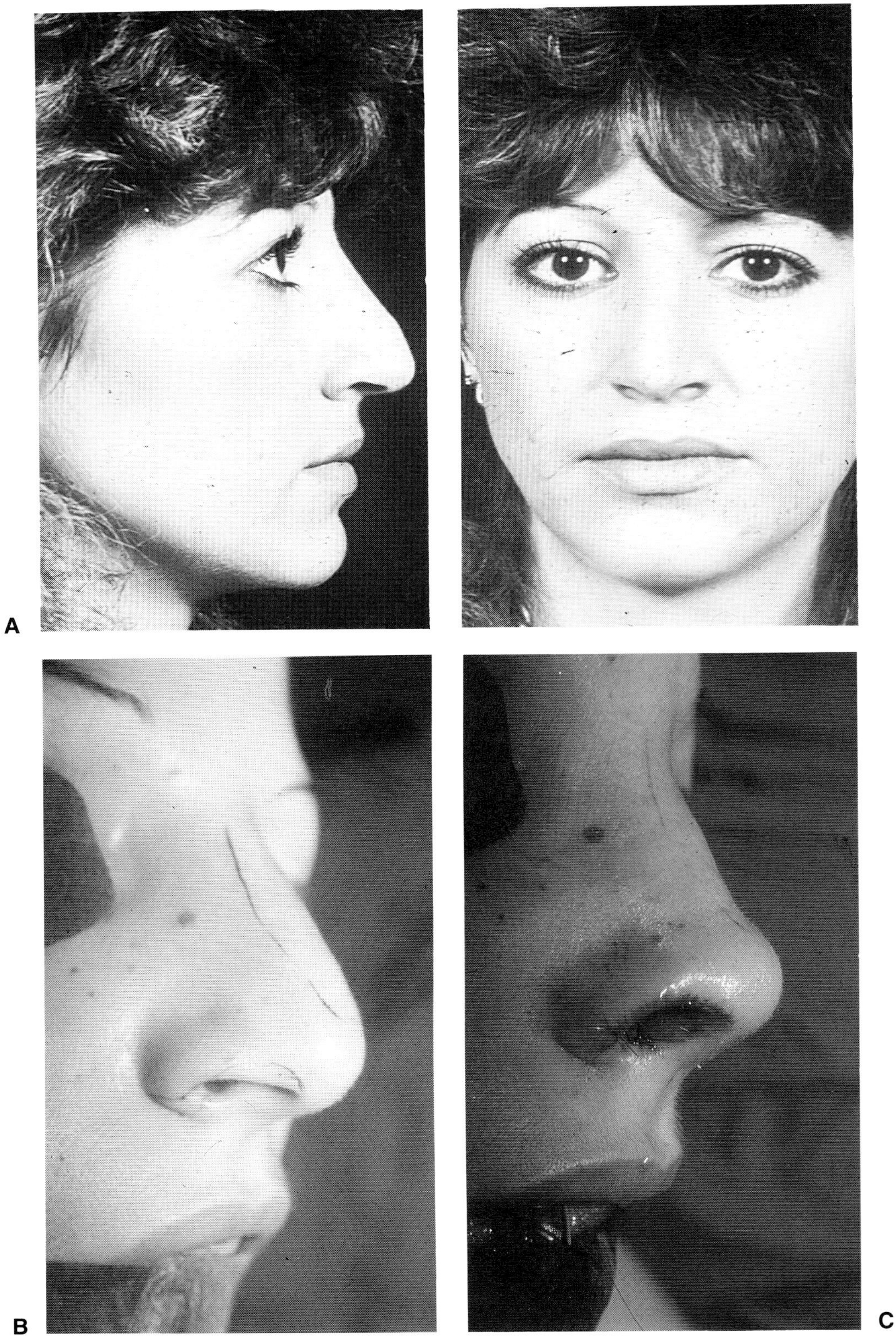

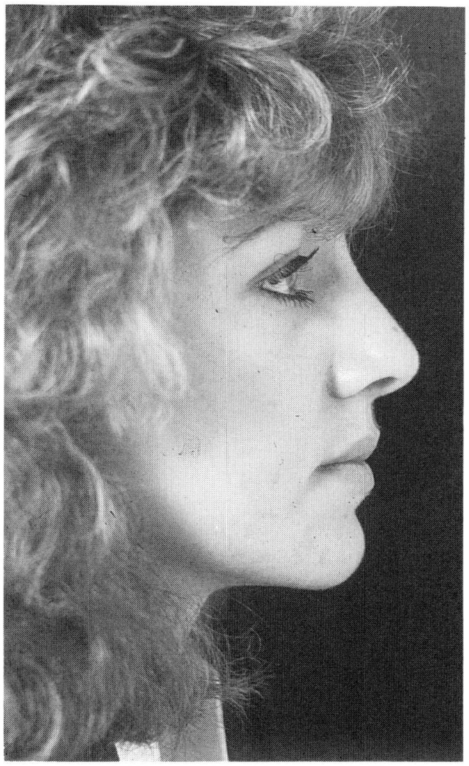

D

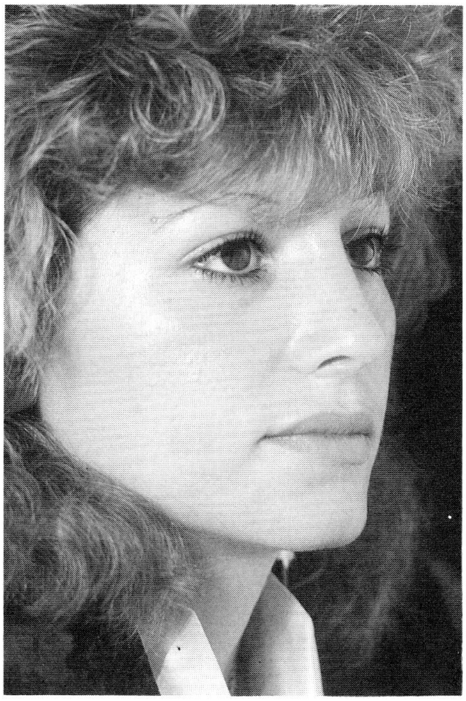

E

Fig. 22-17. A, Hanging alar borders are well demonstrated in this female patient. B, Operative markings of the bilateral marginal resections combined with dorsal hump excision. C, The nose immediately at the end of the operation with the marginal wound meticulously closed using 6-0 monofilament suture. D and E, The final result obtained.

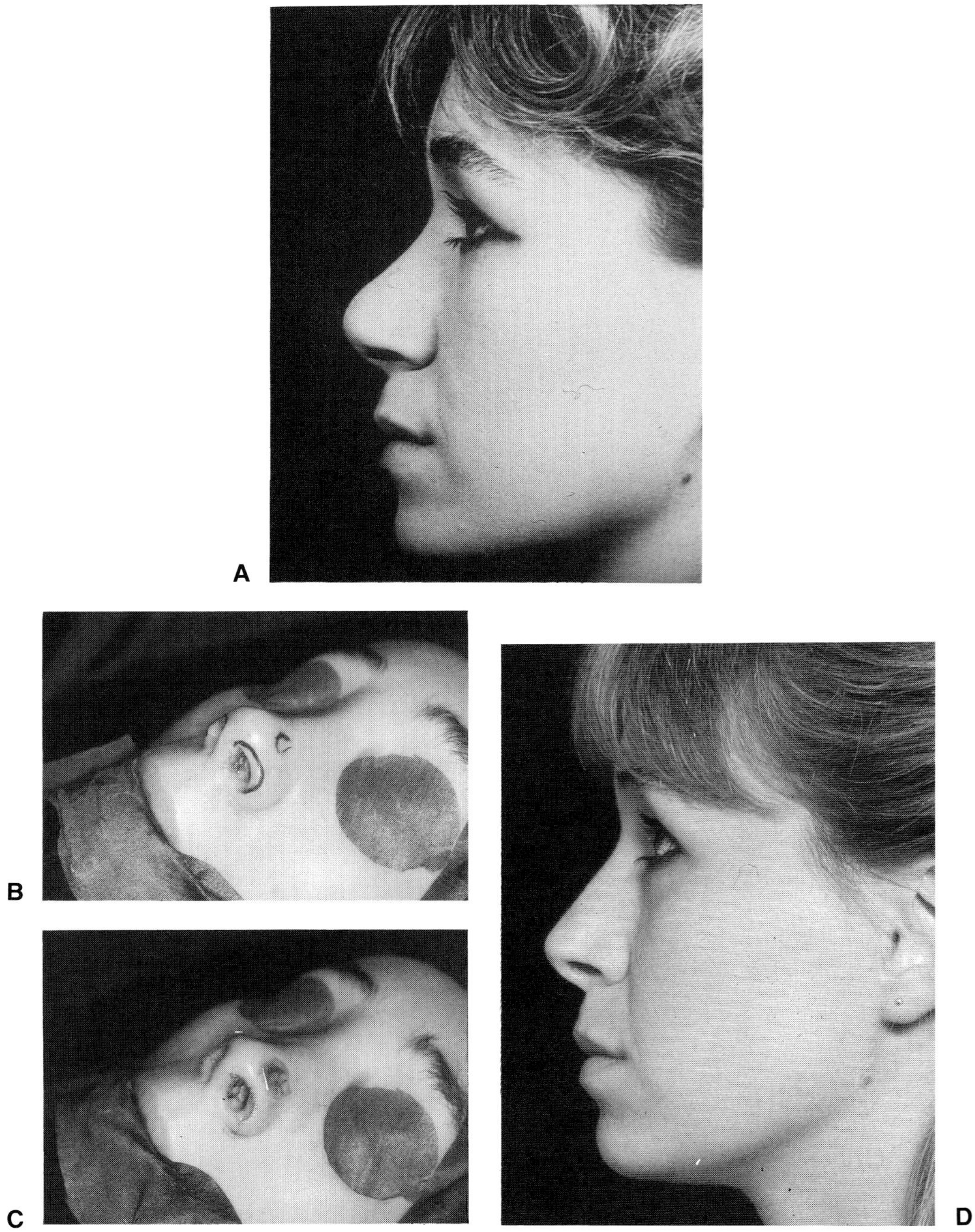

Fig. 22-18. **A,** Hanging ala as a result of a failed primary rhinoplasty well demonstrated. **B,** The preoperative markings; the circle outlined represents a zone of alar collapse. **C,** Operative appearance after marginal resections. Note the fine suture line of over-and-over 6-0 non-absorbable suture. The plastic sheet seen was used to hold a cartilage graft placed to correct the partial alar collapse. **D,** Lateral appearance post-operatively.

Deformities of the Columella

Columellar deformities arising from a primary septo-rhinoplasty may cover a wide spectrum, from a simple asymmetry of the height of the columello-alar angle to the more involved problems of the hidden columella or its corollary, the hanging columella. Asymmetries of height of the columello-alar commissure are simply corrected and balanced by a marginal resection. In certain cases, a marginal resection may be used extensively and bilaterally to actually lengthen the columella (Fig. 22-19).

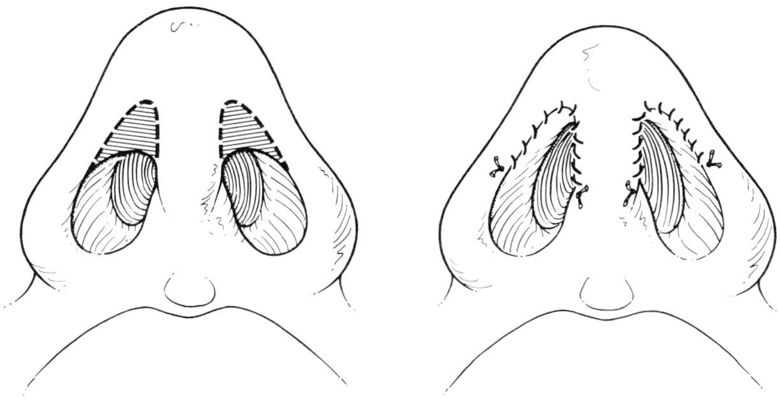

Fig. 22-19. Bilateral marginal resection at the alar columellar commissure (soft triangle of Converse) is readily used to correct a too-short columella.

Hanging Columella

To discover the cause of a *hanging columella* demands a full analysis of the possible contributing structures that may be involved. On one hand, it may be caused by a relative excess of septal length with or without an accompanying anterior bowing of the medial crura. Resection of these elements, as well as a segment of vestibular skin the length of the columella, will correct such cases (Fig. 22-20). On the other hand, retraction of the nostril borders may give the illusion of a hanging columella; in such cases one must reconstruct and repair the retracted alar margins and not carry out a reduction on the columella.

A

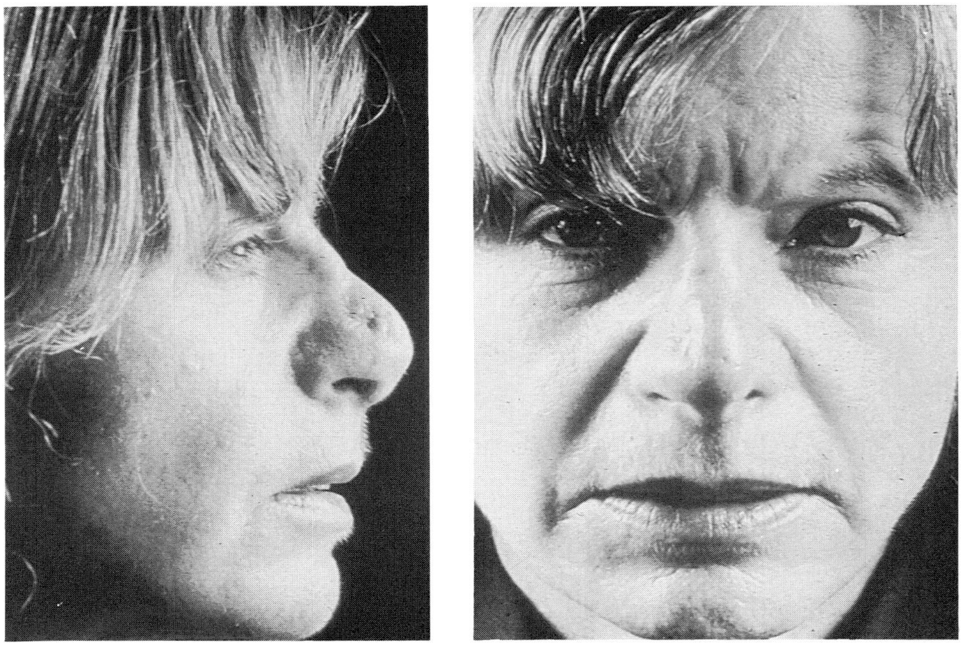

Fig. 22-20. **A**, An example of a poor result with a hanging columella both in the frontal and lateral views. **B**, Planned marginal resections, including portions of the widened columella anteriorly, (as well as vertical segments of vestibular lining and septum posteriorly). **C** and **D**, Postoperative appearance. **E** and **F**, Final result seen after 1 year.

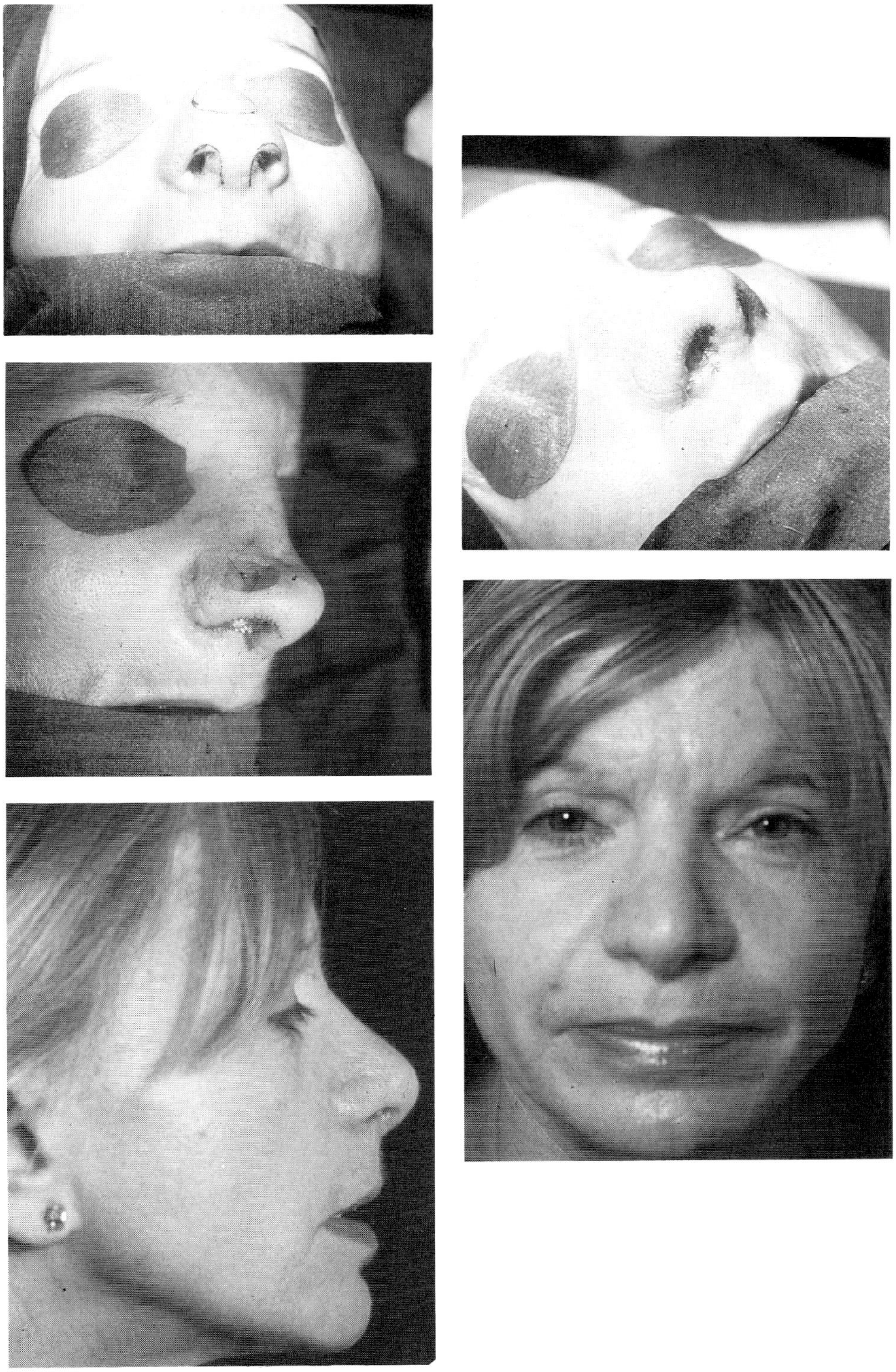

B C D E F

Hidden Columella

The *hidden columella* may result from an over-resection of either the caudal border of the septum or of the vestibular skin located in the same region. The method of correction to be used depends upon the degree of the deformity. In the more basic cases, insertion of a cartilage graft immediately anterior to the remaining caudal border of the septum will allow the columella to "fall" back into its normal position (Fig. 22-21). In cases of vestibular skin insufficiency, a skin graft or possibly a composite skin-cartilage graft may be indicated.

A

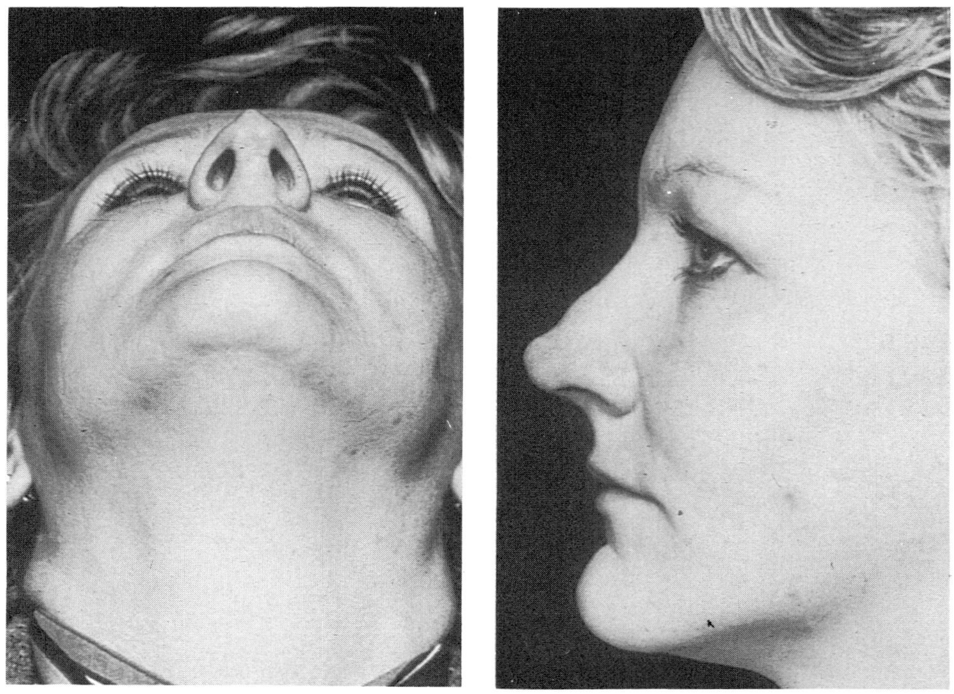

Fig. 22-21. A, This lady had a columellar silicone implant inserted and now presents with an unsightly dorsal projection, as well as a hidden columella. B, Operative markings. C, The silicone implant being removed. D and E, Postoperative result with a smooth dorsal profile and restitution of the columellar projection with cartilage grafts. F and G, Final result.

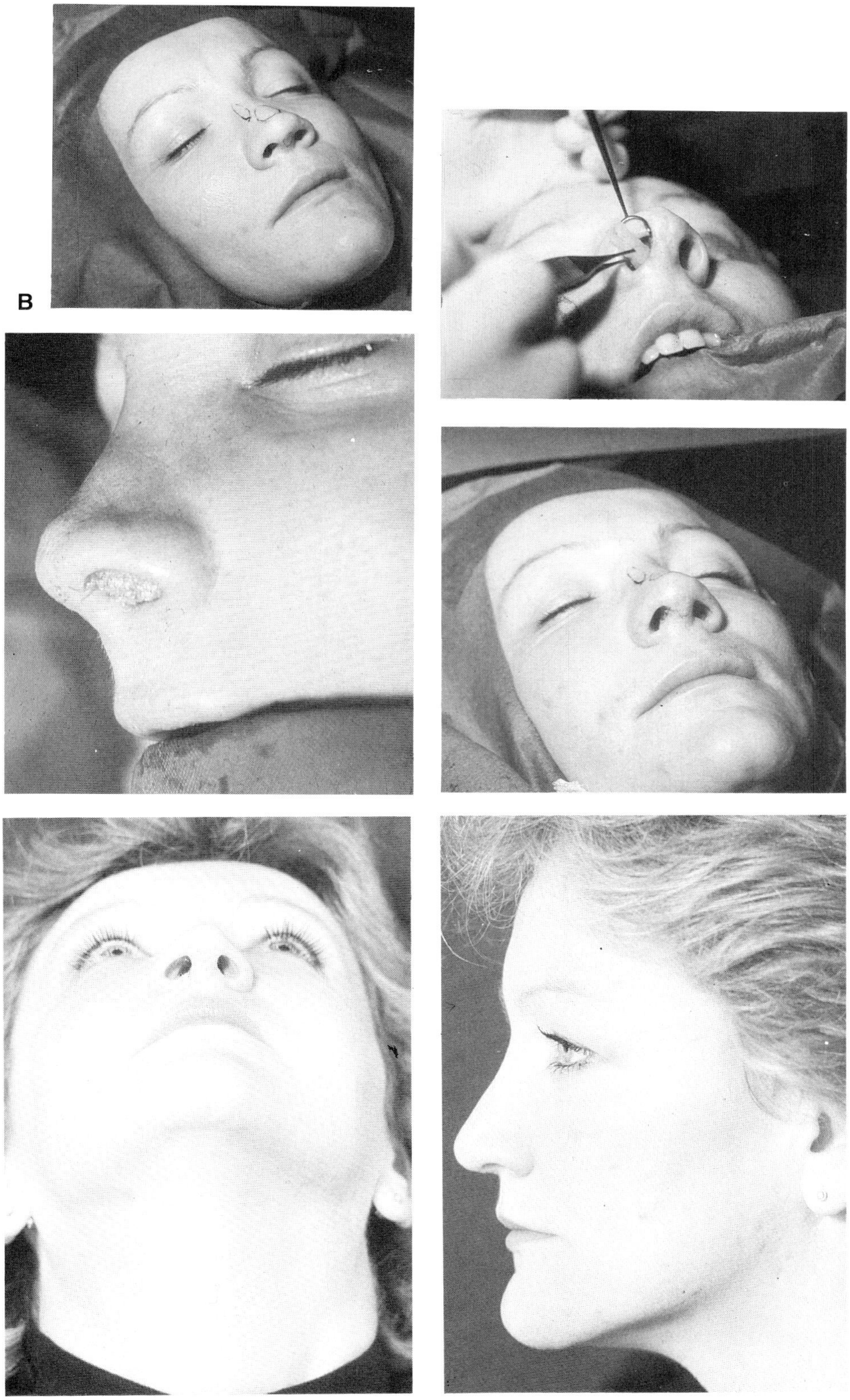

B C D E F G

Another common cause of a retracted columella is the deviated septum, the deflection of the caudal septum directly pulling back on the columella, resulting in a pseudo-hidden columella (Figs. 22-22 and 22-23). Certain cases of columellar retraction and distortion caused by partial resection of the medial crus or by fibro-cicatricial sequelae may justify using the external rhinoplasty technique of Rethi.[13] Such an exposure provides direct visualization of the columellar region, allowing the surgeon to see precisely the area of concern. It also provides a ready access for the insertion of a cartilage graft between the two medial crura if additional columellar support is needed. Additionally, this transcolumellar approach is perfect for complementary fibrous tissue excision along the columella or even V-Y columellar advancement if elongation is necessary.

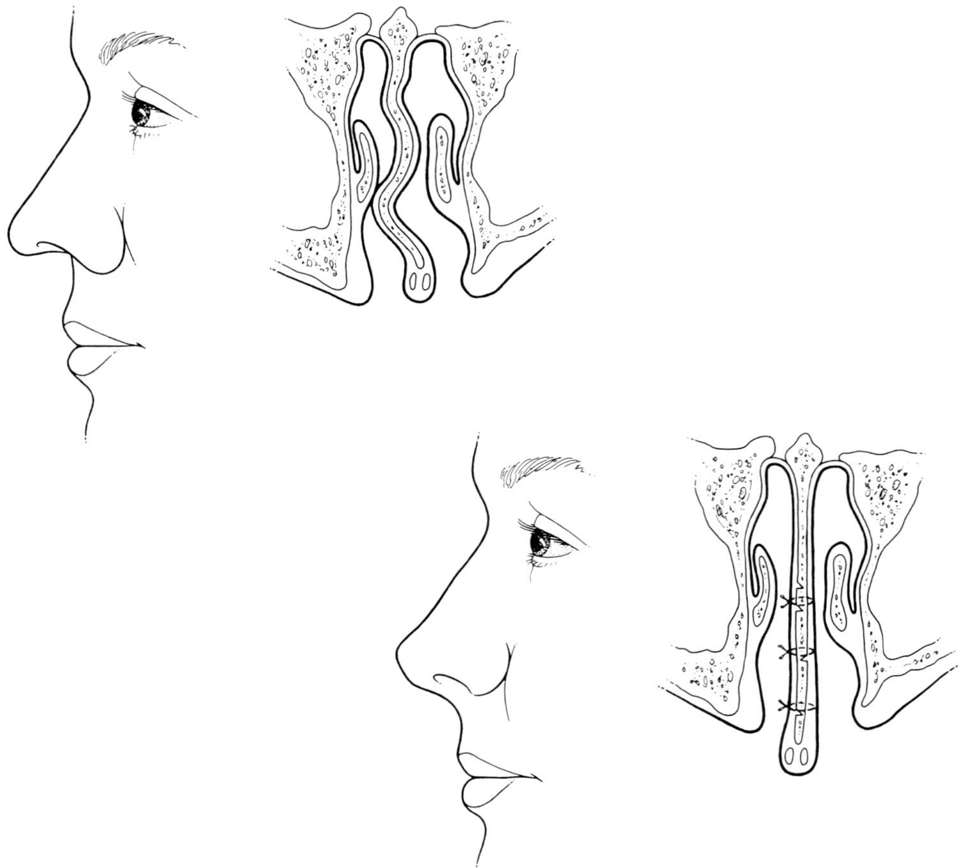

Fig. 22-22. A retraction of the columella can be produced by a severe caudal anterior deviaton of the septal cartilage.

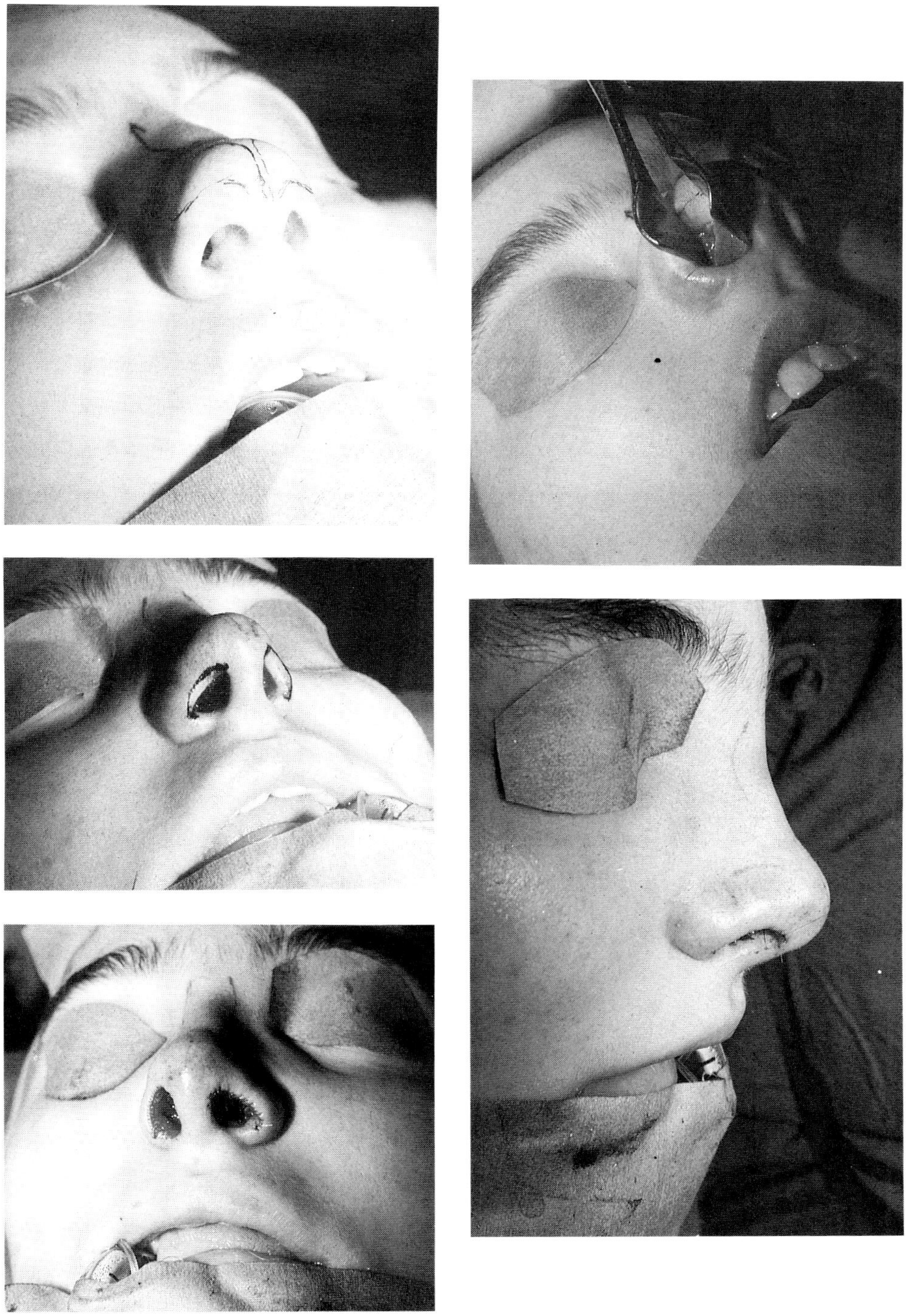

A B C D E

Fig. 22-23. **A,** This patient exhibits the deformity of the columella shown in Fig. 22-22 secondary to deviation of the septum. **B,** Correction of the septum. **C, D,** and **E,** Tip modelling and alar border resection have also been performed.

In certain cases of major columellar retraction it is possible that the entire nasal lobule becomes somewhat dislocated, conferring a pig-snout look to the nose. To correct such a complication, one has to lengthen the nose by sliding the septal mucoperichondrium and mucoperiosteum toward the columella, sectioning the mucoperiosteum obliquely as far posterior as possible. A cartilage graft from the posterior aspect of the septum is then placed at the anterior-inferior border (Fig. 22-24). As for the nasal skin, it is much more easily distended downward and forward. The final remodeling is then fixed in place with transfixion mattress sutures (Fig. 22-25). In extreme cases of columellar retraction the loss of tissue can be filled with one-stage bilateral gingivo-labial flaps covering the advanced quadrangular plate or a cartilage graft placed in the anterior apposition.

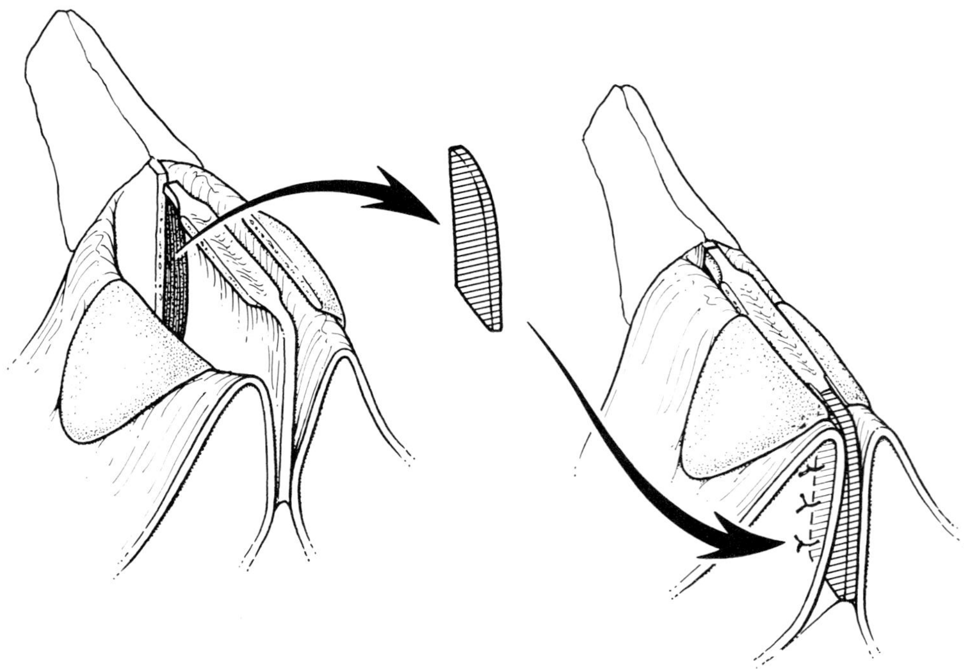

Fig. 22-24. For severe columellar retraction or the "pig-snout" deformity, the mucoperichondrium can be advanced forward using the extramucosal technique, with a strip of posterior septal cartilage transfered anteriorly to lengthen the nose. The dorsal ridge of the donor area should be cut narrowly in order to prevent saddling in that region.

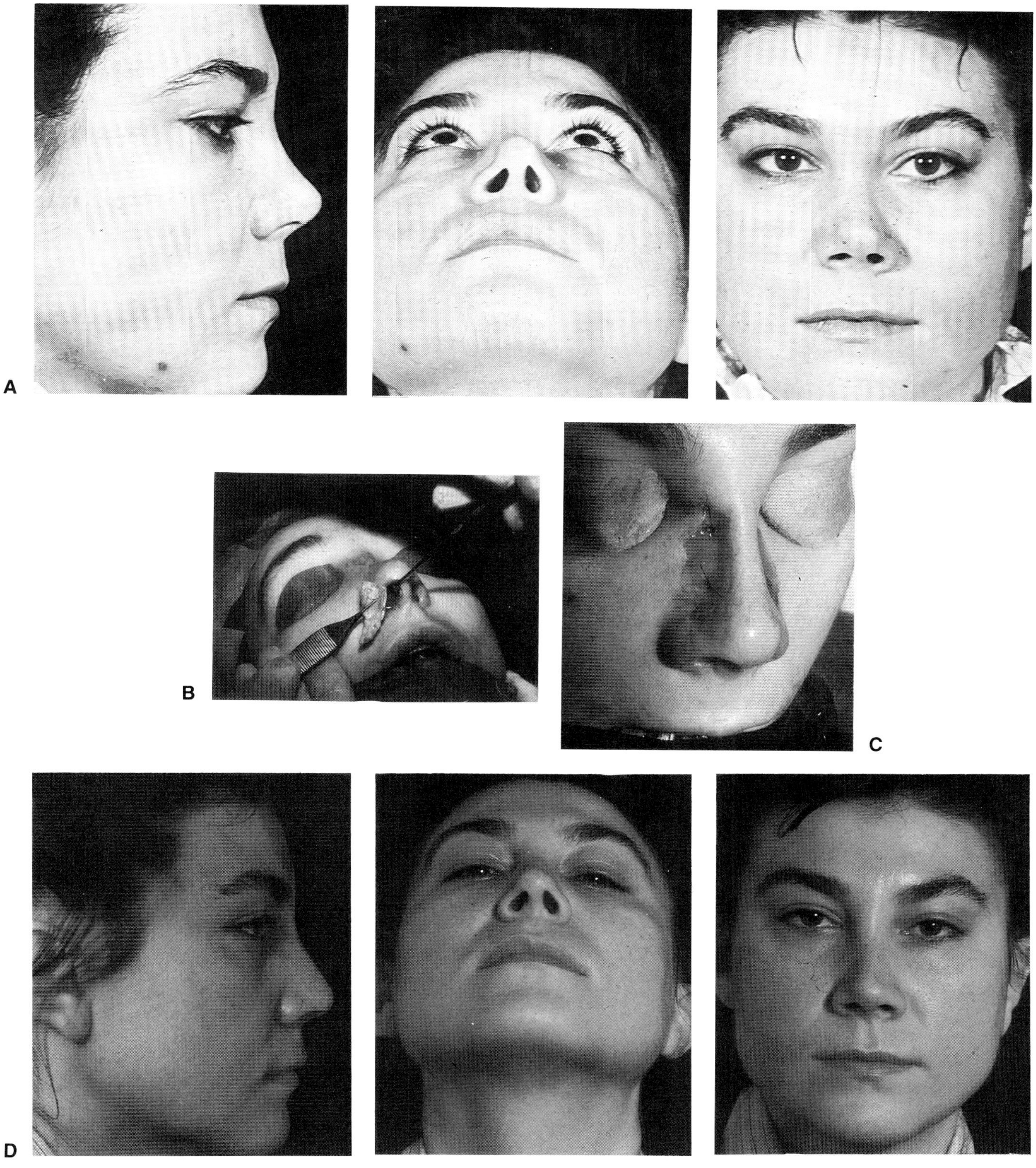

Fig. 22-25. **A**, Pig-snout nose with retracted columella making the nostrils excessively visible when the patient is viewed frontally. **B**, Two auricular cartilage grafts sutured together are about to be inserted to lengthen the nose and project the columella. **C**, Postoperative view after additional osteotomies with transnasal mattress suture placement. **D**, Appearance 1 year later.

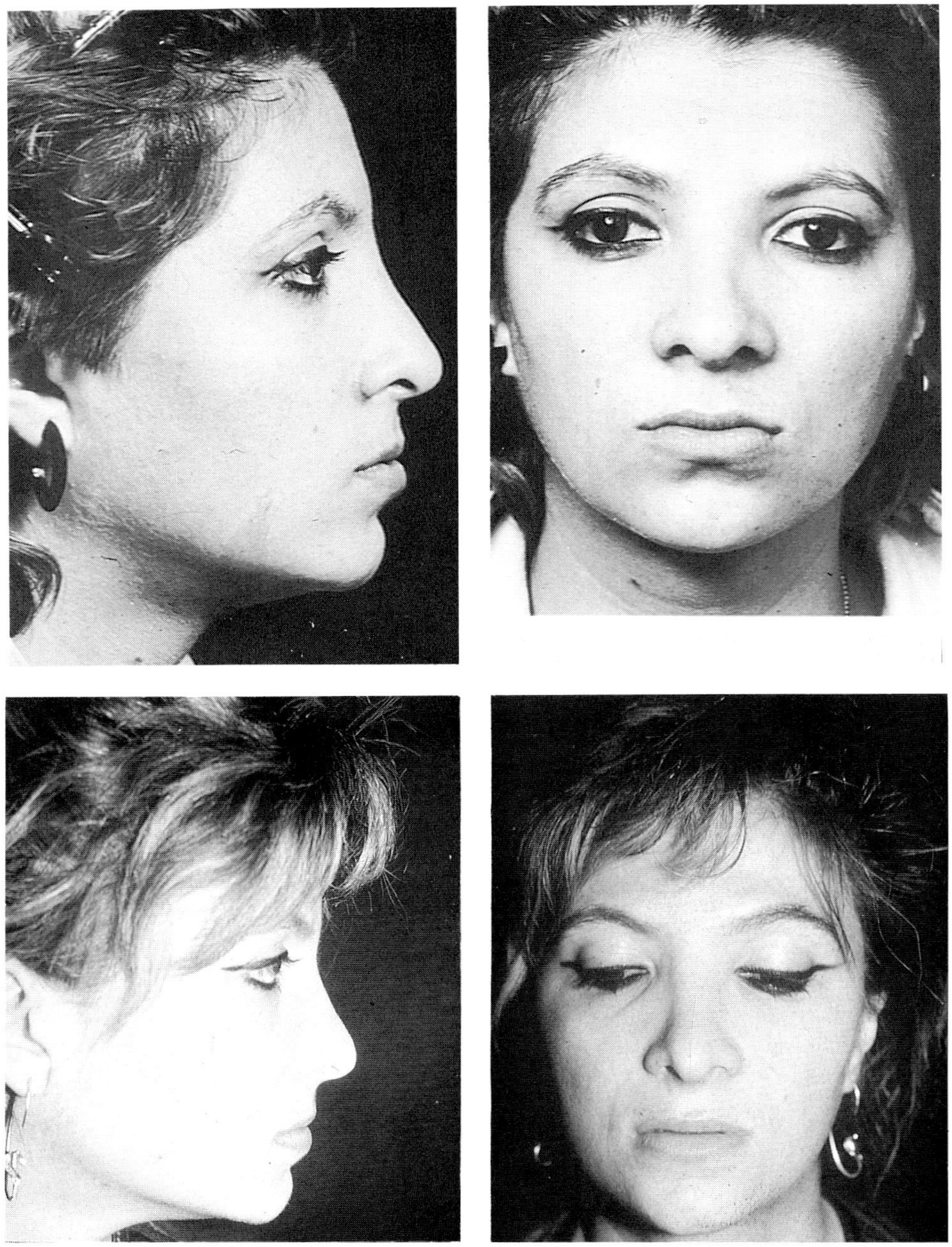

Fig. 22-26. A, Obtuse nasofrontal angle present. B and C, Result obtained after bony resection and deepening of the angle.

Secondary Osseous Deformities

These deformities result from errors in both the placement of the osteotomies and in the manual modeling of the pyramid. We distinguish between minor and major deformities.

Minor Deformities

These deformities are essentially irregularities of the osseous pyramid. Dramatic results may be obtained with small additions or resections of bone such as seen in Fig. 22-26 where the naso-frontal angle has been deepened. Along the line of the lateral osteotomy, one may sometimes find a step-deformity that a second osteotomy, carried out deep to the step, will readily correct (Fig. 22-27). A similar deformity may be encountered secondarily at the transverse osteotomy. To treat this the osteotomy needs to be redone (Fig. 22-28). Irregularities of the nasal dorsum can be treated with the rasp, followed by meticulous aspiration. As for residual dorsal humps, treatment should follow the steps common to a primary rhinoplasty.

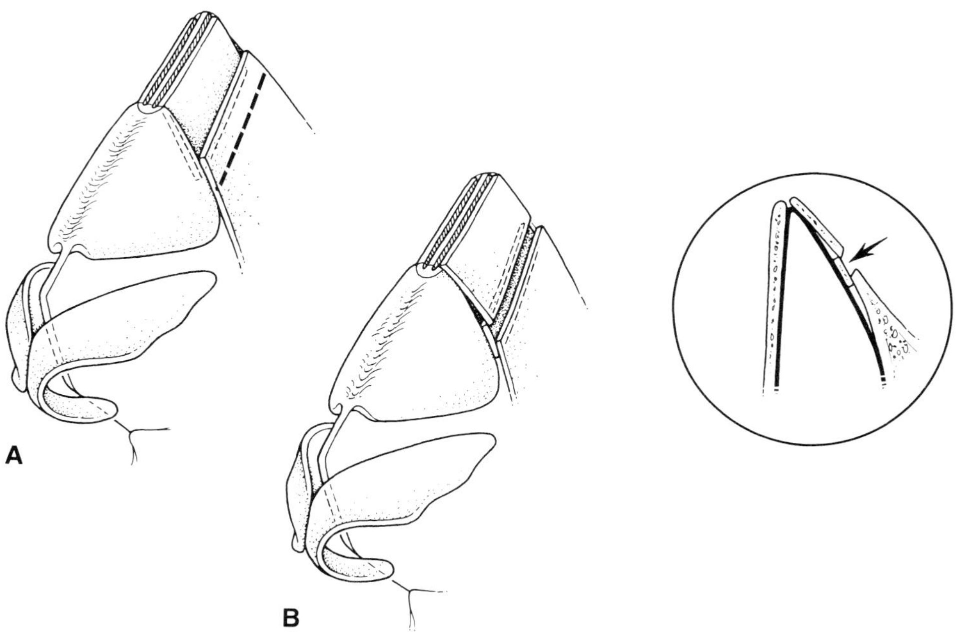

Fig. 22-27. With a palpable step at the lateral osteotomy line a repeat osteotomy should be undertaken. **A**, Outline of the new osteotomy. **B**, New osteotomy shown in section view. The resultant strip of bone is then pushed towards the lumen.

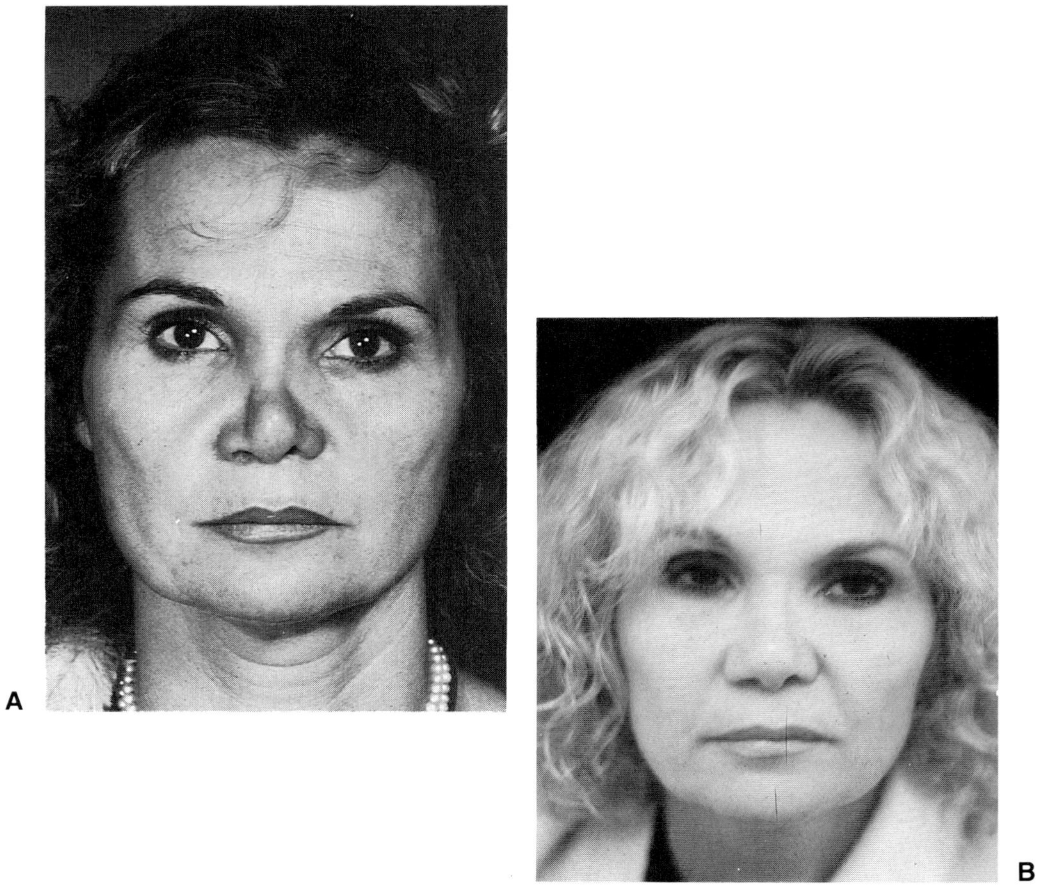

Fig. 22-28. **A,** Postoperative result after primary rhinoplasty; there are many bony irregularities present with a lateral step deformity along with obvious tip asymmetry. **B,** Result after re-osteotomy, remodeling, and rasping the bony contour.

Major Deformities

These deformities mostly encompass those errors associated with the excessive resection of the nasal hump, namely open roof and saddle nose defects.

Open roof. Apart from the non-aesthetic appearance of a squared nasal dorsum, one should also emphasize that most patients also complain of increased nasal sensitivity. A repeat of the osteotomies, taking care to remove a triangle of juxtafrontal bone should permit the two bony leaves of the nasal bones to be re-approximated. In case a residual open roof is left, a morselized cartilage graft can be inserted along the dorsum with gratifying results (Fig. 22-29).

Saddle nose. In general, the saddle nose results from a loss of septal support associated with a defect of the upper lateral cartilages. For those cases of a saddle nose with intact columellar support, correction may be achieved by the insertion of a bone, or a septal or conchal cartilage graft either through an incision made in the nasal vestibule or one carried out at the columellar base. If by chance we find that there is an associated loss of tip support in a saddle nose, we prefer to insert a "L-shaped" cartilage graft via a columellar base incision and transfixion incision giving an elephant trunk-like elevation to the columella and thus restoring the dorso-columellar support (Fig. 22-30). This is usually accompanied by the addition of bilateral longitudinal struts of cartilages used to equilibrate the tension of the L-shaped graft. These grafting procedures are, in our hands, the most effective treatment methods used for major saddle nose correction after having tried all sorts of alloplastic materials and autograft and homograft combinations.[8]

If the saddle nose is a sequela of an excessive hump removal or other hyper-reduction and malpositioning of the nasal bones, then the secondary correction concerns itself only with the nasal dorsum. In these cases we use an iliac bone graft anchored at the glabella. If necessary, we place supplementary longitudinal bilateral fine struts of bone for additional support. For particularly advanced shrunken saddle nose cases, we resort to using a combination of a dorsal bone graft under which is added an additional L-shaped costal cartilage graft that acts to support the first graft and prevent subsequent scar contraction. We have also noted less resorption of the transplanted material when this technique is used. It is important to take into account that often saddle noses involving the middle third of the dorsum are also accompanied by perturbations in nasal valve function.

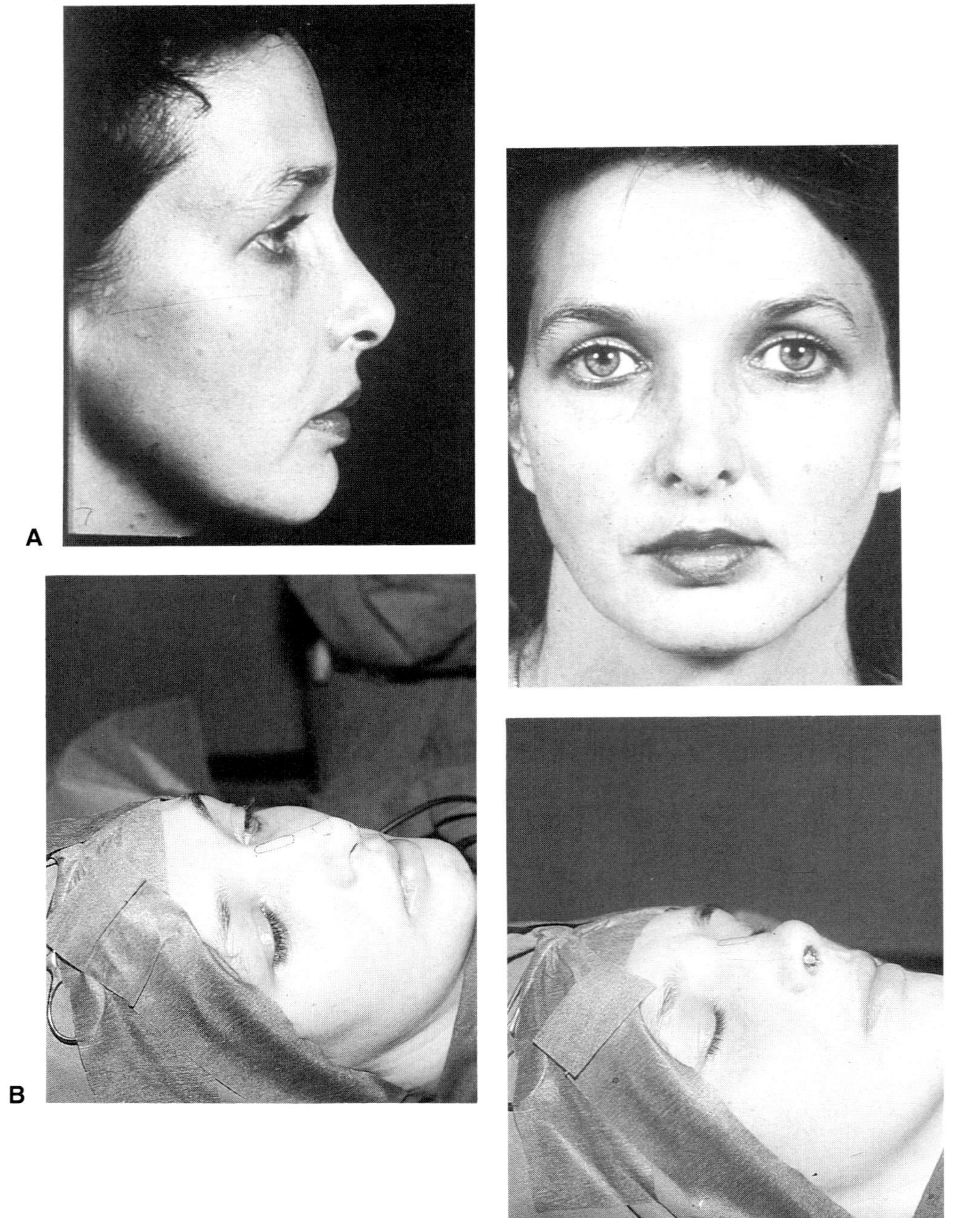

Fig. 22-29. **A,** Patient with an "open roof" defect after a primary rhinoplasty. **B,** Immediately preoperatively. **C,** Immediately postoperatively after dorsal cartilage grafting. **D** and **E,** Result seen one year after the surgery.

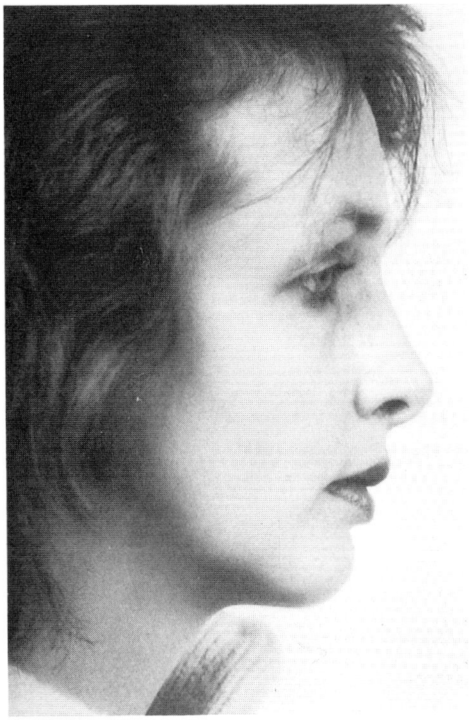

D

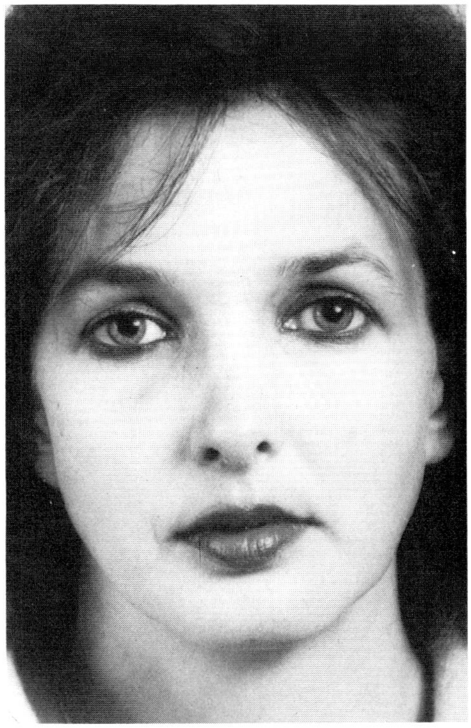

E

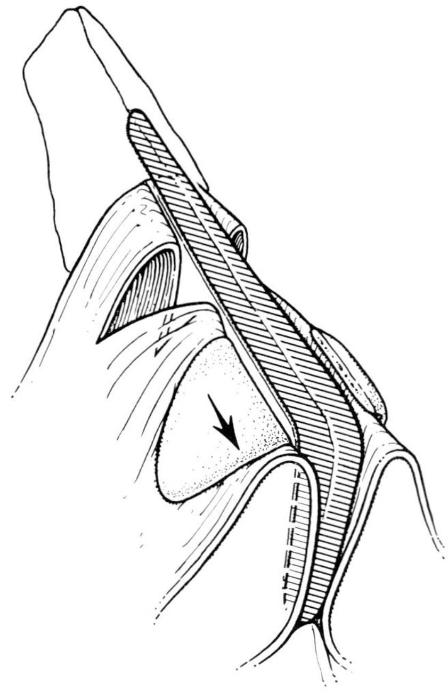

Fig. 22-30. Diagram of saddle nose deformity corrected by L-shaped cartilage graft placement. To allow the mucoperichondrium and mucoperiosteum to cover the supporting cartilage framework a releasing incision can be made in the posterior mucoperiosteum.

Vestibular Stenosis and Valvular Insufficiency

The essential goal of surgery undertaken to correct these pathological conditions is to restore normal respiratory physiology, and then, if possible, often as a further stage, to correct the aesthetic problem. The treatment for vestibular stenoses secondary to excess scarring is to excise all the pathological tissue and to reconstruct the nasal lining using local tissue flaps or grafts if possible, especially if the cartilaginous skeleton is intact. If this is not the case, a composite conchal graft is placed in the resulting defect after fibrous tissue excision. As for secondary nasal valve problems, these generally stem from fibrous tissue, which acts to retract the valve, diminishing the cross-sectional area of the vestibular port and impeding the proper action of the nasal valve. Treatment once again consists of excising all the pathological fibrous tissue, and then restoring valve support by means of a tailored septal cartilage graft held in place with some mattress sutures as already described for collapsing ala treatment. Apart from the anterior stenoses, it is important to rule out the existence of posterior stenoses of the nasal fossa with the resultant blockage of these narrowed passages. Such narrowing can be surgically enlarged by displacing the nasal antral bone laterally towards the maxillary sinus; the inverse of the procedure is used to surgically treat ozena. For treatment of vestibular stenosis we advocated[6] a paranasal semilunar skin flap transferred to the lateral aspect of the floor through a tunnel located at the alar base or with access gained simply by means of alar base sectioning (Figs. 22-31 and 22-32).

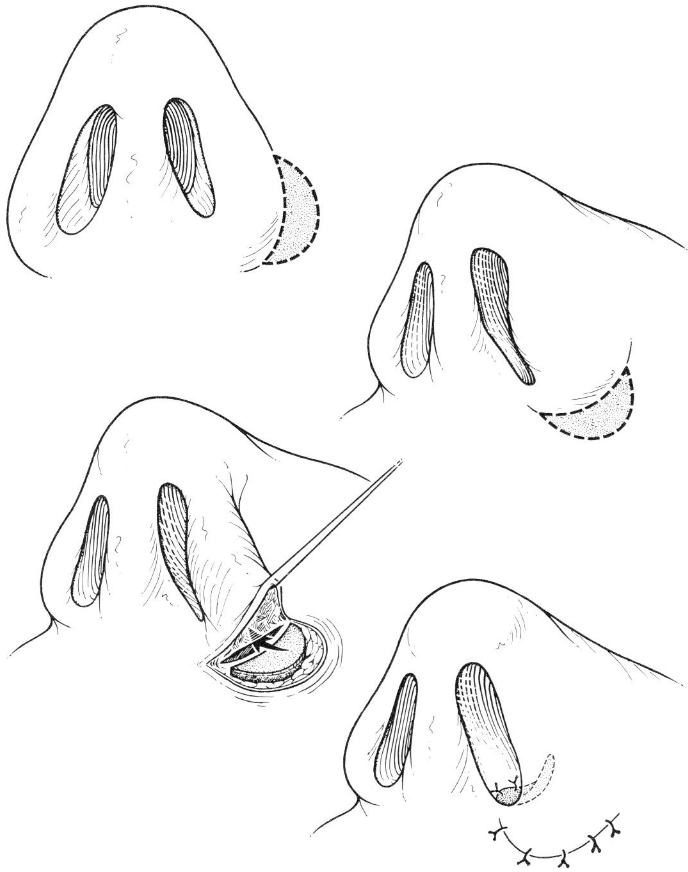

Fig. 22-31. The paranasal island flap used in the patient shown in Fig. 22-32 may also be transferred to the vestibular floor by means of a tunnel fashioned at the alar base.

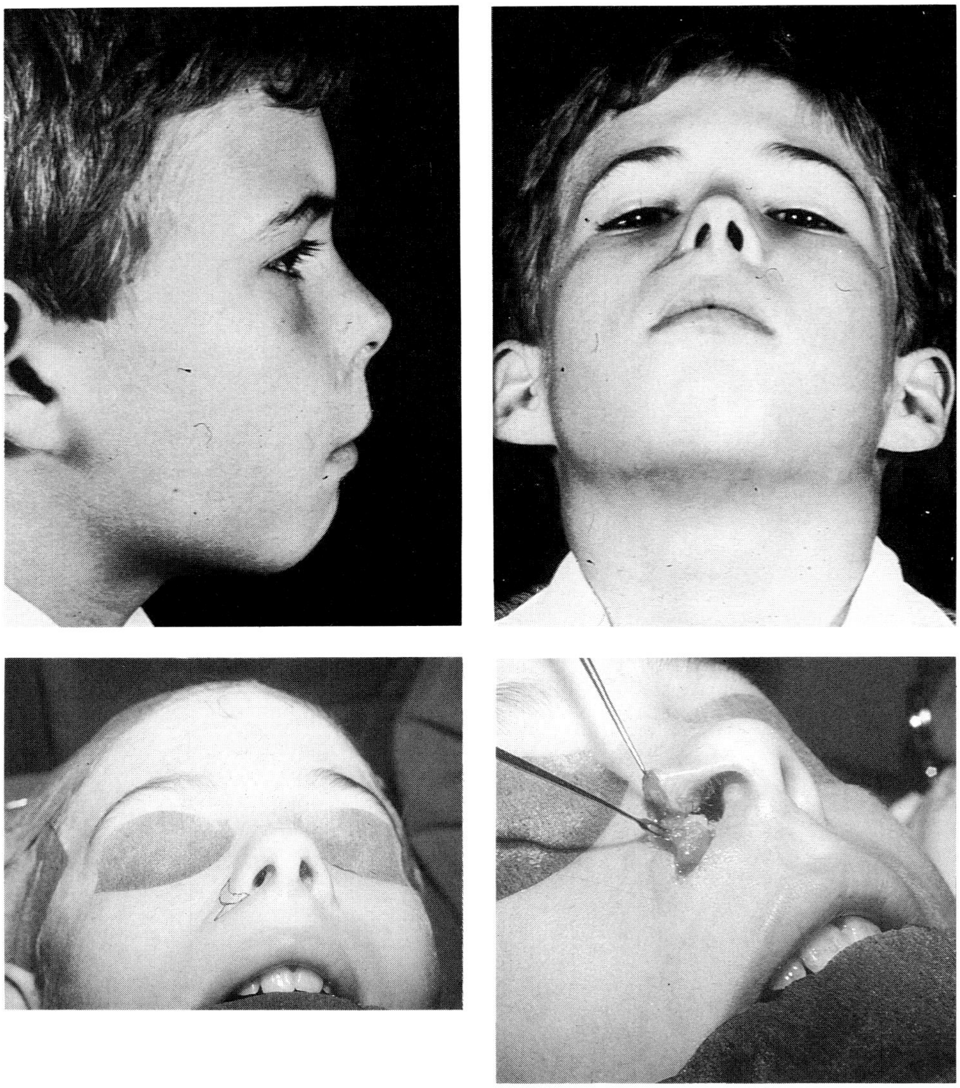

A

B

C

Fig. 22-32. **A**, Right anterior vestibular stenosis with loss of nasal valve function in a young boy. **B**, Local paranasal island flap marked out to be used to reconstitute the lost lining after lateral alar repositioning. **C**, Transfer to the vestibular floor in progress. **D**, Auricular composite graft harvested from the helical crus to be used to provide alar rigidity and restore the nasal valve. **E**, Immediate postoperative appearance. A contralateral alar base wedge excision was performed to further balance the two sides. **F** and **G**, Patient seen after 18 months.

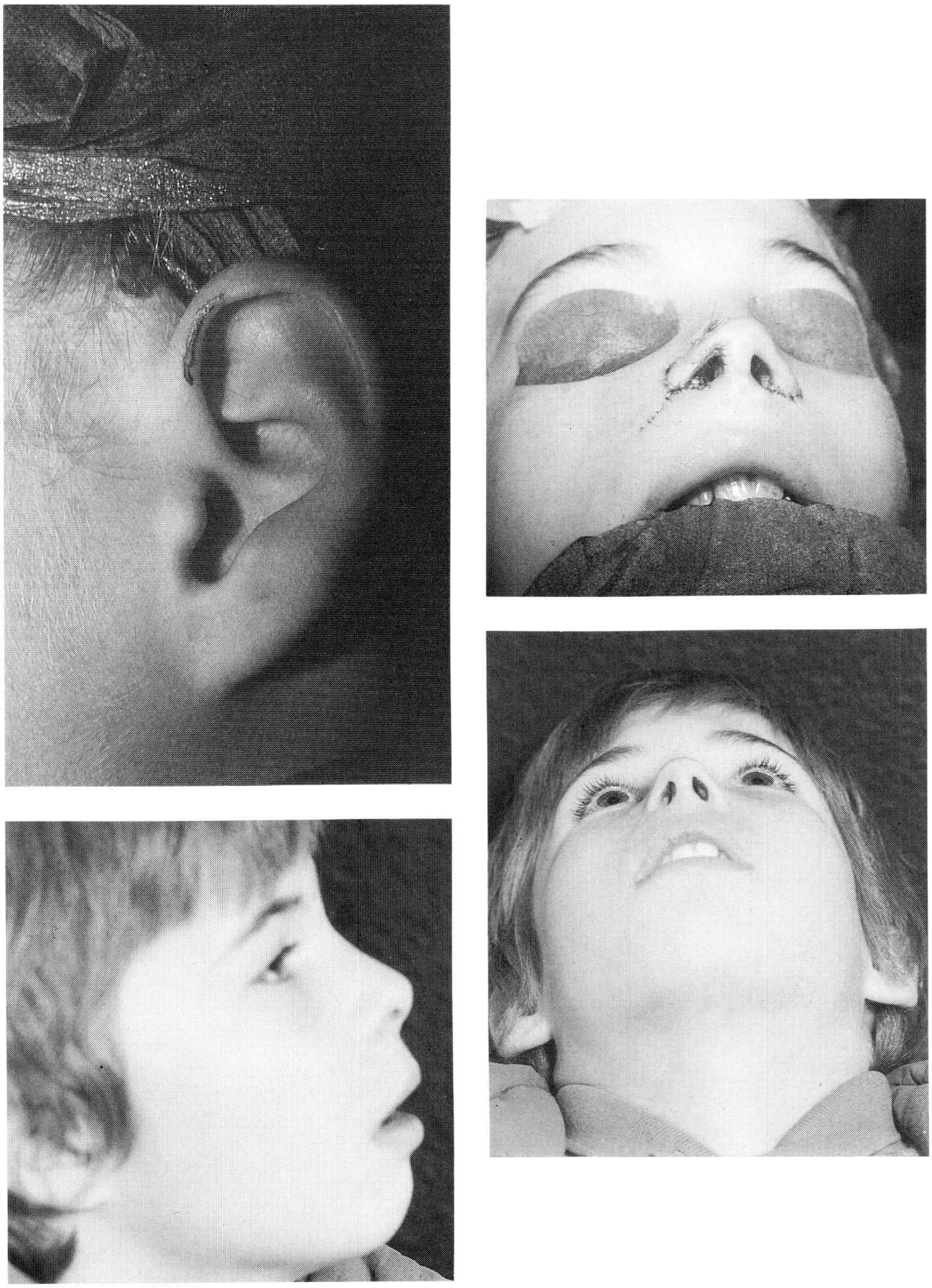

D E F G

Septal Perforation

To surgically treat septal perforations larger than 1 cm^2, it is recommended that a basal columellar incision be used. It facilitates the perfect submucoperiosteal elevation of the nasal floor, which when added to the full submucoperichondrial and periosteal dissection of the septum allows "exteriorization" of the resultant flap. This flap is easily delivered from the nose much in the same fashion that a shirt sleeve comes through the armhole of a vest, making it much easier to suture the septal perforation. For the more simple cases involving the closure of smaller perforations, elevation and mobilization of the mucoperichondrium using the extramucosal approach usually suffices (Fig. 22-33). Certain larger septal perforations may be closed in the same way with addition of simple bilateral one-stage labial flaps, the transfer and suturing of which is carried out through a pre-spinal tunnel (Figs. 22-34 and 22-35).

A

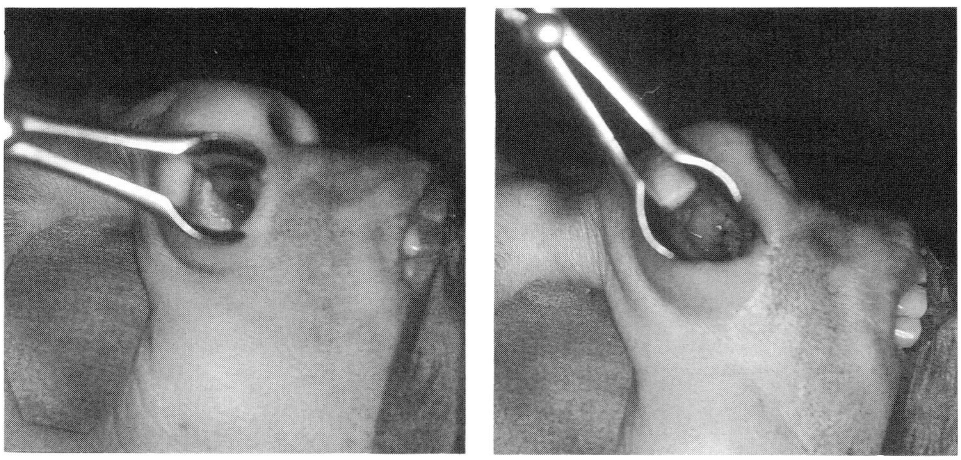

B

Fig. 22-33. **A,** Medium-sized septal perforation after septoplasty. **B,** Closure of the perforation in an oblique line after local mucoperichondrial flap elevation.

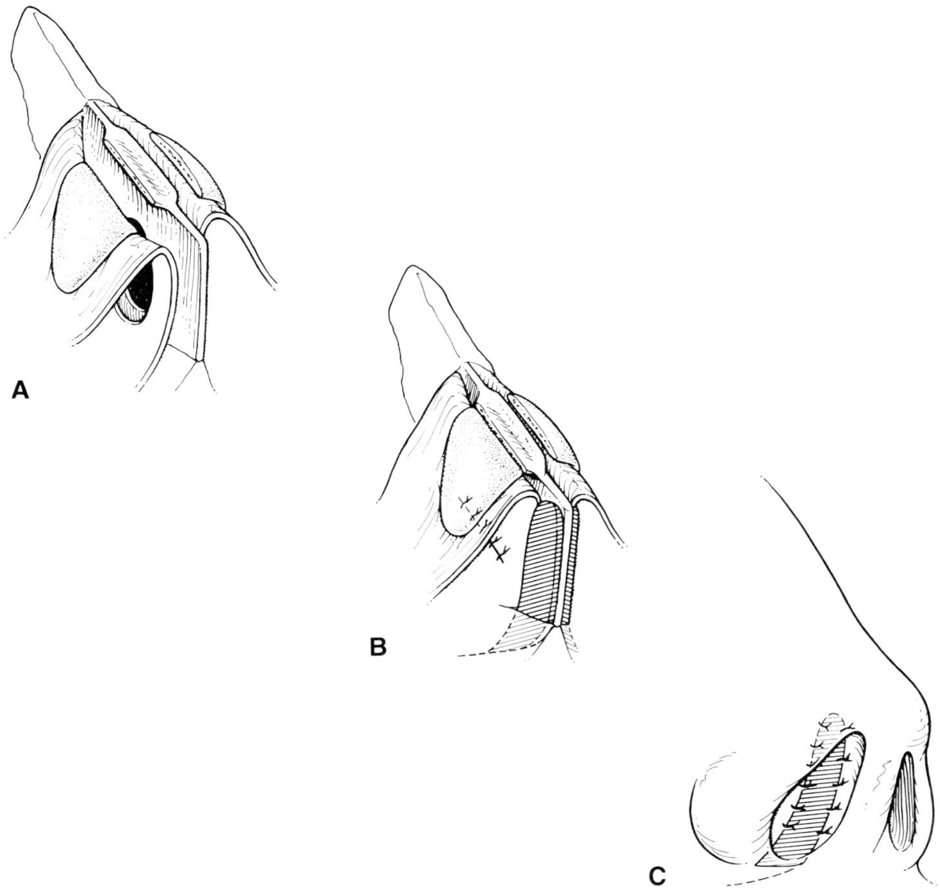

Fig. 22-34. For closure of the large septal perforation as shown in **A,** local mucoperichondrial flaps are elevated using the extramucosal technique, and the hole closed in an oblique line. Because of the degree of advancement of the local flaps, a dehiscence over the anterior septum is produced, **B,** Primary closure of this zone would produce a severe columella retraction, and so a tunneled buccal flap can be used to provide lining **c.** In our experience, with wide extramucosal elevation of the mucoperichondrium it is rare that this buccal flap is required.

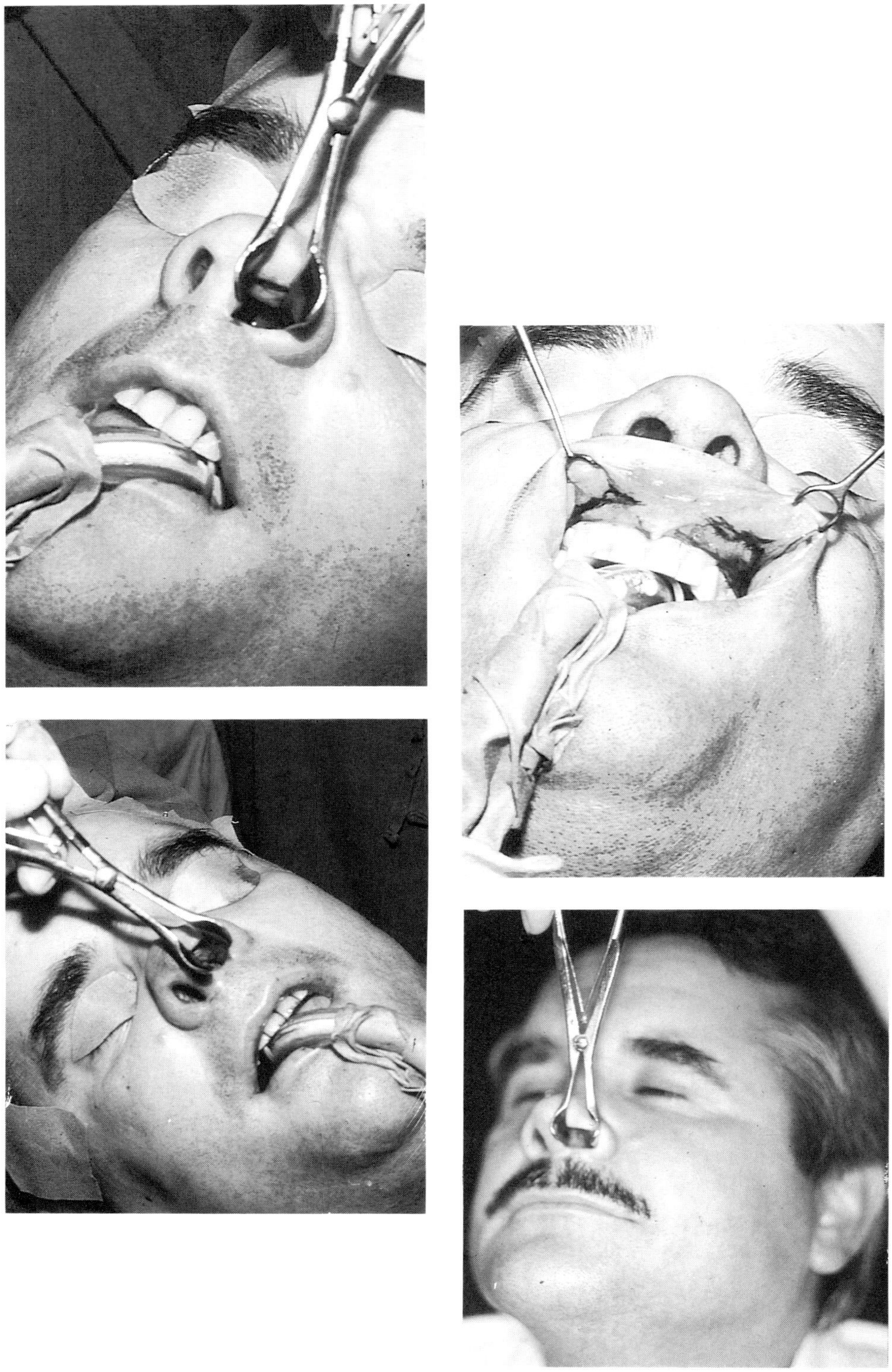

A B C D

Fig. 22-35. **A,** A large septal perforation approximately 3 cm in diameter is seen. Closure obtained using local mucoperichondrial flaps after wide submucous elevation. The perforation is entirely closed but a secondary dehiscence over the anterior septum is left after flap advancement to close the perforation. **B,** Bilateral buccal flaps outlined for tunneling into the base of the nose and lining the area of dehiscence. **C,** Final result after flap insertion. **D,** Result after 1 month.

Perforations larger than 4 cm in diameter require a more complicated procedure involving a three-stage reconstruction beginning with the placement of a conchal cartilage graft in an endo-buccal pocket forming a three-layered spoon-shaped flap followed by transfer at the second stage. To achieve the final desired result it is best to open the nasal base using a basal columellar and/or alar base incision. This allows the surgeon to easily transfer and position the flap, something which would otherwise be rather difficult (Fig. 22-36 and 22-37).

Thus with these two methods, the one-stage procedure with extended extramucosal dissection with or without labial flap transfer and the three-stage procedure with buccal flap, one is able to close every kind and size of septal perforation.[6,10] In addition, by combining the gingivo-buccal flap with a fronto-temporal flap, an entire septo-columellar loss can be repaired in three stages.[9]

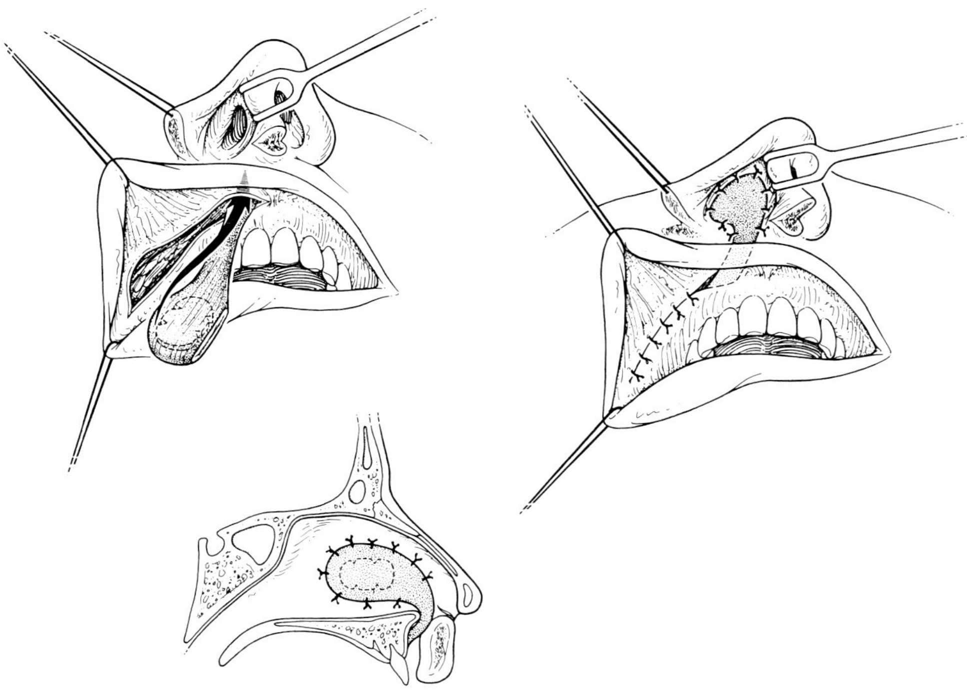

Fig. 22-36. Closure of large septal perforation in a three stage procedure with gingivo-buccal flap. In the first stage, a conchal graft is harvested and buried in a superficial submucosal pocket with the distal end of the buccal flap turned behind the cartilage and placed in a deeper submucosal pocket. In the second stage of the procedure the compound flap is mobilized and ready to be introduced into the nasal cavity. Transfer of the flap to the septal defect occurs through a tunnel in the nasal spine. The flap is sutured into the septal defect. The pedicle can be sectioned and discarded in the third stage.

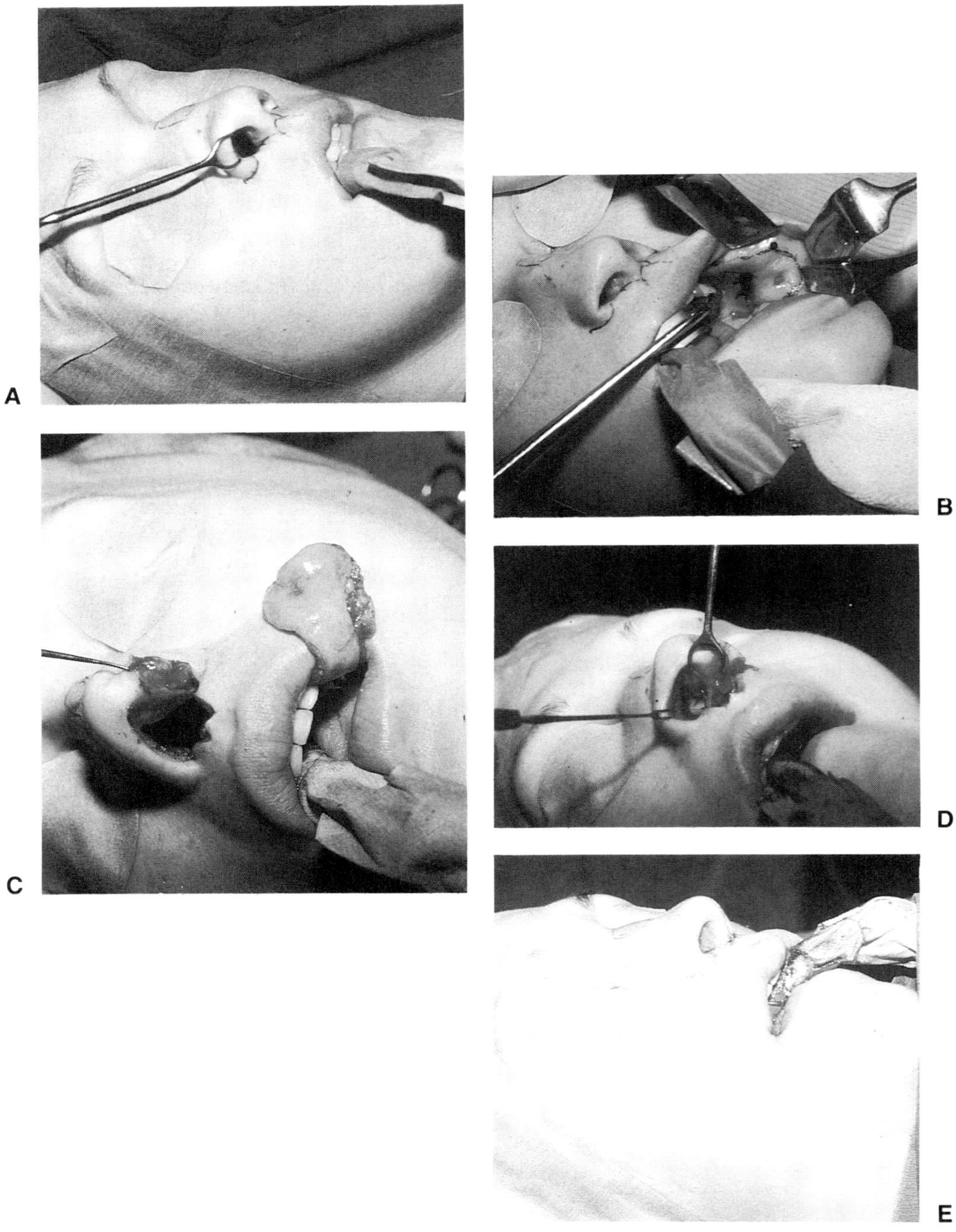

Fig. 22-37. Three-stage procedure is shown in preoperative views in the case of a young female with a 6 cm long perforation involving the anterior two-thirds of the septum. **A**, Anterior part of the perforation visible at the beginning of the second stage before closure. **B**, Outline of the prepared buccal flap before elevation and transfer during the second stage. **C**, Flap detached ready for transfer through the pre-spinal oro-nasal tunnel. The columellar and the membraneous septum are sectioned at the base for facilitating the insertion of the flap. **D**, Suture of the flap into the septal defect on both sides. **E**, End of the operation with reinserted septocolumellar pillar.

REFERENCES

1. Anderson JR: The dynamics of rhinoplasty. Proceedings of the Nineth International Congress in Otorhinolaryngology Excerpta Medica, International Congress Series 206. Amsterdam, 1969, Excerpta Medica.
2. Denecke HJ and Meyer R: Plastische Operationen an Kopf und Hals. Berlin, 1964, Springer-Verlag.
3. Denecke HJ and Meyer R: Plastic surgery of head and neck: rhinoplasty, vol 1, Berlin, 1967, Springer-Verlag.
4. Eitner E: Kosmetische Operationen Wien: Kosmetische Korrekturen im Bereiche der Nasenspitze und ihrer Umgebung. Z. Laryng Rhinol Otol (Stuttg) 26:46, 1935.
5. Jost G: Correction du défaut de projection de la pointe du nez, Ann Chir Plast Esthet 17:245, 1972.
6. Meyer R: Nasal-septal perforation and nostril stenosis. In Goldwyn RM, editor: The unfavorable result in plastic surgery, Boston, 1972, Little, Brown & Co Inc.
7. Meyer R and Kesselring UK: The unusually short nose, Aesthetic Plast Surg 1:271, 1977.
8. Meyer R and Kesselring UK: Sculpturing and reconstructive procedures, Clin Plast Surg 4:1, 1977.
9. Meyer R and Kesselring UK: Reconstructive surgery of the nose, Clin Plast Surg 8:435, 1981.
10. Meyer R and Kesselring UK: Secondary rhinoplasty. In Regnault P and Daniel RK: Aesthetic plastic surgery, Boston, 1984, Little, Brown & Co Inc.
11. Peck GP: Onlay graft for nasal tip projection, Plast Reconstr Surg 71:27, 1983.
12. Pollet J and Baudelot S: La rhinoplastie extra-muqueuse. Ses indications, Ann Chir Plast Esthet 15:1, 1970.
13. Rethi A: Operation to shorten an excessively long nose, Rev Chir Plast 2:85, 1934.
14. Robin JL: La rhinoplastie extramuqueuse, Communiqué Soc Franç Chir Plast et Reconstr 23 mai 1970.
15. Sheen JH: Achieving more nasal tip projection by the use of a small autogenous bone or cartilage graft, Plast Reconstr Surg 56:35, 1975.

NOTE: For more extensive information about revision surgery we would refer the reader to the recent book "Secondary and functional rhinoplasty: the difficult nose" by R. Meyer, published by Grune and Stratton, Inc and Saunders and Co.

23

Closure of Nasal Septal Perforations

W. Douglas Appling and William K. Wright

Closing a nasal septal perforation is sometimes frustrating and always difficult, but excellent results are possible and patients are grateful to have an intact septum. Although some patients are asymptomatic, a nasal septal perforation can be the source of many problems for others. When crusting, obstruction, bleeding, and whistling become severe, consideration should be given to closing the septal perforation. We favor surgical closure over the use of Silastic buttons, provided the patient is medically fit and able to undergo surgery. Using the external septo-rhinoplasty approach to enhance exposure of the septum, we elevate septal flaps. We close the two separate flap perforations with intranasal bipedicled advancement or anterior-based or posterior-based rotation flaps and interpose a graft of mastoid periosteum between the flaps. To protect the healing flaps from drying postoperatively, we place Silastic splints on either side of the septum. Using this method,[1,13] we have achieved results that match any other report in the literature for perforations 3 cm or smaller. Closing perforations larger than 3 cm is very difficult no matter what technique is used.

Although the perforation is usually related to prior nasal surgery, cauterization, or trauma, other conditions can present with a septal perforation. These include factitious ulceration, intranasal cocaine use, intranasal topical corticosteroid therapy, Wegener's granulomatosis, lupus erythematosus, sarcoidosis, tuberculosis, syphilis, and carcinoma.[6,14] As with any patient, a thorough history and physical examination should be conducted prior to surgery.

In addition to the patient who is medically unfit for surgery or whose disease makes permanent closure impossible, there are other patients who are relatively poor candidates for septal perforation closure. The untreated or relapsed cocaine addict is one. Another is the patient who is bothered more by the external appearance of the nose than by the perforation. A patient who has a dorsal saddle and a retracted columella from loss of the caudal septum and who also has a septal perforation should be aware of the possibility that perforation closure can lead to further retraction of the columella as the flaps heal. If we are able to insert a cartilage graft to replace the caudal septum, then we can close the perforation without compromising our efforts to improve the patient's appearance. In most cases, uncomplicated hump and tip work can be readily combined with perforation closure. We also hesitate to close a septal perforation in a patient who requires reconstruction of severely scarred and stenotic nasal valves. If the perforation cannot be closed easily without tension, we confine our work to opening the nasal airways, which is a challenging enough task in itself.

Surgical Technique

Because elevating and closing the flaps is tedious and time-consuming and requires the patient to lie still for as long as two or more hours, we prefer general anesthesia. After securing the endotracheal tube, we pack the pharynx with a 3-inch Kling dressing to prevent blood from collecting in the patient's stomach during the procedure, which causes nausea and vomiting postoperatively. With general anesthesia, we have not noted any excessive bleeding using a 1:100,000 epinephrine solution without lidocaine, which we prepare by adding 0.1 ml of 1:1,000 injectable epinephrine to 10 ml of sterile normal saline. Prior to prepping the patient's nose, face, ear, and post-auricular area, approximately 10 ml of the 1:100,000 epinephrine solution is infiltrated where the marginal rim and transcolumellar incisions are made, at the nasal spine, along the dorsum, and into the mastoid periosteal graft donor site. After the patient is prepped and draped, both sides of the septum are injected with the 1:100,000 epinephrine solution; we use a 25-gauge, 2-inch needle to reach the posterior septum. Decongestion of the nasal cavities by topical application of a cocaine solution is helpful, but not always necessary.

External Septo-Rhinoplasty Approach

First, we mark the transcolumellar incision with a horizontal line across the columella at slightly above the midpoint, above the feet of the medial crura. Next, we make a short incision in the lateral columella caudal to the medial crus extending down to the level of the transcolumellar line. We then position a 10-mm Joseph double hook in the alar rim with one prong in the skin at the midpoint of the alar rim and the other in the soft tissue facet. Everting the vestibular lining with the ring finger of the hand holding the hook, we palpate the caudal edge of the lateral crus with the bevel of a # 15 scalpel blade and make an incision along its caudal border just long enough to insert the tips of the scissors. We insert the tips of the Joseph scissors in the incision, making sure we can get around the caudal edge of the lateral crus; then we undermine on top of the lateral crus toward the dome. Next, we snip the vestibular skin along the caudal edge of the lateral crus, advancing the double hook medially along the alar margin to keep the incision centered between the tongs of the hook. With the ring finger pushing on the tip, everting the vestibular skin in the dome region, we undermine and connect the lateral incision with the one in the columella, carefully following the caudal margin of the lateral crus, which may be buckled in this area. By putting the tissues on stretch and slowly advancing the incision with scissors, we can follow the caudal margin of the lateral crus, even in patients who have thick skin and flimsy or buckled cartilages.

Having made marginal rim incisions, we connect them with a transcolumellar incision. Before cutting through the skin of the previously marked transcolumellar incision, we undermine the columellar skin with scissors, making sure the scissors are anterior to the medial crura. We usually wait until both marginal rim incisions are completed before connecting them with the transcolumellar incision, except when the caudal edges of the lateral crura are difficult to identify. In this situation, we make the transcolumellar incision first and then extend the incision along the caudal edge of the medial and lateral crus under direct vision. We use a straight horizontal incision across the columella and find that it heals as well as or better than an inverted "V" incision.

Elevating Septal Flaps

With the incisions completed, the skin is undermined with scissors in a plane just above the perichondrium of the lower lateral and upper lateral cartilages. We undermine over the nasal bones, then stop and insert a strip of half-inch plain Nu-Gauze packing soaked with 1:1,000 topical epinephrine into the elevated pocket to control bleeding while we proceed to identify the caudal septum, nasal spine, and pyriform openings. We divide the fibrous tissue attachments joining the medial crura until the caudal margin of the septum and the nasal spine can be seen. Then, using a Cottle nasal speculum for retraction, we sweep the muscle fibers from the bone of the premaxilla with a Cottle elevator, which exposes the pyriform openings. Bleeding in this area is stopped, again with the use of topical epinephrine on Nu-Gauze packing, while we return to the septal angle and begin elevating mucoperichondrial flaps.

Retracting the nasal skin with a Parkes retractor, we start elevating mucoperichondrial flaps at the septal angle. Getting under the perichondrium before starting to dissect the mucosal flap from the cartilage is so obvious that we mention it precisely because it is so critical. With scarring, the septal perichondrium and/or periosteum can be surprisingly hard to identify and to stay under with an elevator, but remaining under it for as long as the available cartilage or bone permits is essential to avoid tearing or perforating the flap. Further, it is important to be in the proper plane before continuing to separate the septal flaps beyond the limits of the remaining cartilage and bone. Once the proper mucoperichondrial planes are established on either side of the septum, we divide the upper lateral cartilages from the dorsal septum intraseptally and begin to separate the flaps superior, anterior, and posterior to the perforation. When it is difficult to find mucoperichondrial planes at the septal angle, the mucoperichondrial space on either side of the dorsal septum can be entered by first dividing the upper lateral cartilages from the dorsal septum. Although we may choose to do so on one side later, we do not divide the mucosa beneath the upper lateral cartilages from the mucosa on the septum. Regardless of the loss of septal cartilage from prior surgery or trauma, usually some cartilage can be exposed along the dorsum with the external septo-rhinoplasty approach, and elevation of mucoperichondrial flaps can be started.

After elevating the mucoperichondrial flaps from either side of the remaining caudal septum, we return to the area of the previously exposed premaxilla and nasal spine and cut the fibrous attachments of the septal flaps to the nasal spine and anterior maxillary crest with scissors, trying to avoid buttonholing the flaps. Before the mucosa can be elevated from the floor of the nose, it must be lifted from the crest of bone at the pyriform opening. A tear in the flap at this point can jeopardize the pedicle of an anterior-based flap. Since it is more direct, the sublabial approach may make this elevation easier. Once this maneuver is accomplished, the mucosa along the floor of the nose and in the inferior meatus usually elevates easily. Having created inferior tunnels bilaterally, we continue to elevate mucosa from the floor of the nose superiorly onto the maxillary crest. If the patient has a bony spur, the mucosa must be elevated carefully from it without creating another fenestration. Sometimes the septum is membranous inferior to the perforation, which makes blunt dissection of the mucosal flaps superiorly from the inferior tunnels difficult. In this situation, we stop and go back to elevating the flaps superior, anterior, and posterior to the perforation. When the limits of the residual cartilage or bone are reached, we continue the separation of the flaps superior, anterior, and posterior to the perforation with a # 15 blade, looking back and forth intraseptally and intranasally, to gauge the position of the blade and the thickness of the flaps. When we reach the edges of the perforation, we divide the septal flaps trying to include the mucosal lining of the perforation with one flap, thus decreasing the size of the perforation on that flap while increasing the size of the perforation on the other flap (Fig. 23-1). The smaller mucosal perforation is easier to close and the suture lines are at different levels on each side. After freeing the perforation edges, we have two septal flaps, each with a large hole. If we did not separate the flaps inferior to the perforation earlier, we do it at this time. Often this is done with a knife for a short distance until we can connect the separated flaps with the previously elevated inferior tunnels.

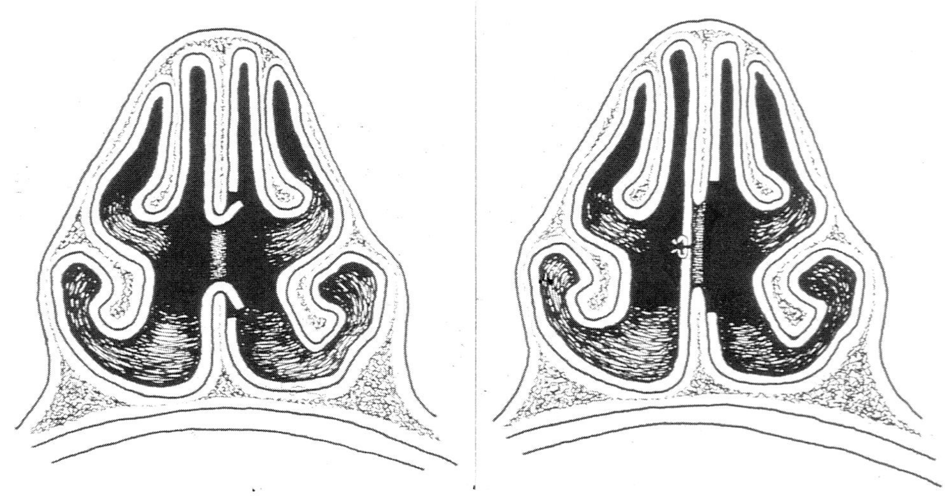

Fig. 23-1. Right and left septal flaps are divided at perforation so that right flap includes cuff of mucosa around left side of perforation. This decreases size of right septal flap perforation at expense of left side. (From Kridel RWH, et al: Septal perforation closure utilizing the external septorhinoplasty approach, Arch Otolaryngol Head Neck Surg 112:168-172, 1986.)

Approximating Perforation Edges

After the flaps are completely elevated, we try to approximate the edges of the perforation in an effort to decide what types of flaps are necessary. Perforations smaller than 0.5 cm can often be closed directly, but larger perforations require relaxing incisions to create bipedicled advancement flaps. In cases with perforations larger than 1.5 cm from superior to inferior edge, the inferior bipedicled flap must be released either posteriorly or anteriorly in order to allow the flap to rotate and close the perforation.

If we cannot close the perforation primarily and it is less than 1.5 cm, we make a relaxing incision in the inferior meatus. Posteriorly, we curve the incision toward the septum; anteriorly, we extend it along the pyriform opening toward, but not actually to, the nasal spine. If the edges almost come together or do so with a small amount of tension, we obtain additional release on that side by incising the mucosa along the superior dorsal septum. This superior relaxing incision, which is longer than the perforation and curved inferiorly on either end, is made only on one side to prevent exposure of cartilage in corresponding areas that might lead to another septal perforation. We do not worry about the bare area left along the nasal floor because mucosa grows over it quickly. These two bipedicled flaps usually close one side of a perforation up to 1.5 cm (Fig. 23-2). We like to close both septal flaps, but if we can only approximate the perforation edges on one side, and a periosteal graft is placed between the sides, the second side eventually heals. Even with an intraseptal graft, if we cannot close the second side com-

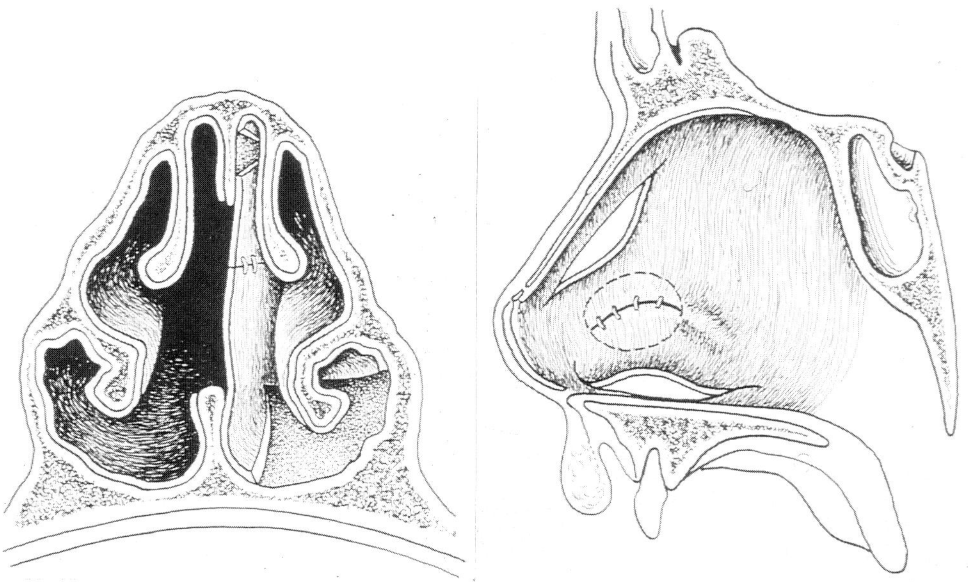

Fig. 23-2. Left superior and inferior bipedicled flaps are advanced, allowing closure of left septal flap perforation with interrupted sutures. (From Kridel RWH, et al: Septal perforation closure utilizing the external septorhinoplasty approach, Arch Otolaryngol Head Neck Surg 112:168-172, 1986.)

pletely, we try to cover the area of the suture line on the first side with mucosa from the second side. Sometimes we accomplish this with an inferior bipedicled flap and at other times with a rotation flap. If two bipedicled flaps do not advance far enough to bring the mucosal edges together on the first side, we use a rotation flap to close at least one side.

For mid or posterior septal perforations that are greater than 1.5 cm from their superior to inferior edges, a posterior-based flap of mucosa from the inferior meatus can be rotated to cover the hole. With a posterior-based flap, we make an incision down the inferior meatus, extend it anteriorly along the pyriform opening and curve it back into the perforation (Fig. 23-3). Posteriorly based flaps may be too short to close an anterior perforation. In this situation, we still use a flap of mucosa from the inferior meatus, but we base it anteriorly on the skin of the nostril floor. Unlike a posterior-based flap, an anterior-based flap can reach the caudal 1 cm of septum. With the anterior-based flap, we make our lateral incision as high as possible in the inferior meatus and our medial incision along the junction of the septum with the nasal floor extending it onto the septum to the posterior edge of the perforation. We cut the posterior mucosa in the inferior meatus between the lateral and medial incisions of the anterior-based flap with a small curved scissors or a right-angled blade.

To rotate and close the perforation without tension, both the posterior-based and the anterior-based flaps must be longer than the perfora-

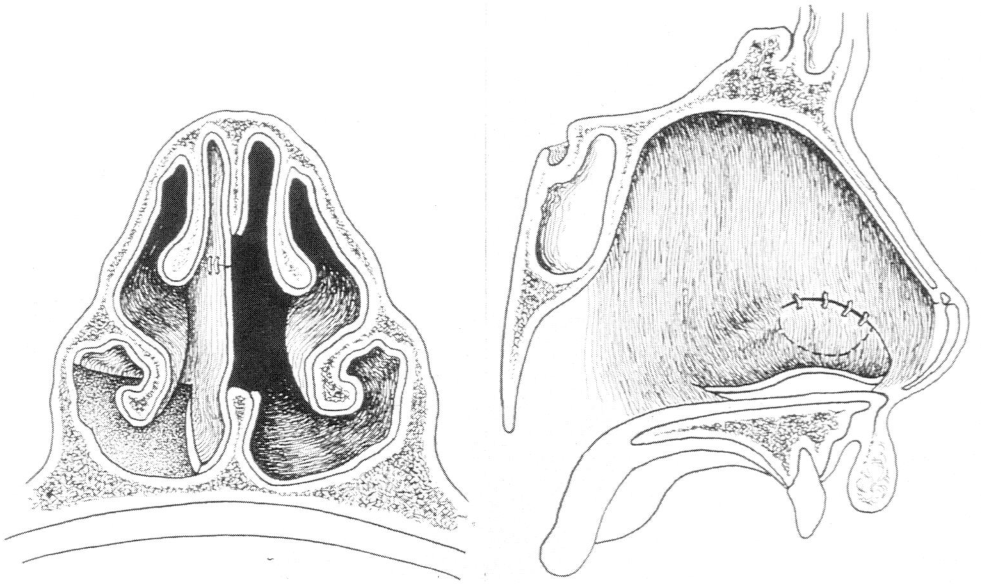

Fig. 23-3. Right posterior-based septal flap is rotated and sutured in place to close right perforated septal flap. When anterior margin of perforation extends to within 1 cm from caudal end of septum, anterior-based flap must be used. (From Kridel RWH, et al: Septal perforation closure utilizing the external septorhinoplasty approach, Arch Otolaryngol Head Neck Surg 112:168-172, 1986.)

tion is from its anterior to its posterior end. Obtaining this extra length is essential and does not result in as much bunching as might be imagined, even with the anterior-based flap. Because we include the septal mucosa beneath and to one end of the perforation with our anterior-based or posterior-based flaps of mucosa from the nasal floor, rotating these flaps into place can leave a bare area on the septum inferior and to one end of the perforation. To avoid creating opposing donor defects, which can lead to another perforation, we do not raise similarly based rotation flaps on either side of the septum unless they can be taken entirely from the floor. Sometimes this means that we can close only one side of the perforation.

To sew the flap edges together, we work within the septum, using interrupted 5-0 coated Vicryl sutures on a P-1 needle. We put a piece of colored metal suture wrapper between the lateral nasal wall and the septal flap to prevent catching the inferior turbinate with a loop of suture. The assistant retracts the nasal skin superiorly with a Converse retractor while pulling the upper lateral cartilage down and away from the dorsal septum with a Parkes retractor, and the surgeon is then able to use both the Webster needle holder and the Cottle insertion forceps to approximate the flap edges from within the septal pocket. We think that this approach is easier than working intranasally and that it represents a major advantage of the external septo-rhinoplasty approach.

Inserting Periosteal Graft Between Flaps

After we have separated the two septal flaps and closed at least one side, preferably both, we place a graft of mastoid periosteum between the flaps to provide both bulk and a platform on which the mucosal edges can heal. We like to tack the graft to any residual septal cartilage to prevent it from becoming dislodged (Fig. 23-4).

To harvest the graft, we make a curved incision that is 4 to 6 cm long, starting on the posterior concha of the ear and extending back along the hairline. This incision, which is essentially a small limb of a facelift incision, affords adequate exposure and leaves the patient with a cosmetically acceptable scar. We elevate the skin in a subcutaneous plane, cut the sternocleidomastoid muscle superiorly from the temporal bone for a short distance, and remove a piece of mastoid periosteum and attached soft tissue that is between 0.5 to 1 cm larger in diameter than the perforation. When the septum is mainly membranous and the perforation can easily be enlarged by the elevation of the septal flaps, we wait until the end of the procedure to take the graft when the true size of the perforation is known. Although excess soft tissue and muscle is removed from the graft, some bulk is an advantage in preventing the thinning that tends to occur when closed septal flaps heal in direct contact with each other, without an intervening filler. We close the postauricular wound in layers using a 3-0 chromic suture subcutaneously and a 5-0 Vicryl suture intradermally. Usually, we do not drain the

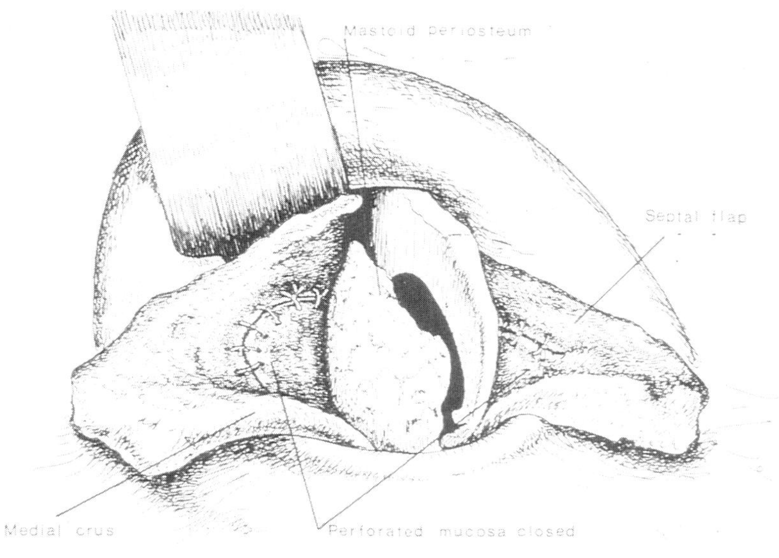

Fig. 23-4. Mucosal perforation is sutured from inside septum. Periosteal graft is then sutured in place to separate closed septal flap perforations. (From Kridel RWH, et al: Septal perforation closure utilizing the external septorhinoplasty approach, Arch Otolaryngol Head Neck Surg 112:168-172, 1986.)

wound, but we do apply a mastoid dressing at the end of the procedure, which we leave on for 24 hours.

Splinting, Packing, and Closing

To complete the procedure, we insert splints, made from 0.02-inch Silastic sheeting, on either side of the nasal septum, securing them at their caudal end with two 4-0 Prolene mattress sutures. Then we pack the posterior nasal cavities with flattened 2 × 8 cm strips of moistened Gelfoam. We close only the marginal rim incisions to ensure that the lateral crura remain tucked beneath the caudal edge of vestibular skin. Usually, one or two 5-0 plain sutures on a side suffice. After we close the marginal rim incisions, we approximate the transcolumellar incision with interrupted 6-0 mild chromic sutures, beginning laterally and working toward the midline. We do not suture the marginal rim incisions in the dome areas, but rather pack them closed with Gelfoam. We pack the anterior nostrils with half-inch Nu-Gauze impregnated with Cortisporin ointment and tape and splint the nose.

Postoperative Care

On the first postoperative visit, which is usually between the third and the fifth day postoperatively, we remove the anterior Nu-Gauze packing from both nostrils and gently suction out enough Gelfoam from each side of the nose to allow some nasal air flow. Although it will eventually dissolve on its own, we prefer to suction out the remaining Gelfoam on succeeding visits. We remove the tape and splint dressing at the end of the first week and take out any remaining transcolumellar sutures, but we leave the intranasal splints in place for at least 6 weeks to keep the septal flaps from drying out. Keeping the flaps from drying out, especially if only one side can be covered, is vital even if the splints must be left in place for months. In one such case in which only one side could be closed and there was concern about a recurrence of the perforation, we felt that leaving the splints in place for 3 months greatly contributed to a successful result. The use of saline nasal sprays and crust removal as needed in the office help patients tolerate the extended use of intranasal splints. In our experience, failure of the perforation to close is evident usually within the first few months postoperatively, but it can occur even years after the operation. Fortunately, these recurrent perforations are usually asymptomatic probably because they are smaller and more posterior.

Discussion of Technique

Based on our experience, we advocate closing symptomatic nasal septal perforations by elevating septal flaps and using mucosal advancement or rotation flaps to approximate the perforation edges on either side of the septum. We also believe in the importance of inserting a graft of mastoid periosteum in the septal space between the flaps and keeping the flaps covered with Silastic splints for at least 6 weeks postoperatively. We also prefer the external septo-rhinoplasty approach because it facilitates elevating and suturing the mucosal flaps. Our technique combines the ideas of many other surgeons[3,4,6-12,15] in a manner we find successful for closing perforations as large as 3 cm in diameter. Although successful, this method of closing septal perforations is difficult and demands patience and a meticulous technique.

Some special situations may require special handling. For very anterior perforations, posterior-based flaps do not reach far enough to allow closure. These perforations, however, can be closed by the anterior-based flaps described by Karlan.[11,12] For very large perforations, the surgeon should consider the extra wide anterior-based flap described by Belmont.[2] Since flap failures occur at the distal end of the flap; the anterior-based flap, even if it is a partial failure, moves the perforation posteriorly where it tends to be asymptomatic. Karlan's method has the additional advantage of closing septal perforations reliably without separating the septal flaps. The hardest and most time-consuming part of the procedure is separating the septal flaps. We often ask ourselves whether we could close perforations as dependably without elevating septal flaps. Certainly, there would be less contraction of the columella in the patient with little remaining caudal septum, and it would eliminate the problem of trying to divide a thin membranous septum without enlarging the perforation. Of course, there are cases in which flaps should be elevated. For example, when the airway is obstructed by deviating or overlapping pieces of cartilage, septal flaps must be elevated before cartilage and bone can be removed and the perforation closed. With the exception of the crooked septum, using a flap or graft without separating the septal flaps would greatly simplify perforation closure. Composite grafts and pedicled flaps from the inferior turbinate and from the labial-buccal area are described,[5,16,17] and although technically easier, they lack the extremely high success rate of procedures that use septal flap elevation. Karlan's[11,12] report of using anterior-based flaps without elevating septal flaps suggests a method that may prove as successful as closure with flap elevation, especially with membranous perforations, where flaps are very hard to divide, and healing following flap dissection is often accompanied by unwanted contracture.

In addition to closing the perforation with mucosal flaps, we think an interpositional graft is critical. Without it, even if both sides are closed, the septum tends to thin out, which often leads to another perforation. When only one side can be closed, periosteum is a better interpositional graft than cartilage or bone, because periosteum sustains the growth of the mucosal edges toward each other on the side that is not closed. If the exposed graft and surrounding septal mucosa are kept moist by covering them with a thin piece of Silastic sheeting, the perforation will heal. If a periosteal graft is placed between elevated septal flaps and neither flap perforation is closed, both sides will eventually heal if the perforation is small and the patient is willing to leave the septal splints in for many weeks.[18] Unless elevation shreds both flaps making their closure impossible at the time of the operation, we fail to see the advantage of just inserting a graft between separated flaps and not using advancement or rotation flaps to close at least one side of the perforation. Fascia also supports the mucosal flaps, but we prefer periosteum because it is thicker and does not curl when wet. Increasing the thickness of the septum by inserting the periosteal graft is usually not a problem unless the patient has markedly hypertrophied inferior turbinates or narrow nasal openings. If the nose is too narrow, the nasal bones can be fractured or refractured and packed out, while the inferior turbinates can be trimmed judiciously even at the time of perforation closure.

Even with both sides closed and a graft in between, we still place thin Silastic sheets on either side of the septum to prevent drying and crusting while the flaps heal. We think their early removal leads to a recurrent perforation in one specific case, so we do not hesitate to leave them in place for 6 weeks or more.

Regardless of what technique is used to elevate mucosal flaps, including the sublabial route, the external septo-rhinoplasty approach makes sewing the flaps in place easier. It adds little if any time to the procedure, and closing is fast and uncomplicated. In addition, we have better exposure for any hump or tip work that we combine with perforation closure. Even though the external septo-rhinoplasty approach may facilitate elevating and suturing the flaps, we still believe that closing a nasal septal perforation is a difficult and at times frustrating operation, requiring patience and careful attention to detail in order to achieve good results.

REFERENCES

1. Appling WD and Wright WK: Nasal septal perforation. In Gates GA, editor: Current therapy in otolaryngology-head and neck surgery-3, Toronto, BC Decker Inc, 1987.
2. Belmont JR: An approach to large nasoseptal perforations and attendant deformity, Arch Otolaryngol Head Neck Surg 111:450-455, 1985.
3. Climo S: The surgical closure of a large anterior perforation of the nasal septum, Plast Reconstr Surg 17:410-414, 1956.
4. Cottle MH: Nasal atrophy, atrophic rhinitis, ozena: medical and surgical treatment: repair of septal perforations, J Int Coll Surg 29:472-484, 1958.
5. Denecke HJ and Meyer R: Plastic surgery of the head and neck: corrective and reconstructive rhinoplasty, vol 1, New York, 1967, Springer-Verlag.
6. Fairbanks D: Closure of nasal septal perforations, Arch Otolaryngol Head Neck Surg 106:509-513, 1980.
7. Fairbanks DNF and Chen SCA: Closure of large nasal septum perforations, Arch Otolaryngol Head Neck Surg 91:403-406, 1970.
8. Fairbanks DNF and Fairbanks GR: Septal perforation. In Gates GA editor: Current therapy in otolaryngology-head and neck surgery 1984-1985, Toronto, 1984, BC Decker Inc.
9. Gollum J: Perforation of the nasal septum: the reverse flap technique, Arch Otolaryngol Head Neck Surg 88:518-522, 1968.
10. Goodman WS and Strelzow VV: The

surgical closure of nasoseptal perforations, Laryngoscope 92:121-124, 1982.
11. Karlan MS, Ossoff R, and Cristu P: Reconstruction for large septal perforations, Arch Otolaryngol Head Neck Surg 108:433-436, 1982.
12. Karlan MS, Ossoff RH, and Sisson GA: A compendium of intranasal flaps, Laryngoscope 92:774-782, 1982.
13. Kridel RWH, Appling WD, and Wright WK: Septal perforation closure utilizing the external septorhinoplasty approach, Arch Otolaryngol Head Neck Surg 112:168-172, 1986.
14. Schoelzel EP and Menzel ML: Nasal sprays and perforation of the nasal septum. JAMA 253:2046, 1985.
15. Strelzow VV and Goodman WS: Nasoseptal perforation: closure by external septorhinoplasty, J Otolaryngol 7:43-48, 1978.
16. Tardy ME: Septal perforations, Otolaryngol Clin North Am 6:711-713, 1973.
17. Tipton JB: Closure of large septal perforations with a labial-buccal flap, Plast Reconstr Surg 46:514-515, 1970.
18. Wright WK: Closure of large nasal septum perforations (letter), Arch Otolaryngol Head Neck Surg 91:492-493, 1970.

Part IV

RECONSTRUCTIVE NASAL SURGERY

24

Nasal Related Craniofacial Surgery

Stanley J. Behrman and David A. Behrman

Each practitioner interested in facial aesthetics will tend to focus on his or her area of expertise: the rhinologist will focus on the nose, the ophthalmologist on the eyes and orbits, the oral and maxillofacial surgeon on the jaws, and the dentist on the teeth. Certainly the nose, that prominent midline protuberance, can be considered the most dominant facial feature. Yet, others have stated that ". . . nothing affects the facial appearance more than the position of the teeth and their supporting structures."[20] Understandably, there was a time when it was acceptable if a particular feature was viewed as "standing alone" as there was little possibility of correction on a larger scale. However, in today's era of essentially limitless reconstructive potential this tunnel vision is no longer acceptable. No isolated feature can be seen as an independent unit but must be viewed, analyzed, and corrected as part of a larger complex—the face. Not only must every aspect of the face in every dimension be evaluated when considering corrective surgery, but every practitioner must be cognizant of what his colleagues can accomplish in those regions outside of his own selected area of expertise.

There are three general classifications of facial features that must be addressed during the development of any treatment plan. First are those features that *cannot* be changed, or *are* changed but rarely because of the extensive and heroic nature of the surgery. An example of a feature that cannot be changed, except in rare cases, is the width between the eyes, as in Crouzon's Syndrome. The second classification is of those features that can, but may or may not be, altered by a colleague. The third classification is of those anatomical features that can be altered, revised, or corrected by the practitioner himself. The overall aim should be one of achieving balance and harmony between the various parts. Each surgeon must ask himself a number of questions: How can I make this face most pleasing to its possessor? What can others do to correct its abnormal or unattractive parts? How can what I do balance those aspects of the face that cannot be altered? How can what I do emphasize the positive features or detract from any other unattractive features? How can I accomplish all of this with the least amount of surgery? The purpose of this chapter is to indicate the facial changes that the oral and maxillofacial surgeon can accomplish and to demonstrate one such surgeon's method of "designing" a face.

History of Orthognathic Surgery

Orthognathic surgery (*ortho*—to straighten; *gnathic*—jaws) as we know it today is little more than two decades old. The first surgical correction of mandibular prognathism was performed by Hullihen[11] in 1848, more than 30 years before John Orlando Roe[17] performed the first endonasal reduction rhinoplasty prior to 1887. Perhaps oral and maxillofacial surgeons could be forgiven for not considering facial features other than the mandible because, until the early 1960s, all they could effectively do was move the mandible *back* into a reasonable occlusal relationship with the maxilla, thus correcting the prognathic or pseudo-prognathic jaw. A great variety of procedures were used for this, some on various parts of the vertical ramii[3,16,21] and others on parts of the horizontal body.[4,8] Except for one body technique performed both intraorally and extraorally (with an interval of several weeks between the two approaches)[7] and a couple of very rarely performed intraoral methods,[14] all of these procedures were done through extraoral cutaneous incisions. These same techniques were either not applicable at all or, if applicable, were of limited value in advancing the mandible to correct retrognathia or micrognathia.

Similarly, perhaps rhinologists could be excused from concerns about a long or prominent anterior maxilla, what Gustav Aufricht[1] called a "gummy smile" (Fig. 24-1, *A*). After all, until the mid-1960's all that their oral surgical colleagues could do was extract the prominent teeth, excise the protrusive alveolus, and have a fixed or removable prosthesis inserted by the patient's dentist. Attempts at maxillary corrective procedures such as LeFort I movements either failed[6] or, if made up of dento-alveolar segments, were so controversial as to be minimally utilized.

As with Jacques Joseph in rhinoplastic surgery, our Western European colleagues were ahead of us in orthognathic surgery. Kole,[12] Wassmund,[25] and Schuchardt[18] were performing and reporting maxillary segmental surgery in the 1950s. Trauner and Obwegeser were moving back and successfully advancing the mandible in the 1950s, and were doing this via an intraoral approach. They presented an extensive report of their work in the American literature in 1957.[24] However, this seemed so radical to American oral surgeons that a comprehensive survey in the late 1960s indicated that their procedure had been performed only rarely before 1967.[2] Although it was Aufricht and Safian who brought Jacques Joseph's rhinoplastic techniques to America, it was Obwegeser himself who truly introduced his and other European techniques to American surgeons at a historic conference at Walter Reed Hospital in July 1966.[15] This marked the *real* beginning of orthognathic surgery in the United States. Soon, fundamental research in blood supply, animal experimentation, and American ingenuity produced an explosion of surgical procedures, instrumentation, and techniques. Today, both jaws, the mandible and maxilla, can be moved and repositioned, tilted and torqued, in whole or in segments, up and down, forward and back, in any direction, and to almost any extent. The middle and lower thirds of the face can be sectioned, segmented, and repositioned like a jigsaw puzzle. And, the oral and maxillofacial surgeon can do all of this via intraoral approaches. Only when the nose is to be moved along with the maxilla (LeFort II movement),[5,9] or when portions of the orbit are to be repositioned (LeFort III or craniofacial movements),[23] are extraoral incisions used.

Corrective Surgical Movements

It is important to remember that what we see when we look at a face is soft tissue supported by bone. If the surgeon wants to produce changes in the basic structural appearance, the underlying supportive hard tissues must be moved either physically or by simulation, as with an implant. Although a soft-tissue procedure, such as a rhytidectomy, can counteract the effects of aging, it can do little to change the basic facial architecture. It is important to know what changes surgical movements can accomplish.

The body of the mandible, which is a horseshoe-shaped arch containing the teeth, can be moved back to correct prognathism, forward to correct retrognathism, and rotated to either side to correct laterognathia. It can be torqued (rotated) up in front to close an open bite or brought down to correct a deep, closed bite. If the maxilla is brought up to shorten a long face, the mandible can autorotate up or be brought up into proper contact with the maxilla (Fig. 24-1, *B-D*). It can rotate or be brought down when the maxilla is lengthened to correct a short "middle-third." The mandible can be widened or narrowed anteriorly or posteriorly. Although total mandibular sub-apical alveolar movements are not too successful, tooth-containing segments can be repositioned in any direction within certain constraints of distance. The non-tooth-bearing portions of the mandibular body can be moved as well. The bone of the chin may be advanced or retruded, raised or depressed, made wider or narrower, and be moved to the right or left. The lateral bony borders and the angles may be trimmed or augmented.

Although Tessier developed techniques to move the entire maxilla including even the orbits (LeFort III),[23] these will have minimal application to most surgeons doing rhinoplasties. Their interests should be di-

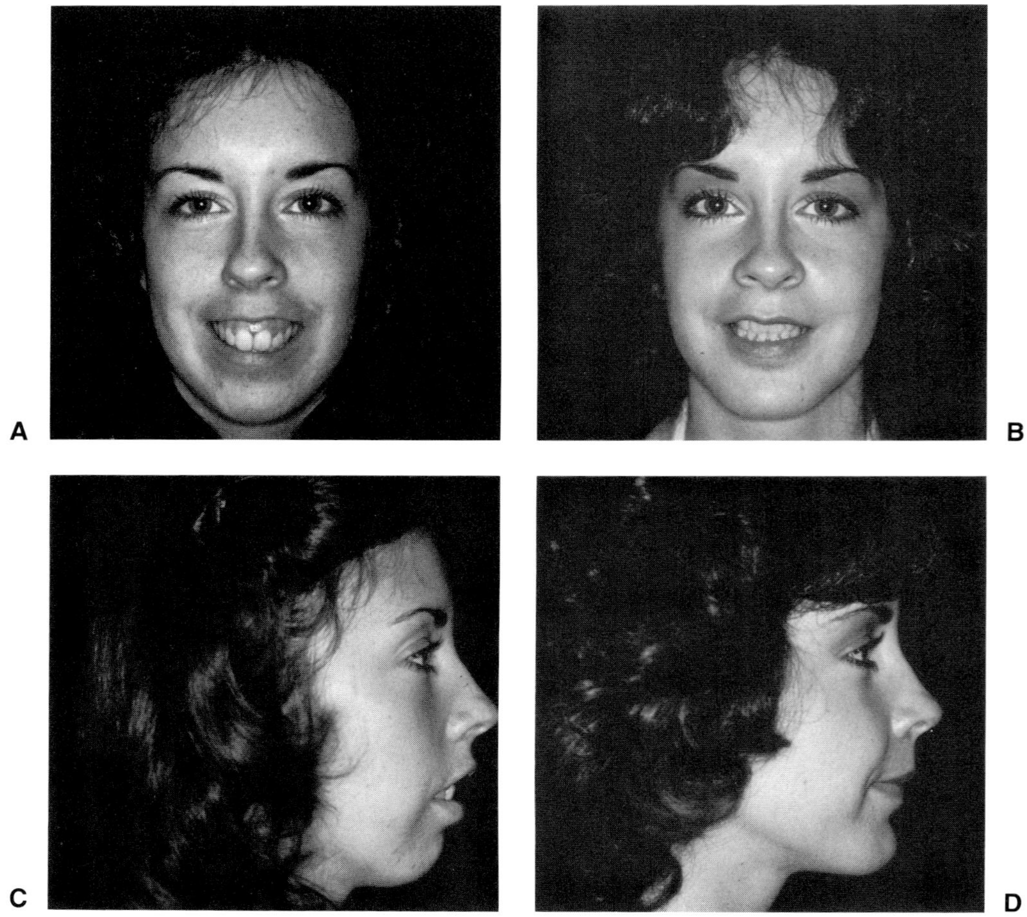

Fig. 24-1. **A** and **C**, A 22-year-old female with a "gummy" smile (vertical maxillary excess) and excessive interlabial gap. **B** and **D**, Moving the maxilla up and forward as the mandible autorotates in the correct occlusion corrects the problem. Moving the chin up and forward aids in reducing the interlabial gap and improves the profile.

rected to what can be accomplished by dento-alveolar segmental movements as well as LeFort I and LeFort II types of changes. We have found the LeFort II movements particularly useful for advancing the middle third, the maxilla and the nose, which has been depressed secondary to trauma and subsequently healed in an uncorrected or incompletely corrected position. The LeFort II advancement can be modified by simultaneous LeFort I movement in any direction. However, it is the LeFort I movements, those of the maxillary dental arch with or without the palate (the latter to minimize any changes in nasal respiratory volume), as a unit or in segments, that have the principal application to rhinoplastic surgeons. These are the movements that can correct Aufricht's "gummy smile", change the naso-labial angle, advance or retrude the upper lip, broaden or possibly soften the alar bases, or raise or lower the tip of the nose (see Figs. 24-1 and 24-2). Each of these movements and their effect on the soft tissue must be considered individually.

The role of the orthodontist and the prosthodontist must not be forgotten. Through their "non-invasive" techniques they can change the lip support and contour, affect the naso-labial angle, and lengthen or shorten the anterior teeth in relation to the lips. Newer methods of bonding, of fastening facings onto the labial surfaces of the teeth, can make interesting and significant changes without removing tooth structure.

The precise degree of response—the millimeter movement of the soft tissues responding to movement of the underlying teeth and bone—will vary depending upon the texture, thickness, and type of support of the soft tissues. When the mandible is set back, it carries the overlying soft tissues—the lip and chin—back in a 1 : 1 ratio. When the mandible is brought forward the chin responds in a 1 : 1 ratio while the lower lip may advance 60% to 70%. Soft-tissue response to an anterior segmental movement usually is about 75% of hard-tissue movement. An anterior mandibular six-tooth segment can be brought back, carrying the lip with it, to 'create' a chin that was not evident before. The segment can be torqued, tilting its base forward, diminishing a too-deep mento-labial sulcus.

Probably no extra-nasal structures affect the appearance of the nose as much as do the upper lip and the paranasal tissues. If these are protruded, the nose will appear small; if they are retruded, the nose will appear large (Fig. 24-2, *A*). Altering the size of the nose will change its independent appearance but may not improve the total facial aesthetics or correct the underlying structural problem. A thin, flat upper lip will detract from an otherwise aesthetically pleasing nose as will a too-full upper lip with a markedly acute naso-labial angle. The six-tooth anterior maxillary segment can be tilted forward to support a thin, flat lip, or can be brought back to help flatten a too-curved or prominent lip. Soft-tissue response will be about 75% of the tooth movement.

The amount of upper anterior teeth shown in repose or when smiling must be taken into consideration. A 'gummy' smile is both unattractive and unhealthy (see Fig. 24-1, *A*). The patient with an excessive interlabial gap, whose perioral muscles must strain to get a lip-seal in order to swallow, often will have xerostomia, with periodontal problems as a frequent consequence. Not showing teeth with the lips at repose is a sign of aging. The maxillary anterior segment can be raised or lowered to change the amount of teeth and gingiva seen at repose or when smiling. Of course, all of these segmental movements, both mandibular and maxillary, are predicated upon obtaining a good functional occlusion.

The LeFort I movement is an extremely versatile procedure with repositioning possible in all directions (see Figs. 24-1 and 24-2). These movements, up and down, forward and back, etc., can be in various

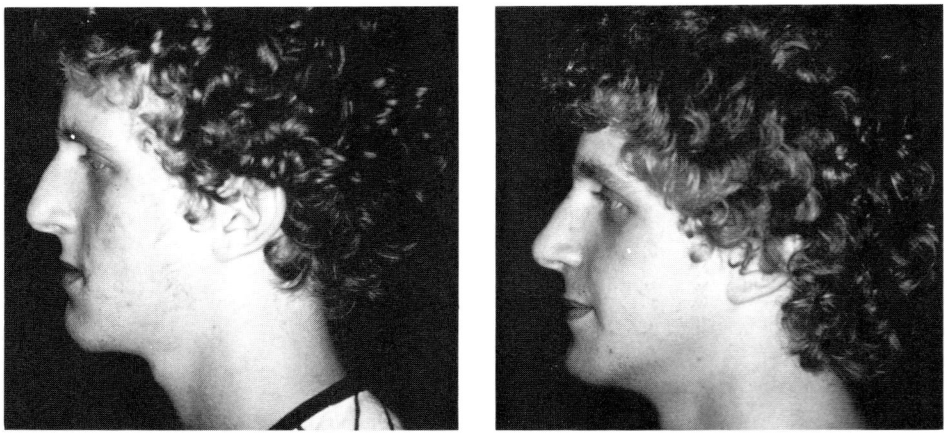

A B

combinations and three-dimensional planes. All will have different and cumulative effects on the overlying soft-tissue. Some generalities of response can be noted. The upper lip often follows superior LeFort I movements in a ratio of approximately 1:5, soft-tissue to hard-tissue; there is minimal lip lengthening in response to inferior repositioning. Forward movements usually bring the soft-tissue forward between 50% and 75%, but this can vary greatly. Backward LeFort I repositioning usually causes the soft tissue to follow about 50% to 75% and allows the upper lip to fall slightly. That portion of the lip supported by the incisors will move more than the tissue approximating the anterior nasal spine. The LeFort I may be "high" or "low", relating to the height of the bony cuts. The higher they are the more soft tissues of the paranasal and cheek areas will be affected.

Of importance is that superior and forward LeFort I movements will cause elevation of the nasal tip relative to the degree of movement and treatment of the anterior nasal spine. There will also be an increase in the fullness of the cheeks lateral to the nose and broadening of the alar bases (see Figs. 24-1 and 24-2). Use of an alar cinch suture can help minimize the widening of the alar bases. There always will be variations of change related to the degree of movement, soft-tissue volume, texture, consistency, and suturing technique. A consequence of the horizontal vestibular incision and release of the paranasal musculature is a thinning of the upper lip. A "V-Y" suturing closure can be used to restore bulk to the lip if this thinning is not desirable.[19]

The knowledge that so many facial changes are possible places a new burden on the rhinological specialty surgeon—the face must be seen differently. Features that previously may have been omitted from his conscious purview because nothing could be done about them must now be seen, perhaps measured, and evaluated. The surgeon must also bring these areas of potential change to the patient's attention. Because

Fig. 24-2. A 17-year-old male with a prominent nose, **A,** and with a malocclusion, **C,** which can be corrected by moving his mandible back or his maxilla forward. Either way the occlusion will be the same, **D.** He has a Profile Angle of 81° and his lips are well behind the Profile Line. Moving the maxilla forward (LeFort I) makes the nose appear smaller, **B.** The Profile Angle remains at 81°; the lips are in better relationship to the Profile Line.

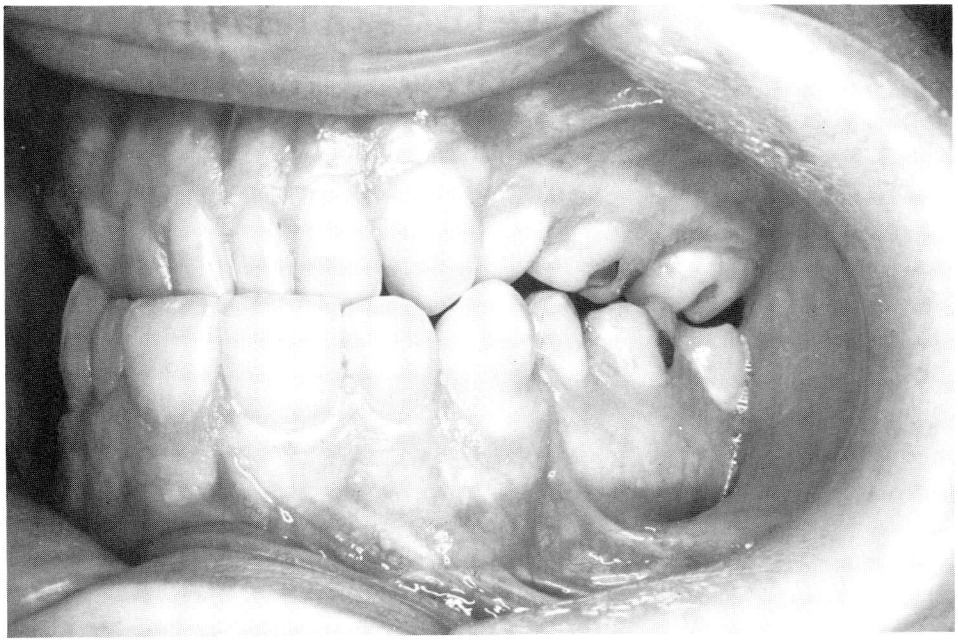

C

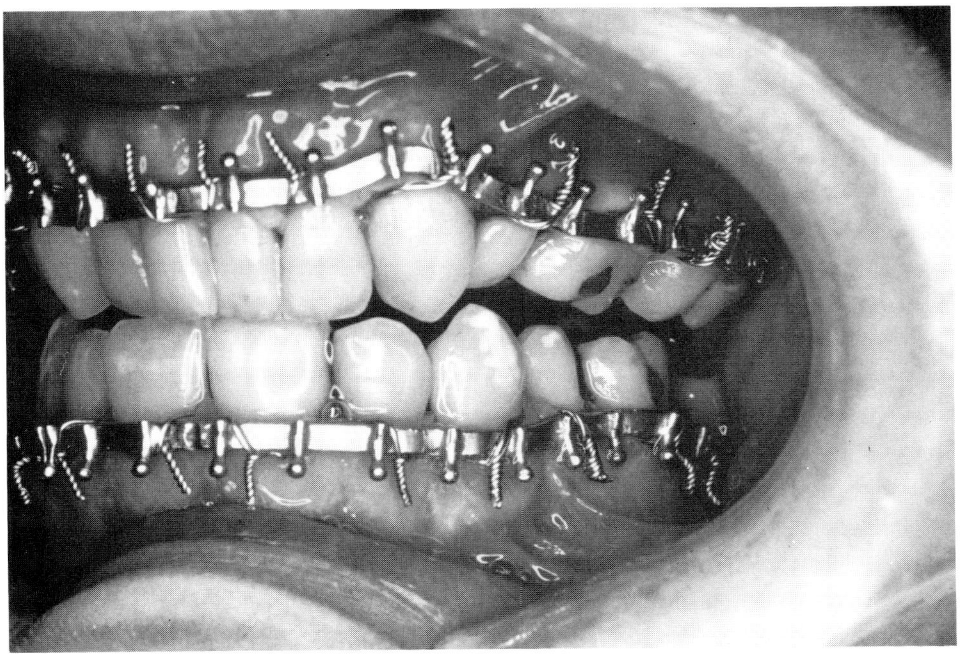

D

patients have no idea that these deformities can be rectified, they frequently will claim that certain unattractive facial features are not bothersome. Once they learn that correction is possible, they reveal their true feelings. Alternative treatment plans may have to be developed to provide the patient with sufficient information to make a rational choice. Questions such as rhinoplasty versus other surgery, rhinoplasty with other surgery, and the timing and sequencing of these procedures must be addressed.

Facial Planning

With very rare exceptions, every face has two eyes set high and lateral to a midline nose with a horizontal oral orifice below. The entire face is not much larger or smaller than a hand. Yet, with so few features to consider is it not remarkable that of the billions of people on this earth, except for the occasional zygotic twin, no two people are facially identical? What, then, is facial beauty? What comprises an attractive face? What makes someone "good-looking?" These are age-old questions. To the philosopher, good looks may be the inner beauty shining through. To others, facial beauty may influence many aspects of personal development or achievement.

Are there standards of attractiveness? Of course there are. And they vary from time to time, place to place, and individual to individual. Concepts of attractiveness are affected by ethnicity, culture, age, and even occupation. The professional beauty, the photographer's model, shows a different face in *Vogue* or *Harper's Bazaar* than she does in *Good Housekeeping* or *Ladies Home Journal.* In each publication the typical model presents a different appearance today than she did twenty years ago or will twenty years from now.

It is very misleading to propose that there are fixed determinants of facial beauty. One study involving the reactions of 150 males at a midwestern college to pre-selected photographs of beauty contestants purported to determine the perfect face by analyzing such things as height of the eyebrows and width of the nostrils. It should be obvious that this rather uniform group of males had concepts of facial beauty that had been culturally determined by exposure to television, motion pictures, and other media. The study really showed what *that* group at *that* time thought were the best looking of those pre-selected photographs. Another group at a different place may have seen things differently. Most significantly, of what value are standards that state such things as, ". . . the width of the mouth should be aligned with the pupils?" Neither the location of the eyes nor the width of the mouth can be changed readily, even with today's skills. Why should the alae of the nose be aligned with the inner canthi of the eye? Must the face be divided into equal thirds? Must the patient with an unusually long middle-third (measuring from the nasion to the anterior nasal spine) which cannot be changed be advised to have an equally high forehead and long lower third? The surgeon's own bias towards beauty must also be taken into account. Personal and subconscious views cannot and should not be eliminated. However, a conscious effort always must be made to consider the patient's desires paramount when "designing" a new face.

Craniofacial Analyses

Cephalometric Evaluation

Orthodontists have studied the facial skeleton for many years. Using lateral head radiographs—cephalograms—taken in a fixed, natural-head position, multiple analyses were developed expressing various anatomical relationships. These analyses were devised as aids in treatment planning and in predicting the pattern of facial growth and development. However, orthodontists were treating pre- and post-adolescents and were emphasizing the hard tissues. To make certain that the teeth were in occlusion the lips were held tightly shut. Thus, if the soft tissues were visible, they were distorted. The orthognathic surgeon operates on the hard tissues, but he must be completely aware of the soft tissues. He needs to see the soft tissues at repose for two reasons. First, aesthetic changes are a very important part of the treatment plan. Second, because a common presenting complaint is the lack of a lip seal, the circum-oral tissues must be evaluated without any strain to facilitate plans for correction. Therefore, for orthognathic purposes, a lateral cephalogram must be taken with the head in a natural position and with the teeth in contact and the lips at repose.

Initially, oral and maxillofacial surgeons adopted those standard cephalometric relationships that they found to be of value. In turn, new analyses were devised with recent increasing emphasis on soft-tissue evaluation. Anyone doing a considerable amount of surgery will find that all analyses are applicable when the basic facial skeleton is "normal" or near normal. "Normal" in this context is based on the "usual" measurements of "attractive" people. However, these systems falter if one or two of the fundamental components are askew. For example, the line SN, drawn from sella (the midpoint of the sella-turcica) to nasion (the junction of the nasal and frontal bones) represents the base of the skull. Many systems use angles drawn from this line to determine whether the mandible and maxilla are protruded or retruded from the norm.[22] However, if SN, the base line, is itself in an unusual position, very flat or extremely angulated, the system falls apart. The face may be very attractive, but the angles from the base line are abnormal and indicate otherwise. Similarly, when the length of SN is used as a basis, the system works best when it is "normal." Our emphasis is first on the unattractive soft-tissue relationships and then on the underlying skeletal structures that produced them. We are not interested in the analyses or their "numbers." Our treatment plan is to move the underlying structures in order to produce the desired *soft tissue* changes while providing or maintaining a functional occlusion. If the occlusion is good and the face is pleasing, the cephalometric skeletal values are supportive.

Profile Evaluation

All these analysis systems use lateral or profile projections. The orthognathic surgeon, like the rhinoplastic surgeon, must evaluate the profile. For the former it is important because, to date, all known dimensional change measurements are based on profile studies (with the exception of changes in nasal base width). For both surgeons the relationship between the nose, the chin, and the lips is a critical one, perhaps *the* critical one, in analyzing and planning a face. The rhinoplastic surgeon knows this better than anyone. Of course, all recognize that facial evaluation must be a three-dimensional one, "viewing" the face from all perspectives. However, until such time as the computer will allow the

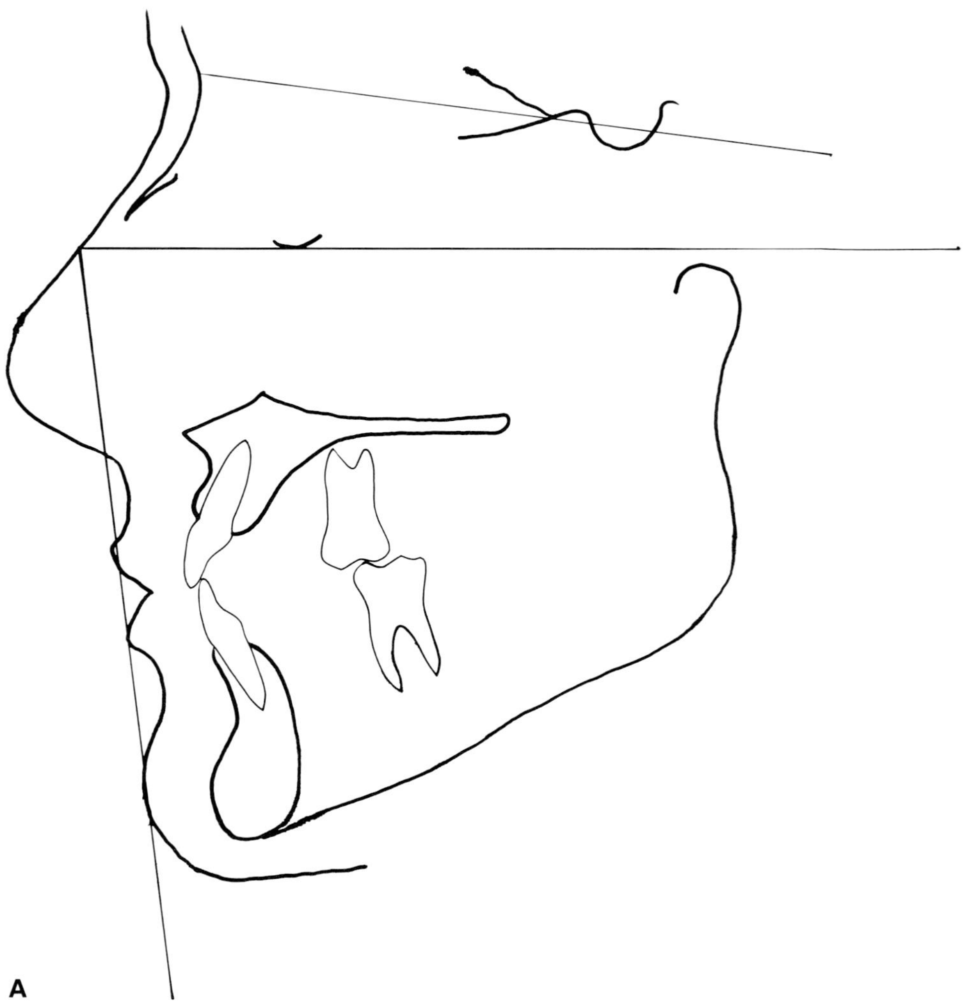

A

Fig. 24-3. The Profile Line and the Profile Angle. **A,** A tracing of an aesthetically pleasing profile: a 22-year-old model (Ford model) and actress. The Profile Angle is 83°, typical of the high-fashion model. **B,** A low Profile Angle (69°) can indicate either an over-projected nose or a retruded lower third of the face. **C,** A high Profile Angle (86°) can indicate either an under-projected nose or a protruded lower third of the face.

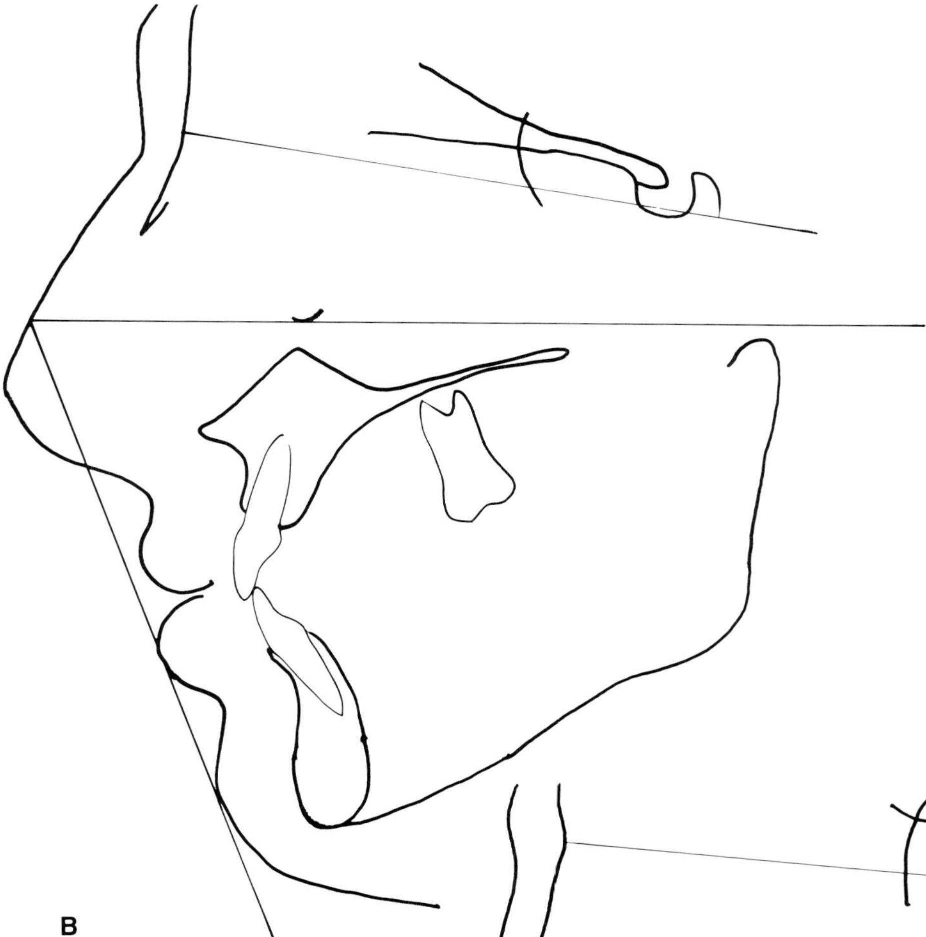

B

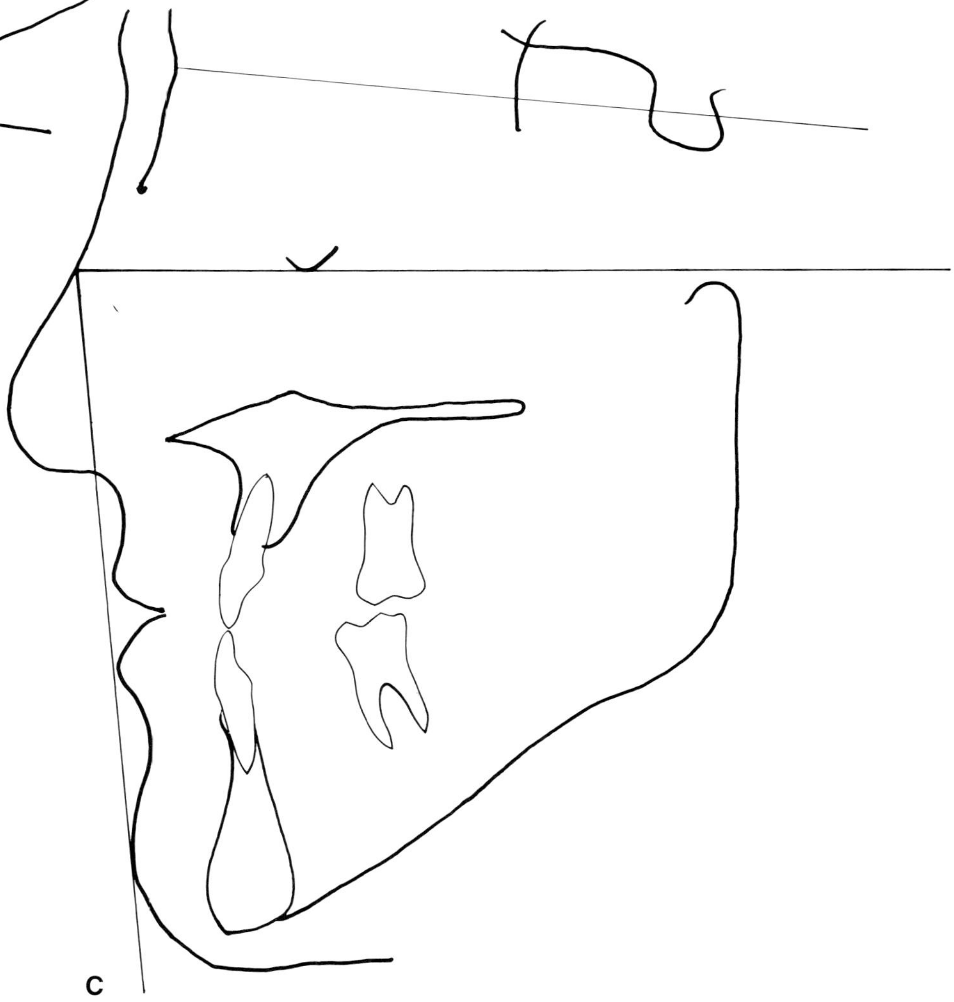

C

facial image to be rotated and soft-tissue response to skeletal movement to be visualized, it is the profile projection with which we must work.

There are two lines and the angle between them that we find most effective for evaluating the relationship between the nose, the lips, and the chin (see Fig. 24-3).

The profile line. The Frankfort Horizontal is a standard anthropological line. It is drawn from the most superior point of the external auditory canal to the base of the bony orbit. In our analysis, the Frankfort Horizontal is extended to intersect with the soft tissue of the nose. A line is drawn from this intersection tangential to the most prominent point of the soft-tissue chin. This line is the "profile line".* In an attractive profile the lips usually are just about on the profile line, or a little

*This is a modification of Merrifield's Profile Line[13] which, in turn, was a modification of Holdaway's H Line.[10] Our analysis of professionally judged attractive faces (models, actresses, actors) produced the above values.

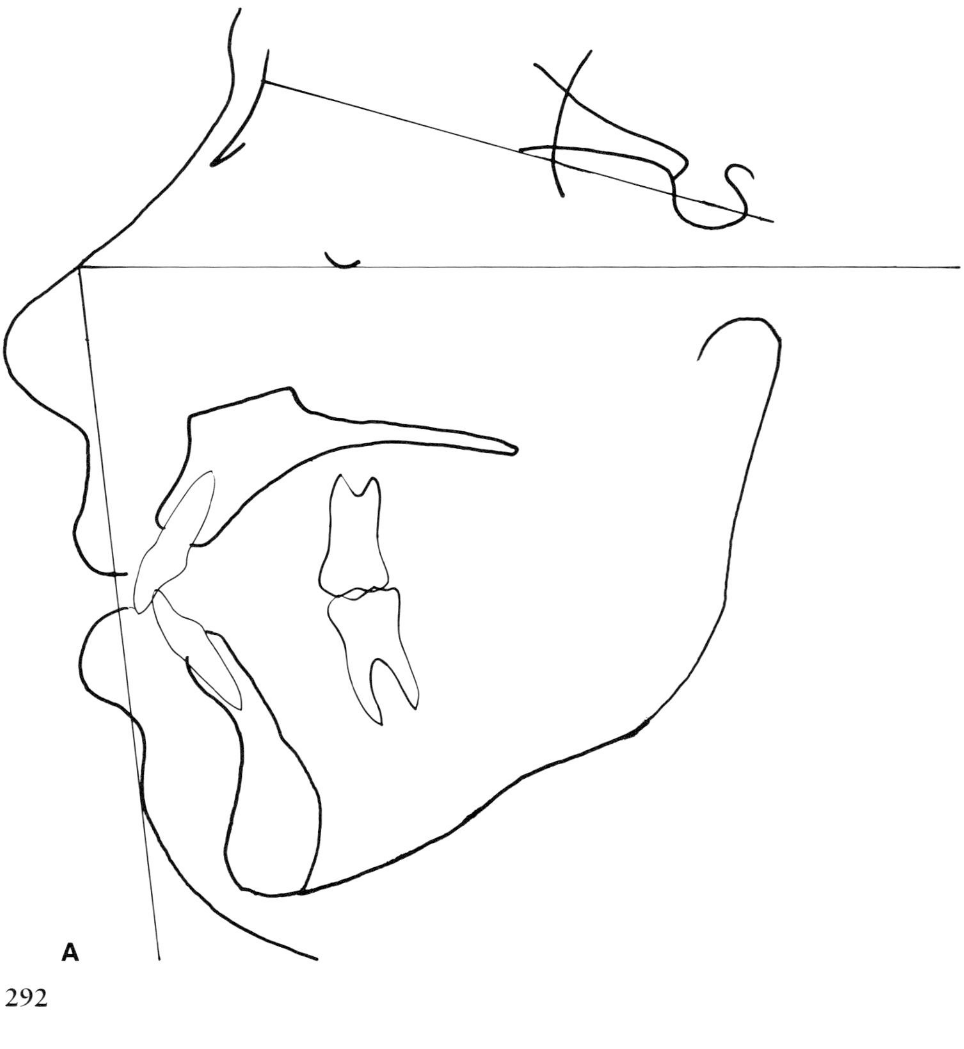
A

Fig. 24-4. The relationship of the lips to the Profile Line. The lips usually should be just in front of, on, or just behind the Profile Line with the upper lip a bit more forward than the lower. (Also see Figs. 24-3, *A*, and 24-5, *E*.) Both patients have a Profile Angle of 83°. **A,** The lips are well in front of the Profile Line, giving a bimaxillary protrusive appearance. **B,** The lips are well behind the Profile Line, giving the face a "dished-in" appearance.

bit forward or a bit behind (Fig. 24-3, A). The upper lip usually is a bit more forward than the lower. If the lips are too far forward of the line, a bimaxillary protrusive appearance will be present (Fig. 24-4, *A*). If the lips are too far behind the line, the face will appear concave or "dished-in" (see Figs. 24-4, B and 24-2, *A*). Ethnic features must be considered when developing any analysis or treatment plan, particularly as it concerns the position of the lips forward of the profile line.

The profile angle. The angle between the Frankfort Horizontal and the profile line is the "profile angle." An aesthetically pleasing profile is usually present when this angle is in the range of 80 to 83 degrees (see Fig. 24-3, A). The two facial features that have the most effect on the profile angle are the nose and the chin (see Figs. 24-3 and 24-5). The prominence of the nose is inversely proportional to the degree of the profile angle; the prominence of the chin is directly proportional to the degree of the profile angle. Reducing the prominence of the nose (Fig. 24-5, B) or advancing the chin (Fig. 24-5, C) will have the same effect on

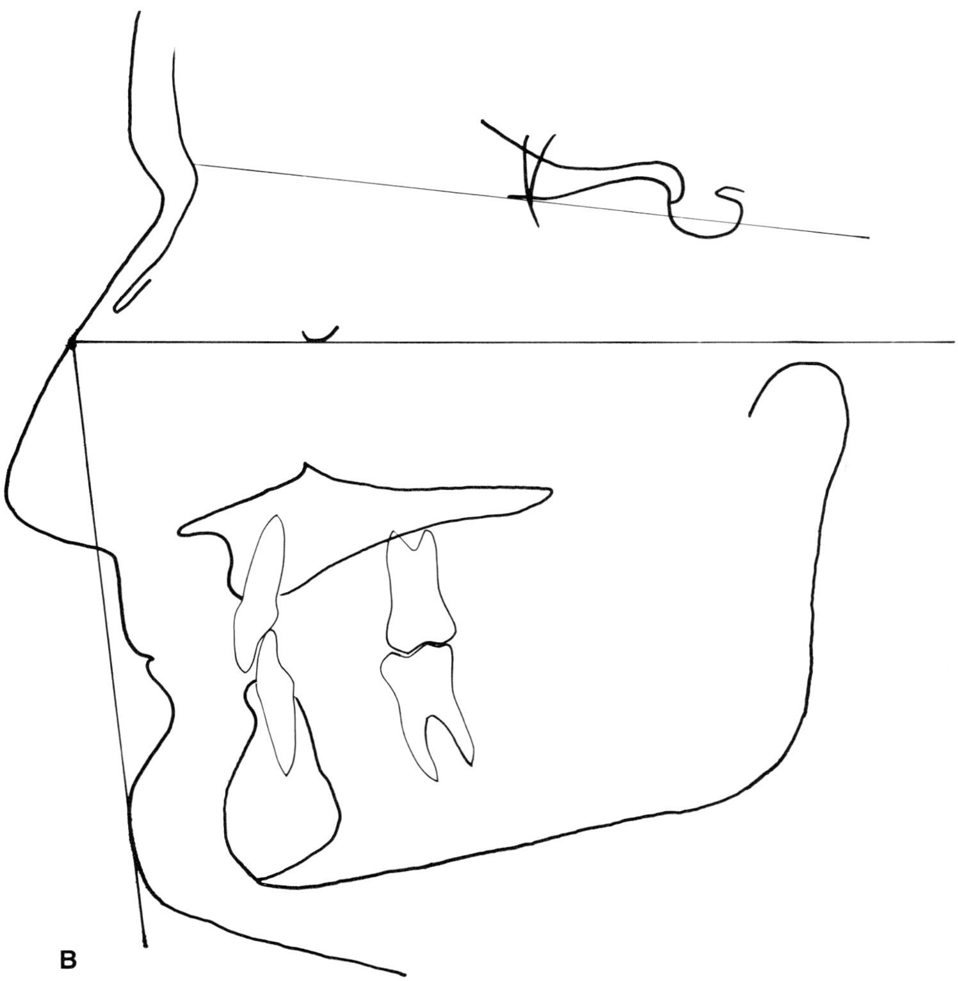

B

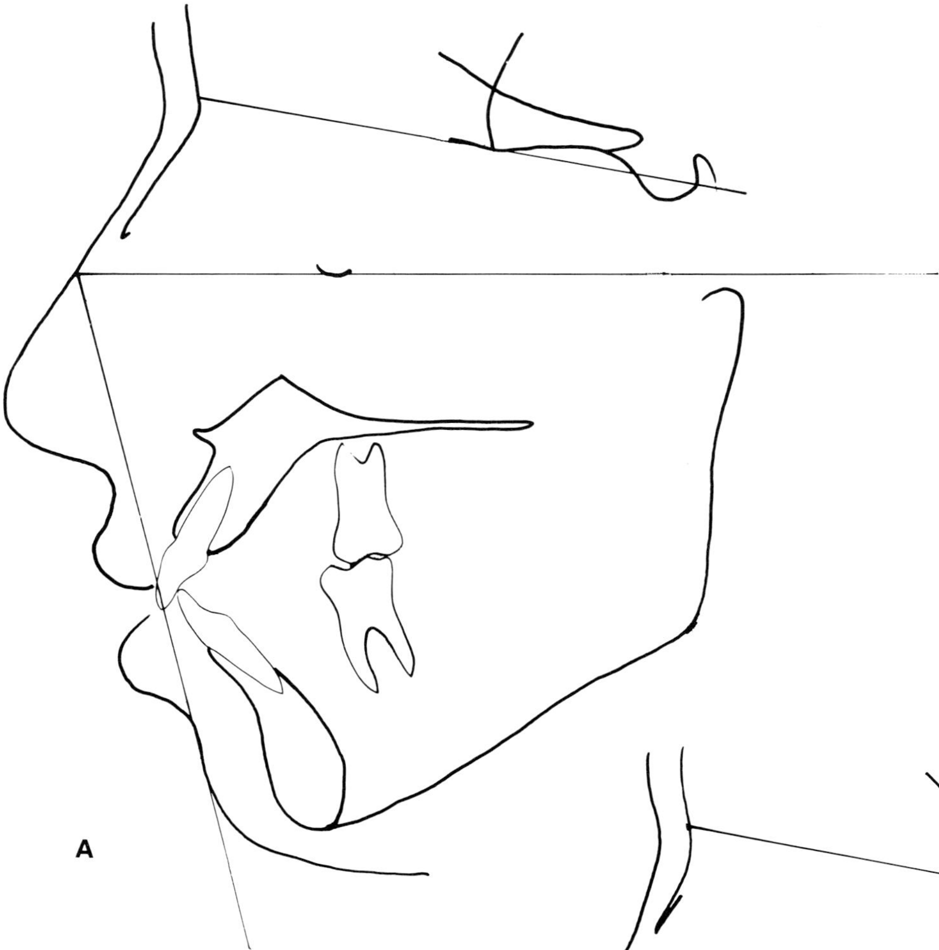

A

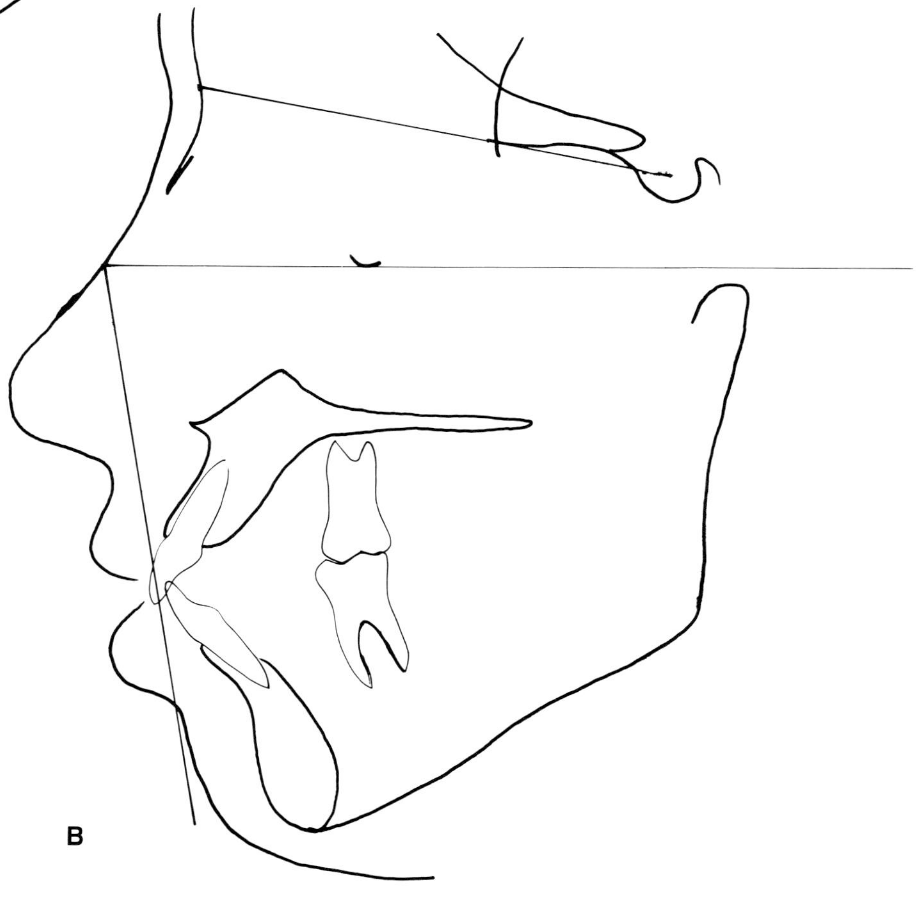

B

Fig. 24-5. Treatment planning: how the Profile Line and Profile Angle can help in selection of surgical procedures. **A,** The tracing of a 24-year-old medical student with a Profile Angle of 75° and her lips well in front of the Profile Line. **B,** Reduction rhinoplasty improves the Profile Angle to 80°, but the lips remain too far forward of the Profile Line.

Fig. 24-5, cont'd. C, Advancement genioplasty or chin augmentation also improves the Profile Angle to 80°, but the lips are still too far forward of the Profile Line. **D,** Reduction rhinoplasty plus chin advancement or augmentation advances the Profile Angle to 83°. The relationship of the lips to the Profile Line is improved, but the lips are still too far forward.

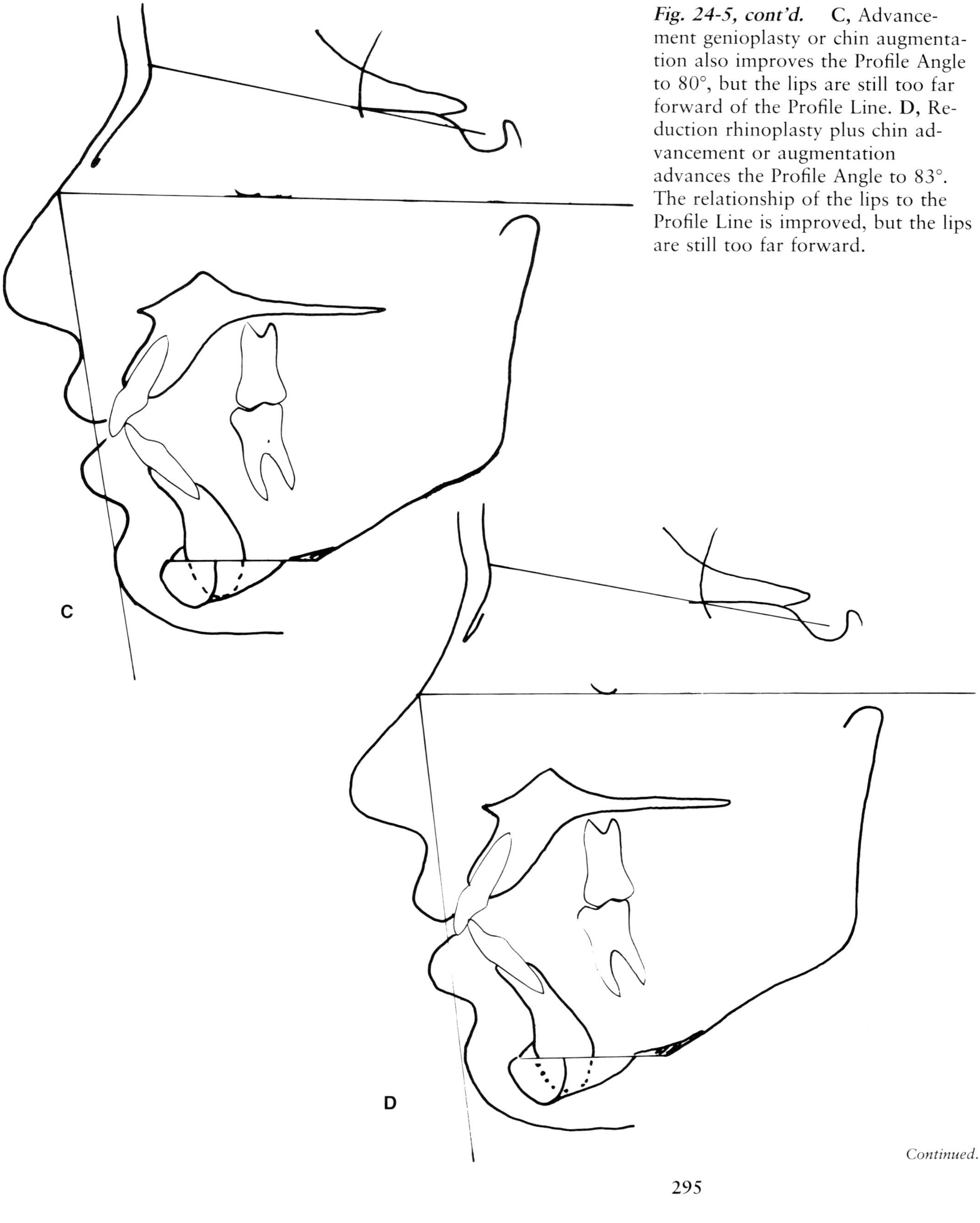

Continued.

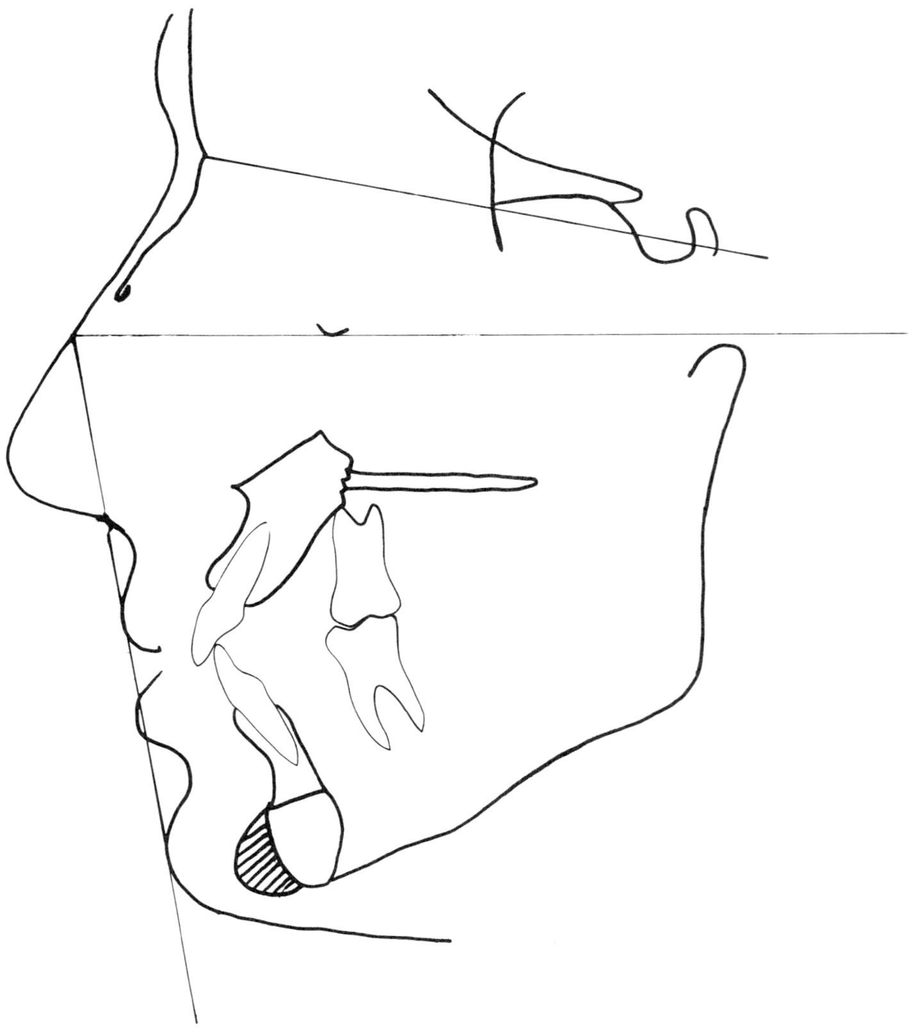
E

Fig. 24-5, cont'd. E, Chin augmentation advances the Profile Angle to 80°. Moving the anterior maxillary and mandibular segments back brings the lips to a good relationship with the Profile Line. This provides the most pleasing result.

the profile angle—that of increasing it. But each will have a different effect on the profile line. Reducing the prominence of the nose will bring the profile line closer to the lips; advancing the chin "moves" the profile line away from the lips. Thus, rhinoplastic, genial, and other orthognathic surgical procedures can be used to provide a pleasing aesthetic appearance using the profile line and profile angle as a guide for nose-lip-chin harmony (Fig. 24-5, *E*). Generally, a masculine profile looks good if the lips are slightly behind (see Fig. 24-2, B) or barely touching the profile line and the chin is well defined. Good balance between the nose and chin relative to the profile line may call for a slightly "stronger" nasal prominence and chin position, with a profile angle in the high-to-normal range. Conversely, the female profile line may call for a bit more nasal reduction, slightly fuller lips, and a less defined chin, with a profile angle in the low-to-normal range.

To the orthognathic surgeon, a low-profile angle usually connotes a retruded mandible (see Fig. 24-3, A), a high angle a protruded mandible or chin (see Fig. 24-3, C). To the rhinological surgeon, a low-profile angle may indicate a too-prominent nose (see Fig. 24-3, *B*), while a high angle may indicate a small, deficient nose (see Fig. 24-3, C). Each surgeon must evaluate the profile in its entirety if an appropriate treatment plan is to be developed with the best interests of the patient as its goal (see Fig. 24-5). For example, if the profile line traverses 6 or 7 mm of the upper lip area, it usually indicates maxillary protrusion. Reducing the prominence of the nose will only worsen that appearance. Advancing the chin will bring the profile line more forward, but may yield an unacceptable aesthetic appearance. Too frequently, we see a patient with a prominent maxilla who has had nasal reduction that emphasizes the already unattractive protrusion. Often, this is aggravated by the failure to remove premolars and to orthodontically retract the anterior teeth, which would have reduced the protrusion. Difficult problems such as this could be avoided if every practitioner viewed the entire face and established ideal treatment goals. It would be better still if we all could work in concert.

Other Evaluations

Although a lateral head cephalogram is ideal for developing a treatment plan, it is by no means the only projection possible. Acetate overlays can be taped over a photograph; the floor of the orbit can be approximated and the Frankfort Horizontal drawn tangential to it from mid-tragus to the nose. The profile line can then be drawn and the profile angle measured. This can be done on photographs of the patient or on pictures from magazines.

Vertical plane relationships and ratios also deserve consideration. For these purposes, upper facial height is measured from the point of junction of the frontal and nasal bones (point N) to the anterior nasal spine (ANS). Lower facial height is measured from anterior nasal spine (ANS) to the most inferior aspect of the chin (menton). Total anterior facial height extends from N to menton. In attractive faces, lower facial height usually is 43% to 45% of the total facial height. Because upper facial height cannot be changed significantly, almost all vertical correction must be made in the lower face. The maxilla (LeFort I) can be raised or lowered; the chin can be raised or lowered. As with all "values," there should be exceptions to the 43% to 45% ratio. A patient with a high forehead and a very long facial upper third does not *have* to have a long lower third. It certainly might be shortened to be 47% or 48% of the face and still be attractive.

The dimensions of the space between the lips at repose must also be analyzed. An interlabial gap of 3 to 4 mm will permit a facile and comfortable lip seal that is necessary for easy swallowing. A larger gap requires considerable strain of the perioral and mentalis muscles, as well as abnormal tongue function, to facilitate swallowing. In any patient with vertical maxillary or mandibular excess or deficiency, careful treatment planning is necessary prior to any surgical procedure. Vertical shortening of the nose in a patient with vertical maxillary excess will only worsen the "toothy" or "gummy" appearance. Raising the nasal tip to give the patient the turned-up nose she thinks she wants will exaggerate the gingival excess present and may create a problem for the patient where one did not exist before. Conversely, raising the nasal tip in instances of vertical maxillary deficiency will give the illusion of increased maxillary height.

The patient seeking help from the rhinological surgeon obviously feels there is something "not right" about his or her nose. This may or may not be valid. The nose may be abnormal in size or shape and may indeed not be "right" for an otherwise well-featured face. But the nose may not appear attractive because of some other aberrant facial feature. It is therefore the responsibility of any facial surgeon to be aware of the treatment potentials offered by the various surgical sub-specialities and of how these could affect the patient, and then to integrate these modalities into the treatment plan and its presentation to the patient.

REFERENCES

1. Aufricht G: In Stark RB: Aesthetic plastic surgery, Boston, 1980, Little, Brown, & Co Inc.
2. Behrman SJ: Complications of sagittal osteotomy of the mandibular ramus, J Oral Surg 30:554, August 1972.
3. Caldwell JB and Letterman GS: Vertical osteotomy of the mandibular ramii for correction of prognathism, J Oral Surg 12:185, 1954.
4. Cameron JR and Stetzer JJ: Bilateral resection of the mandible to correct prognathism, J Oral Surg 6:69, 1948.
5. Converse JM, Horowitz SL, Valauri AJ, and Montaudon D: The treatment of nasomaxillary hopoplasia. A new pyrimidal naso-orbital maxillary osteotomy, Plast Reconstr Surg 45:527, 1970.
6. Conway H, Smith JW, Behrman SJ: The late reduction of facial fractures, Am Soc Plast Reconst Surg 46:325, Oct 1970.
7. Dingman RO: Surgical correction of mandibular prognathism: an improved method, Am J Orthod 30:683-692, 1944.
8. Harsha WM: Bilateral resection of the jaw for prognathism, Surg Gynecol Obstet 15:51, 1912.
9. Henderson D and Jackson JT: Nasomaxillary hypoplasia: the LeFort II osteotomy, Br J Oral Surg 11:77, 1973.
10. Holdaway RH: A soft-tissue cephalometric analysis and its use in orthodontic treatment planning. I, Am J Ortho 84:1-28, July 1983.
11. Hullihen SP: A case of elongation of the underjaw, Am J Dent Sci 9:157-165, 1849.
12. Kole M: Surgical operation of the alveolar ridge to correct occlusal abnormalities, Oral Surg 12:277, 1959.
13. Merrifield LL: The profile line as an aid in critically evaluating facial esthetics, Am J Ortho 52:204-22, Nov 1966.
14. Moose SM: Correction of abnormal mandibular protrusion by intra-oral operation, J Oral Surg 3:304, 1945.
15. Obwegeser HL: Comprehensive Conference on Oral Surgery. Sponsored by The American Society of Oral Surgeons. Walter Reed Army Medical Center, Washington, DC, June 1966.
16. Robinson M: Mandibular prognathism corrected by overlapping open vertical osteotomies of the ramii. Report of 71 Cases, Am J Surg 98:894-897, 1959.
17. Roe JO: The deformity termed "pug nose" and its correction by a single operation, Med Rec 31:621, 1987.
18. Schuchardt K: Experiences with the surgical treatment of abnormalities of the jaws: prognathia, micrognathia and open-bite. In Wallace AG, editor: Sec-

ond Congress of the International Society of Plastic Surgeons, London, 1959, E & S Livingstone.
19. Schendel S and Williamson LW: Surgical maxillary superior repositioning and the facial muscles, J Oral Maxillofac Surg 41:235-240, 1983.
20. Shira R: Comprehensive Conference on Oral Surgery. Sponsored by The American Society of Oral Surgeons. Walter Reed Army Medical Center, Washington, DC, June, 1966.
21. Spilka CJ: Surgical correction of mandibular prognathism, Oral Surg 9:1255, 1956.
22. Steiner CC: Cephalometrics in clinical practice, Angle Orthod 29:8-29, 1959.
23. Tessier P: Total osteotomy of the middle third of the face for faciostenosis for sequelae of LeFort III fractures, Plast Reconst Surg 48:533, 1971.
24. Trauner R and Obwegeser HL: Surgical correction of mandibular prognathia and retrognathia with consideration of genioplasty. I. Surgical procedures to correct mandibular prognathia and reshaping of the chin, Oral Surg 10:677, 1957.
25. Wassmund M: Lehrbuch der Praktischen Chirurgie des Mundes und der Kiefer, Bd I Leipzig, 1935, Meusser.

25

Cosmetic Rhinoplasty on the Cleft Lip Patient

Howard W. Smith

The cosmetic surgeon performing rhinoplasty may be faced with his greatest challenge when a patient presents with a repaired cleft of the lip, seeking improvement in the appearance and function of the nose. It is essential that the cosmetic surgeon approach the patient with great caution and with a fundamental background in the pathological anatomy of the cleft lip nose. Routine rhinoplasty techniques may create limited improvements that ignore some defects. These improvements may be based on a distorted platform and may not result in an overall improvement.

Two basic types of cleft lip nasal deformity exist: those associated with the single cleft lip and those associated with the bilateral cleft lip. The nose is markedly deformed in both but in a very different manner. Added to the basic nasal defects associated with cosmetic rhinoplasty are those related to the repaired lip both in the primary repair and secondary procedures. A working knowledge of both the primary and secondary techniques is helpful since some primary repair techniques attempt to improve the nose while other techniques avoid working on the nose other than to effect a satisfactory closure of the nostril floor, equalization of the nostril size, and elimination of the connection between the mouth and internal nasal passages.

The entire face must be taken into consideration in evaluating the cleft lip nasal deformity. A frontal view of the nasal deformity in a single cleft lip patient differs markedly from that of the bilateral cleft lip nasal deformity. An acceptable frontal view of the repaired lip may present a very different perspective from a lateral view. The length of the columella, the height of the tip, the naso-labial angle, the relationship of the upper lip to the lower lip, the sublabial crease, and the chin tip are seen best in a profile view. It is on the profile view that the bilateral cleft lip nasal deformity is also shown to greatest advantage. In contrast, the frontal view is of greater importance in the single cleft lip nasal deformity.

Basic analysis lines are drawn on photographs of the patient and facial symmetry is analyzed in the frontal view, in the normal (Fig. 25-1, A), single cleft (Fig. 25-1, B), and bilateral cleft (Fig. 25-1, C).

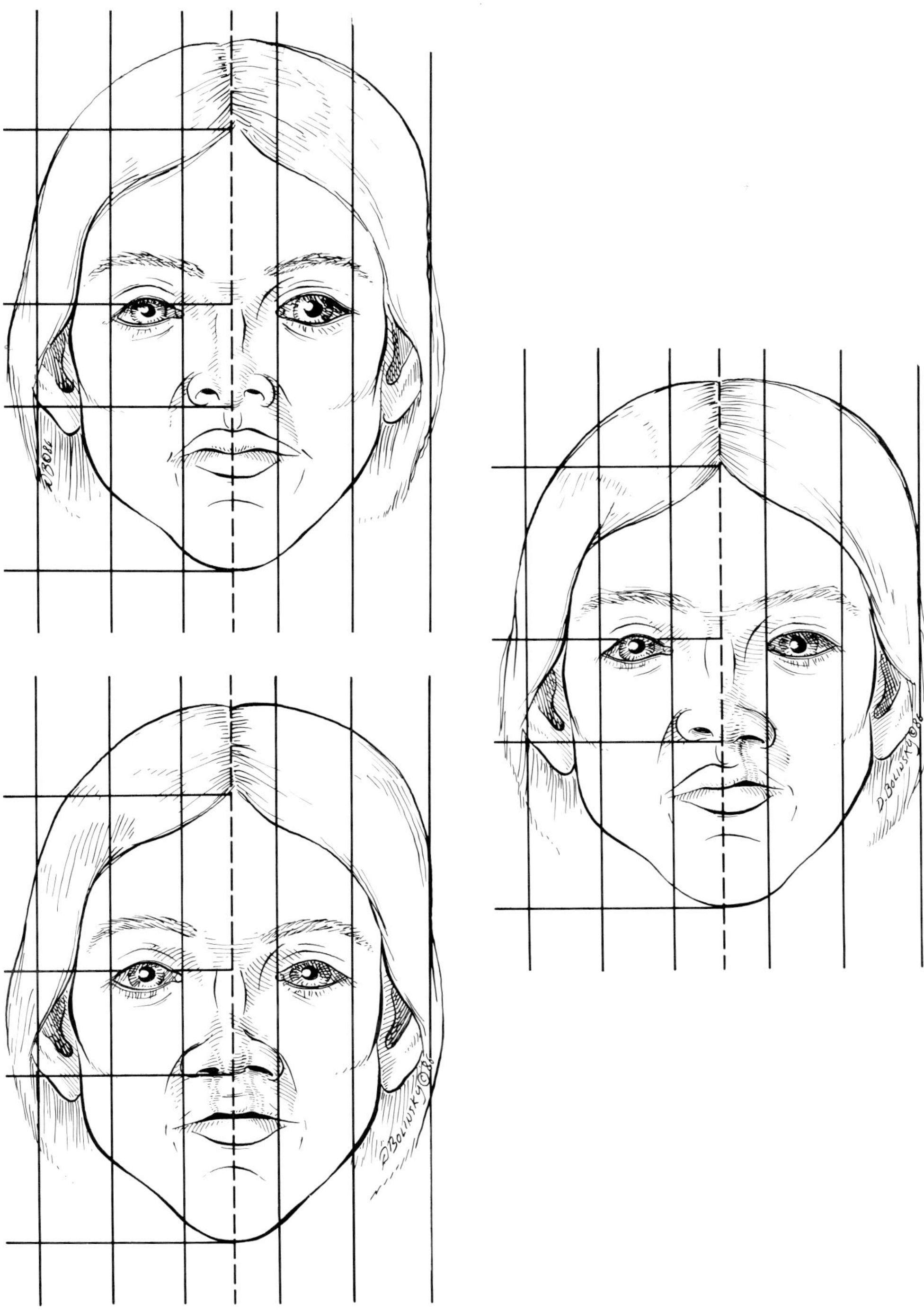

Fig. 25-1

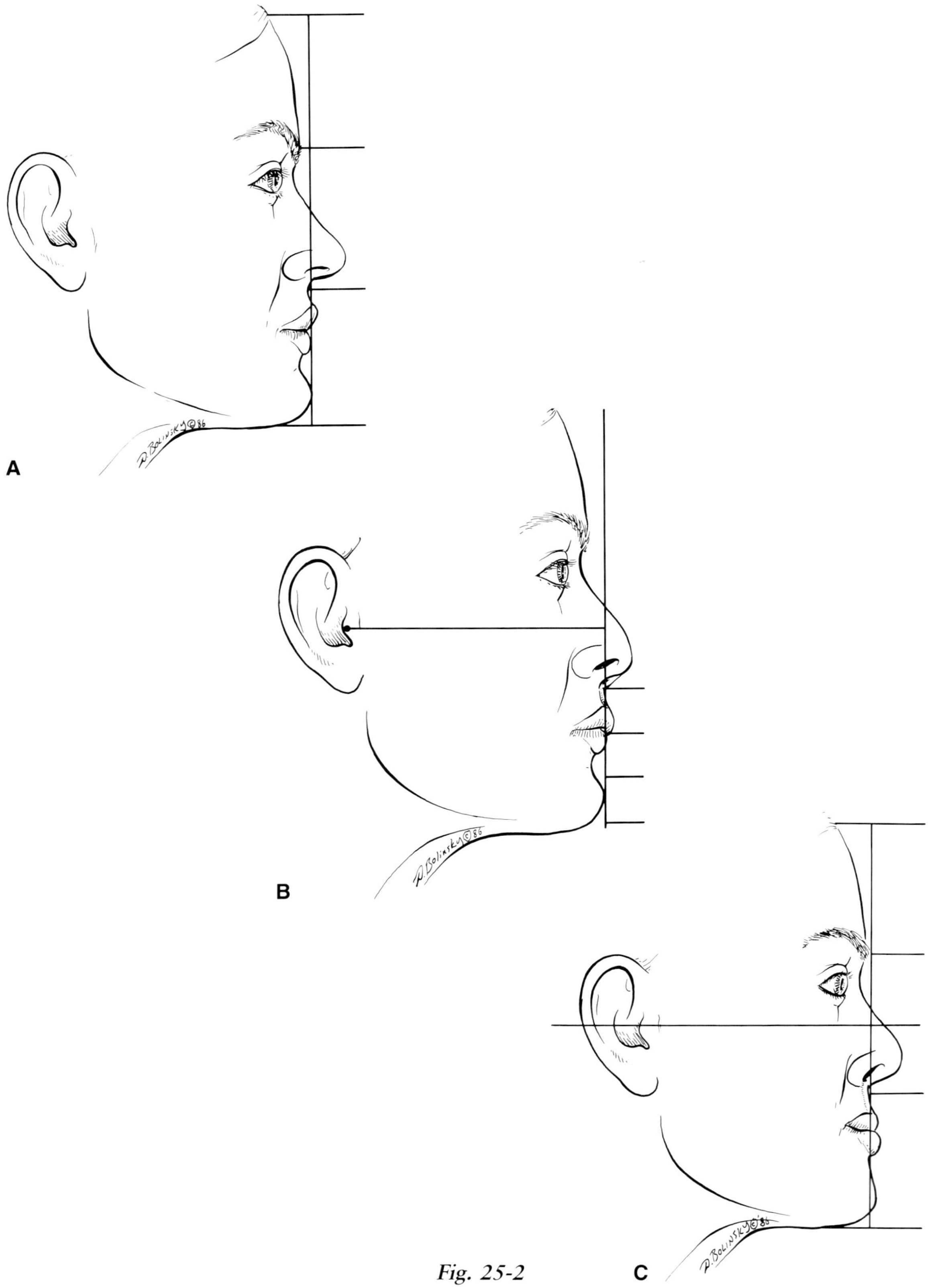

Fig. 25-2

The nasal problem is further analyzed on the profile view, using a perpendicular line drawn from the Frankfort horizontal line passing through the subnasali, normal (Fig. 25-2, A), single cleft (Fig. 25-2, B), and bilateral cleft (Fig. 25-2, C).

The three-quarters base view is analyzed in a similar manner: normal (Fig. 25-3, A), single cleft (Fig. 25-3, B), and bilateral cleft (Fig. 25-3, C).

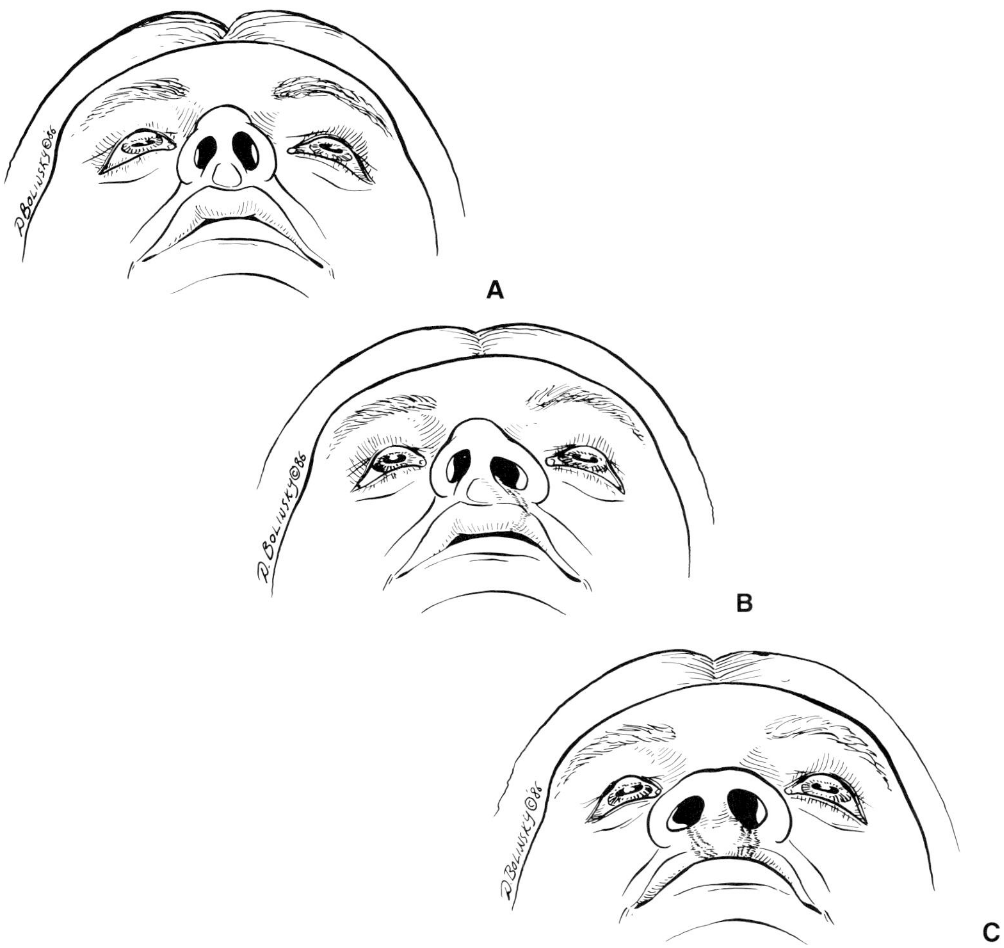

Fig. 25-3

Effect of Primary Repair of the Single Cleft Lip on the Nasal Defect

Regardless of the technique used, single cleft lip repair aims to close the floor of the nose and reduce the cleft in the lip. At this primary lip procedure, the repair in the floor of the nose is accomplished in the pre-alveolar and alveolar portions of the cleft. To enable these flaps to reach each other anteriorly and bridge the gap in the prealveolar area, it is necessary to release the lateral lip element from its cleft position so it can be brought medially to join with the noncleft portion of the lip. This involves making an incision in the depth of the cleft side labial sulcus, and to a lesser degree, in the labial sulcus of the non-cleft side. Undermining is done laterally over the maxilla and under the alar on the cleft side so that the freed lip elements can be brought toward each other in the midline. The cleft edges have to be pared to expose the muscle and create a mucosal edge, a muscle edge, and a skin edge for a three-layer lip closure. The mucosal edge of the lip becomes continuous with the mucoperiosteum covering the nasal and oral walls of the cleft in the pre-alveolar and alveolar areas.

In a manner similar to the lip, the mucosa over the nasal walls have to be freed so that they will meet in the midline. To do this it is essential to incise medially along the junction of the vomer mucoperiosteum with the oral periosteum and along the lateral border of the cleft to raise flaps along the vomer in the midline and along the nasal side of the cleft laterally (Fig. 25-4, A & B). These flaps are raised to allow the cut edges to approximate in the midline of the cleft where they can be stitched together, thus forming a floor for the anterior portion of the nose (Fig. 25-4, C).

It is readily appreciated that moving the cleft lip element medially allows the pre-alveolar flaps to approximate without tension. Thus, it is possible to easily close the floor of the nose with everting mattress sutures to create a single layer closure. The lip is then closed in layers. This is the simplest concept of cleft lip closure and it is also readily appreciated that very little has been done to the cleft-related defects in the nose.

A few surgeons interested in cleft lip-cleft palate surgery have developed techniques over the years to improve the appearance of the nose at the time of primary closure of the lip. Other surgeons have limited the primary cleft lip closure to simply closing the floor of the nose and approximating the nostrils.

Regardless of the technique used, all were aimed toward closing the nasal floor, creating nostrils of equal size, and producing as good a lip repair as possible. The effect of closing the lip allows the alveolar segments to come together and permits the nose to grow, without exaggerating the primary defects with added scar tissue.

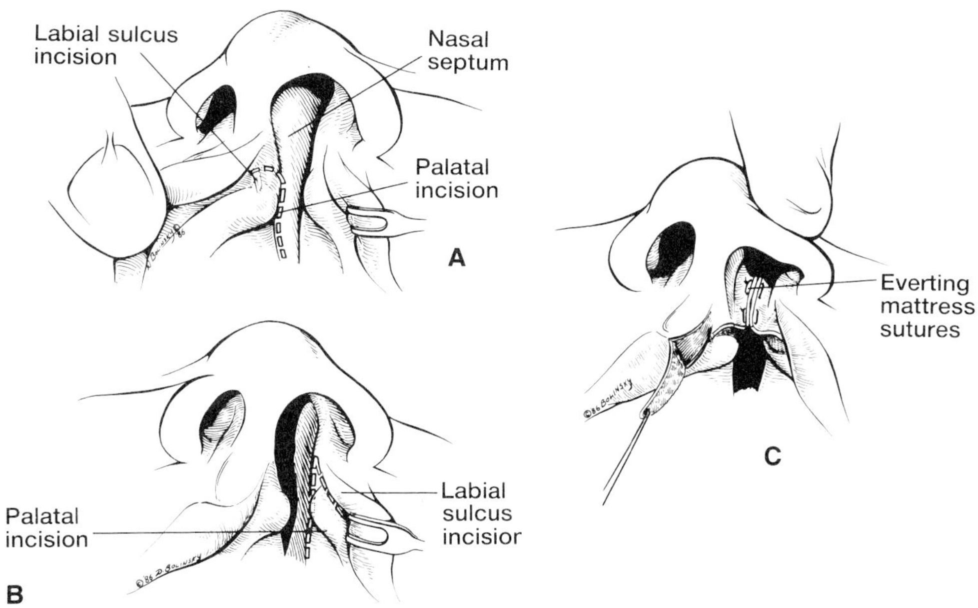

Fig. 25-4

The aim of operating on the nose at the time of primary closure of the lip is to make the nose more acceptable in appearance so that the growing patient could skip the period of secondary repairs (at the age of 6 to 8 years) and present at the age of 15 to 18 years for final cosmetic nasal surgery. At this later time it was felt that the entire problem could be addressed with essentially adult structures altered only in form and in position.

During the time lapse between the primary surgery within the first three months and the definitive nasal surgery between the age of 15 to 18, many patients are cast adrift from a particular plan unless cared for by a multispecialty team or in an age-staggered surgical group practice setting. Additionally, in our mobile society, the patient is quite likely to be in a different community at the age of 15 to 18 and is also likely to seek the services of a local cosmetic surgeon highly skilled in rhinoplasty, but not necessarily skilled in cleft lip and cleft palate repair, or inexperienced in treating nasal defects related to a cleft lip deformity.

Rapid advances in rhinoplasty technique also demand that the surgeon, who may be skilled in cleft lip and cleft palate repair, keep up with the advances in cosmetic rhinoplasty to possess these new skills that may be applied with benefit to the small number of cleft lip cases in his ongoing practice.

So it seems that the cosmetic surgeon specializing in rhinoplasty also needs to know what to do with a patient presenting for nasal surgery with a cleft lip background, since such a surgeon is likely to have more of the necessary skills to improve this type of nasal deformity.

Contributions to nasal improvements made at the time of primary closure are apparent in several techniques such as Skoog,[19] Millard,[13] Wynn,[24] Tennison,[21] McComb,[15] Sayler,[17] Schultz[18] and others. Since the lip scars are a good indication of the technique used,[7,13,19,21,24] the cosmetic surgeon can reasonably assume what was done with the nose at the time of primary closure or intermediate surgery. Since records are usually not retained by operators or institutions after a ten-year period, it is possible that the original records may have been destroyed. Often the record simply states what procedure was performed and does not give any of the minute details regarding what was done to various aspects of the pathological anatomy. The following techniques are of significance for the nose:

1. *Rose Thompson.* This is a simple straight-line surgical lip closure technique. The defect in the floor of the nostril is sutured, the nostril rims are made about equal in size, and the lip is simply closed in a straight line approximating the mucosa, vermilion, muscle, and skin (Figs. 25-5, A & B).

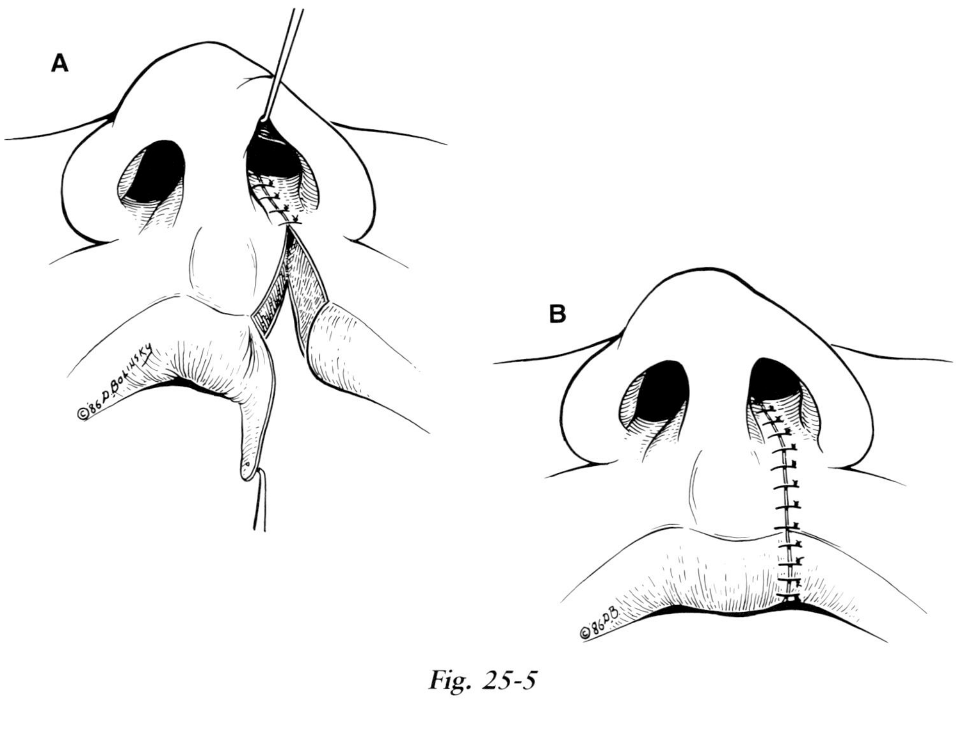

Fig. 25-5

2. *Tennison—Triangular Flap (Randall Modification).* This technique brings a triangular flap from the cleft lip element to augment the non-cleft portion of the lip in the lower one third (Figs. 25-6, A-C).

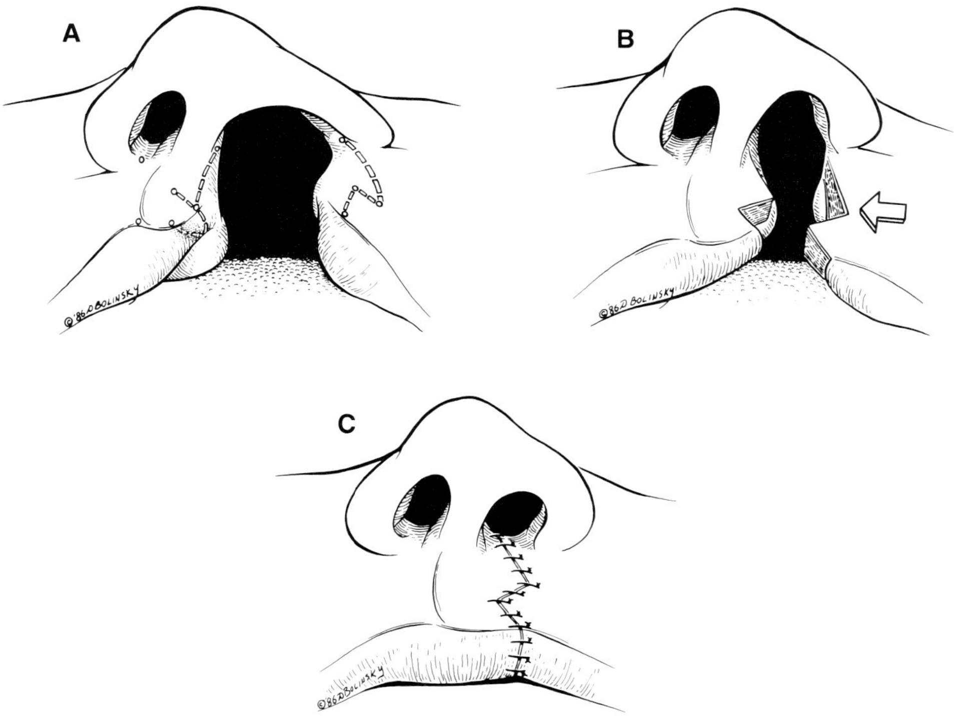

Fig. 25-6

3. *LeMesurier—Quadrilateral Flap (Wang Modification).* In this technique the lip is closed with a step-off similar to the triangular flap by adding a square piece of lateral lip element to the medial lip in the lower one third (Figs. 25-7 A & B).

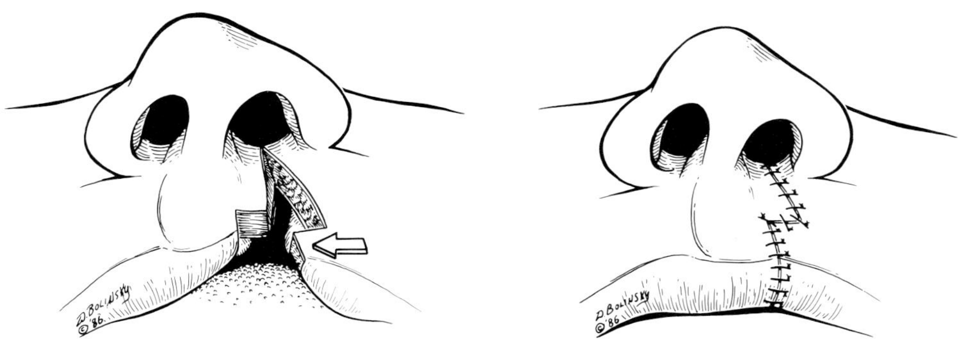

Fig. 25-7

4. *Millard Rotation Advancement.* This technique provides an advancing triangle of lateral lip element into the upper one third of the lip-base of the columella to raise, straighten, and support the depressed columella on the cleft side (Fig. 25-8).

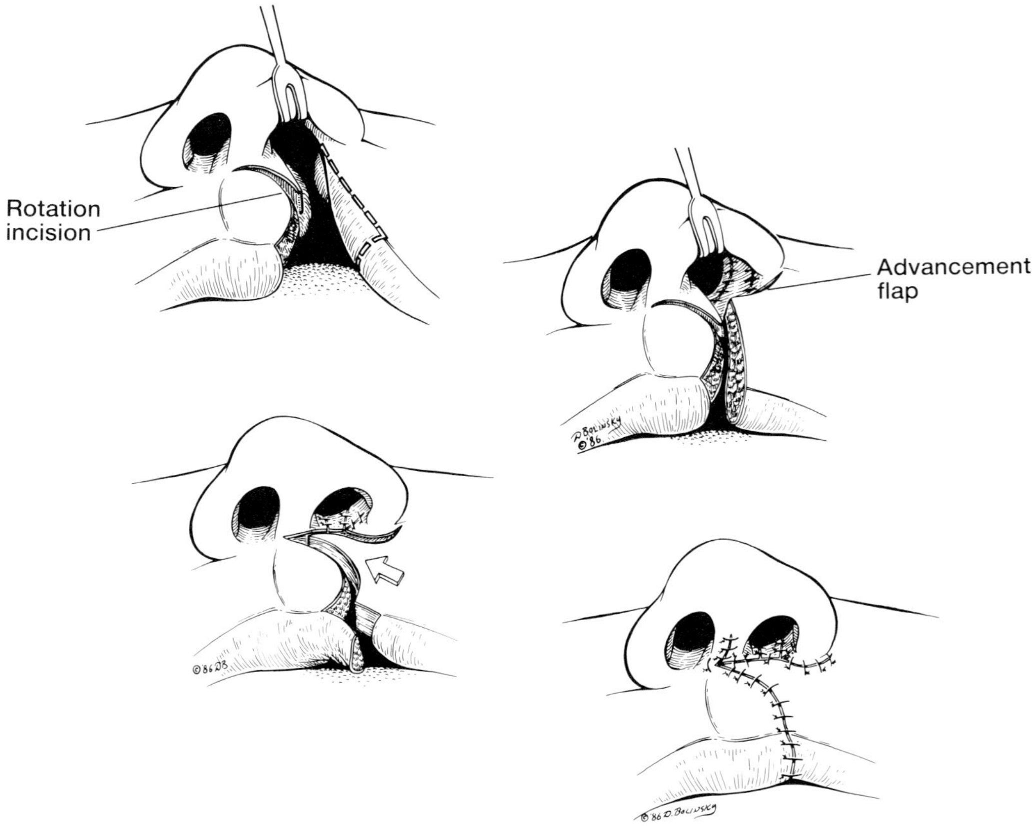

Fig. 25-8

5. *Skoog*. This technique provides a double triangle of tissue from the cleft side into the non-cleft side in the lip and columella areas to improve the nose (Fig. 25-9, A & B).

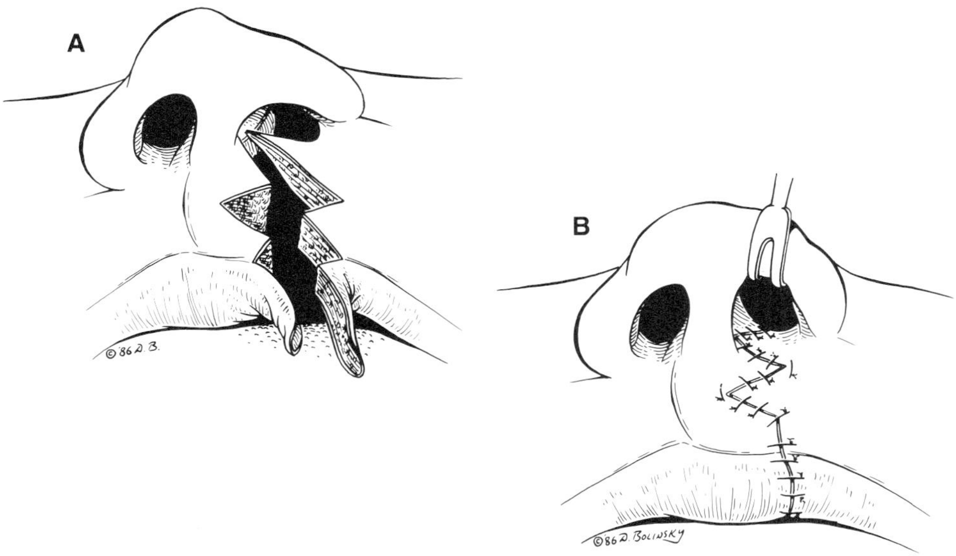

Fig. 25-9

6. *Wynn*. This technique uses a double triangle technique augmenting the non-cleft side at a lower level than Skoog (Fig. 25-10, A & B).

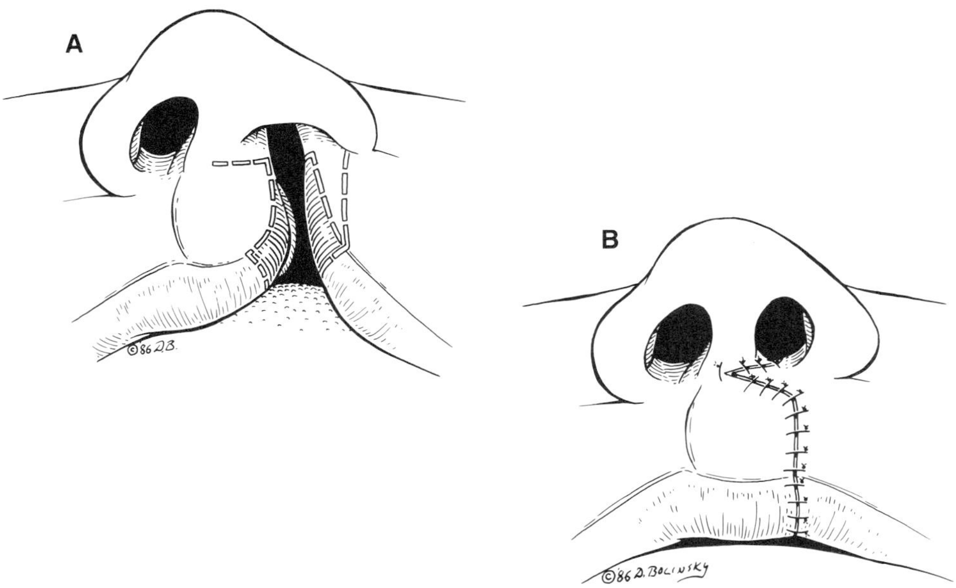

Fig. 25-10

Examination

The single cleft lip nasal deformity presenting in patients between the ages of 15 to 18 years or older must be examined carefully. Photographs are taken and prints are made to record the defects observed at examination for later study and postoperative comparison. For routine rhinoplasty procedures, the various parts of the nose, dorsum, lobule, and septum, must relate normally with each other. In the single cleft lip nose, the nose must relate to the cheeks, the upper lip, and the underlying maxilla even more than the nose considered for routine cosmetic rhinoplasty.

The experienced rhinoplasty surgeon realizes that he cannot create perfection, but he should be able to determine if he can effect improvement in some of the following defects.

A. Bony Supporting Structures

1. Hypoplasia of the cleft side of the maxilla involving the pyriform aperture.
2. Malocclusion or irregularity of the maxillary arch.
3. Lowered nasal floor on the cleft side.
4. Nasal spine displaced from the midline toward the non-cleft side.
5. Total nose deviated and directed toward the non-cleft side with respect to the rest of the face.
6. Flattening and possible shortening of the cleft side nasal bone.
7. Flattening of the alveolus in the region of the roots of the cuspid and lateral incisor teeth on the cleft side.
8. Missing teeth.
9. Collapsed dental arch.

B. Lip

1. Irregularity of the vermilion.
2. Prominent lip scars.
3. Tightness of the lip in the upper one-half.
4. Malposition of the base of the columella.
5. Elongation of the lip on the cleft side.
6. Scars below the cleft side alar.

C. Lower One-Half of the Nose

1. Cleft side alar base low, recessed, malformed, and inadequately rotated.
2. Nostril floor on the cleft side may be higher or lower than the normal side.
3. Unequal nostrils, drooped and retruded on the cleft side.
4. Rotation of the long axis of the nostrils toward the horizontal plane.

5. Tip of the columella tilted toward the cleft side with the base directed toward the non-cleft side.
6. Alar rim on the cleft side thin and possibly buckled.
7. Top of the nostril rim is low on the cleft side.
8. The dome of the nose is flat on the cleft side, displaced laterally with some degree of bifurcation. The tip is hooked down over the lip.
9. Palpable separation of the lower lateral cartilage from the upper lateral cartilage on the cleft side.
10. Shortening and flattening of the cleft side upper lateral cartilage with cartilage directed toward the non-cleft side.
11. Lower position of the lower lateral cartilage medial crus in the columella on the cleft side.
12. Angulation of the cartilaginous dorsum toward the non-cleft side with variation in the profile height.
13. Rotation or flattening of the cleft side lower lateral cartilage to produce a wall or baffle at the nasal valve area.

D. Septum

1. The anterior nasal spine is displaced toward the non-cleft side.
2. The quadrilateral cartilage presents in the non-cleft nostril and tilts toward the cleft side at the dome.
3. Deflection of the nasal septum at the junction of the quadrilateral cartilage with the perpendicular plate of ethmoid bone into the cleft nasal passage.
4. Displacement of the quadrilateral cartilage from the vomer groove into the non-cleft nasal passage with blockage of one or both airways.
5. Deflection of the vomer into the non-cleft passage and perpendicular plate of ethmoid bone to the cleft nasal passage.

Techniques

It is not possible to deal effectively with every defect in the nose associated with single cleft lip deformity. In some instances, tissue changes, tissue loss, or scar contractures are beyond correction. In most instances, however, it is possible to make cosmetic and functional improvements and erase many of the stigmata that cause one to instantly recognize a cleft lip nose.

Before working on the nose, it is desirable to evaluate the nose and lip as is done at the time of primary lip surgery. The lip is dried with acetone to degrease it and both the lip and the nose are marked out with Bonney's Blue Dye with either a sharpened applicator stick or pen. The following landmarks are identified (Fig. 25-11, A & B):

1. Midline of the lip (lowest point of Cupid's Bow).
2. Peak of Cupid's Bow on the non-cleft side.
3. Peak of Cupid's Bow on the repaired cleft side.
4. Midline of the nose at the base of the columella.
5. Base of the columella as it approaches the floor on the normal side to meet the philtral line.
6. Base of the columella on the repaired side as it approaches the nostril floor.
7. Termination of the alar roll on the normal side.
8. Termination of the alar roll on the repaired side.
9. Outline of lower lateral cartilage.
10. Proper height of nostril rim.

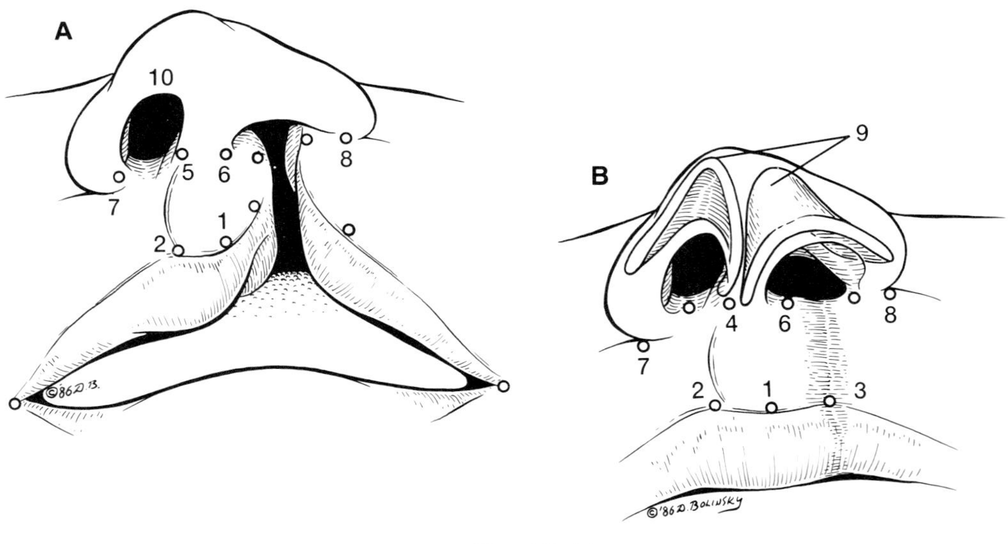

Fig. 25-11

The proper width of the nostril can be determined by using the normal side as a guide and taking the distance between 5 and 7 and comparing it with the cleft side markings between 6 and 8.

Although it presents many problems, the single cleft lip nasal defect can be studied and the defects sorted out. It appears that a routine rhinoplasty can correct many of the following defects:

1. Nasal hump.
2. Deviated nose.
3. Deviated columella.
4. Nasal spine displacement.
5. Septal deflections with nasal obstruction.

What a routine rhinoplasty does not correct are the following:

1. Hypoplasia of the maxilla.
2. Low, recessed, malformed, and inadequately rotated alar base.
3. Malposition and shape of the cleft side lower lateral cartilage.
4. Nostril asymmetry.
5. Buckled alar rim.

It is these nasal defects that take away from an otherwise acceptable lip repair. Most of all, they are the defects that the patient sees constantly and are the ones that will remain unless skilled surgery is applied to the areas not amenable to routine rhinoplasty techniques.

The technique described and illustrated here will be grouped to demonstrate methods available to augment the maxilla, correct the alar base, improve rim rotation, restore the lower lateral cartilage to an acceptable position, and thereby reduce or eliminate most of the nasal asymmetry.

Maxilla

It is essential to build a suitable and stable platform for the corrected nose to rest on. This means placing the anterior spine of the maxilla in the midline and adding substance to the pyriform aperture of the cleft side to create a suitable degree of symmetry.

Direct observation of the spine and both pyriform apertures can be achieved through an oral labial sulcus incision (Fig. 25-12). A hip graft, an irradiated cartilage graft, or a hydroxylapatite bone grafting material may be placed as necessary to raise the low pyriform aperture or build out the anterior nasal spine. Care must be exercised here to avoid recreating an oral nasal fistula, since the floor of the nose may be extremely low. Augmentation can raise the nostril floor as well as the alar base. The nasal spine can be chiseled free and slid over to the cleft side, thus placing the columella base in the midline (Fig. 25-13).

A more extreme approach has been described by Black et al.[3] It uses three incisions, one in each nostril and one in the buccal sulcus. The nasal vestibular incision starts at the base of the columella and goes up the side to follow along the anterior and lateral rim of the vestibule to the floor of the nostril at the alar base. To prevent contracture of this near-total rim incision, a V-plasty is placed in the nostril floor from the medial and lateral aspects of the incision, with the apex of the "V" placed back into the nostril floor. Through the nostril incisions the skin is elevated from the cartilages and bone of the nose. The third incision is in the depth of the labial sulcus from one bicuspid tooth to the other. The soft tissues are elevated from the maxilla. This elevation connects with the elevation carried out through the nostril incision so that the entire framework of the nose can be visualized after retracting the soft tissues upward to the glabella.

Through this exposure, the anterior nasal spine can be placed in the midline by chiseling it free and wiring it in a new position. The skin is now re-draped over the nose. The nostril rims are closed with 6-0 plain catgut sutures, and the oral incision is closed with 4-0 chromic catgut interrupted sutures.

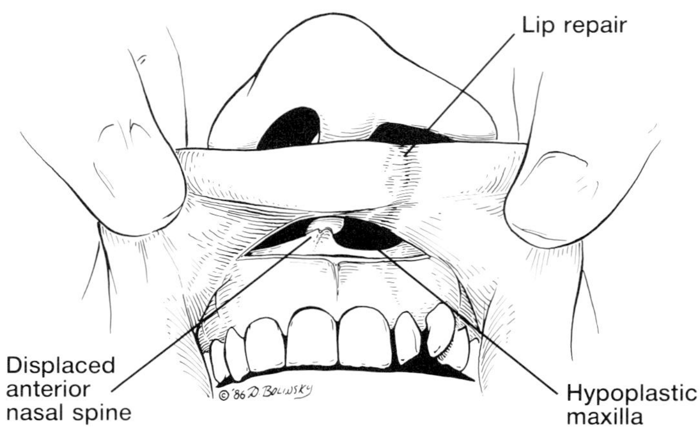

Fig. 25-12

A less extensive exposure is described by Farrior,[10] who works through an incision at the alar base to create a pocket beneath the periosteum for implantation of bone or aloplastic material (Fig. 25-14).

Ariyan et al.[1] describes a simple technique for raising the alar base by simply incising deeply around the alar fold, detaching the alar, and then closing the deficit underneath, which actually raises the alar base to give it a higher platform (Fig. 25-15).

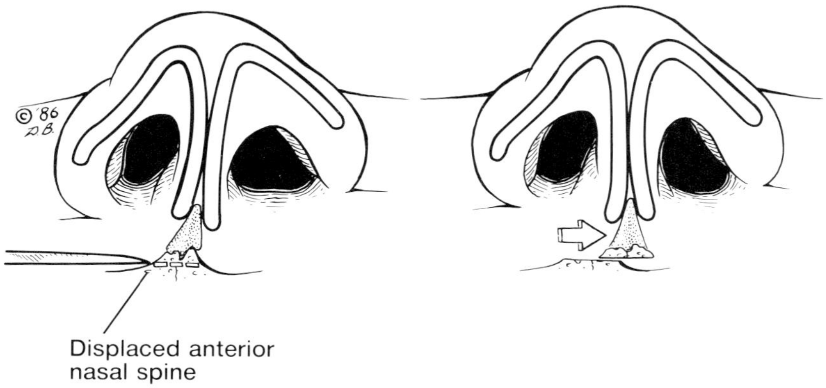

Fig. 25-13

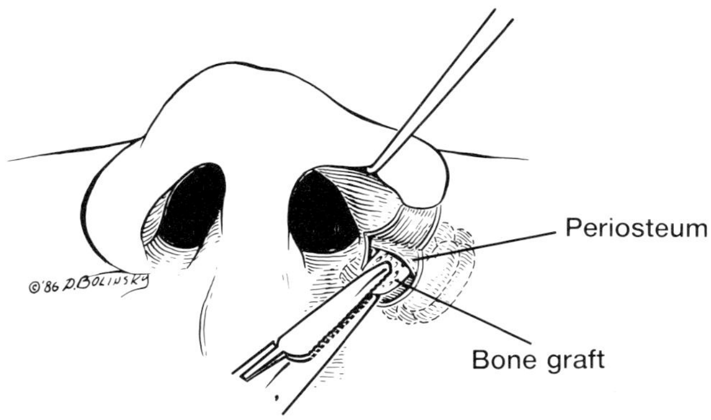

Fig. 25-14

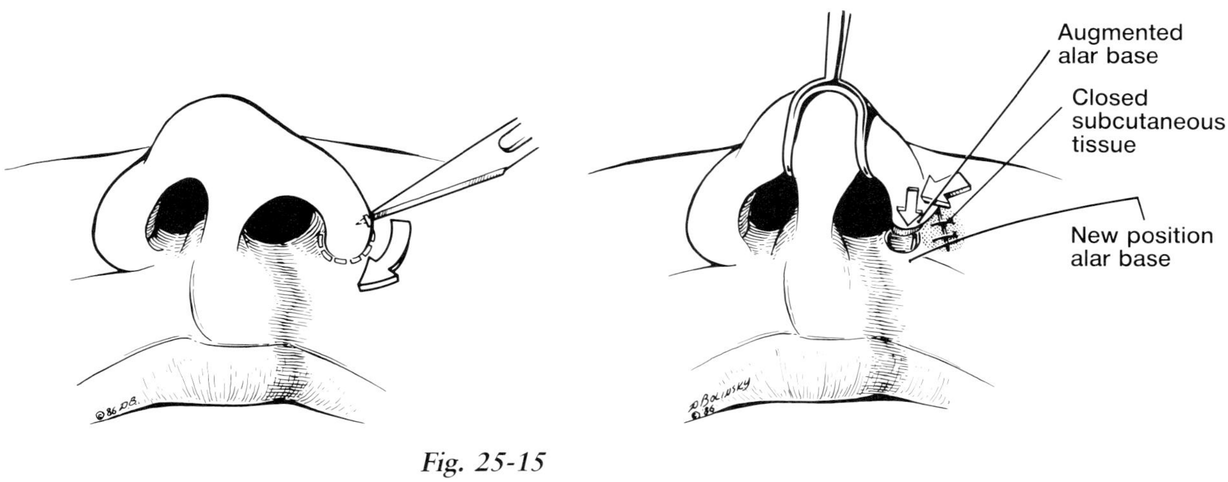

Fig. 25-15

Alar Base

The position of the cleft side alar base, once raised by augmentation of the maxilla and by raising the floor of the nostril, needs to be measured from the midline of the columella and compared to the opposite nostril width and non-cleft alar base position. The nostril is often too wide.

Excess width correction involves excising a wedge or a diamond of tissue or advancing the alar base. This may require wide uncovering to free up the scar tissue and possibly to revise a large portion of the lip scar. If there are holes through the nostril floor into the vestibule of the mouth, the lining of the hole must be brought into the nasal cavity by releasing the skin lining the hole. This is accomplished by placing a small hook in the hole and cutting a full thickness of tissue around the hole from below in the labial sulcus area. This is a difficult area to work in and it may be necessary to take down the upper two thirds of the lip repair and widely undermine the tissue underneath the alar area in a similar manner to the primary closure. This may not be successful, and if the nostril is excessively narrow, a small flap from the cheek lateral to the alar may be rotated into place to plug the hole. This same flap may be required when the nostril floor is at a lower level compared to the normal side, or when the nostril floor is too narrow.

The nostril floor may be deficient or low or narrow and in such instances, the alar base may need to be positioned outward with a single Z-plasty incision (Figs. 25-16, A & B). Millard[12] pulls the alar base in by denuding a portion of it and inserting it into the columella base (Figs. 25-17, A-C).

Lack of bulk on the cleft alar base may be augmented by a free graft (composite) from the alar base of the non-cleft side (Figs. 25-18, A, B).

The everted, furled, and displaced edges of the alar wing may be a symptom of inadequate tissue growth at the lateral portion of the alar cartilage. To create a symmetrical alar maxillary junction, Vecchione[23] takes a section of the cleft side alar facial fold and inserts it into the deficient cleft side ala (Figs. 25-19, A & B). This is combined with a diamond-shaped excision in the cleft side nostril floor when the floor is too wide.

The alar base may be simply advanced if the floor is of adequate height by removing skin only and advancing the base (Figs. 25-20, A & B).

With the facial platform level, the columella base in the midline, and the nostril floor adequately positioned, concerns for the lower lateral cartilages, septum, and dorsum of the nose can be considered.

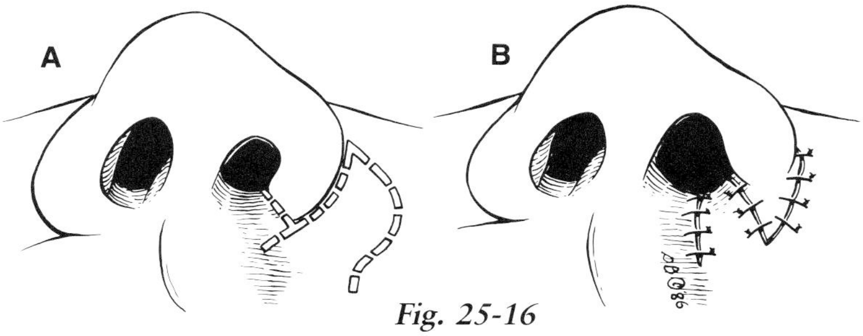

Fig. 25-16

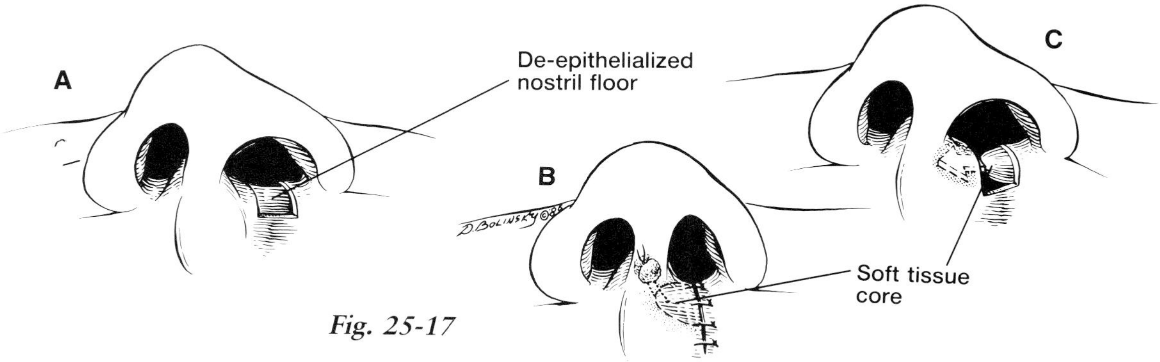

Fig. 25-17

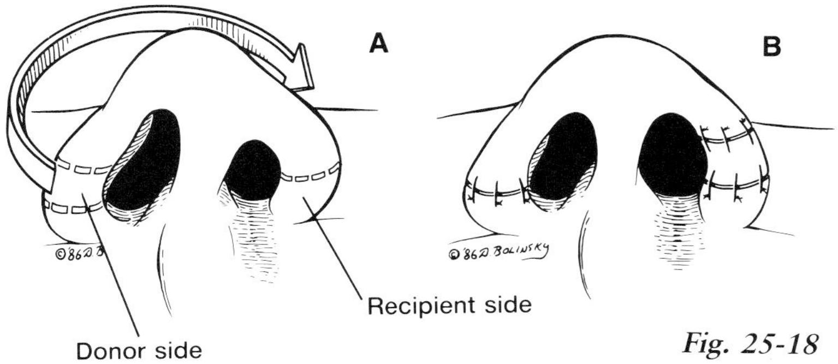

Fig. 25-18

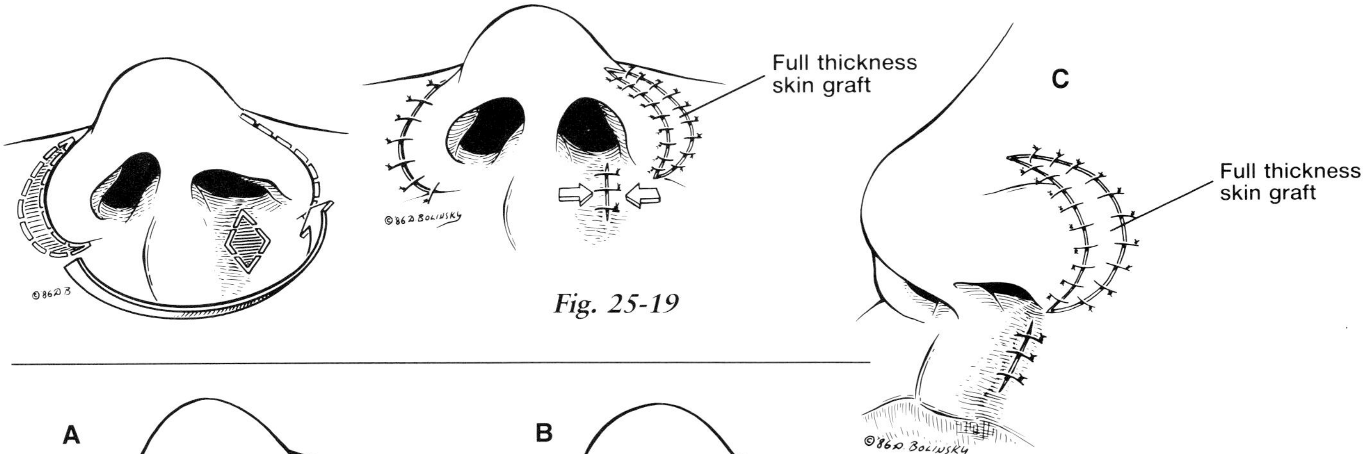

Fig. 25-19

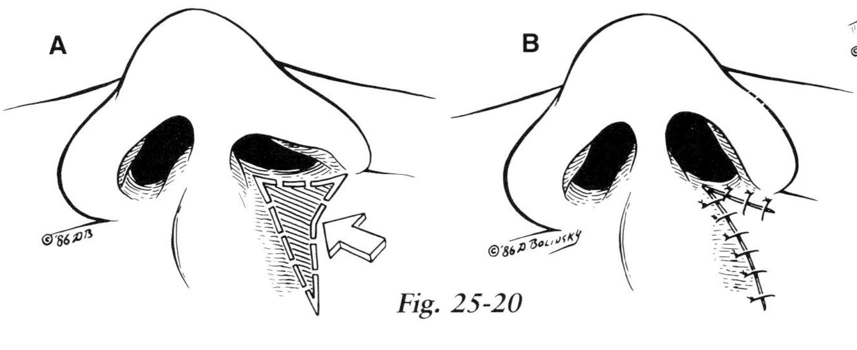

Fig. 25-20

Cleft Side Lower Lateral Cartilage

This defect along with the alar base constitutes the major recognizable defects that cause one to immediately recognize a cleft lip nasal defect. Although the alar base has been given separate attention, these two defects may have to be surgically combined. Many excellent techniques are available for this phase of the surgical correction. Some of these are now being used in the primary closure of the lip but are also available at the time of definitive rhinoplasty.

The Blair[5] columella-splitting incision (Fig. 25-21) is as widely accepted today as is open rhinoplasty. The columella is incised either horizontally or vertically and entry to the dorsum is made between the medial crura. The object here is to raise the lowered portion of the medial crus on the cleft side. A more extensive use of this principle was advocated by Dr. Berkley,[2] but may not be as acceptable cosmetically because of scarring, since the incision extends over the dome of the nose (Fig. 25-22).

As an alternate to the Berkley technique of raising the medial crus with a columella incision, Millard[14] emphasizes an incision in the alar skin designed to match the non-cleft rim, and through this incision frees up the medial two-thirds of the lower lateral cartilage and places it in a higher position in the dome. The entire lower lateral cartilage is freed from the overlying skin and then sutured high in the dome along with its attached vestibular skin (Fig. 25-23, A & B).

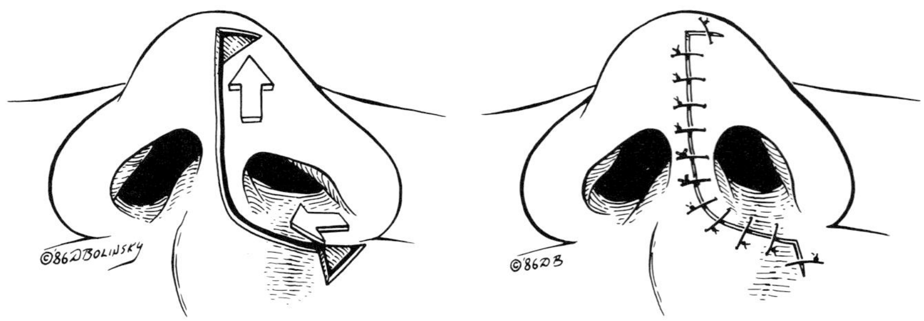

Fig. 25-21

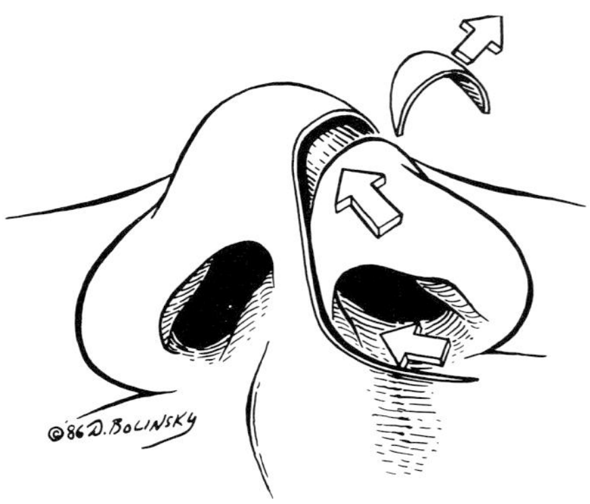

Fig. 25-22

Through a rim incision of variable length and shape, a number of operators have freed the cleft side lower lateral cartilage and sutured it to the upper lateral cartilage, the septum, and the dome of the non-cleft lower lateral cartilage.

In an extensive review of the unilateral cleft lip nose problem, Farrior[10] used both an intercartilaginous and an alar margin incision to gain access to the area. His intercartilaginous incision was extended farther laterally than usual to gain access to the tail of the cartilage. The alar margin incision was also made to extend farther laterally. The dorsal skin was elevated over the lateral crus and lower border of the upper lateral cartilage and in between the medial crura. The vestibular skin is completely freed from the lateral crus, the dome, and the upper portion of the medial crus (Fig. 25-24). This extensive freeing allowed the lower lateral cartilage to be placed wherever desired.

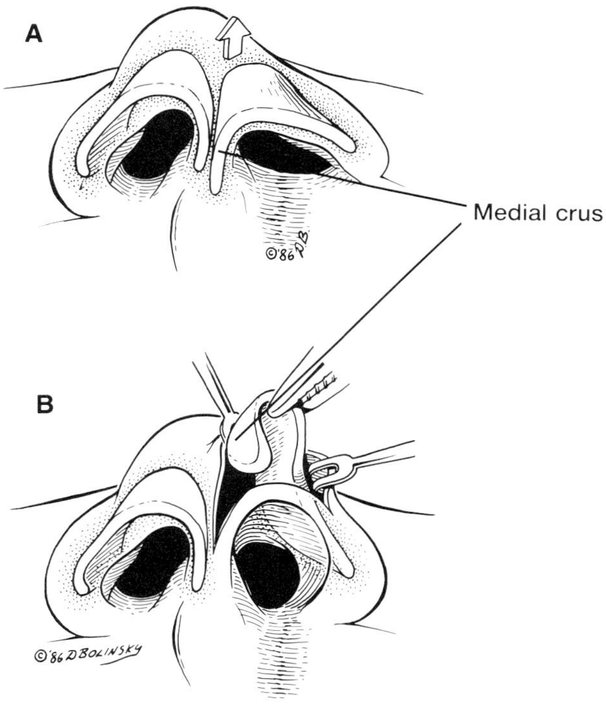

Fig. 25-23

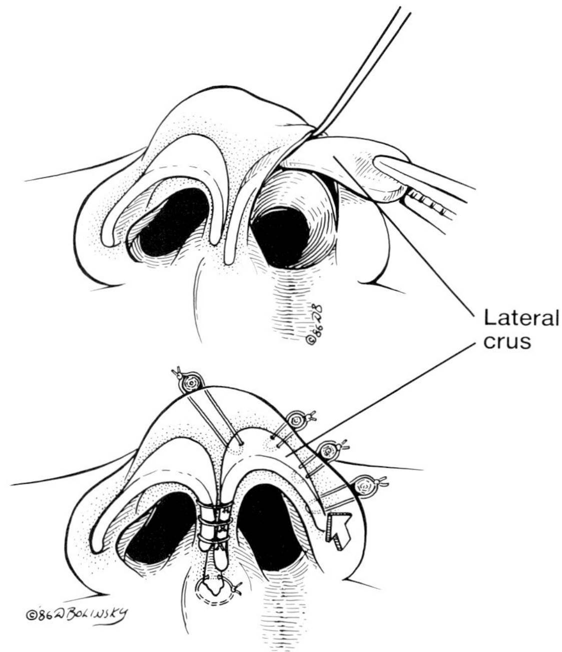

Fig. 25-24

Tajima[20] used a reverse-U incision to approach the cleft side lower lateral cartilage (Fig. 25-25, A & B). The incision line is marked after pushing the cleft side alar base medially to raise the dome of the depressed cartilage and make the bases somewhat symmetrical. This incision starts medially in the vestibular skin but crosses the external skin at the top of the nostril at a level that simulates the normal nostril but is slightly lower and ends laterally in the vestibular skin. Through this incision the skin is separated over the lower two thirds of the nose. The vestibular skin remains attached to the lateral cartilage. The cleft side lower lateral cartilage is attached to both the upper lateral cartilages and to the opposite lower lateral cartilage.

McComb[15] observed that the nose was longer on the cleft side in the unrepaired single cleft lip deformity of infants. He further observed that the nose on the cleft was too long in adults who had single cleft lip repair. He studied the growth of the nose in the patient who had more radical correction of the nose at the time of primary repair and found that there was no interference with growth.

His technique in the infant was to use the incisions already existing at the time of primary lip closure to free the skin over the lower two-thirds of the nose and suspend the cleft side lower lateral cartilage with mattress sutures passing from the vestibule underneath the nasal skin to emerge at the glabella (Fig. 25-26, A & B). Bolsters were used at both ends of this mattress suture. The vestibular skin was not elevated from the lower lateral cartilage. Additional local mattress sutures were tied on as bolsters through the lower lateral cartilage area to eliminate dead space. McComb[16] felt that intercartilaginous incisions carried a significant risk of stenosis in the infant. His sutures remained for five days.

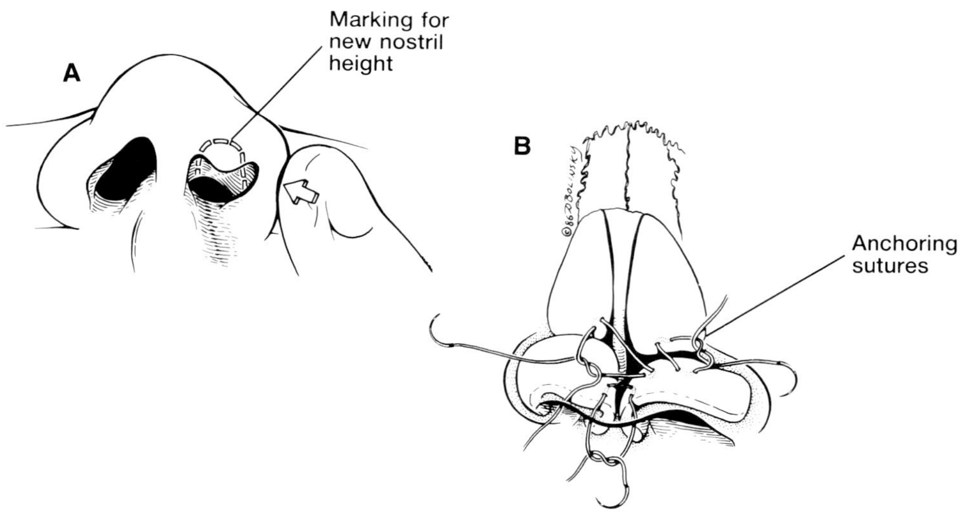

Fig. 25-25

Blackwell et al.[4] describe a less extensive method of equalizing the domes on adults by harvesting cartilage from the cephalic border of one or both lower lateral cartilages and placing multiple onlay grafts in layers over the cleft side lower lateral cartilage (Fig. 25-27, A & B). This delivery technique deals only with the inequality of the dome area, but does not correct defects such as alar rim buckling or nostril asymmetry. Thompson[22] uses cartilage from the ear as an onlay graft and rotates the excess nostril rim to augment the columella.

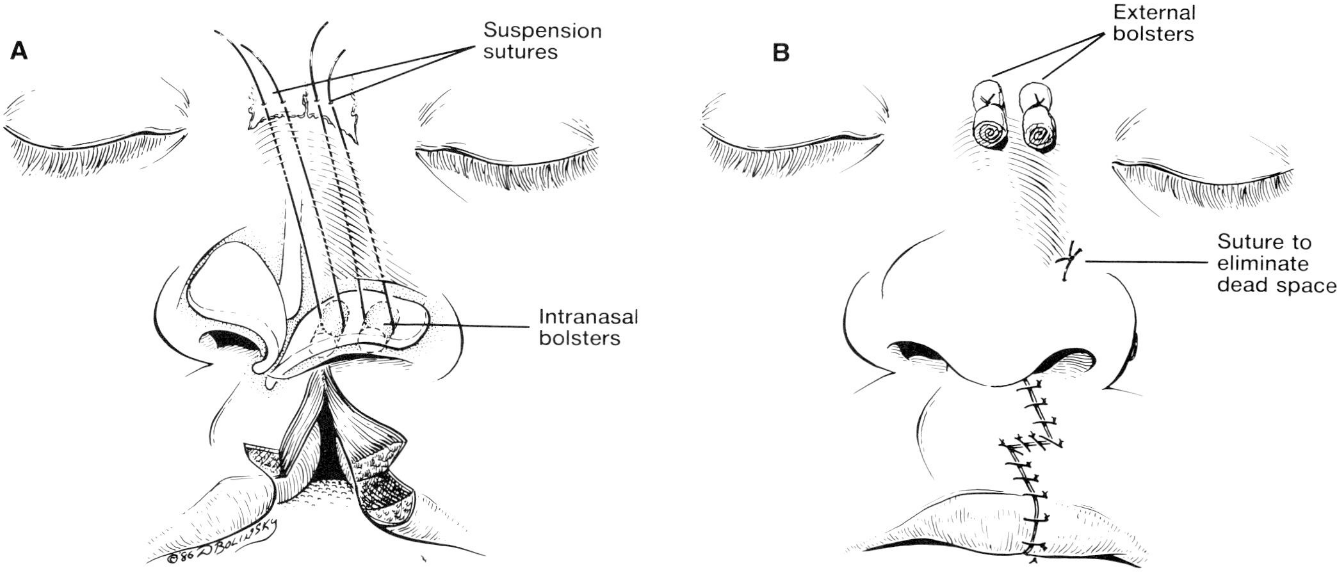

Fig. 25-26

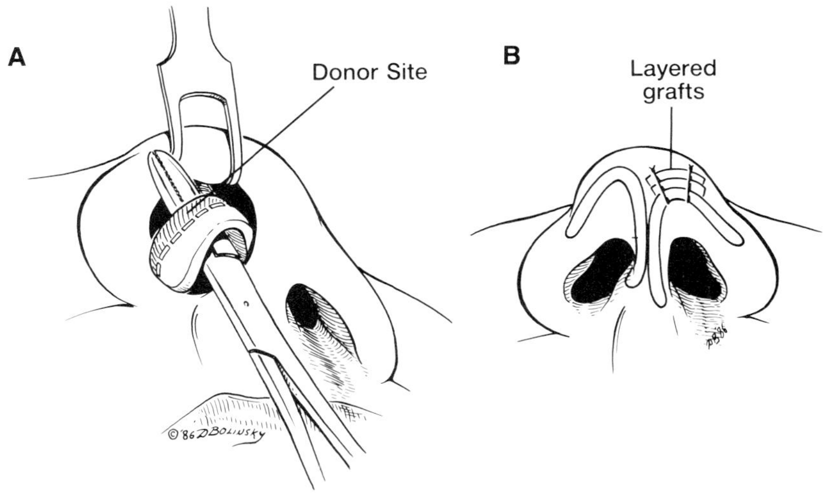

Fig. 25-27

Open Rhinoplasty

The technique of open rhinoplasty has been practiced for many years by cosmetic surgeons dealing with defects of the nose associated with a repaired cleft lip. This technique has gained wide acceptance in recent years among surgeons specializing in adult rhinoplasty. The early work in the direct-exposure technique was often performed along with secondary repairs of the lip scars between the ages of 6 to 8 years.

Elevation of the overlying skin immediately exposes the superior surface of the unequal lower lateral cartilages. Through this incision the whole lateral crus can be separated from the vestibular skin and brought up to a normal height with respect to the normal dome. If necessary, a piece of septal or irradiated cartilage can be placed between or just behind the medial crura for support and the cephalic border of the lateral crus can be sutured into an overlap position with the cleft side upper lateral cartilage (Fig. 25-28). Once the cartilage is in the proper position, the vestibular skin can be reattached to the cartilage with absorbable sutures such as 4-0 Vicril or 4-0 Dexon.

The medial portion of the skin incision has been varied from a simple gull type (Erich)[9] (Fig. 25-29) to those lower in the columella with the ascending and lateral limbs completely within the nostril in the vestibular skin (Figs. 25-30, A & B). Ecker[8] recommended lateral extensions beyond those used by Erich and Schultz.[18] Fujimori et al.[11] added an island flap to the external incision and used it to correct alar buckling in addition to directly repositioning and anchoring the displaced cleft side lower lateral cartilage (Fig. 25-31, A-E).

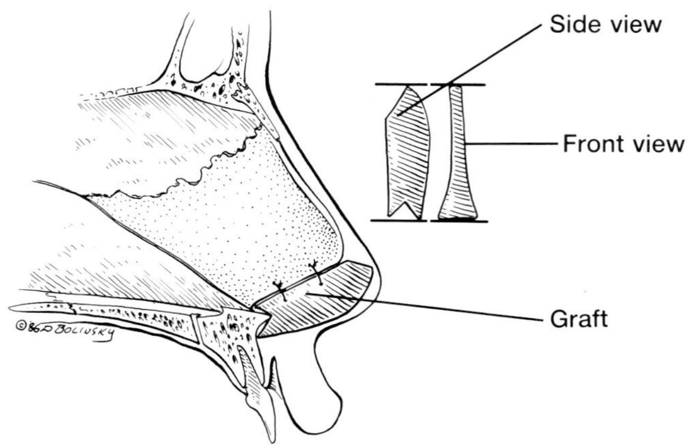

Fig. 25-28

Black[3] described a radical exposure of the whole nose from the labial sulcus to the glabella. After correction of the alar base and spine, the cleft side lower lateral cartilage can be repositioned. Vestibular skin is elevated under the lower lateral cartilage dome of the non-cleft side to allow sutures through the dome. The cleft side medial crus is freed in the midline but is left attached to the vestibular skin to allow upward movement at the dome and rotation upward to an overlap relation with the cleft side upper lateral cartilage. In this position it can be sutured to both the septum and the upper lateral cartilages. Thus, relief of the curled lateral crura tip will aid in reduction of the web or baffle effect in the lateral vestibule.

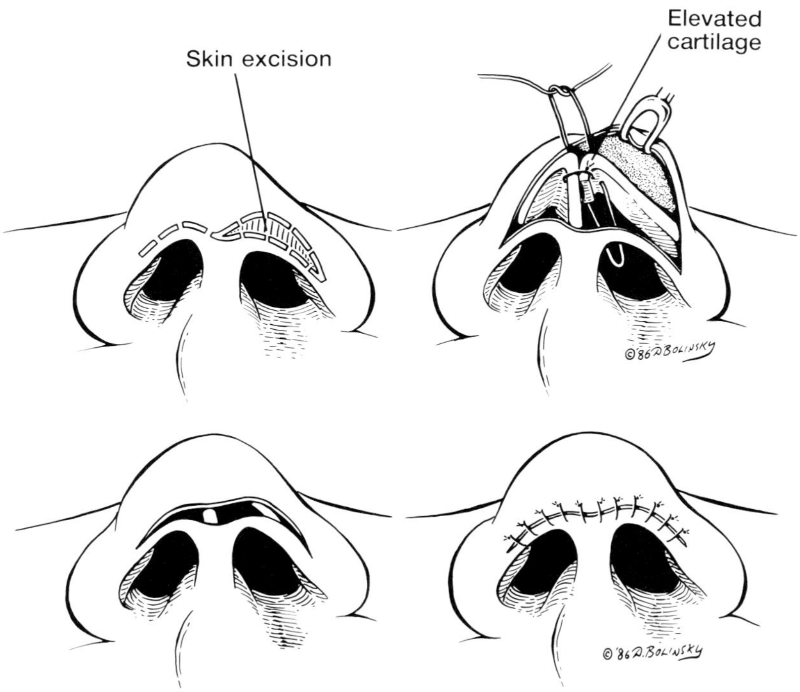

Fig. 25-29

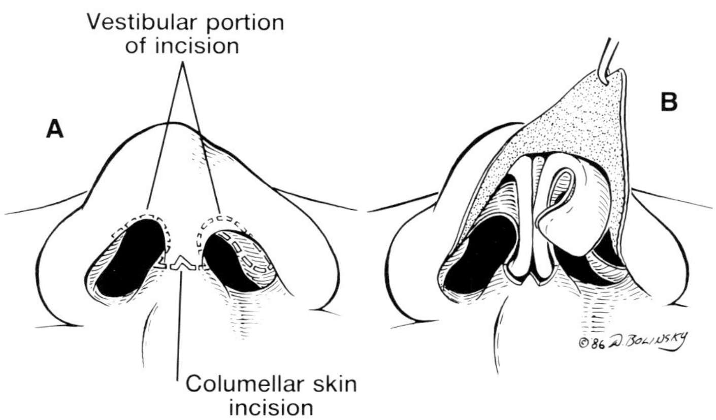

Fig. 25-30

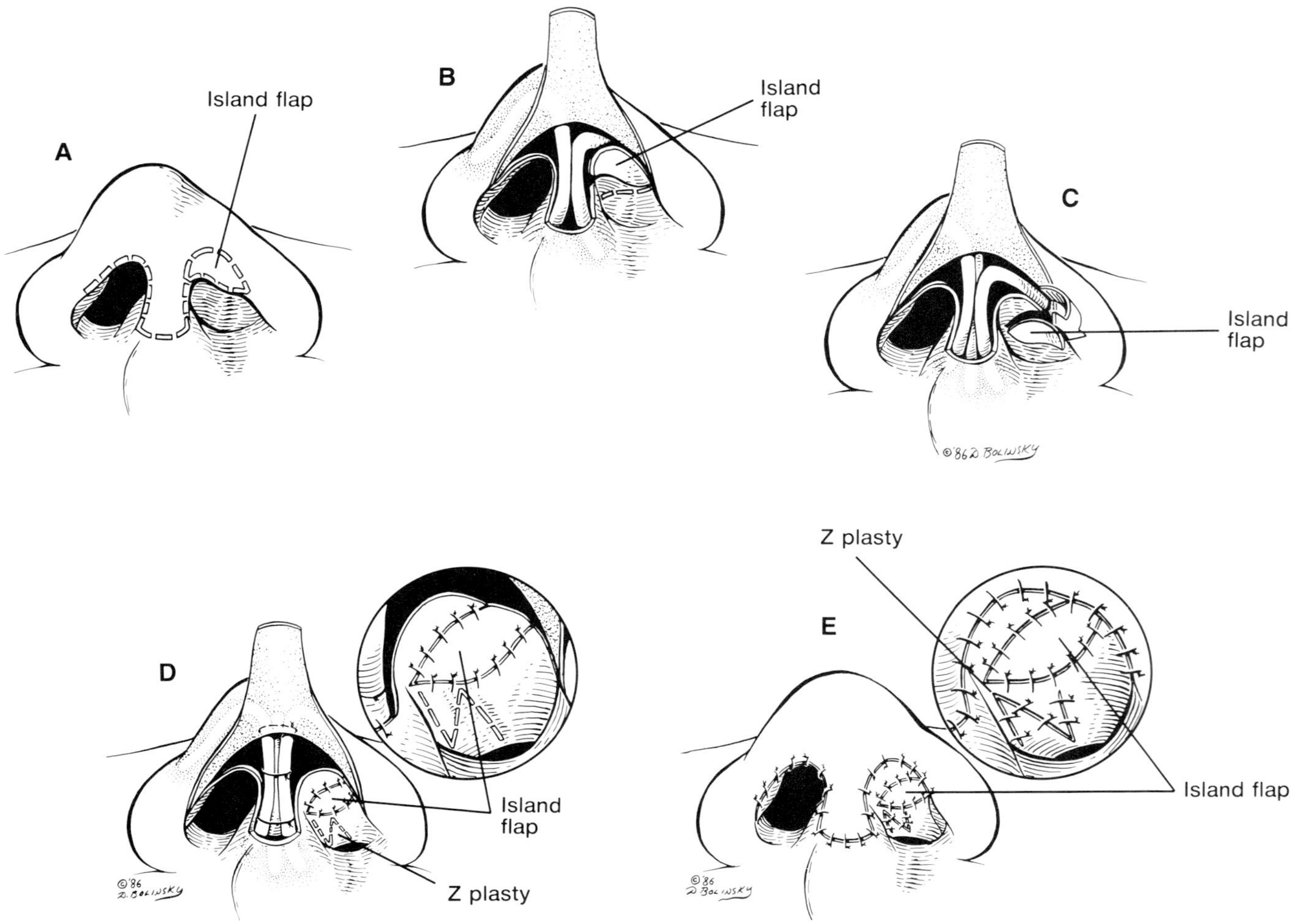

Fig. 25-31

The buckled or collapsed lateral crus can be corrected with a boxed mattress suture in the cartilage (Fig. 25-32).

Refinements of the cleft alar cartilages of all types have been recommended such as onlay grafts, flip-over grafts using portions of the normal lower lateral cartilage to the cleft side, moving the cephalic border of the lateral crus to the midline, and unequal division of the cartilages (Fig. 25-33).

It appears that the single cleft lip nasal deformity can present a variety of defects that do not lend themselves to a single, compact, straightforward, step-by-step procedure. Each defect has to be evaluated on its own and as part of the adjacent defect. By separating those procedures that can be handled by a routine rhinoplasty, one is left with essentially two major concerns: the alar, with respect to its position and height, and the lateral crus on the cleft side. Proper position of these two major defects will improve the nostril floor, the size and shape of the nostril, correct the columella slant, and equalize the inequality at the tip.

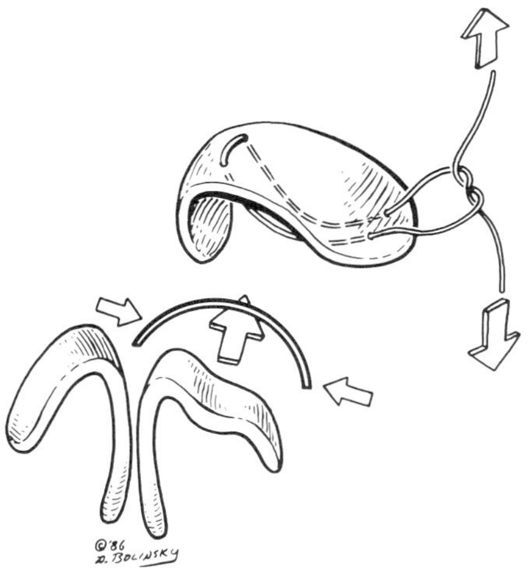

Fig. 25-32

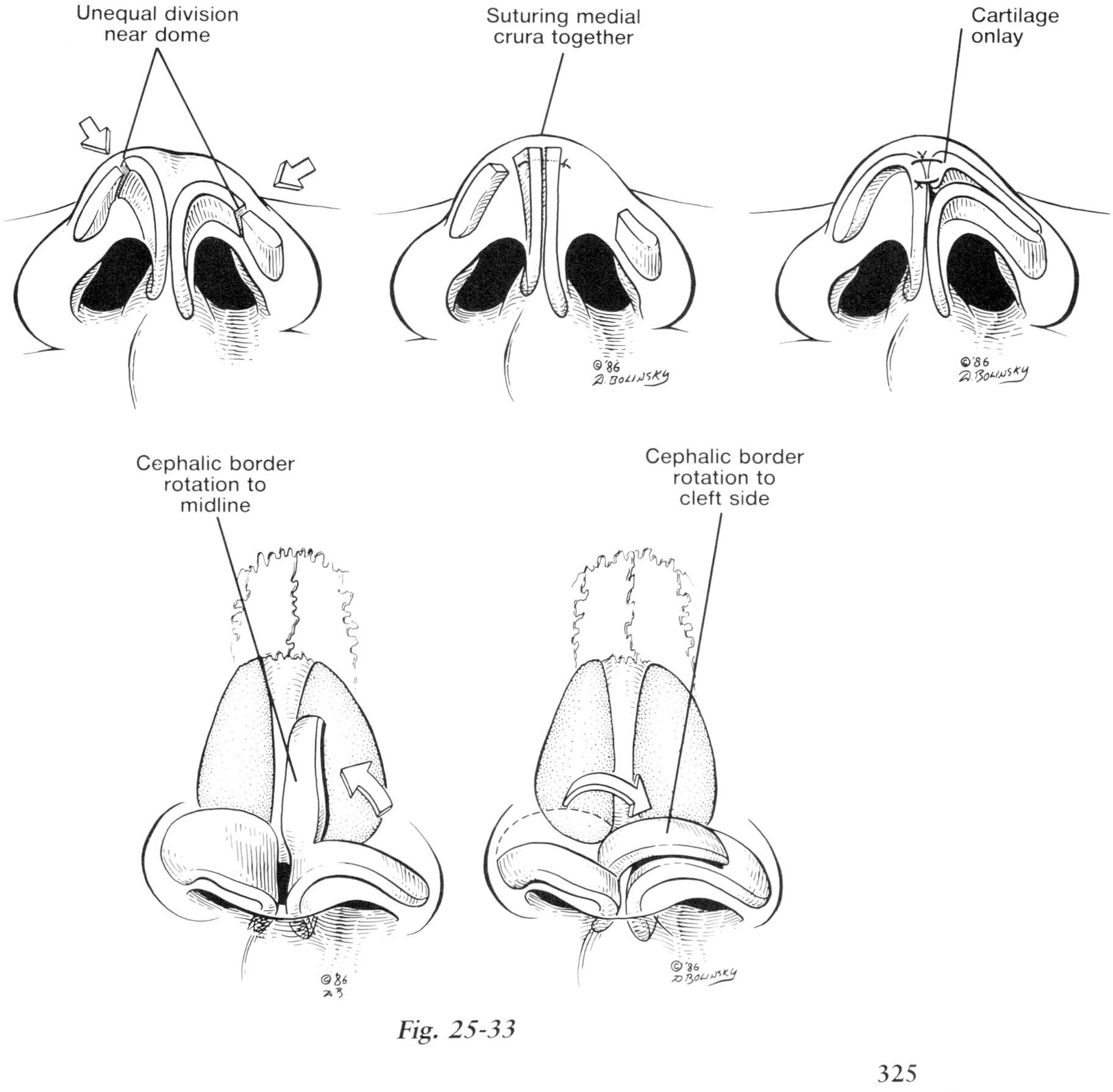

Fig. 25-33

Closed Approach

This technique may be used by those less experienced with the open rhinoplasty technique. Satisfactory results may be obtained, but with some limitations. The operation starts with the hemi-transfixion, using a Cottle[6] or Metzenbaum incision along the caudal end of the quadrilateral cartilage (Fig. 25-34). The mucoperiosteum is elevated on the incision side over the area of intended cartilage removal. A 1 cm strip of quadrilateral cartilage is left in place and a dorsal strip of quadrilateral cartilage, about 1½ cm in height is also left in place so that an L-shaped piece of quadrilateral cartilage remains (Fig. 25-35). Depending upon the degree of deflection, the quadrilateral cartilage may be detached from the vomer and allowed to swing toward the cleft side like a barn door without extensive removal of quadrilateral cartilage (Fig. 25-36). Grafts for the columella and the dorsum may be harvested at this time from the inferior border of the quadrilateral cartilage.

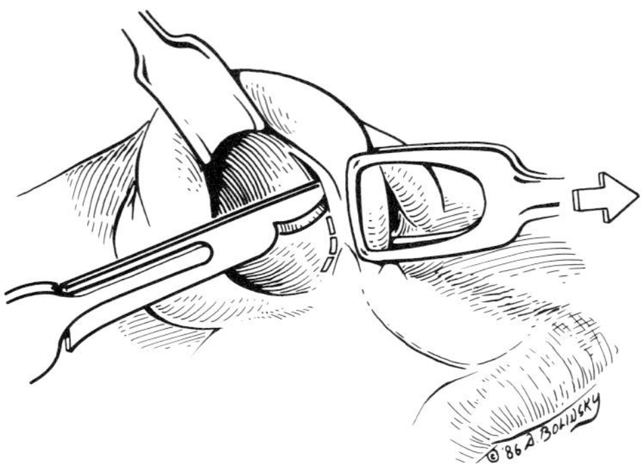

Fig. 25-34

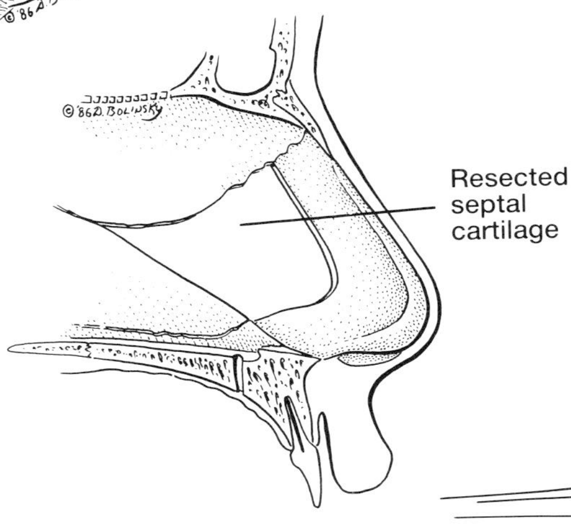

Fig. 25-35

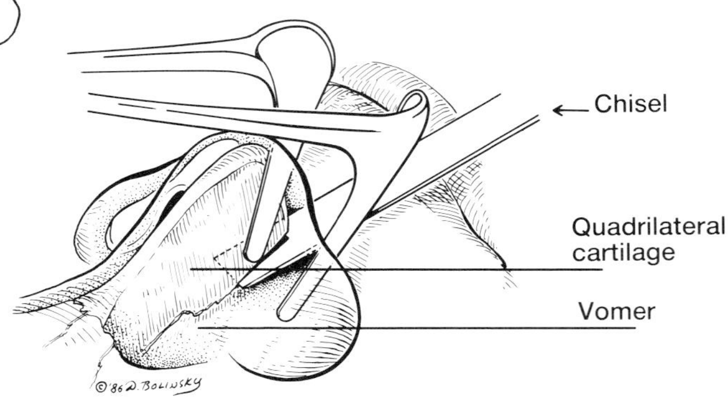

Fig. 25-36

With the septal work completed, intercartilaginous incisions are performed (Fig. 25-37) stopping at the dome area instead of continuing with a complete transfixion incision. If, however, the septum is straight and a septal reconstruction is not desired, the operation can begin with an intercartilaginous incision followed by a complete transfixion incision (Fig. 25-38). Through this incision sufficient work can be done on the septum if so desired.

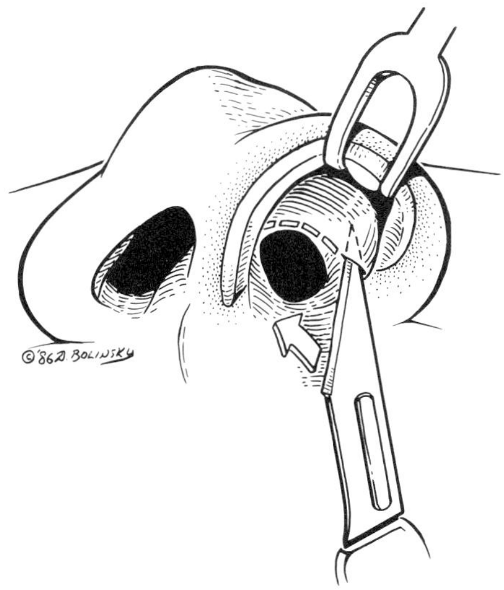

Fig. 25-37

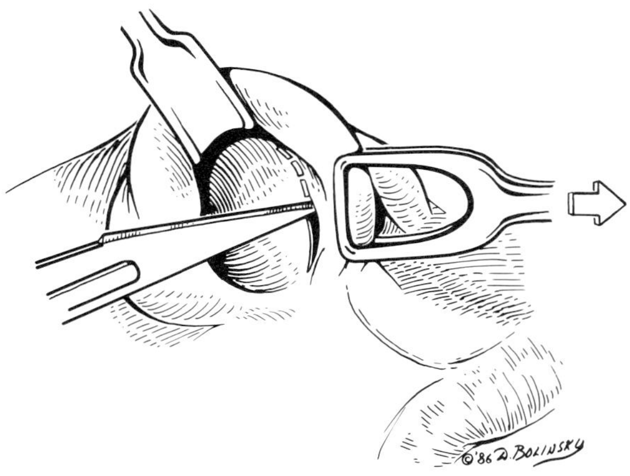

Fig. 25-38

The rim incision is performed along the anterior border of the lateral crus and extends down the medial crura for about 3 to 4 mm (Fig. 25-39, A & B). These two incisions (intercartilaginous and rim incisions) leave the lateral crura in a bipedicle flap. The overlying skin is separated from the lateral crura bilaterally (Fig. 25-40). The vestibular skin is also separated bilaterally (Fig. 25-41), which makes it possible to deliver both lateral crura at the same time for comparison (Fig. 25-42). By delivering these cartilages, it is possible to raise the left side lateral crus and suture it to the opposite crus at the dome. It is also possible, through intercartilaginous incisions, to suture the cephalic border of the cleft lateral crus cartilage to the inferior border of the upper lateral cartilage (Fig. 25-43). A small batten or graft of septal cartilage or irradiated cartilage can be placed between the medial crura for support, prior to suturing at the dome (Fig. 25-44). The vestibular skin on the cleft side lateral crus can be resutured to the crura with 4-0 Vicril or 4-0 Dexon to raise the nostril rim.

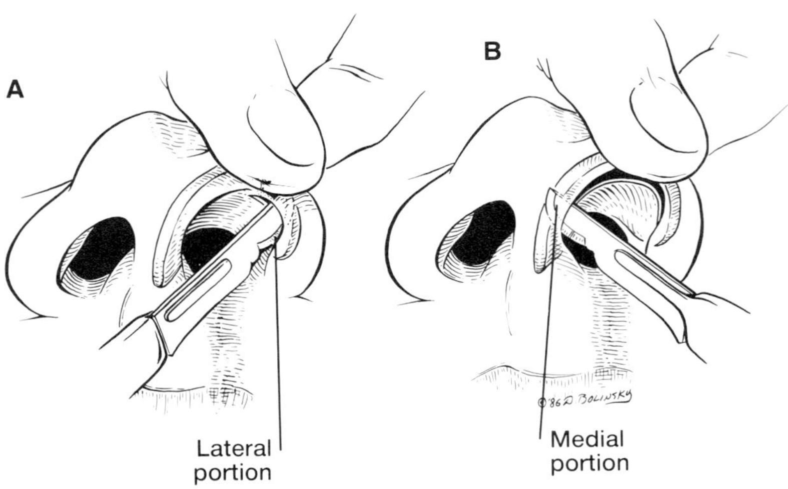

Fig. 25-39

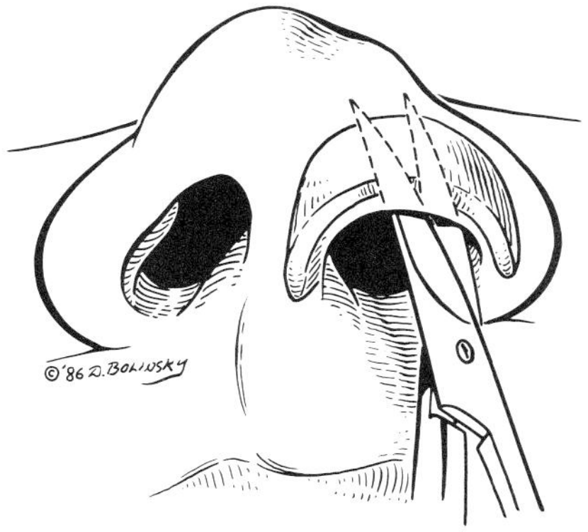

Fig. 25-40

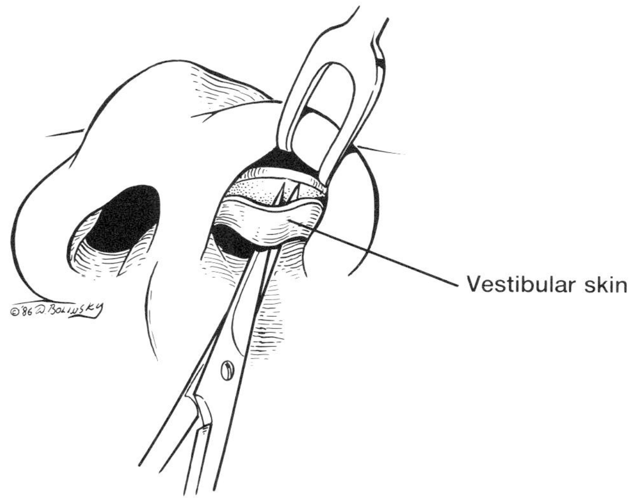

Fig. 25-41

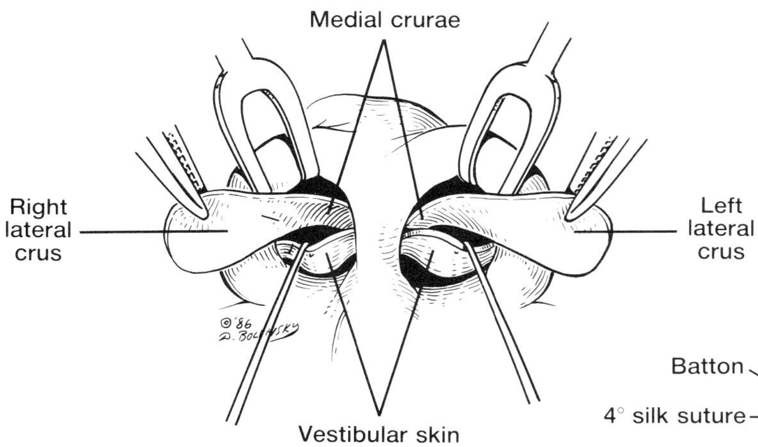

Fig. 25-42

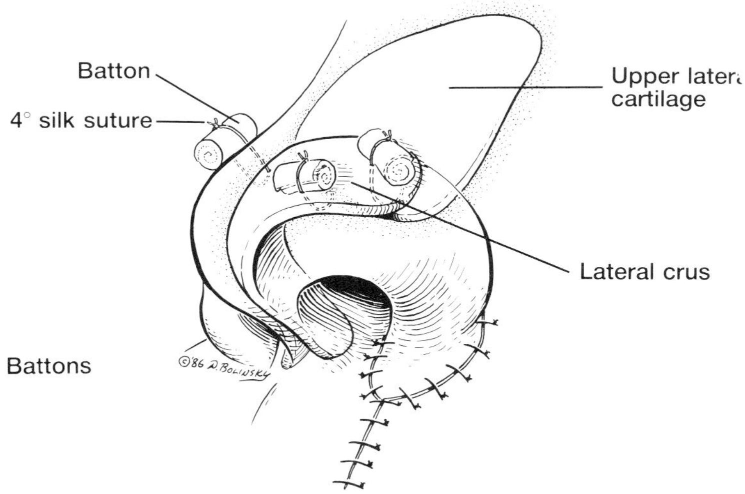

Fig. 25-43

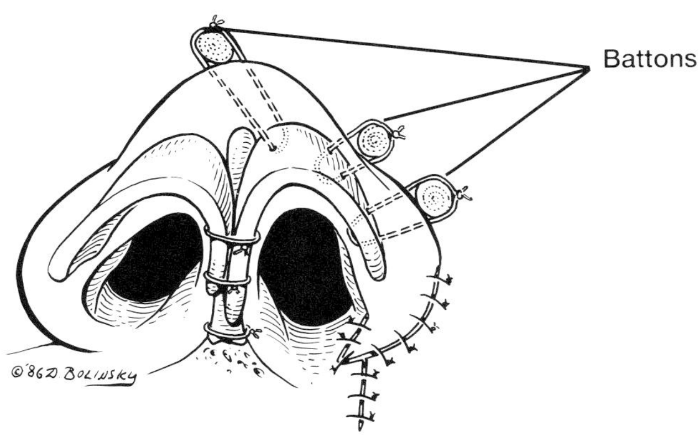

Fig. 25-44

As an alternative to the lower lateral cartilage technique, the lower lateral cartilages may be delivered for inspection without elevation of the vestibular skin. The non-cleft side cartilage is divided at the dome, including the vestibular skin. The cleft lateral crus is divided lateral to the dome for about 3 to 4 mm. These two medial crura are delivered into one nostril and sutured together with or without a batten placed between them (Fig. 25-45). This technique corrects the asymmetry of the dome of the nose but does very little for nostril asymmetry and the laterally rotated long diameter of the cleft nostril (Fig. 25-46). Discrepancies not readily correctable with these procedures on the lower lateral cartilages may be helped by the placement of auricular cartilage graft onlays.

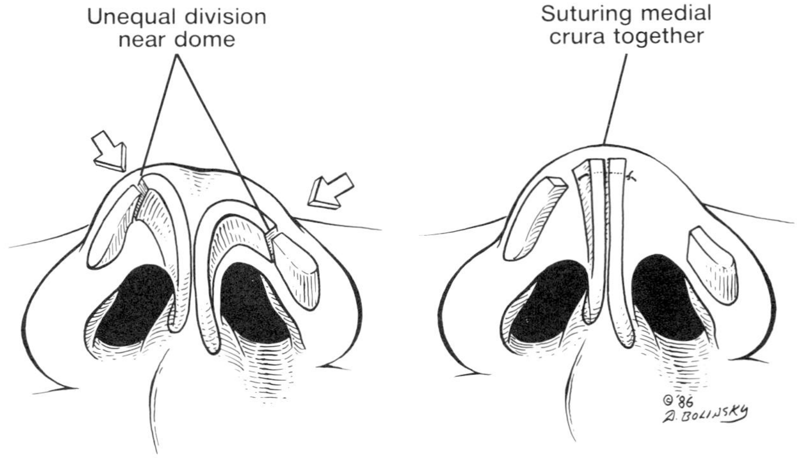

Fig. 25-45

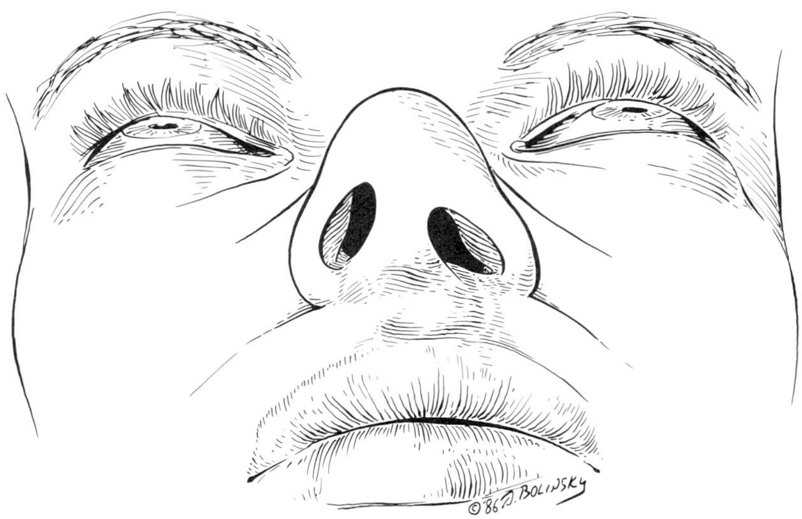

Fig. 25-46

With the tip completed, the cartilage and bony dorsum can be adjusted via the intercartilaginous incision. Lateral osteotomies are performed via vestibular incisions with or without medial osteotomies as desired. The nasal spine of the frontal bone may need to be chiseled to allow the whole nose to be set into the midline. The rim incision is closed with 4-0 chromic catgut. Packing is placed in the nose as desired and the nose is splinted. It is essential to pack the vestibule with a half-inch salvage gauze impregnated with Bacitracin ointment if the lower lateral cartilages have been divided. This packing is needed to splint the lateral crura in position to avoid distortion. An external splint of the operator's choice can be placed in the usual manner.

REFERENCES

1. Ariyan S and Drizek TJ: A simplified technique for correction of the cleft lip nasal deformity, Ann Plast Surg 1:568, 1978.
2. Berkeley WT: The cleft lip nose, Plast Reconstr Surg 23:567, 1959.
3. Black PW, Hartram PF, Carl J, and Beegle P: Cleft lip type nasal deformity: definitive repair, Ann Plast Surg 12:128, 1984.
4. Blackwell SJ, Parry SW, Roberg BC, Huang TT: Onlay cartilage graft of the alar lateral crus for cleft lip nasal deformities, Plast Reconstr Surg 76:395, 1985.
5. Blair VP: Nasal deformities associated with cleft of the lip, J Am Med Assoc 84:185, 1925.
6. Cottle MH and Loring RM: Surgery of the nasal septum: new operative procedures and indications, Ann Otolaryngol 57:707, 1948.
7. Cronin TD: A modification of the tennison type lip repair, Cleft Palate J 3:376, 1966.
8. Ecker H: A direct approach to the more severely deformed cleft lip nose, Plast Reconstr Surg 67:369, 1981.
9. Erich JB: A technique for correcting a flat nostril in cases of repaired hare lip, Plast Reconstr Surg 12:320, 1953.
10. Farrior RT: The problem of the unilateral cleft lip nose, Laryngoscope 72:289, 1962.
11. Fujimori R and Hirita Y: Elongation of the nostril and columella using an island flap, Br J Plast Surg 35:171, 1982.
12. Millard DRJ: A radical rotation in single hare lip, Am J Surg 95:318, 1958.
13. Millard DR Jr: Cleft craft, vol 1, Boston, 1976, Little, Brown & Co Inc.
14. Millard DR Jr: Earlier correction of the unilateral cleft lip nose, Plast Reconstr Surg 70:64, 1982.
15. McComb H: Treatment of unilateral cleft lip nose, Plast Reconstr Surg 55:596, 1975.
16. McComb H: Primary correction of unilateral cleft lip nasal deformity: a ten year review, Plast Reconstr Surg 75:791, 1985.
17. Sayler KE: Primary correction of the unilateral cleft lip nose: a 15-year experience, Plast Reconstr Surg 77:558, 1986.
18. Schultz RC: Improving the cleft lip nose, Plast Reconstr Surg 71:148, 1983.
19. Skoog T: Plastic surgery, Philadelphia, 1974, WB Saunders Co.
20. Tajima S and Maruyama M: Reverse U-incision for secondary repair of the cleft lip nose, Plast Reconstr Surg 60:256, 1977.
21. Tennison CW: The repair of the unilateral cleft lip by stencil method, Plast Reconstr Surg 9:115, 1952.
22. Thompson HG: The residual unilateral cleft lip nasal deformity: a 3-phase correction technique, Plast Reconstr Surg 76:36, 1985.
23. Vecchione TR: Repair of the unilateral cleft lip nose using contra-lateral alar crease grafts, Ann Plast Surg 14:148, 1985.
24. Wynn SK: Lateral flap cleft surgery technique, Plast Reconstr Surg 26:509, 1960.

26

Surgical Correction of the Nasal Deformity Secondary to Double Cleft Lip Repair

Howard W. Smith

It is impossible to consider cosmetic surgery on the bilateral cleft lip nasal deformity without paying strict attention to the lip and its underlying alveolar structures. To fully understand the peculiarities of this type of nose, it is essential to have a working knowledge of the original defect and the possible selection of the primary repair technique and the extent of secondary measures that are almost uniformly required. This is so because there may still be a need to borrow from the lip to improve the nose and even a further possibility of borrowing from the lower lip to compensate for the flap taken from the upper lip and placed in the nose.

The bilateral cleft lip is not only a single cleft lip times two, it tends to be more severe, and there is a true deficiency of the columella tissue. The midline structures are not twisted to one side as in a single cleft lip nasal defect and the septum is straight, but there is forward protrusion of the central segment of the alveolus (premaxilla) and sitting on top of this is a small, undeveloped prolabium (center of the upper lip) that is thin and contains no muscle (Fig. 26-1). The central segment seems to be attached to the columella, which is very short and almost absent. This central structure is surrounded by two large nostrils that communicate freely with the mouth. There are, of course, variations, but the complete bilateral cleft is most common.

The lip deformity is covered by the depressed and wide tip of the nose, and laterally by two arches, which hook over to the lateral lip elements (Fig. 26-2). Thus, the tip of the nose is broad and flat and the alar are far apart as though they have been squashed down and allowed to spread laterally. The clefts individually tend to be wider than the single complete cleft lip. There is a real shortage of columella and the prolabium is far behind the other elements in growth, but is has the potential to catch up, thus rendering unnecessary the need to augment the prolabium at the time of primary closure.

The type of primary closure most often used is the Veau type III[12] (Figs. 26-3, A & B) which makes no attempt to augment the columella. The edge of the clefts are pared. The lateral flaps are folded in from the prolabium to provide a mucosal layer and the vermilion flaps from the lateral lip elements are preserved and used to augment the vermilion at the free edge of the prolabium. A three-layered closure is not possible since the prolabium has no muscle. The floor of the nose is closed and continuity of the nostril rim is achieved along with lip closure.

Details of how the premaxilla is treated before and after closure will not be discussed, except to say that when contemplating rhinoplasty on patients between the ages of 15 to 18, the position of the maxilla relative to the mandible must be considered along with an opinion from an orthognathic surgeon regarding the possibility of repositioning the whole maxilla prior to performing cosmetic rhinoplasty.

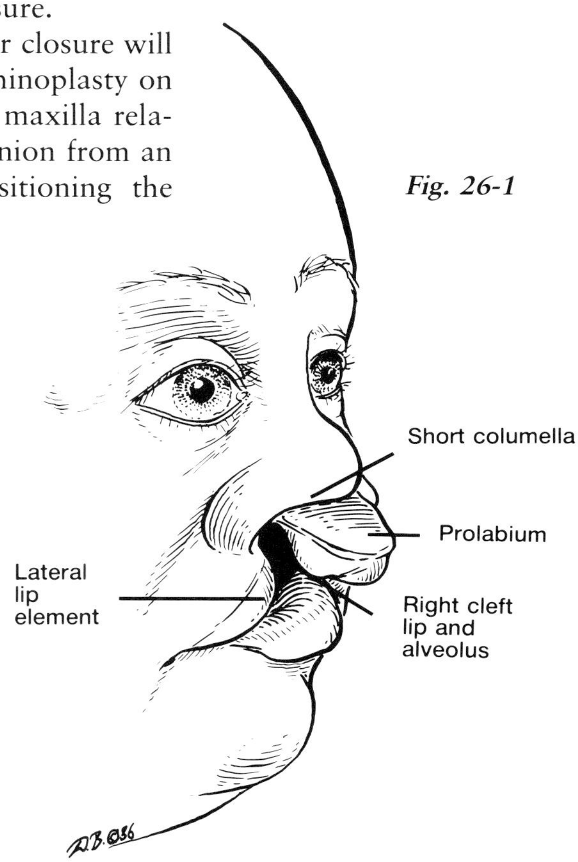

Fig. 26-1

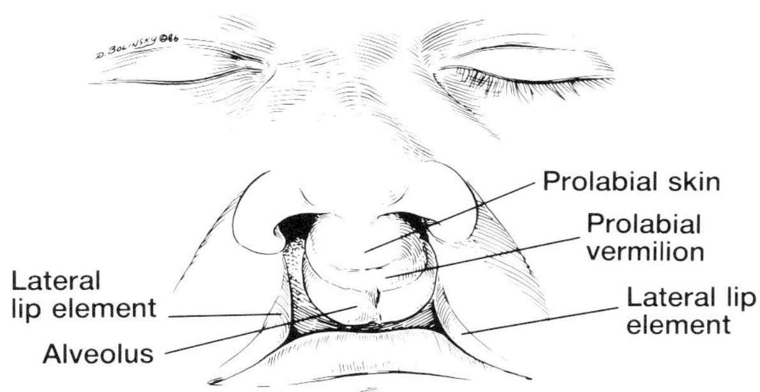

Fig. 26-2

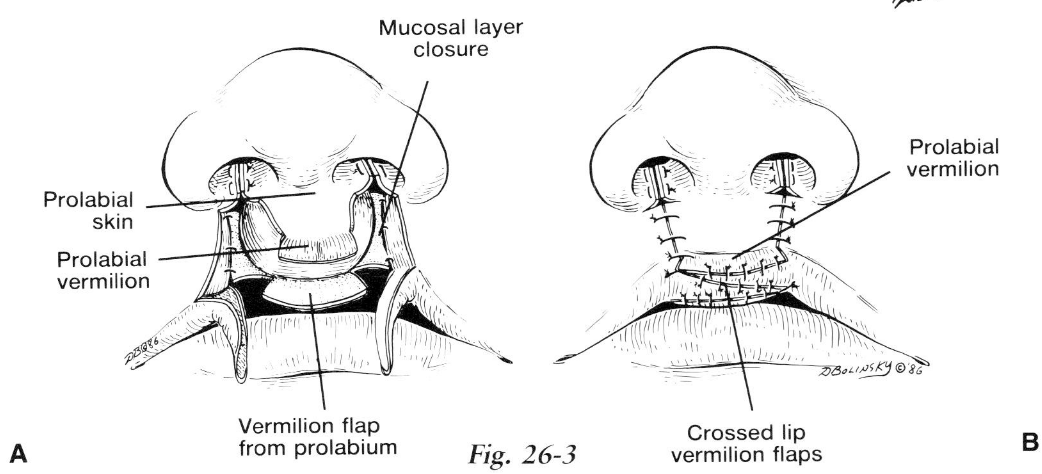

Fig. 26-3

Closure Techniques

Other techniques of bilateral cleft lip closure include those used by Skoog,[11] Millard,[8] Wynn,[13] and many others. These techniques, in part, can be used to augment the columella in an attempt to avoid secondary columella lengthening in patients at the early age of 4 to 6 years.

Skoog (Figs. 26-4, A-C) used a portion of the lateral prolabium skin and rotated it into an incision in the base of the columella. The bilateral cleft was closed as a two-stage procedure three months apart, starting the first closure at age three months. The defect created in the lateral prolabium is augmented by a flap from the lateral lip element at each stage.

Millard (Fig. 26-5, A & B) has promoted the rotation advancement flap for incomplete bilateral cleft lips.

The Z-plasty technique[5] (Fig. 26-6, A & B) has been used by a number of others with the idea of improving the fullness of the vermilion border centrally in the prolabium.

Wynn (Fig. 26-7, A & B) used a triangular flap to augment the columella base similar to Skoog but obtained the tissue from the lateral lip element. The closure was also done in stages, about three months apart.

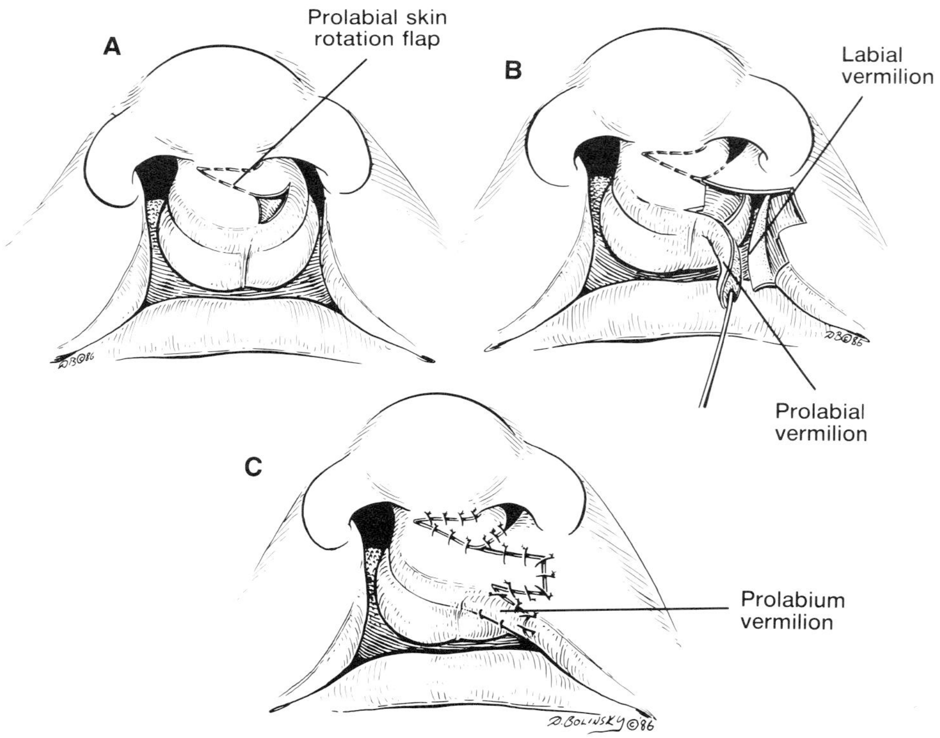

Fig. 26-4

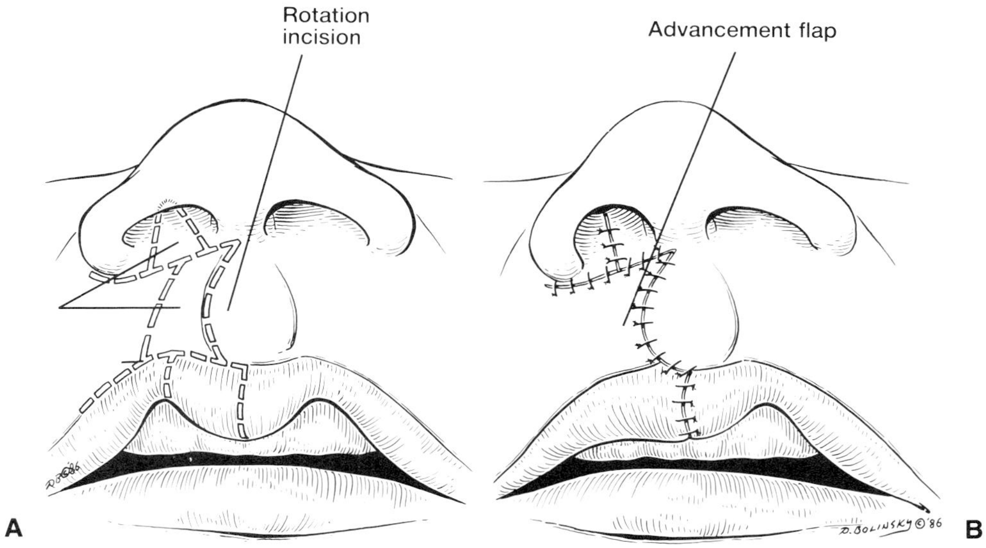

Fig. 26-5

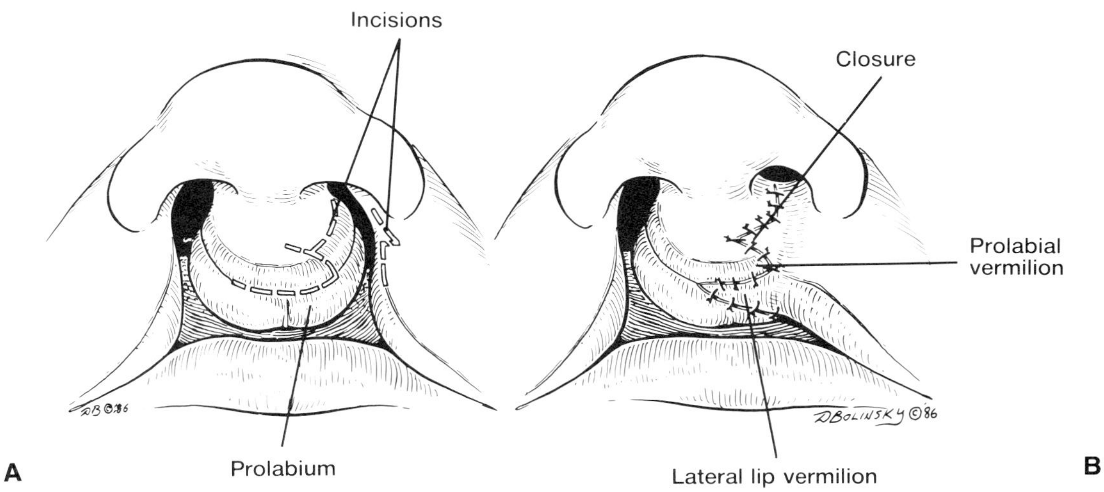

Fig. 26-6

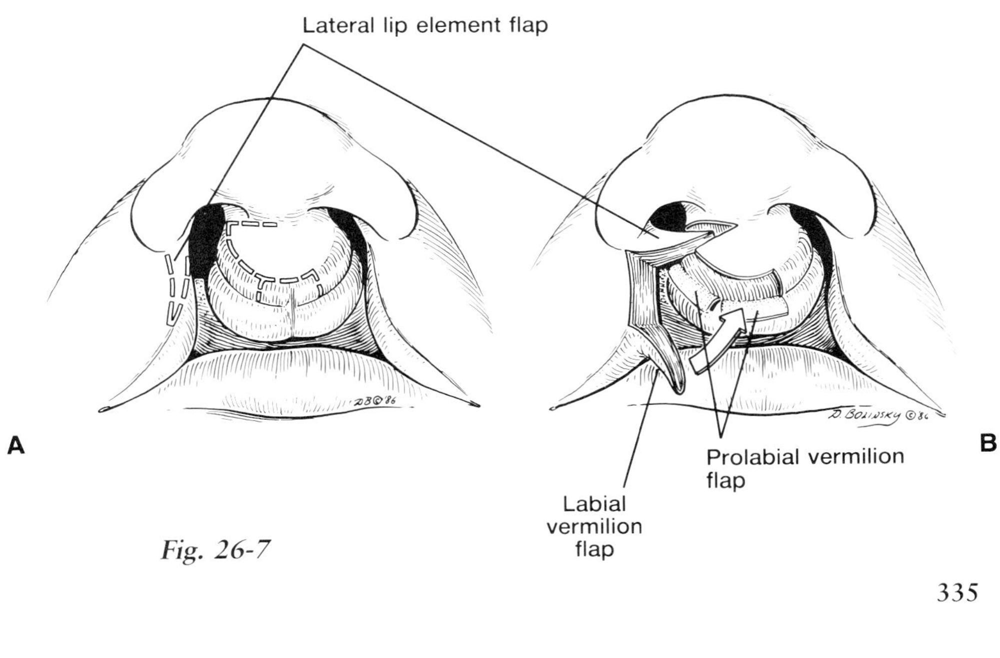

Fig. 26-7

The Veau type III single stage bilateral cleft lip closure leaves lip scars that can be used in the secondary repair to augment the columella in a manner similar to an open rhinoplasty. At the time of this secondary surgery, the lower lateral cartilages are reshaped to increase the height of the nose.

With this background, patients presenting between the ages of 15 to 18 years for cosmetic rhinoplasty with a history of bilateral cleft lip repair constitute a very different problem than those having a single cleft lip nasal defect and so require a different approach. There is a likelihood that the maxilla is deficient and that the lip is tight at the columella base. The nasal tip remains wide, alar bases are far apart, with nostrils presenting with a horizontal orientation of their greatest diameter.

Techniques for secondary repair are often performed on patients between the ages of 7 to 9 years or even earlier. If a snubbed-down nose situation develops, one which raises the upper lip and exposes the upper teeth, the procedure may be done between the ages of 4 to 5 years. These same techniques are available between the ages of 15 to 18 years. The secondary procedures may not have been performed and can also be applied at this age.

Elongation of the Columella

The Millard Forked Flap Technique[8] is available for adults as well as children (Fig. 26-8, A to C). It releases the columella, which is augmented by suturing the paired lip scar flaps together. In instances of a very tight lip, the central skin of the prolabium can be used to augment the columella and raise the depressed tip. The upper lip is then divided completely through to the alveolus in the midline, allowing the divided

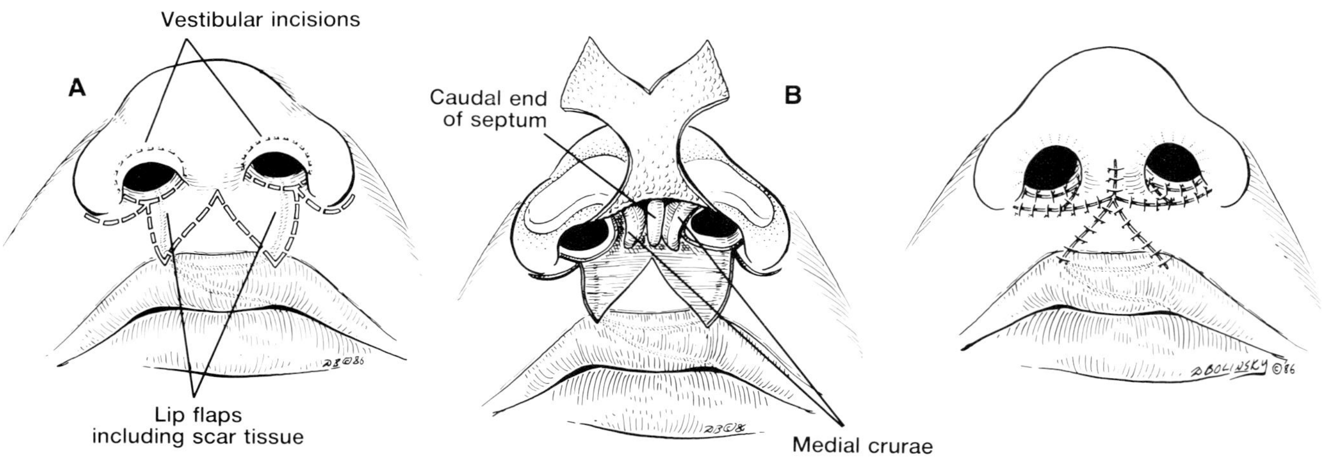

Fig. 26-8

lip to hang in a normal manner by making back cuts laterally toward the alae. The defect is measured and is filled in by a cross-lip flap[1] (Fig. 26-9, A to F). There is disagreement on the amount of lower lip to be used in this procedure, but generally the range is from half to full replacement, depending upon on how much the lower lip can spare.

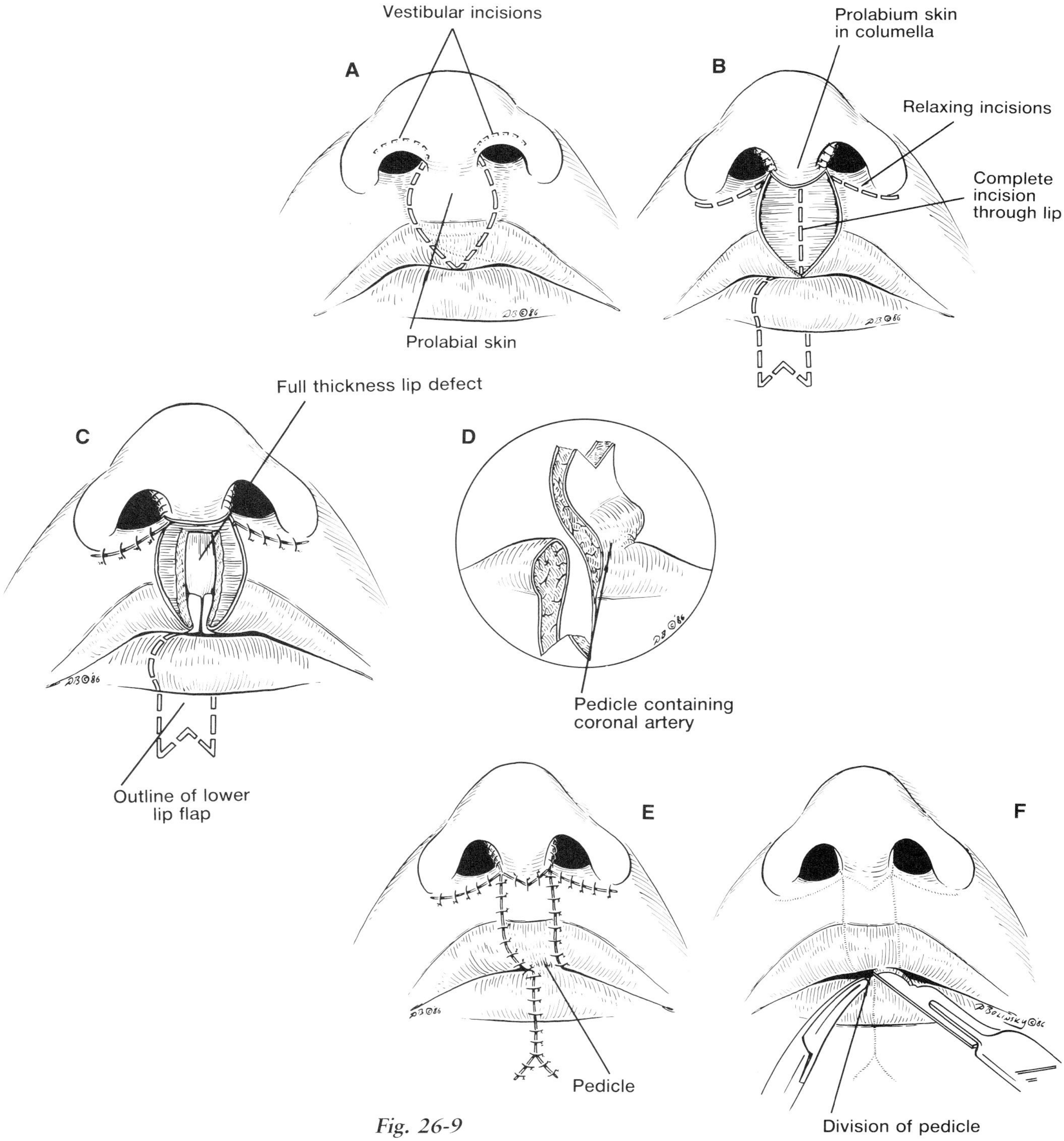

Fig. 26-9

The Cronin refinement of the Carter Technique[4] (Fig. 26-10, A & B) rotates the alar medially, excises part of the lip scar, and brings tissue into the base of the columella. The V-Y Advancement[9] (Figs. 26-11, A & B) is a similar technique of removing skin from the upper lip and placing it in the base of the columella. This particular maneuver, however, creates a scar in the center of the lip in addition to the ones already present.

A Brown-McDowell square flap[3] is outlined on the upper lip beneath the columella in the remnant of the prolabium. Its length is determined by the amount of tissue needed to get the nasal tip forward. Side wedges or darts are outlined across each nostril floor to provide tissue for the opening created after incising the septum and raising the tip (Fig. 26-12, A & B). The flap is of full-thickness skin and subcutaneous tissue about 2 to 3 mm thick. The membranous septum is cut across behind the columella and up to the top of the septum. The tip is freed by cutting through the septum just below the tip. This frees the tip of the nose. It may be necessary to extend the incisions laterally to allow some free movement. The new flap portion inferiorly is folded upon itself to create a new columella. Wedges excised from the nostril floors move up and are used to fill in the space above the septum. The feet of the medial crura may protrude, and if so, they need to be trimmed to provide a new, smooth columella. The defect in the lip is closed, first by closing the sites of the wedge excisions, then the central portion is pulled down together from above with interrupted sutures. A triangle of tissue may need to be taken out just above the vermilion in order to pull the skin together without making a protrusion in the midline of the upper lip. If the anterior nasal spine is prominent, it may need to be chiseled or drilled down to let the soft tissue of the nasal labial angle settle in.

If the tip is not sufficiently protruding and the cartilaginous dorsum is flat, it may be necessary to insert cartilage from a cartilage bank, irradiated cartilage, or autogenous cartilage. An L-shaped piece of costal cartilage can be placed in patients between the ages of 6 to 9 years with the understanding that it will need to be replaced at a later date.

The bilateral cleft lip nostrils tend to be round and have their greatest diameter in a horizontal orientation. This causes a fixed-snout appearance. This is due in part to the original defect; however, thickening of the skin of the rim of the nostrils occurs with growth and may need to be thinned. This situation is improved by partial excision of the nostril bases.

The techniques illustrated, which use tissue from the lips, have certain limitations. The tissue used may contain hair that is brought into the columella. The use of tissue from the lip may make it unduly tight and effect the lip-columella angle, and the lip tissue does not fit well into the columella, making it thick and irregular.

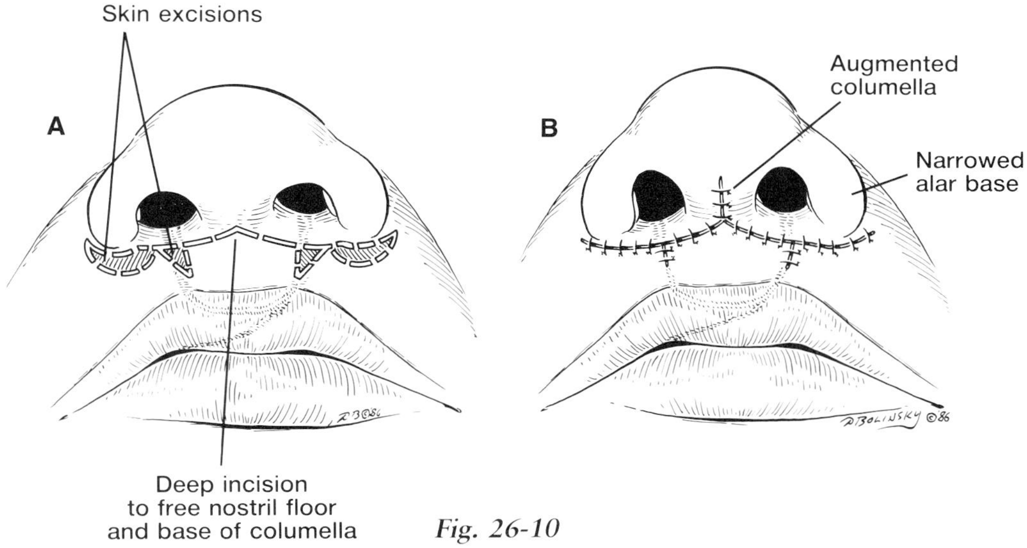

Fig. 26-10

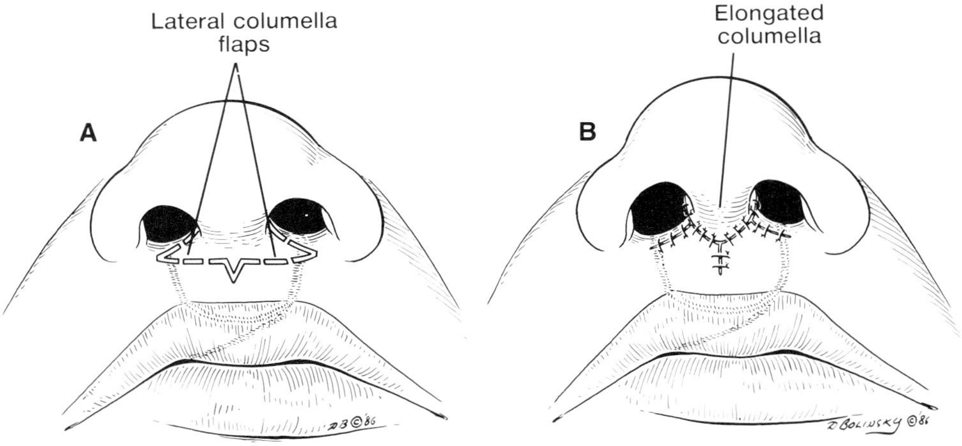

Fig. 26-11

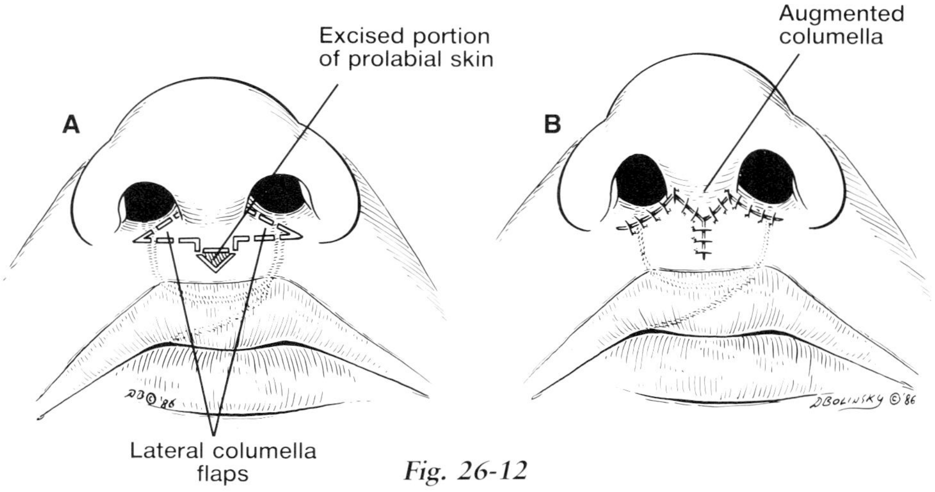

Fig. 26-12

Application of Non-Caucasian Procedures

New procedures arising from a rising volume of non-Caucasian rhinoplasty cases can be applied to the bilateral cleft lip rhinoplasty. Matory[7] (Fig. 26-13, A-D) freed up the alae bilaterally and rotated them medially to elongate the columella, narrow the inter-alar width, and reorient the long axis of the nostrils.

Millard[10] (Fig. 26-14, A-C) describes an alar cinch procedure to improve the flat, flaring nose. The advancing forward edge of the alar roll is denuded and freed by relaxing incisions and is pulled into a pocket created medially beneath the columella so that these alar tips meet in the midline. This causes a narrowing of the nostril floor and improvement in the alar flare.

Gorney[6] has approached the horizontally oriented nostril and depressed dome with a centripetal rotation procedure combined with a columella graft, tip shield, and cartilage onlay graft to the dorsum (Fig. 26-15, A-E).

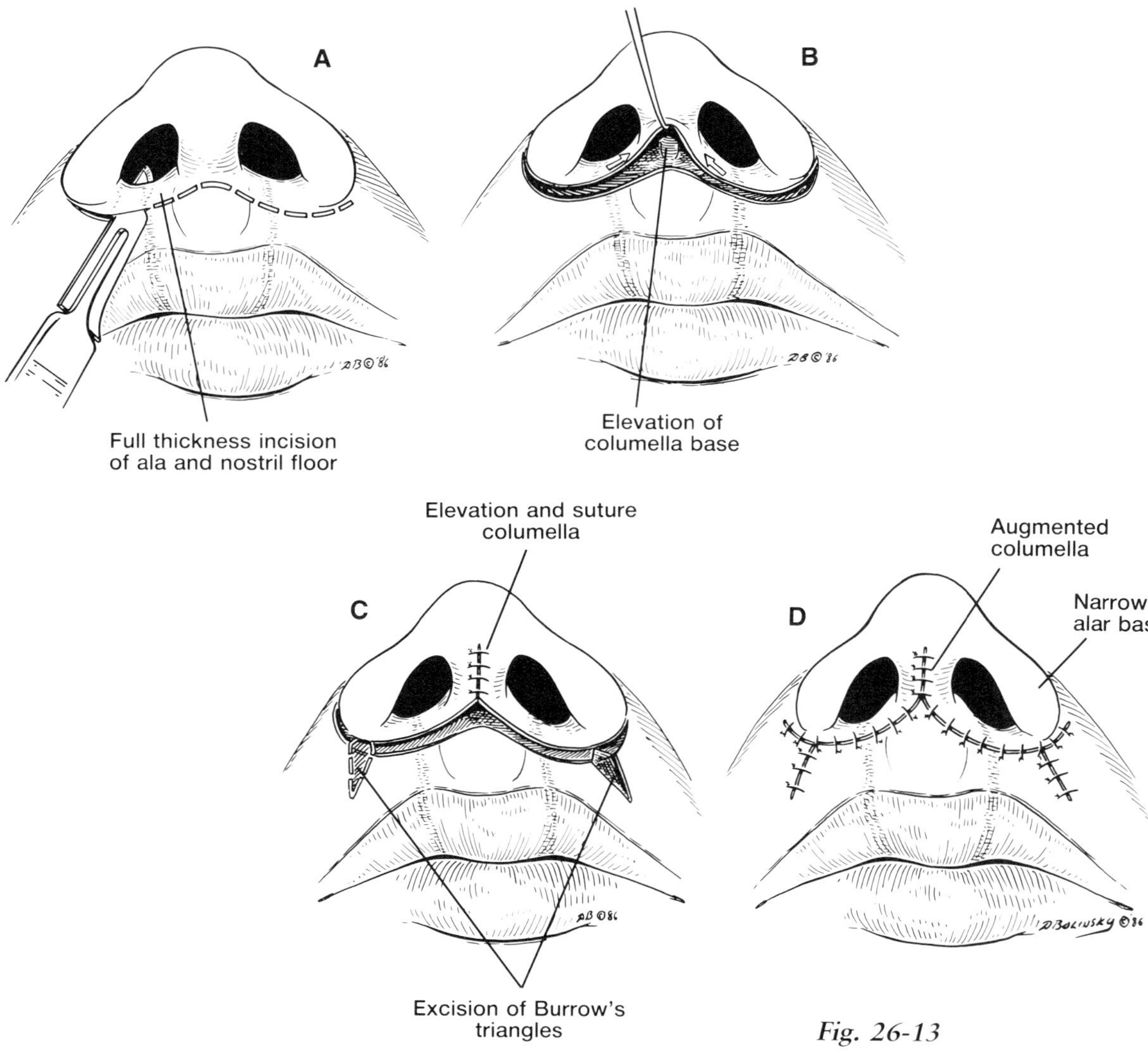

Fig. 26-13

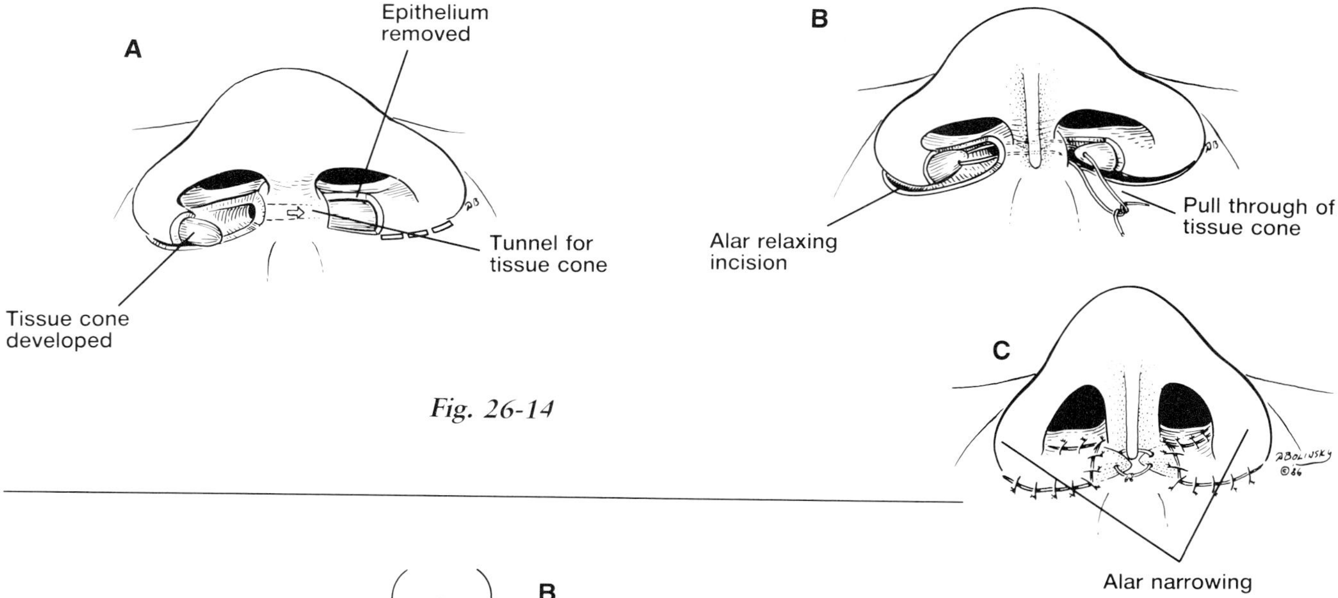

Fig. 26-14

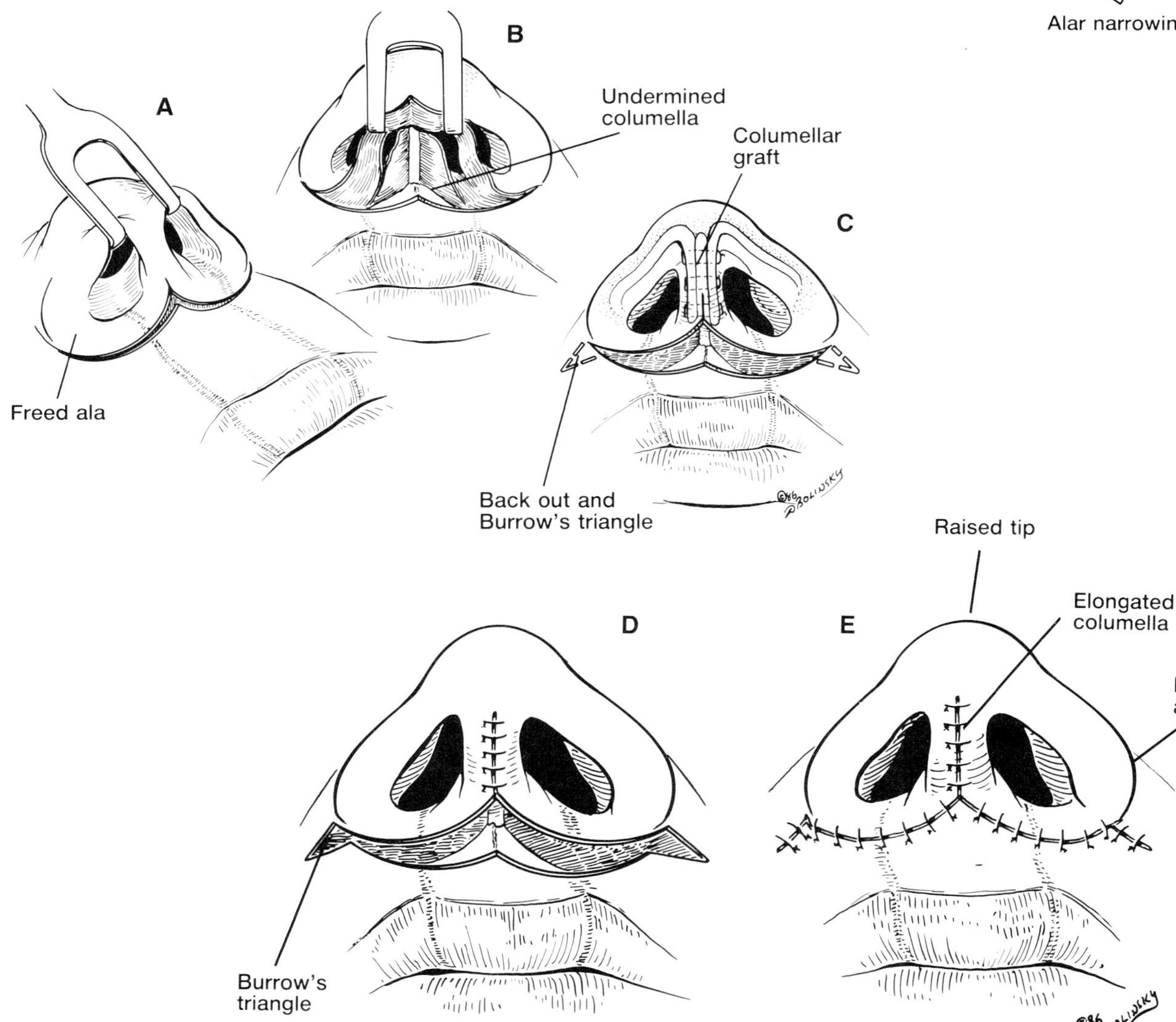

Fig. 26-15

The de-gloving technique (Fig. 26-16, A-E) of Black et al[2] has been used on both single cleft lip noses and bilateral cleft lip noses. Three incisions are used: one in each nostril, and one in the depth of the labial sulcus. The nostril incision is a complete rim incision except for an inverted V-shaped incision at the nostril floor. The incision makes it possible to completely separate the skin from the lower one half of the nose without incising the columella or having a complete circular vestibular incision, thus avoiding scar contracture and vestibular narrowing. The oral incision from bicuspid to bicuspid allows the soft tissue of the anterior maxilla to be freed and the two dissection spaces joined. The whole cartilage and bony framework can be viewed at once after adequate retraction. The lateral crura can be freed and raised laterally by suturing the domes together. The medial crura can be reinforced by replacing a columella graft of septal cartilage. As in all rhinoplasty procedures, the skin redrapes itself to fit over the new cartilaginous and bony framework.

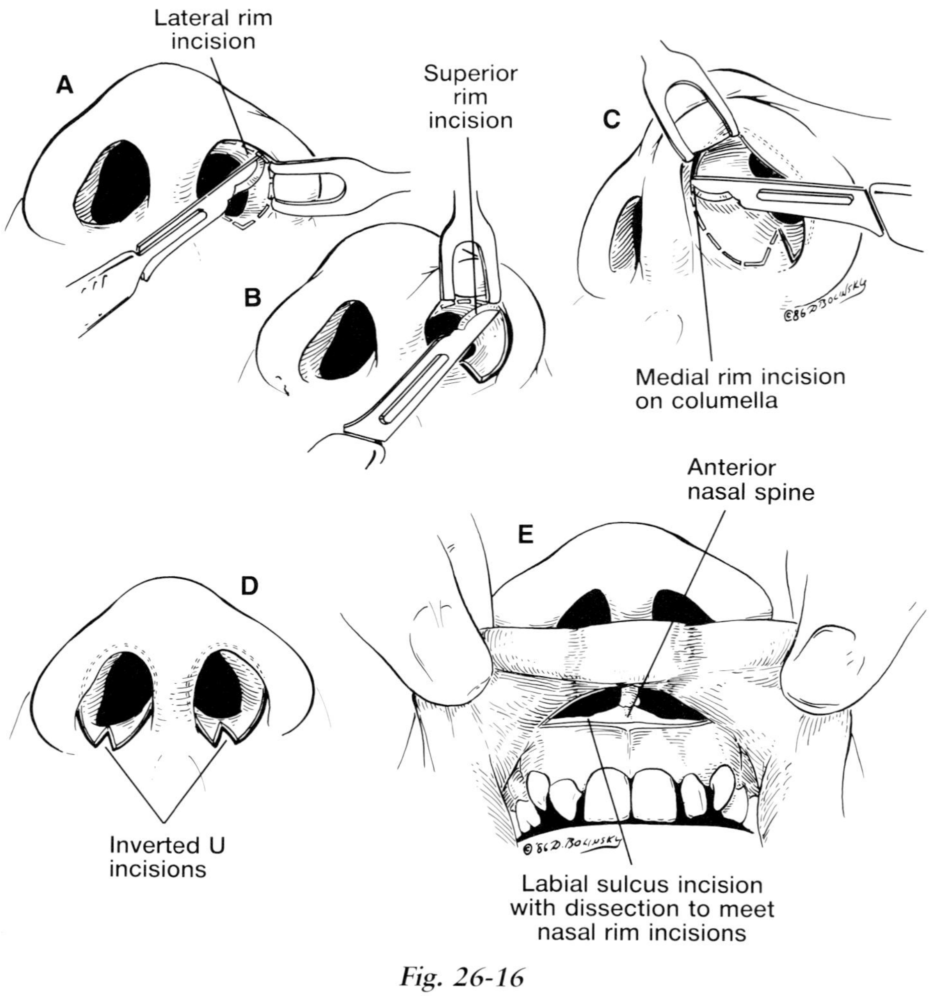

Fig. 26-16

The procedures need to be done after correcting the alar bases and the lower lateral cartilages are those common to most rhinoplasties. The septum may require attention; however, in most instances of bilateral cleft lip, the septum is straight.

The bony and cartilaginous dorsum may be both low and wide. The decision simply may be to perform routine medial and lateral osteotomies to narrow the nose. With a wide and low nose it may be a better choice to simply augment the dorsum with bone, cartilage, or alloplastic material.

REFERENCES

1. Abe R: A new plastic operation for relief of deformity due to double hare lip, Medical Record 53:477, 1898.
2. Black PW, Hartram PF, Carl RJ, and Beegle P: Cleft lip type nasal deformity: definitive repair, Ann Plast Surg 12:128, 1984.
3. Brown JB and McDowell F: Plastic surgery of the nose, Springfield, Ill, 1951, Charles C Thomas.
4. Cronin TD: Lengthening the columella by use of skin from the nasal floor and alae, Plast Reconstr Surg 27:417, 1958.
5. Cronin TD: A modification of the tennison type lip repair, Cleft Palate J 3:376, 1966.
6. Gorney Mark and Rosenberg, HL: Centripetal rotation: advancement for cleft lip deformities, Ann Plast Surg 2:374, 1979.
7. Matory WE and Falces E: Non-Caucasian rhinoplasty: a 16-Year experience, Plast Reconstr Surg 77:238, 1986.
8. Millard DR Jr, Columella lengthening by a forked flap, Plast Reconstr Surg 22:454, 1958.
9. Millard DR Jr: Cleft Craft, vol 1, Boston, 1976, Little, Brown & Co Inc.
10. Millard DR Jr: The alar cinch in the flat flaring nose, Plast Reconstr Surg 65:669, 1980.
11. Skoog T: Plastic Surgery, Philadelphia, 1974, WB Saunders Co.
12. Veau V: Operative treatment of complete double hare lip, Ann Surg 76:143, 1922.
13. Wynn SK: Lateral flap cleft surgery technique, Plast Reconstr Surg 26:509, 1960.

27

Cleft Lip Nose

Rodolphe Meyer and Louis O. Boileau

One of the most challenging, and in turn, most rewarding rhinosurgical procedures is the correction of the cleft lip nasal deformity. Cases differ widely in terms of whether they are associated with unilateral or bilateral lip clefts, depending on the severity of the clefting. With that in mind, an individualized approach appropriate to the patient's deformity should be adopted in each case. It is important for the surgeon to be acquainted with as many of the techniques available for correcting the various facets of the cleft lip nose, and if necessary, to improvise on them.

Timing

Special consideration should be given to timing of surgery. Generally, in the newborn, repositioning of the alar structures by elevating the displaced lower lateral cartilage, freeing it completely, with the possible addition of a trans-alar fixation suture may be undertaken at the time of the original cleft lip repair. The nasal structures, especially the infant cartilage, are very delicate and caution must be exercised in such procedures. Attempts to modify all the contributing factors to the cleft lip nose in infancy may be somewhat presumptive as the effect achieved is not always maintained with the subsequent growth of the child, and, furthermore, excision of tissue and osteotomies may complicate a future rhinoplasty.

If secondary corrections are required, as is often the case in patients with a bilateral cleft lip nose, we believe these should be undertaken prior to the growth spurt of the child. By doing so, one achieves three important goals:

1. Better tissue cosmesis as the abnormal tissue placement is corrected.
2. Improvement of airway function with correction of alar webbing, nostril stenosis, etc.
3. An important psychological boost for the patient and his or her family. This is particularly important for children about to enter school where the abuse generated by peers may severely stigmatize the patient.

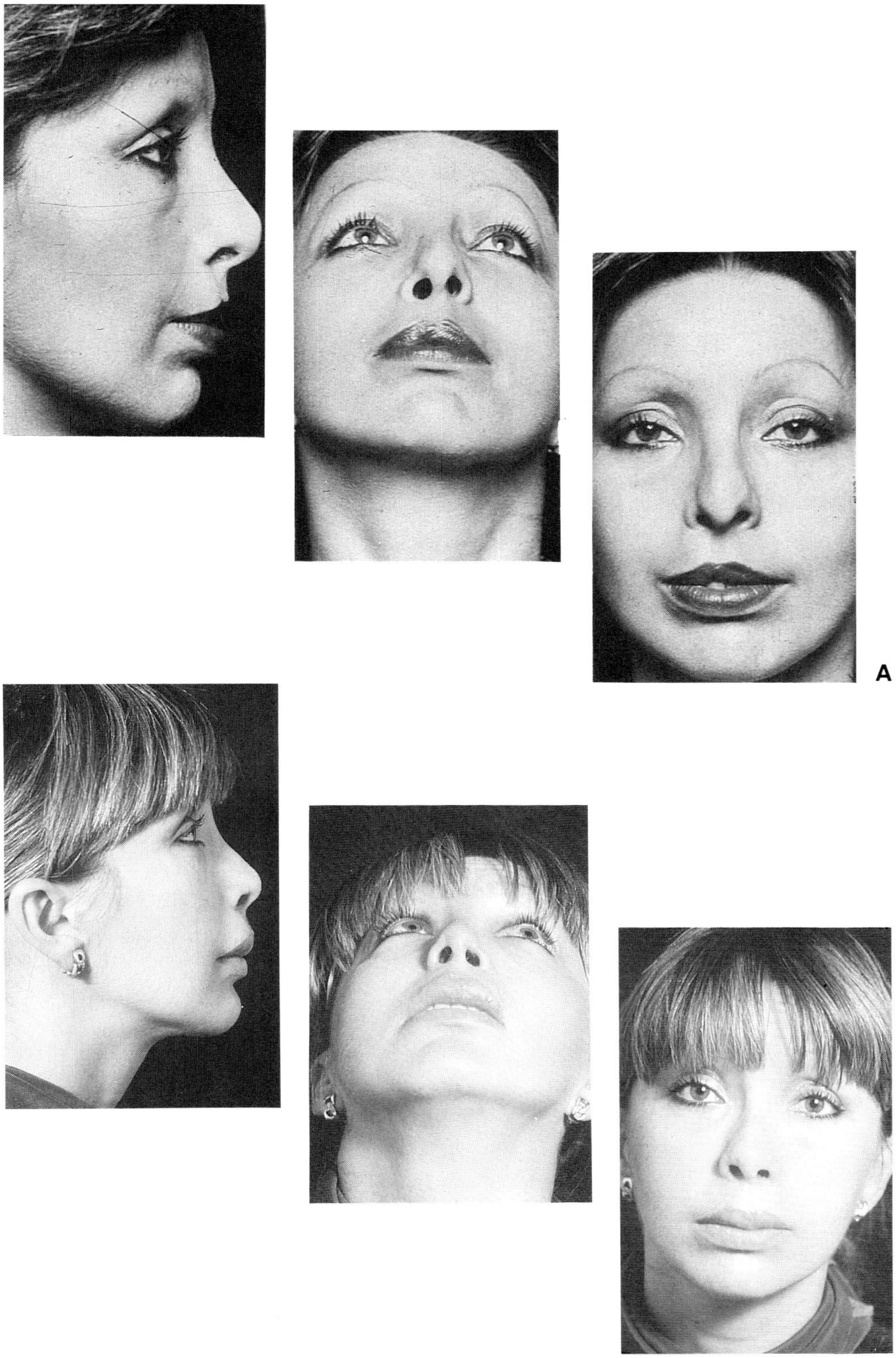

A

B

Fig. 27-1. **A,** A young lady with a repaired right unilateral cleft lip. Nostril asymmetry is present, with a lack of definition to the tip. **B,** One year after undergoing a conventional rhinoplasty.

The aim is to achieve as normal-looking a nose as possible with final refinements, including conventional rhinoplasty with or without osteotomies, hump reduction, and septoplasty reserved for the "adult" nose, i.e., after the age of 15 or 16 years (Fig. 27-1).

Unilateral Cleft Lip Nose

Abnormalities

We have enumerated eleven points requiring correction in individuals with a unilateral cleft. These can be subdivided into abnormalities found on the cleft side, and those more particular to the entire nasal structure.

Involving the cleft side

1. Septo-columellar deviation towards the cleft side.
2. Flattening and caudal displacement of the ala with a resultant loss of dome protrusion.
3. An abnormal insertion of the ala into the naso-labial region.
4. Shortening of the columella border on the cleft side.
5. An advanced anterior commissure of the nostril.
6. A broad nasal floor, located at a different level as compared to the unaffected side.
7. Maxillary hypoplasia in the region of the insertion of the ala.
8. Caudal displacement with inward traction of the lateral crus of the ala.

Involving the whole nose

1. Tendency toward a bifid tip.
2. Asymmetrical upper lateral cartilages.
3. Asymmetrical bony pyramid.

We will consider some of the different techniques available, which we have found of benefit in correcting these various components of the cleft lip nose. Several of the points listed may be properly managed with the surgical technique, and so rather than consider each point specifically, we will discuss some of the surgical options available to reconstruct the nasal base and gain columellar length, as well as those used to obtain tip projection and repair the constricted nostril.

Techniques

Base of the nose. Methods used to correct the alar base have been previously described by Fomon[16] and Meyer.[11,12] Farrior[14] mobilizes a constricted alar base laterally, with an inferior advancement of the membraneous septal skin, completed by a V-Y closure of the vestibular floor. Currently, we prefer to use a paranasal myocutaneous island flap that is transferred into the vestibule by either a tunnel directed beneath the alar foot plate, or more directly positioned after an alatomy (Fig. 27-2).

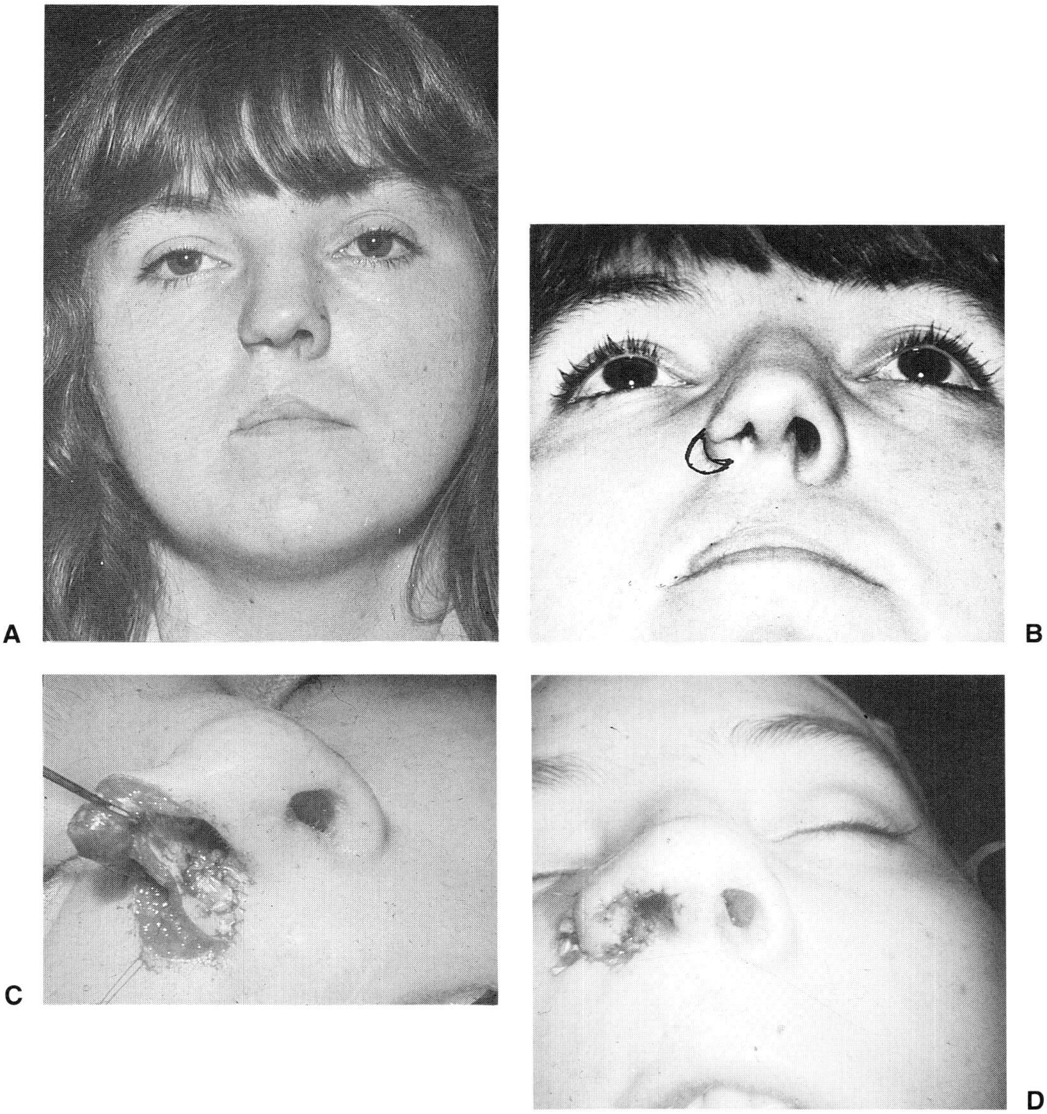

Fig. 27-2. **A,** A young lady with a repaired left unilateral cleft lip who has an anterior vestibular stenosis of the left nostril. **B,** The paranasal island flap is outlined. **C,** The flap has been elevated and inset into the vestibular floor defect after correction of the stenosis. **D,** Immediate postoperative appearance with a slightly overcorrected result.

The depression of the alar base results in nasal asymmetry, which is best corrected by elevating the alar-facial junction to the height of the normal noncleft side by using cartilage onlay grafts to obtain the desired augmentation. Maxillary onlays may be obtained in vivo or from a bone cartilage bank. Work done by Skoog,[27] Ritsila et al.[26], as well as clinical results currently being obtained by Courtemanche,[8] support the role of pure periosteal grafts commonly harvested from off the tibia and applied as a maxillary onlay. The ability to subsequently form bone is preserved, and this serves to build up the depressed nasal base (Fig. 27-3). Most surgery on the base of the nose done for both functional and cosmetic reasons can be carried out during the preschool years. This is not at all deleterious to subsequent soft tissue growth, nor does it preclude any further surgical procedures if they are deemed necessary.

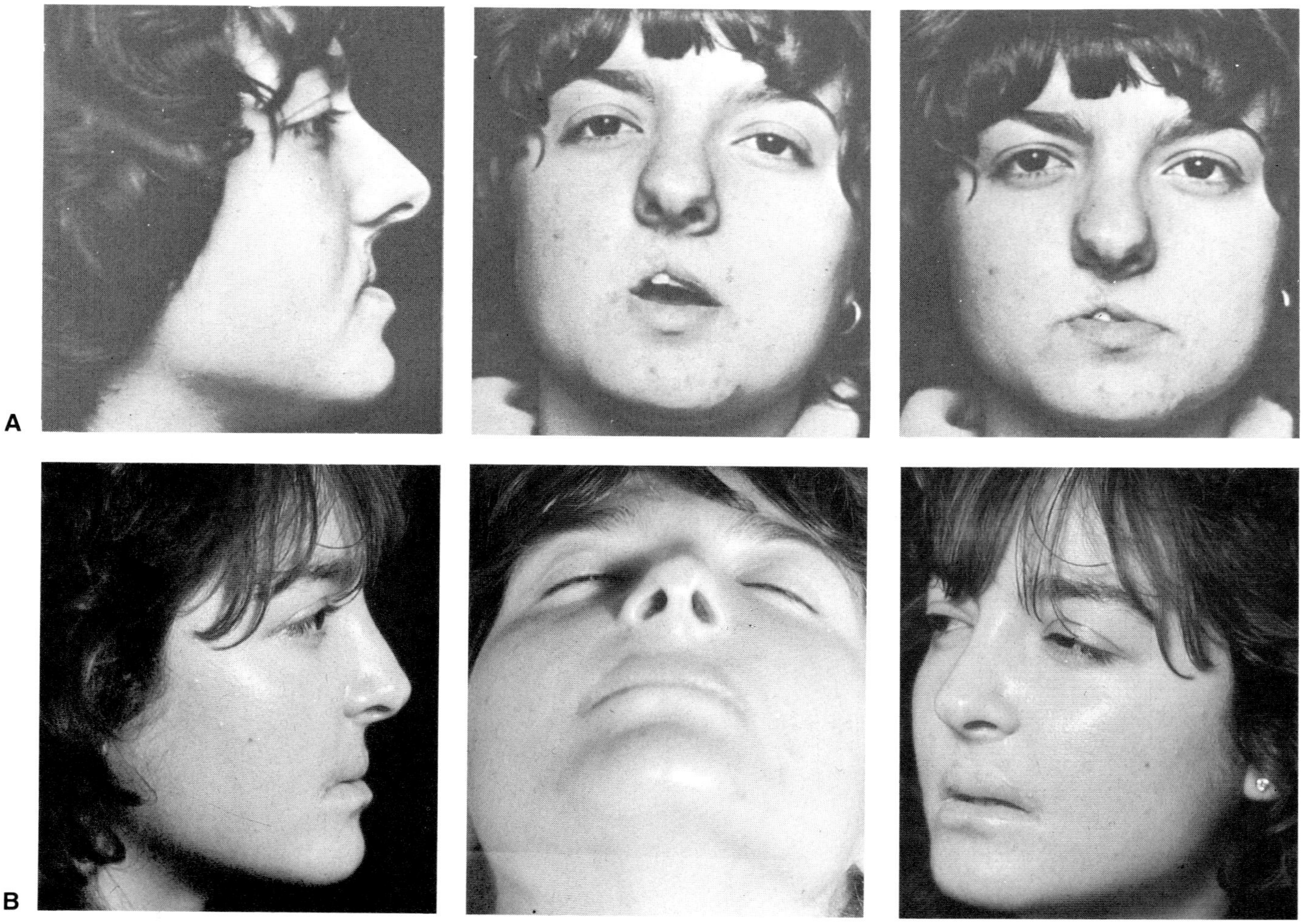

Fig. 27-3. **A,** This patient clearly exhibits a significant degree of upper lip and columellar base retraction in association with a repaired complete left unilateral cleft lip and palate. **B,** Postoperative result after inserting of premaxillary bony onlays and temporal fascial grafts to the upper lip to give additional bulk. The cupid's bow has also been revised.

The columella. The short columella occurs in conjunction with an abnormal position of the rest of the nostril and so many techniques have been elaborated to repair both of these deformities concomitantly. Blair and Brown[2] were the first to split the columella in the midline, the cut swinging outward along the junction of the floor of the nostril with the lip. The whole cleft side nostril then, with its splayed ala, is rotated into a more normal position. Ivy[20] modified the Blair[1] procedure incorporating the constricted nostril into a flap based on the lateral ala, which is then advanced superiorly and medially. The nostril apex is advanced into a defect created by excising a full-thickness wedge of tissue (Fig. 27-4). Such procedures involving the inward rotation and medial repositioning of the lateral alar attachment have proved to be very effective. The need to incorporate an additional labio-vestibular flap to widen the vestibular floor after using such techniques is felt occasionally (Fig. 27-4). In 1964 we further modified the technique by adding a Z-plasty at the columellar base, helping to maintain the rotated hemi-columella in place (Fig. 27-5 and 27-6). No vestibular narrowing was observed. A similar method was also used by us in adults, giving very satisfactory results, and published in 1975. Here the skin of the membraneous septum along with the medial crus of the alar cartilage on the cleft side is rotated with a 1 cm wide strip of vestibular floor skin taken as an advancement flap and used to fill the resultant defect.

An alternative to rotating vestibular skin exists. A half-moon shaped resection is performed in the lobule on the cleft side permitting elevation of the anterior commissure to the level of the unaffected side. Similarly, one may also resect the commisural border, creating a new margin and lining with a composite graft harvested from the inner aspect of the auricular crus helicis (Figs. 27-7 and 27-8).

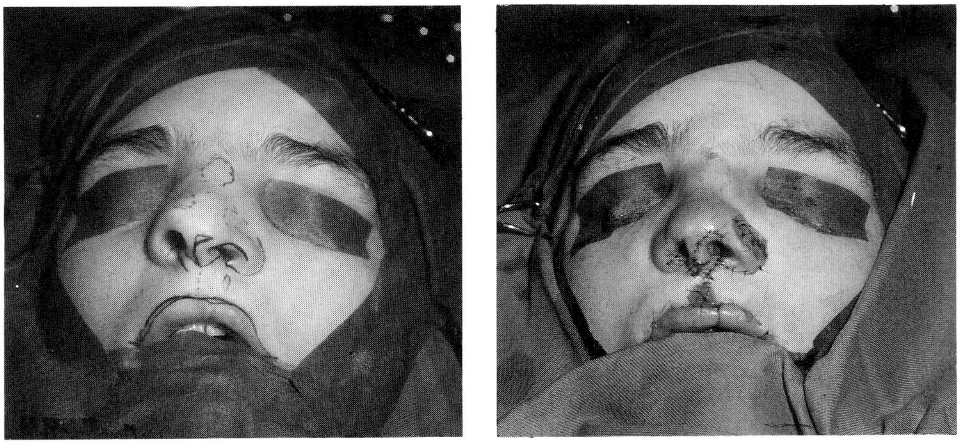

A B

Fig. 27-4. **A,** Example of tip symmetry gained by the columellar splitting incision with hemicolumellar rotation. The preoperative markings are shown. **B,** Immediate postoperative result, which shows that tip symmetry has been established. To balance the columellar base a transposition flap from the left vestibular floor has been inserted into the right nasal floor.

Fig. 27-5. Diagram depicting the technique of hemicolumellar rotation with the addition of a Z-plasty at the columellar base.

A

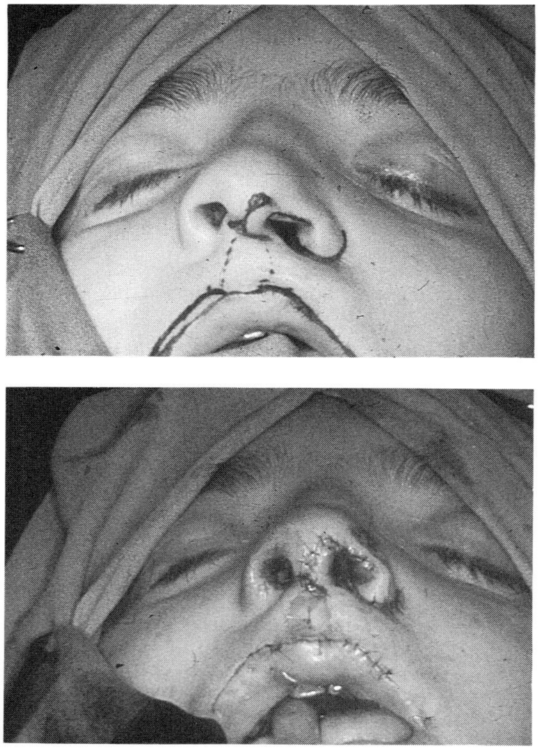

B

Fig. 27-6. A, This child has all the stigmata of a unilateral cleft lip nasal deformity. The preoperative markings are shown with a columellar base Z-plasty included. B, Immediate result obtained postoperatively after hemi-columellar rotation and marginal resection.

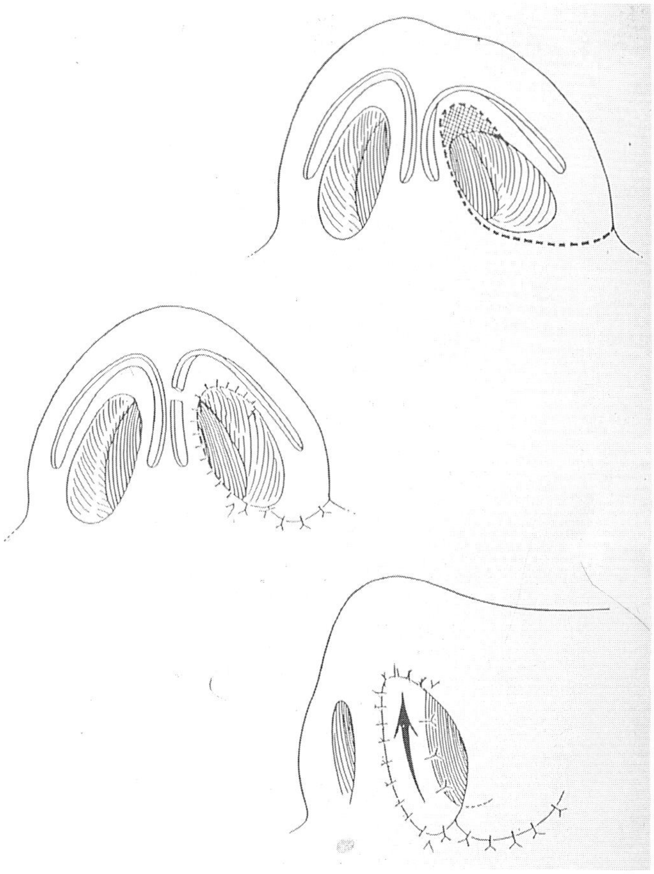

Fig. 27-7. Advancement of the vestibular floor and part of the membraneous septum with sectioning of the medial crus to obtain nasal symmetry. The columella-alar commissure also requires reduction.

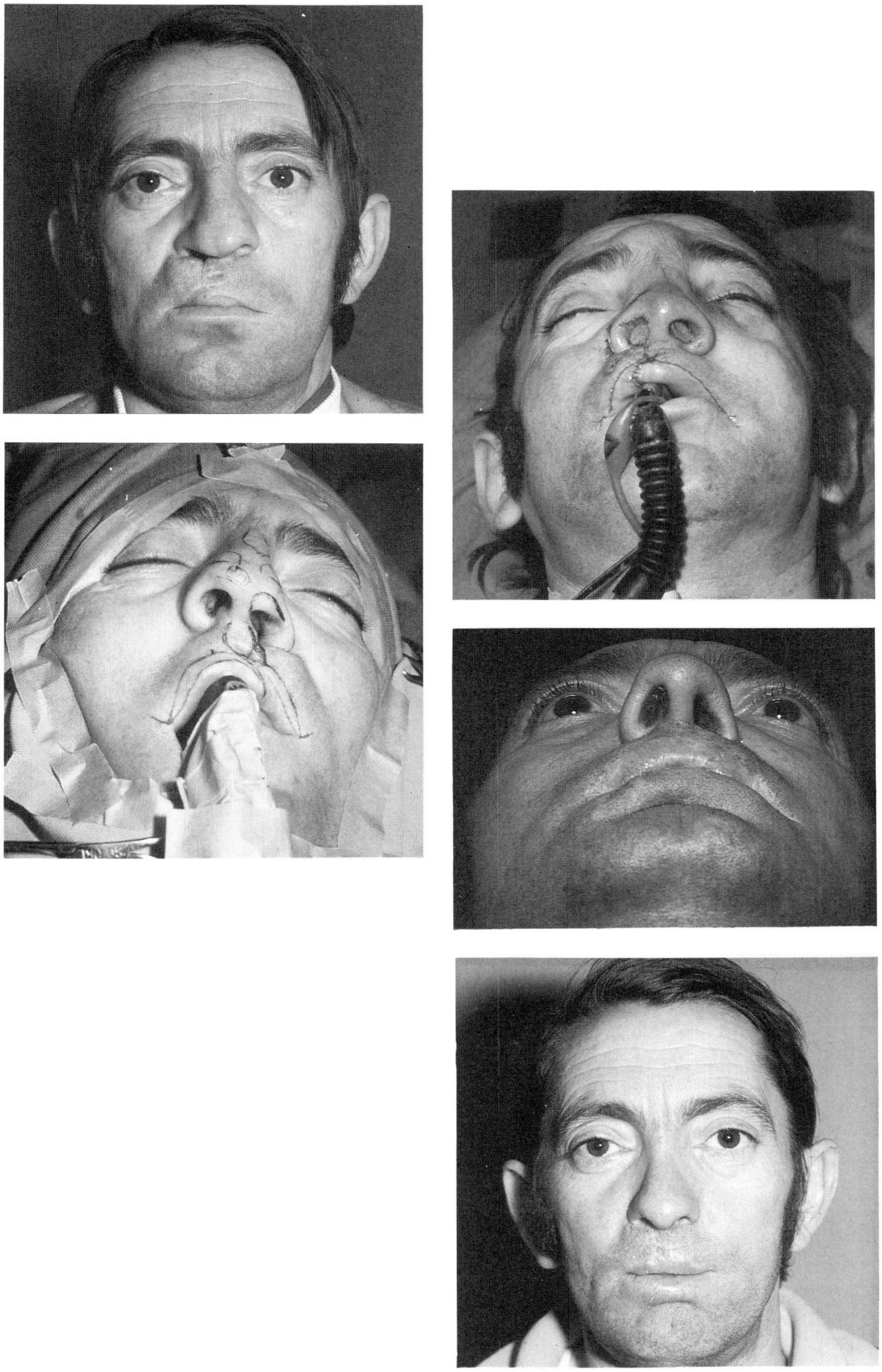

Fig. 27-8. A, Middle-aged patient showing marked nostril asymmetry. B, Preoperative markings for the balancing technique shown in Fig. 27-7. C, Immediate result obtained using the vestibular floor advancement technique with additional lobular and alar cartilage onlays and lip revision with a 3-layer closure. D and E, Result seen at one year in the axial and anterior views.

The nasal tip. Numerous methods have been designed to balance the commissure and alar domes found in the tip region. Many of the previously described techniques used to gain columellar length also have the secondary benefit of achieving better tip symmetry. Using the method of Potter[23] we can obtain an elongation of the columella through a V-Y plasty at its base as well as dome elevation by designing yet another V-Y plasty on the lateral wall of the vestibule. The dome of the cleft side should be elevated to the level of the dome on the non-cleft side, or even better, to a slightly over-corrected position. We tend to cut the medial crus on the cleft side into two, elevating the dome with the superiormost portion of the cut medial crus and fixing it in its new position to the opposite dome using mattress sutures. To maintain proper tip support a cartilaginous strut harvested from the septum or from the contralateral alar cartilage, which is often reduced to further balance the tip, is apposed along the split medial crus (Fig. 27-9).

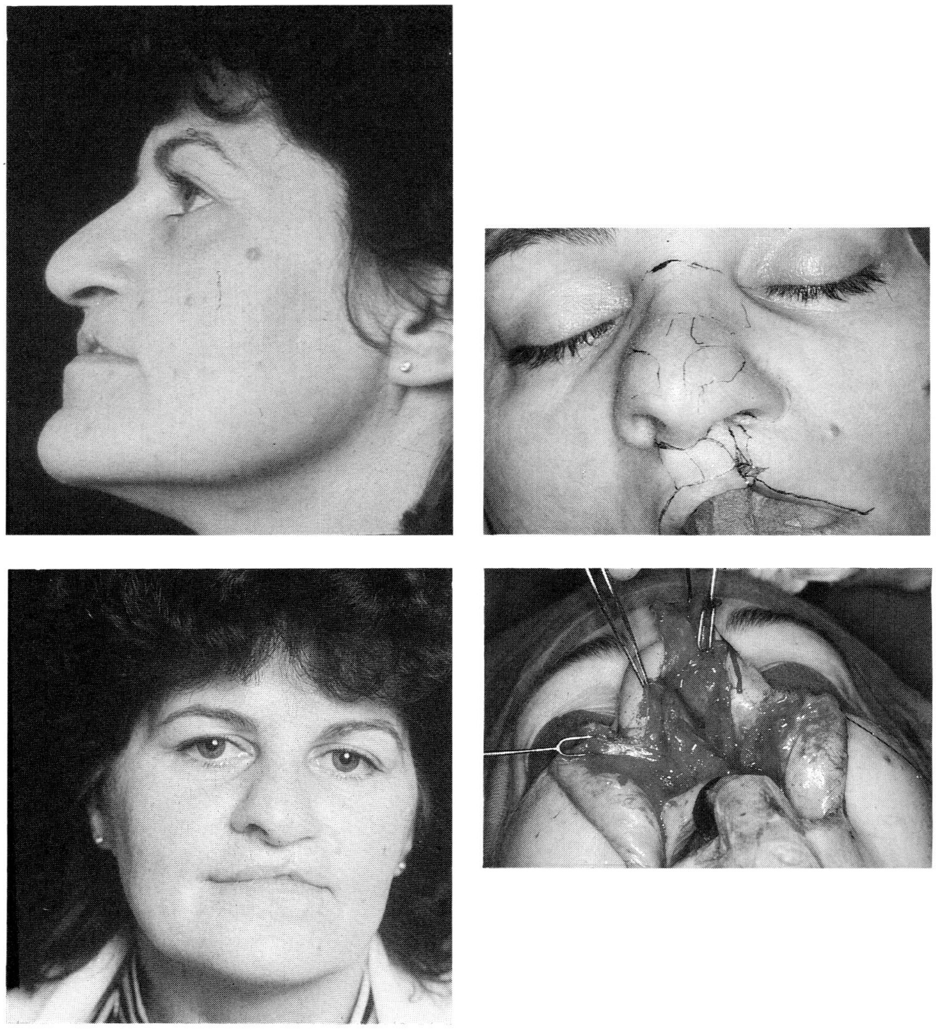

A C D B

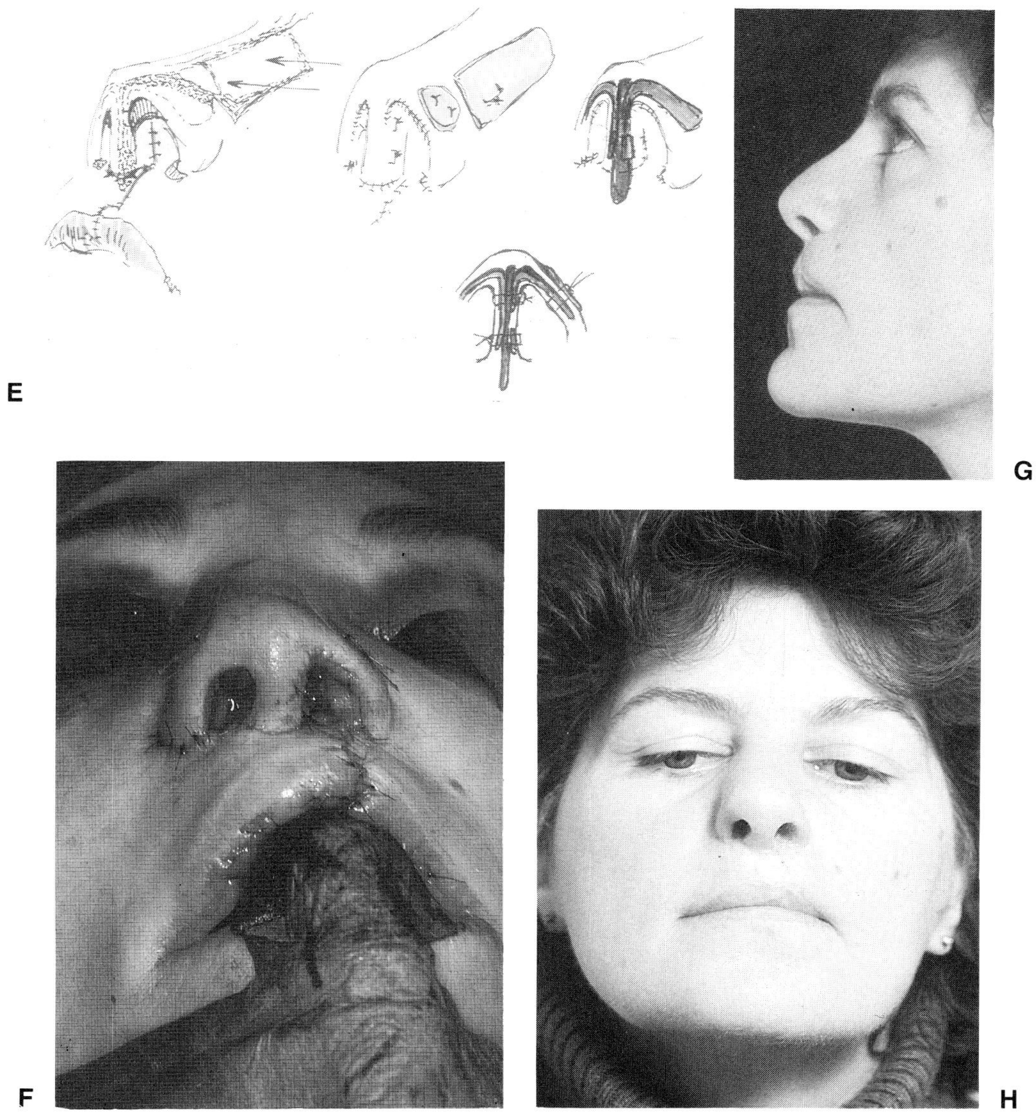

Fig. 27-9. A and B, This patient with a repaired left unilateral cleft lip and palate demonstrates marked tip and alar asymmetry, with deviation of the septum and nasal dorsum. C, Preoperative markings for the Potter columellar base incision, with additional markings for the dome resection and lip revision. D, A view of the intra-operative access gained with the incisions described above. The deviated septum and nasal dorsum are corrected by the bilateral extramucosal dissection of perichondrium. E, Diagram showing the symmetry gained by sectioning the cleft side medial crus and insertion of a cartilaginous strut for support. Our modification of the Potter incision, which includes the medial crura in the elevated columellar flap, is outlined. For balancing the domes, cartilage grafts with trans-alar mattress sutures are used. The transnasal mattress sutures shown are rarely required after proper osteotomies. F, Immediate postoperative appearance with lip sutures, trans-alar and transcolumellar mattress sutures, and sutures along the alar base wedge resection line performed on the non-cleft side are seen. G and H, The patient seen after one year.

Tip augmentation can also be achieved with a turning over of the cranial portion of the non-affected alar cartilage. Tip balance can also be realized with more attention paid to the mobilization of the lateral crus as apposed to that just described involving the medial crus. Rees[24] proposed a medial and superior advancement of the lateral crus with its attached vestibular skin into a more elevated position. Scoring of the cartilage and additional onlay grafts are also effective adjuncts when using this method. Some controversy exists regarding the final suture fixation of the mobilized cartilage.

Holt[19] sutures the mobilized alar cartilage to its ipsilateral upper lateral cartilage. We have found, however, that in the majority of cases the upper lateral cartilages themselves are in an asymmetrical arrangement, and so, we prefer to have the upper and lower lateral cartilages free and independent from one another. We choose rather to suture the two domes together in a somewhat overcorrected position as proposed by Tolhurst.[28] We also believe that trans-alar mattress sutures looped over plastic sheets are important in stabilizing the new convex shape of the ala and in obliterating the potential dead space that exists between cartilage and skin.

We have also obtained good results regarding columellar-tip balance in secondary unilateral cleft lip nose reconstruction using Rethi's[25] decortication technique of open access, which provides excellent exposure for the mobilization of the cartilaginous dome (Fig. 27-10). Other popular incisions include Erich's[13] "listing seagull" and Goodman's modification[18] of the Rethi incision, which is actually much the same as that described in 1952 by Figi.[15]

Fig. 27-10. The Rethi incision.

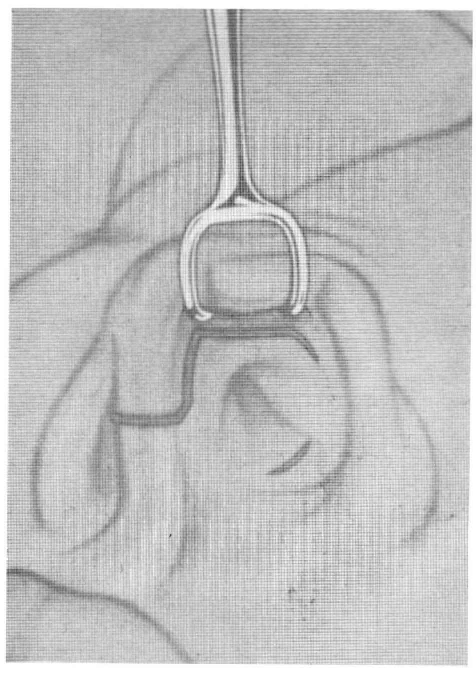

Further tip refinement with nostril balancing can be achieved using other rather straightforward techniques. In the unilateral cleft lip nose, the affected alar border is generally found in a more caudal position than is the unaffected side. A simple in-rolling of the nostril margin of the noncleft side can result in greater nostril/tip symmetry. For obvious reasons, the internal skin should never be rolled out.

Similarly, these marginal resections may be used to give a more canted nostril tilt as opposed to the transverse orientation commonly found on the cleft side, as well as to remove the alar overhang (Fig. 27-11). A Z-plasty placed in the lateral vestibular wall can also alter the level of the alar rim, as well as remedy the collapsing alar fold. If necessary, any lack of lateral vestibular wall lining can be restituted with a composite helical crus graft.

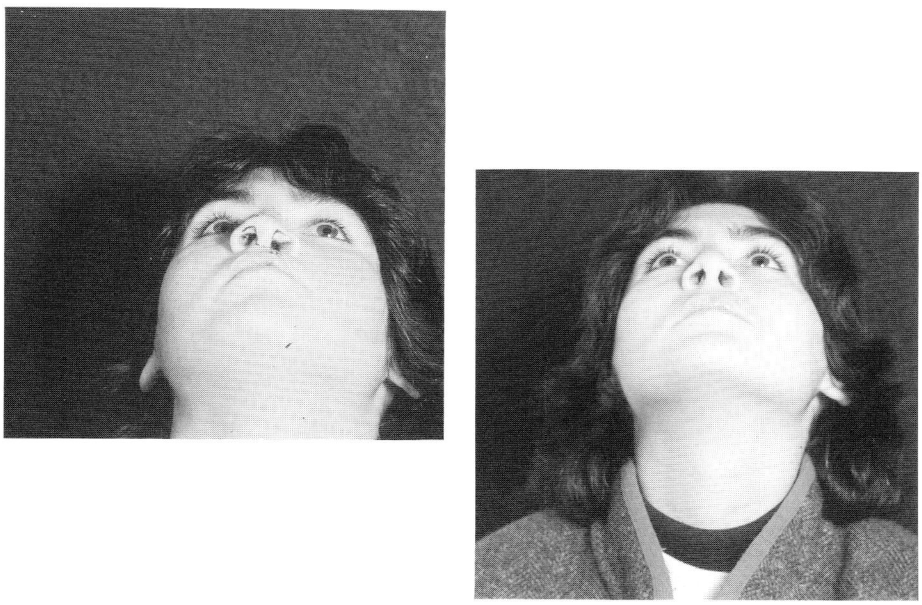

A B

Fig. 27-11. A and B, Alar marginal resection was combined with a conventional tip plasty in this young girl.

Bilateral Cleft Lip Nose

The bilateral cleft lip nose is somewhat of an enigma: on one hand it is rather challenging when one considers the gross deviations characteristic of the deformity; on the other hand, because there is no "normal" side to be compared against because the nose is symmetrically abnormal, surgical intervention can often provide encouraging, dramatic improvements in a patient's appearance (Fig. 27-12). The bilateral cleft lip nose is patho-anatomically just the sum of the parts of two unilateral cleft lip nasal deformities. The points previously discussed in the section on the unilateral cleft lip nose apply equally here. In particular, three aspects of the bilateral cleft lip nose that are important to consider are:

1. There is an excessive shortening of the columella with a loss of tip protrusion.
2. The lobule is broad with the alar domes laterally displaced, giving rise to a bifid tip.

A

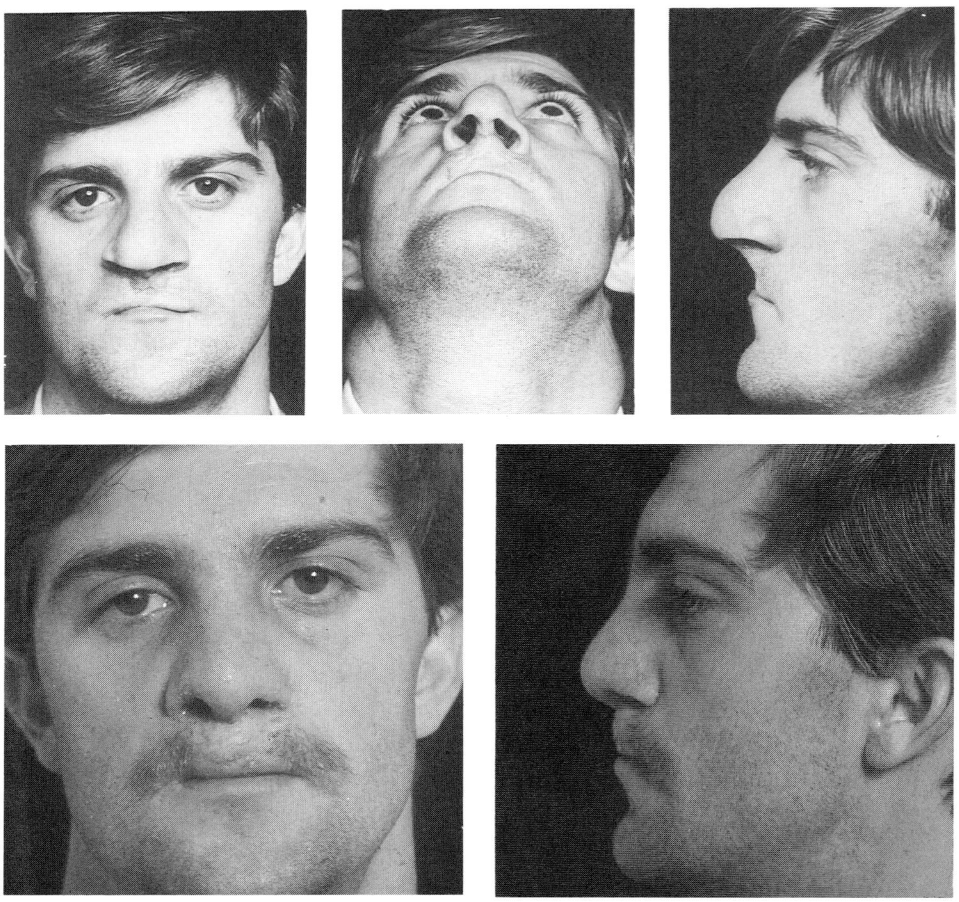

B C

Fig. 27-12. A, B, and C, This young man with repaired complete bilateral cleft lip and palate shows the benefits of a conventional reduction rhinoplasty, along with alar marginal resections. The lip has also been revised with fascial strip transplants and a cupid bow correction.

3. The angles of the lower lateral cartilages are laterally displaced, creating a sharp bend, and producing an oblique oval position of both nares, as well as resulting in a wide nostril floor.

Because of its obvious nature and important contribution to the appearance of a hare-lip nose, we will center our discussion on some of the various methods used to achieve columellar lengthening.

Columellar Lengthening

In children we use the technique of Burian[6] and Millard,[22] both of whom described this method independently. Two lateral prongs are elevated on either side of philtrum, leaving this shield-shaped structure intact—thus the name "fork flap." These flaps are raised and left in their longitudinal position, advanced forward, and sutured together in the midline as columellar skin. This technique also affords the surgeon the opportunity to remove any undesirable lip scarring that may be present (Fig. 27-13). Another technique found beneficial in lengthening the columella in both adolescents and adults is a modification of Potter's[23] method already described in the section dealing with nasal tip construction in cases of unilateral cleft lip nose. The membraneous septum with its enclosed medial crura of the lower lateral cartilages are included to form a columellar flap arising from a bilateral basal V-Y advancement.

For lengthening the columella in adults with a bilateral cleft lip nose we prefer to choose among three popular methods of reconstruction:

1. The fork flap and modifications of it.
2. The basal V-Y plasty of Cronin.[9]
3. The reverse lobule V-Y plasty of Brauer.[3]

Cronin[10] refined and popularized the ingenious principle of shifting nasal floor skin into the columella in a V-Y fashion. Bipedicled flaps based medially on the columella and laterally on the ala are raised. One cut is carried along the groove of the ala with the upper lip, joining in the midline of the middle or upper third of the columella its corresponding incision, and carried out on the contralateral side. The second incision in the vestibule is made nearly parallel to the first incision in order to separate the columella from the septum. This internal incision is not required in every case. The flaps are sutured medially, elevating the columella, and at the same time correcting the excess nostril flare commonly seen in bilateral cleft cases. Maeda[21] and his group of Japanese surgeons described a technique that gives direct exposure to the alar cartilages and achieves columellar lengthening calling upon an amalgamation of both Cronin's[10] technique and Brown and McDowell's[5] method of V-Y advancement of the upper lip.

Another method, proposed by Brauer and Foerster,[4] adapting the double wing flaps of Gillies and Millard,[17] has also proved popular, particularly in cases where the nasal base as well as the philtral region are balanced and do not require secondary correction. Using this technique, two tapered flaps based on the columella take up some of the ex-

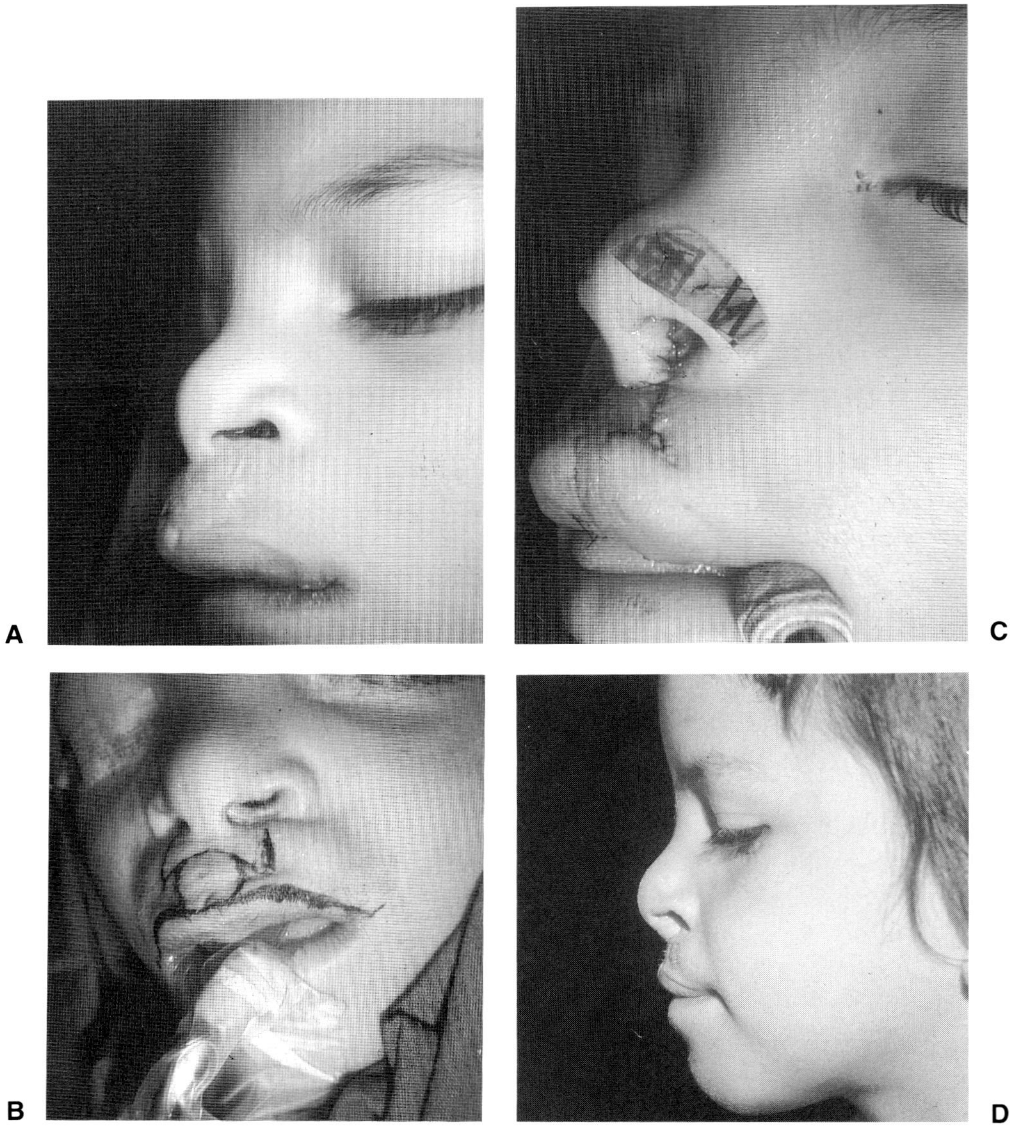

Fig. 27-13. **A,** A young boy who clearly shows the typical shortened columellar, flattened tip, and oblique oval postioning of the nares seen with a bilateral lip deformity. **B,** Preoperative markings of a modified broad fork flap. **C,** Immediate postoperative result showing the increase in columellar length obtained with straightened ala obtained using trans-alar mattress sutures. **D,** Same patient seen one year later.

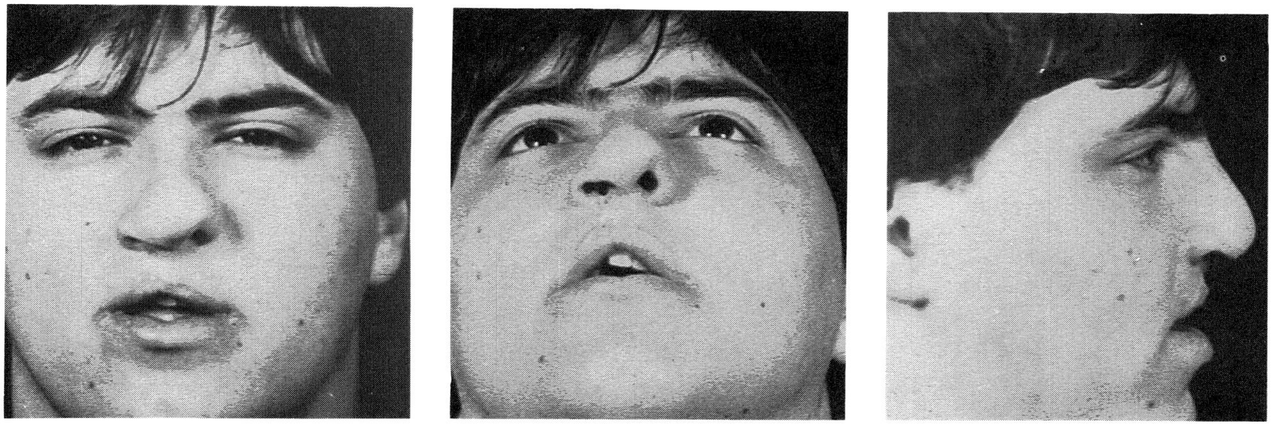

A

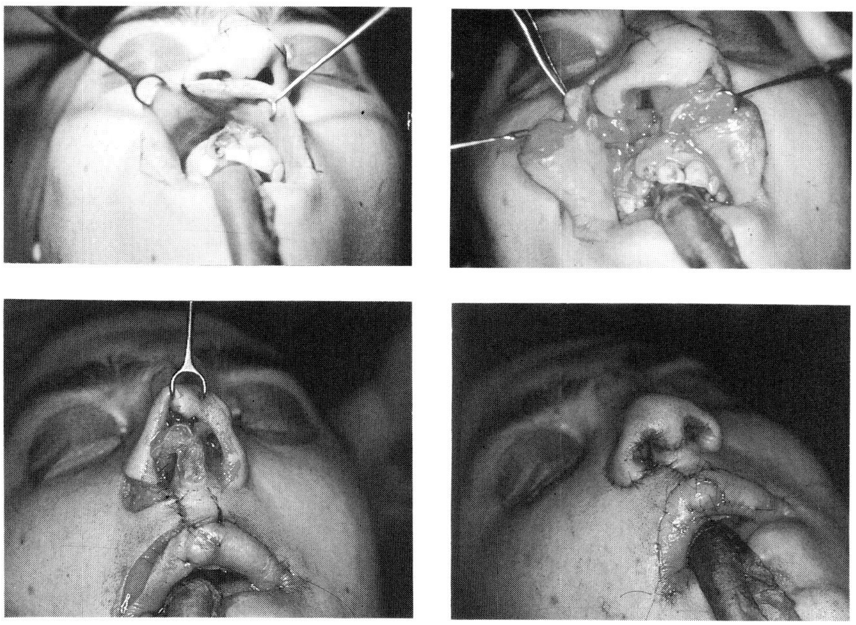

B C D E

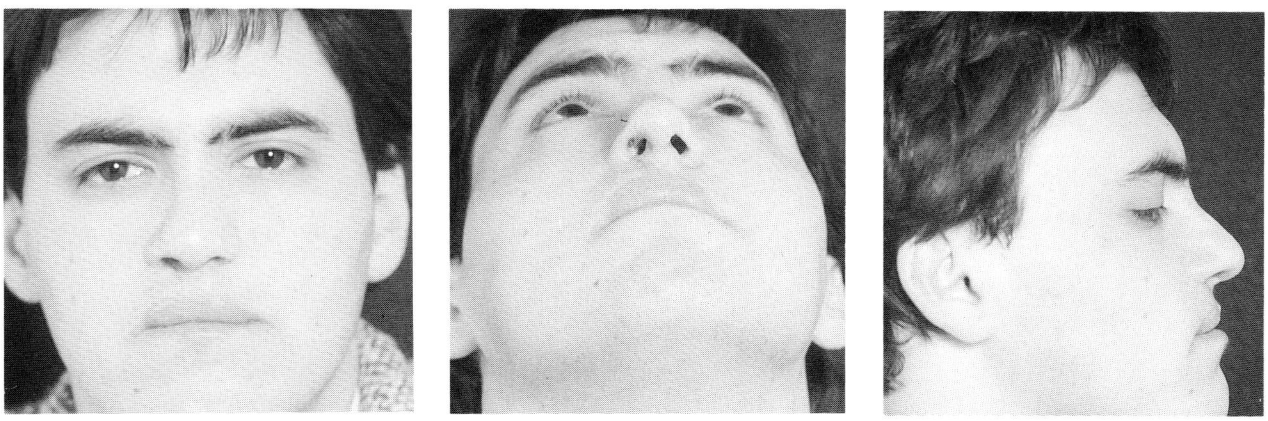

F

Fig. 27-14. **A,** Preoperative view. **B,** Preoperative markings are shown; the Rethi incision and fistula are seen. **C,** Lip opened, de-roofing the fistula. **D,** The Rethi incision allows one to clearly visualize the nasal domes. The cleft side medial crus is sectioned. **E,** Postoperative suture lines. **F,** Final result seen at one year.

cess skin of the tip-lobule complex. Part of the inferior border of the lower lateral cartilage may be included in the flap to give it more support. The soft tissues of the tip must be dissected out over the upper lateral cartilages to release the tip from its tethered or sagging position.

Using a technique described in the book by Denecke-Meyer[11,12] involving the marginal resection of tissue bilaterally in the Converse[7] soft triangle combined with triangular tissue excision at the base of the membraneous septum, we have been able to correct cases of moderate columellar discrepancy above.

With the over-abundance of more or less complicated methods of cleft lip nasal correction at the disposal of the surgeon, one should attempt to familiarize oneself with many of the procedures available in order to be able to "pick and choose" which of the techniques best suits the particular case at hand. This is well illustrated in the following case review.

A 20-year-old male presented with a significant oro-nasal fistula associated with a right unilateral complete cleft lip. Examination revealed that he had several of the stigmata of the cleft lip nasal deformity still present, namely, a stenosis of the right nares, a collapsed alar dome on the right, as well as asymmetrically orientated nostrils (Fig. 27-14, A and B). For such situations we undertake both the closure of the fistula and the correction of the secondary cleft lip nasal deformity at the same time. The lip repair was completely taken down, affording excellent visualization for the subsequent three-layer closure of the fistulous tract (Fig. 27-14, C). To provide equally good exposure for the corrective rhinoplasty a Rethi incision was used, exposing the entire dome region (Fig. 27-14, D). Alar dome balance was achieved with a turnover lower lateral cartilage flap from the noncleft side. Nostril symmetry was achieved using the marginal resection technique, which also provided additional refinement to the tip. Lastly, the stenosis was relieved using the paranasal island flap technique previously described in this chapter (Fig. 27-14, D and E) and in the chapter on secondary rhinoplasty. The result achieved are seen in (Figs. 27-14, F-H) taken one year after surgery. The fistula has also remained closed. Fig. 27-15 shows an intraoperative view of a similar case.

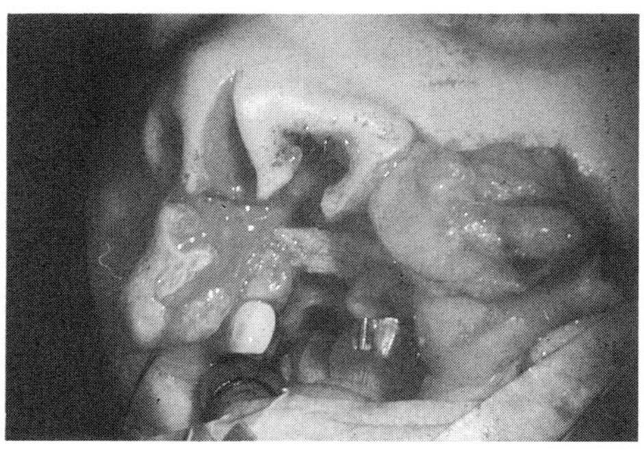

Fig. 27-15. A similar case as described in Fig. 27-14, this time using a columellar-splitting incision rather than the Rethi incision for open access to the nose.

REFERENCES

1. Blair VP: Nasal deformities associated with cleft of the lip, J Am Med Assoc 84:185, 1925.
2. Blair VP and Brown JB: Mirault operation for single hare-lip, Surg Gynecol Obstet 51:81, 1930.
3. Brauer RO: Comparison of the Tennison and Le Mesurier lip repair, Plast Reconstr Surg 23:249, 1959.
4. Brauer RO and Foerster DW: Another method to lengthen the columella in the double cleft patient, Plast Reconstr Surg 38:27, 1966.
5. Brown JB and McDowell F: Secondary repair to cleft lips and their nasal deformities, Ann Surg 114:101, 1941.
6. Burian S: Chirurgie der Lippen und gaumenspalten, Berlin, 1963, Verlog Volk und Gesurdhert.
7. Converse JM: Reconstruction of nasolabial area by composite grafts from concha, Plast Reconstr Surg 5:247, 1950.
8. Courtemanche AD: Personal communication, Vancouver, Canada, 1987.
9. Cronin TD: The V-Y rotational flap for nasal tip defects, Plast Reconstr Surg 11:282, 1983.
10. Cronin TD: Lengthening columella by use of skin from nasal floor and alae, Plast Reconstr Surg 21:417, 1958.
11. Denecke HJ and Meyer R: Plastische Operationen an Kopf und Hals, Berlin, 1964, Springer-Verlag.
12. Denecke HJ and Meyer R: Plastic surgery of head and neck, Rhinoplasty, vol 1, Berlin, 1967, Springer-Verlag.
13. Erich JB: A technique for correcting a flat nostril in cases of repaired harelip, Plast Reconstr Surg 12:320, 1953.
14. Farrior RT: The problem of the unilateral cleft lip nose. A composite operation for revision of secondary deformity, Laryngoscope 72:289, 1962.
15. Figi FA: The repair of secondary cleft lip and nasal deformities, J Intern Coll Surg 17:297, 1952.
16. Fomon S: Cosmetic surgery: principles and practice, Philadelphia, 1960, JB Lippincott Co.
17. Gillies H and Millard R: The principles and art of plastic surgery, vols I and II, Boston-Toronto, 1957, Little Brown & Co.
18. Goodmann WS: Recent advances in external rhinoplasty, J Otolaryngol 10:433, 1981.
19. Holt GR: Management of cleft lip nasal deformity, Facial Plast Surg 3:161, 1986.
20. Ivy RH: Congenital anomalies, Plast Reconstr Surg 20:400, 1957.
21. Maeda K, Ojimi H, and Yoshida T: A new method of secondary correction of the bilateral cleft lip nose, Br J Plast Surg. 40:52, 1987.
22. Millard DR: Columella lengthening by a forked flap, Plast Reconstr Surg 5:454, 1958.
23. Potter J: Some nasal tip deformities due to alar cartilage abnormalities, Plast Reconstr Surg 13:358, 1954.
24. Rees TD: Aesthetic plastic surgery, Philadelphia, 1980, WB Saunders Co.
25. Rethi A: Über die korrektiven Operationen der Nasendeformitäten, Chirurg 1:1103, 1929.
26. Ritsilă V, Alhopuao S, Gylling U, and Rintala A: The use of free periosteum for bone restoration in congenital clefts of the maxilla: a preliminary report, Scand J Plast Reconstr Surg 6:57, 1972.
27. Skoog T: The use of periosteum and surgical for bone restoration in congenital clefts of the maxilla, Scand J Plast Reconstr Surg 1:113, 1967.
28. Tolhurst DE: Secondary correction of the unilateral cleft lip nose deformity, Br J Plast Surg 36:449, 1983.

28

Nasal Flaps and Grafts

Claus Walter

The quest for beauty is as old as mankind. In the tombs of ancient kings and queens have been found jars, utensils, colored creams, and ointments for cosmetic purposes. Therefore, it is not surprising that a great deal of professional interest is devoted to cosmetics and rejuvenation since so much of one's personal well-being and professional success depends on one's appearance.

Besides an increasing interest on the part of the public in cosmetic products and beauty parlors, we also observe an ever-increasing demand for plastic surgery, which now has a well-accepted and important role in the quest for rejuvenation.

It is quite interesting to look back into the history of plastic surgery. Reconstructive rhinoplasty dates back as far as 500 BC. Corrective rhinoplasties to alter the shape of the nose were developed by the American surgeon, O. Roe, and the German surgeon, J. Joseph, at the turn of the century. Early publications show that even in the first quarter of this century, older persons had their noses corrected because of the noticeable growth of the nasal cartilages in post-menopausal women and in men of comparative age groups.

Nasal Reconstruction Principles

The general principles of nasal reconstruction are divided into 9 sections:

1. Free tissue transplantation
   a. Skin
   b. Composite grafts, double layer
   c. Composite grafts, triple layer
2. Horizontal suprabrow flap
3. Island flaps
4. Median or oblique forehead flap
5. Converse scalp flap
6. Visor flap
7. Cheek rotation flap

8. Small flap, rhomboid (bi-lobed)
9. Shoulder flap

Free Tissue Transplantation

Skin. The superficial defect closure is done by full-thickness skin grafts only when all the cartilaginous and bony structures are present. Skin grafts done on soft tissue alone will shrink and distort the appearance. Preferred donor sites are the post-auricular, supraclavicular, and inguinal areas. The disadvantage of this skin lies in the fact that it is thinner than nasal skin. To overcome this, a composite graft is a better alternative.

Composite graft, double layer. This graft is composed of two structures: bone-muscle, skin-cartilage, skin-fat, mucosa-cartilage, etc. In nasal surgery external and endonasal defects must be covered. Here there may be two-layer defects or even the total loss of the organ, in which case a triple layer graft is required. Such grafts offer a multitude of possibilities. The defect closure is quickly achieved and the patients are relieved of the need to undergo multiple surgical procedures.

Grafts need donor sites. In nasal reconstruction, grafts are taken from the nose itself or from the auricle. The ear can offer double and triple layer grafts: from the helix, the concha, the earlobe, anteriorly, and from the post-auricular surface. After some 300 composite graft transplantations, the conclusion is that post-auricular grafts are best suited for external nasal coverage or the columella, and concha grafts with the very adherent skin are best suited for endonasal tissue replacement.[8]

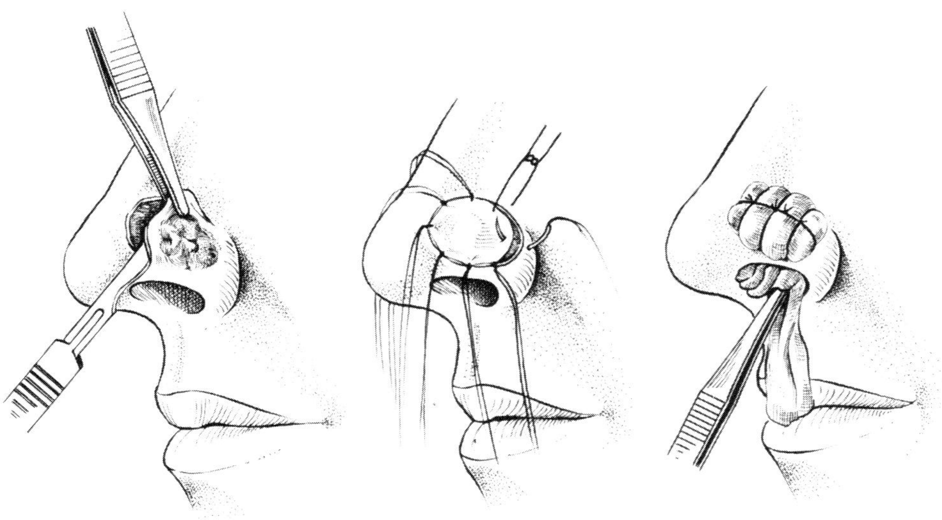

Fig. 28-1. Bolus-type dressing for full skin grafts and composite grafts. (From Survey of the use of composite grafts in the head and neck region, Otolaryngol Clin N Am, vol. 5, no. 3, October 1972.)

There are certain limitations to the size of the graft. It should not extend more than 1 × 2 cm. The defect, which is created at the donor site, can be closed either by direct wound approximation, by a small adjacent flap, or by an island flap that is cut posteriorly and then turned forward as a cover in the case of anterior conchal defects. This technique leaves virtually no appreciable anterior auricular deformity or discernible scar. When suturing the graft into the nasal defect, a bolus type of dressing is applied for a week. Patients are advised to apply ointment for 2 to 3 weeks to keep the tissue soft[1] (Fig. 28-1).

In endonasal strictures the scar is totally excised and the nasal skin is undermined as wide as possible if lengthening is to be achieved, at the same time allowing a downward pull on the nasal tip. This might lead to an enlargement of the endonasal defect. Grafts from the nasal septum or the anterior concha are taken for endonasal use. If the grafts must bridge the top of the nasal septum, a strip of mucosa or skin must be removed corresponding to the septum to avoid a perforation superiorly.

In order to avoid a dislodgment of the graft on top of the septum when bilateral scars have to be replaced, we cut out a rectangular piece of cartilage and remove the mucosa. Into this space the graft is neatly placed and secured by sutures (6.0 Nylon[2]; Fig. 28-2). The nose is

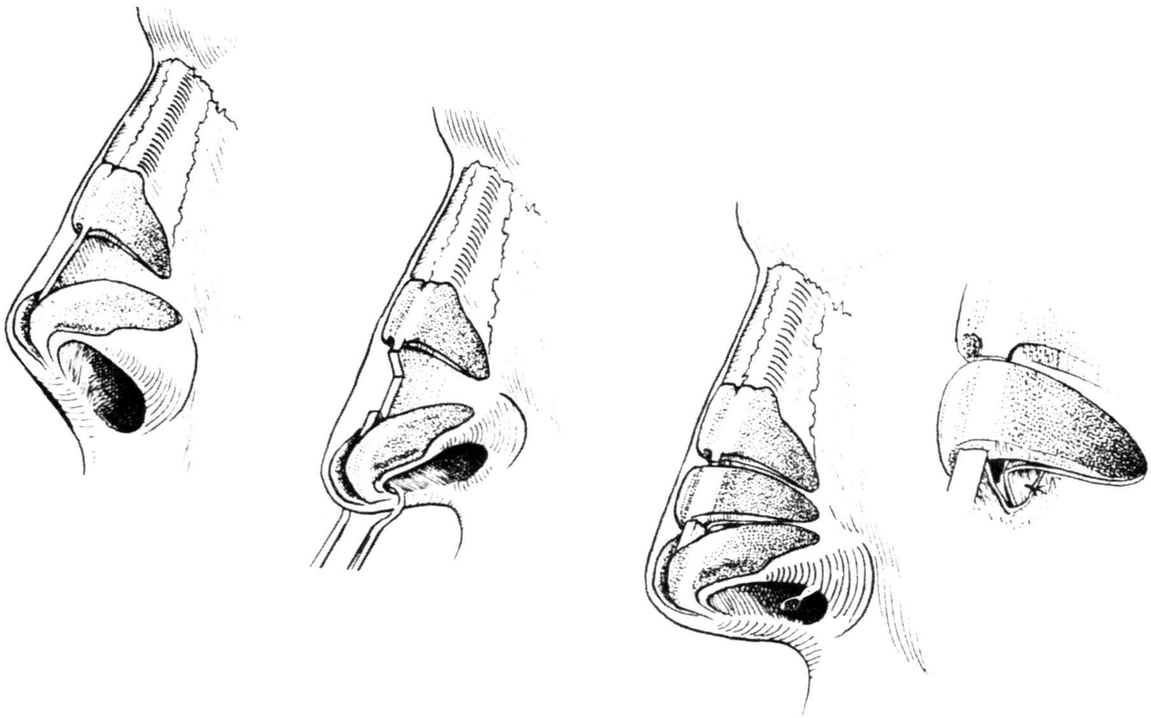

Fig. 28-2. The endonasal placement of a composite graft from the concha. (From Walter C: Composite grafts in nasal surgery, Arch Otolaryngol 90: 622-630, 1969.)

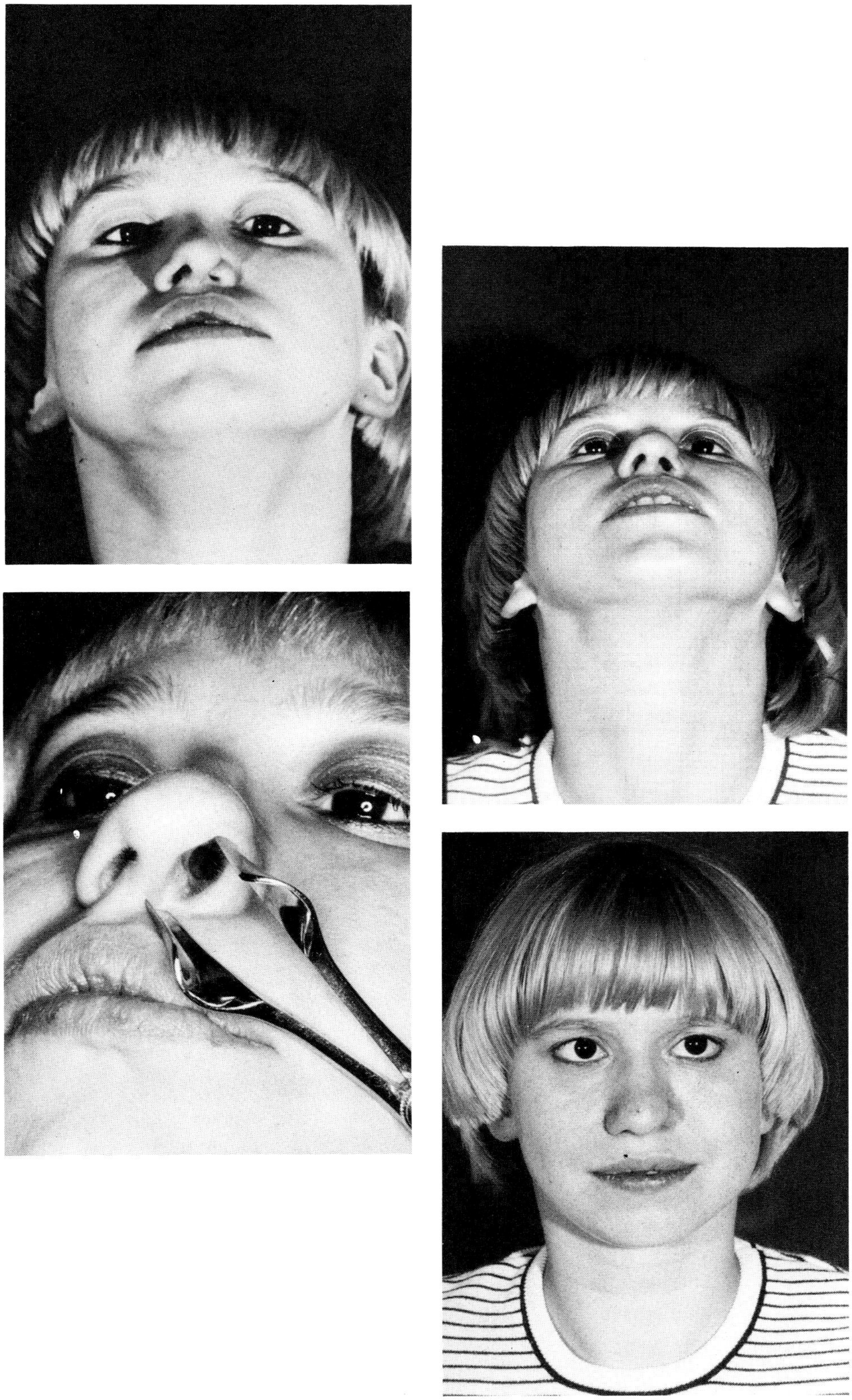

A B C D

Fig. 28-3. Endonasal scarring caused an entrance stenosis. **A**, Preoperative **B** and **D**, Postoperative view one year later. **C**, After inserting a composite graft.

packed for 5 days and mercurochrome is applied to it afterwards. A patent obturator of acrylic is then inserted and left in place for 2 to 3 months to prevent cicatrization. Occasionally the patient applies Volon cream to the stent (Fig. 28-3, A-D). Not only cranially positioned strictures but scarring and obliteration on the floor of the nasal entrance are also treated in this way. In such cases, the graft is pulled through the base of the columella after denuding the center part of skin.

Composite graft, triple layer. This graft is used to replace lost parts of the ala at the tip. Rim sections of the ear or concha serve as a triple-layer graft which is the entire thickness of the auricle. The suturing technique is the same[4] (Figs. 28-4, A-C and 28-5, A-E).

In the columella lengthening, the tissue is divided horizontally, creating either a triangular or rectangular defect. The graft, usually taken post-auricularly, contains a sufficient amount of cartilage to withstand the tendency of tissue to contract. Sometimes the graft is reinforced by inserting additionally septal or costal cartilage into the center of the graft to act as a tent pole. The same bandage technique and nasal packing are applied (Fig. 28-6, A-D).

A double-layer composite graft can be used and folded to serve as a triple-layer graft in lengthening the columella. Elliptical post-auricular skin and cartilage can be transposed as a folded wedge-shaped triple graft with cartilage in between to serve as bilateral coverage, duplicating

A B C

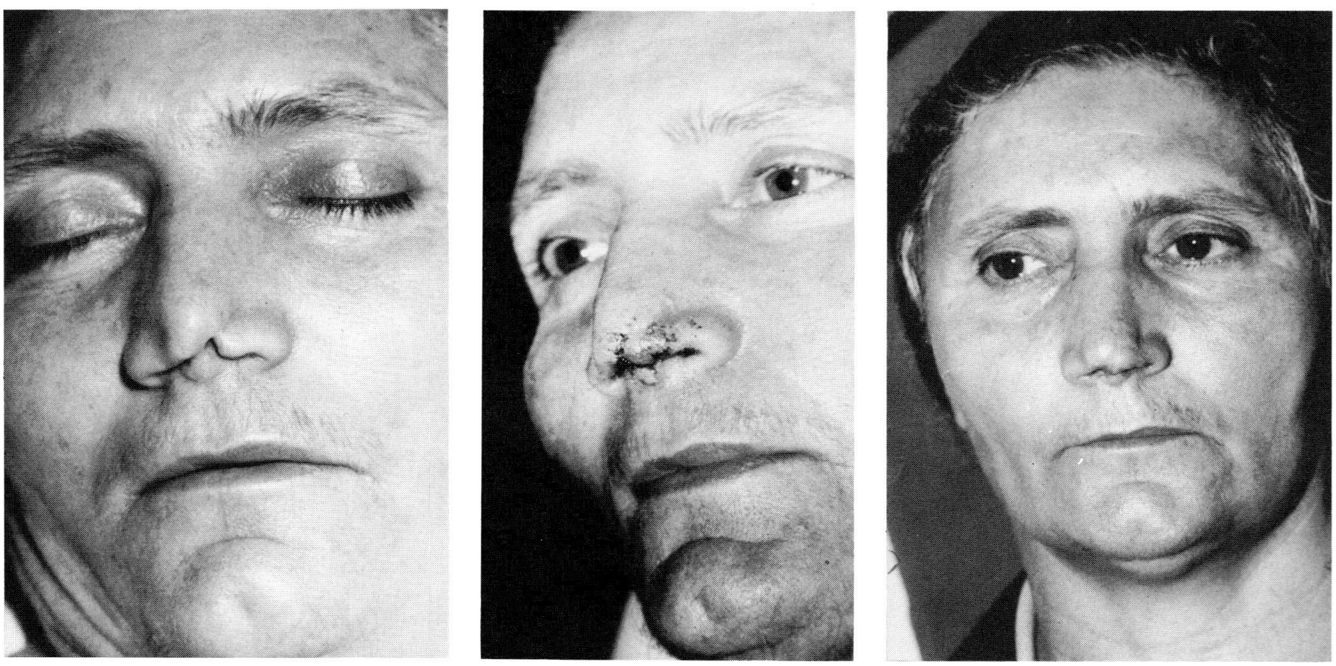

Fig. 28-4. **A,** Traumatic partial nasal tip loss. **B,** Corrected by a composite graft. **C,** Postoperatively.

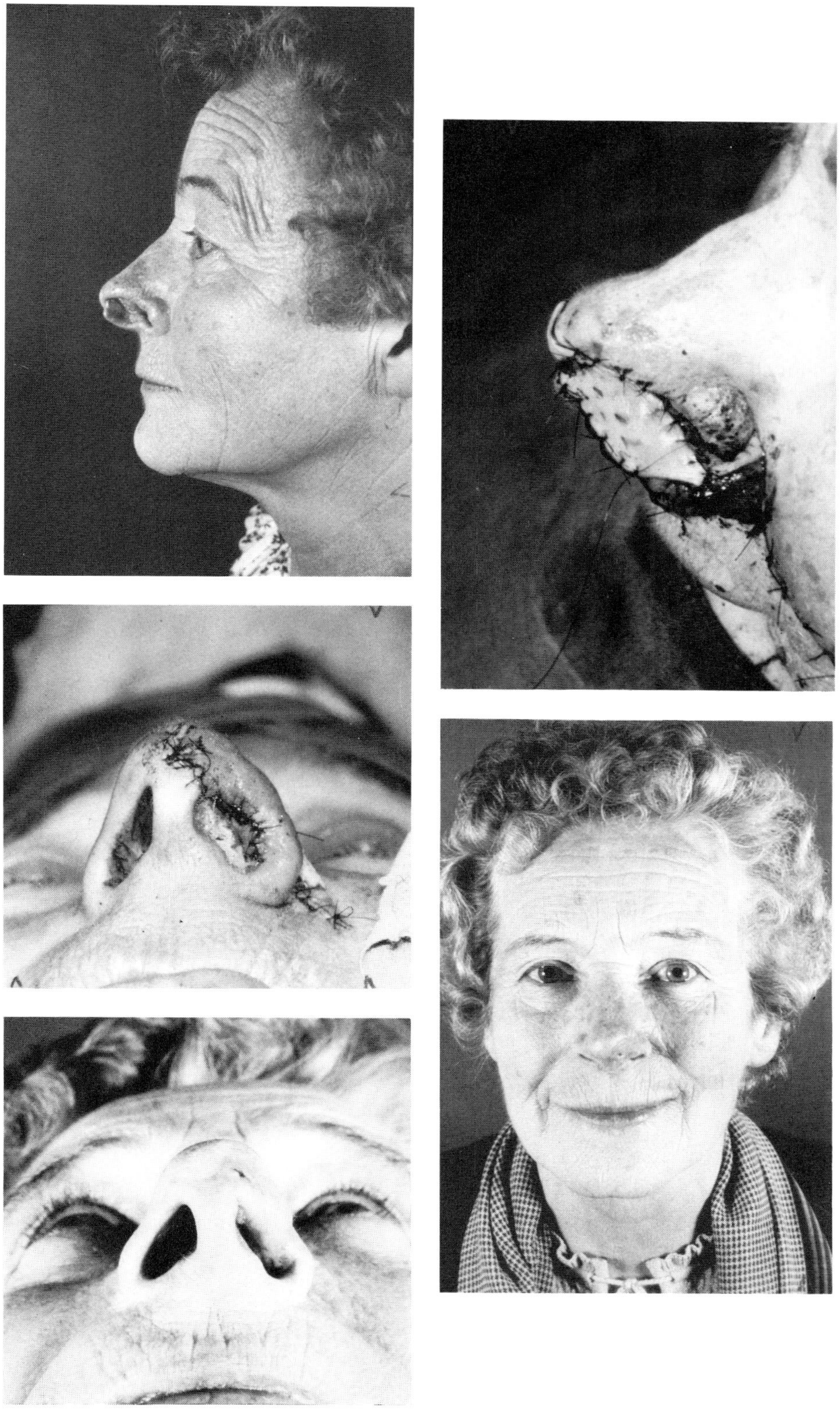

A
B
C
D
E

Fig. 28-5. A, Traumatic tissue loss of nasal ala. B and C, Corrected by a composite graft. D and E, Postoperatively.

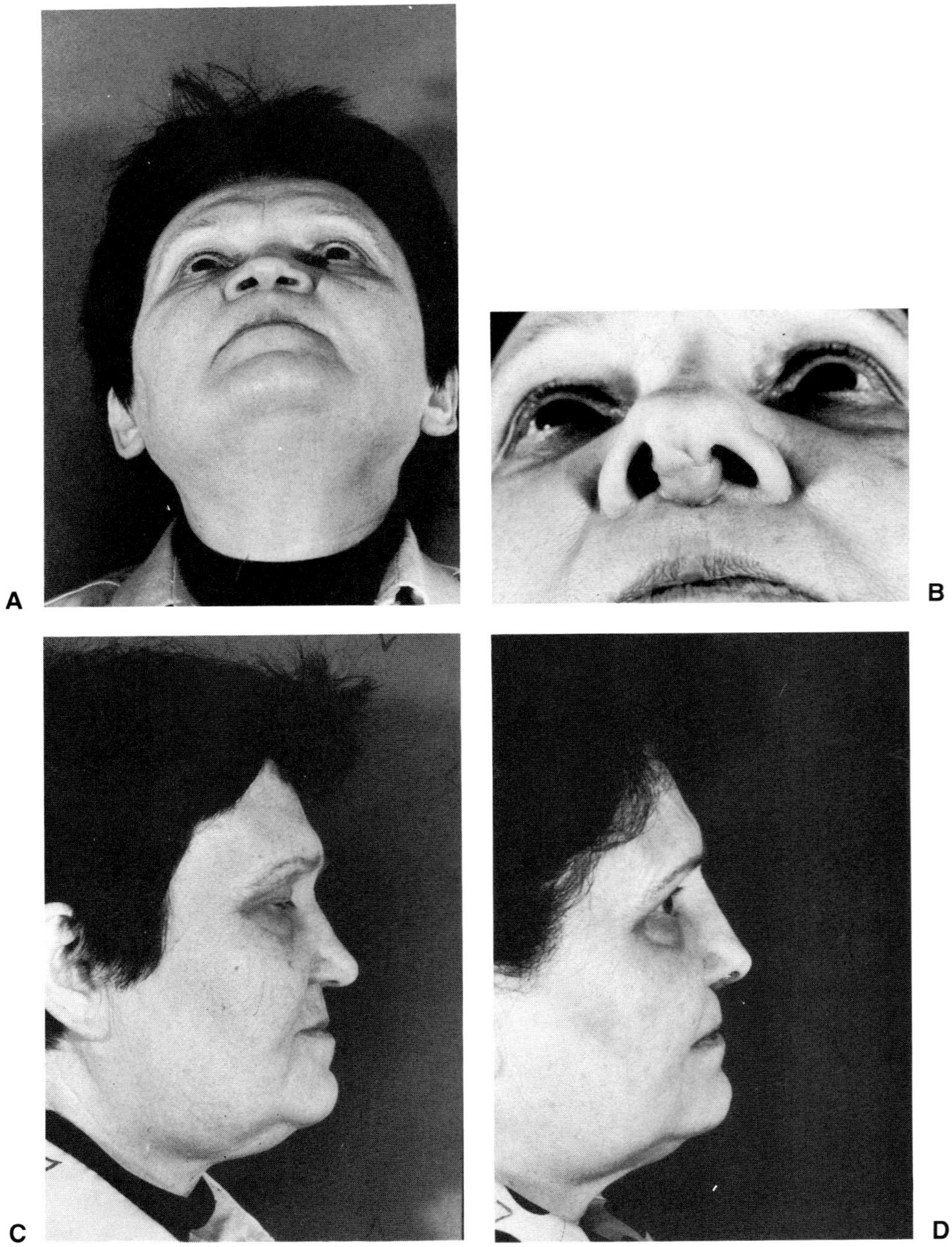

Fig. 28-6. A and C, Preoperative columella lengthening. B, By a postauricular composite graft. D, Postoperatively.

the columella. It has proven advantageous to use an additional strut of cartilage as a tent pole to prevent compression of the graft in the columella. This facilitates the ingrowth of vessels and ensures the survival of the tissues.

Sutures of 7.0 nylon are placed 2 mm apart and packing is used intranasally to prevent any motion of the graft. The patients are advised to speak and laugh as little as possible and avoid extreme movements of the lips for about a week. Protection of the graft from the air current will prevent drying from taking place. Mercurochrome is used instead of ointment (Fig. 28-7, A & B). Besides tissue transfer in nasal reconstruction, a great reliance is placed on flap reconstruction. Although the procedure lasts longer, multistaging makes for greater security in healing. Additional administration of Cortisal for 5 days is very helpful in increasing the chances of a good take.

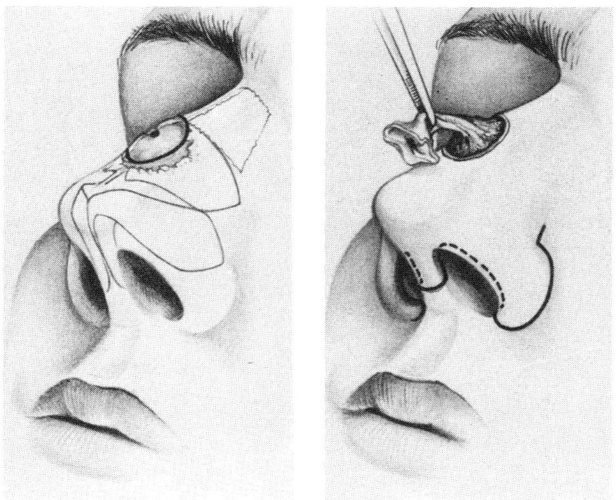

A

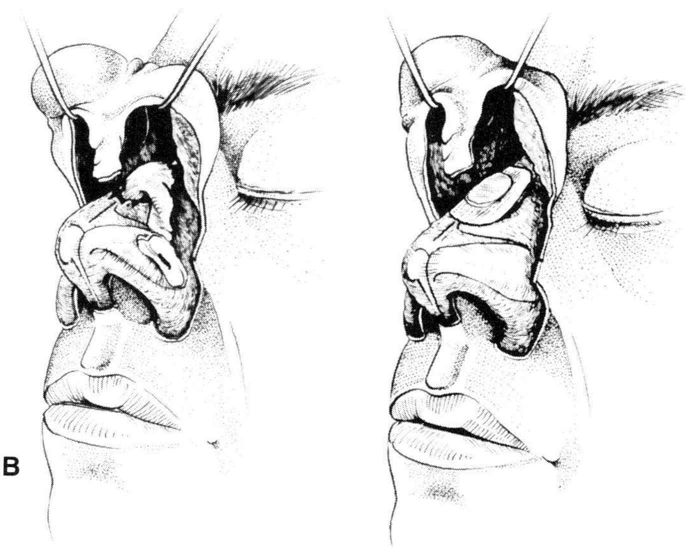

B

Fig. 28-7. **A,** Treatment of a congenital nasal fistula by excision. **B,** Insertion of a composite graft. (From Walter, C: Plast Chirugie im Kopf-und Halsbereich. Herausgegeben von J Berendes, R Link, F Zollner, 2 Band HNO-Heilkunde, Stuttgart, 2. neubearbeitete und erweiterte Auflage, 1977, Georg Thieme Verlag.)

Horizontal Suprabrow Flaps

Next described is the horizontal suprabrow pedicle, which is carried out according to the proposals of Schmid and Meyer. This pedicle flap is a difficult procedure and requires very careful staging. The pedicle is based on the frontal artery and the tissues that serve as part of the newly-made nose are built up in the hair-free region of the temple.

The procedure is carried out in stages. The first stage is circumcision of a horizontal pedicle just adjacent to the eyebrow. This small pedicle is lifted out of its bed and a split-skin graft is wrapped around the circumference. Then, forehead skin is elevated cephalically, the tissue is pulled down, and the incision line closed with PDS sutures that are 4.0 or 3.0 in size. It is important to incorporate in the suture line the periosteum of the suprabrow and supra-orbital rim to avoid pulling the eyebrow cranially. At the same time some cartilage can be taken from the nose or bank cartilage, or a composite graft can be used from one auricle for implantation subcutaneously to create whatever is needed to replace the defects on the nose. The size of the tissue needed is carefully measured in the nasal area. With the composite graft it is possible to bring cartilage and skin to the most distal part of the pedicle.

To ensure blood supply, a bridge of about 1 cm of skin must remain untouched between the horizontal suprabrow pedicle and the temple region, which will become the new nose. Two weeks later this bridge of tissue is incised in continuation with the former skin incisions. This remaining piece of pedicle is then elevated to create a longer pedicle, extending from the center of the forehead to the temple region. One week later the last fibers and tissue connections in the temporal region are severed and the whole pedicle is lifted and brought down to the nose. The surgeon should pay very careful attention to the main blood supply and carefully free the most mesial part in order to avoid necrosis of the pedicle when turning it down into the nose. The most distal end of this pedicle is then carefully fitted into the defect with skin or scar excisions, whatever is necessary. In another two to three weeks the pedicle can be severed and part of it can be discarded (Figs. 28-8 and 28-9, A-D).

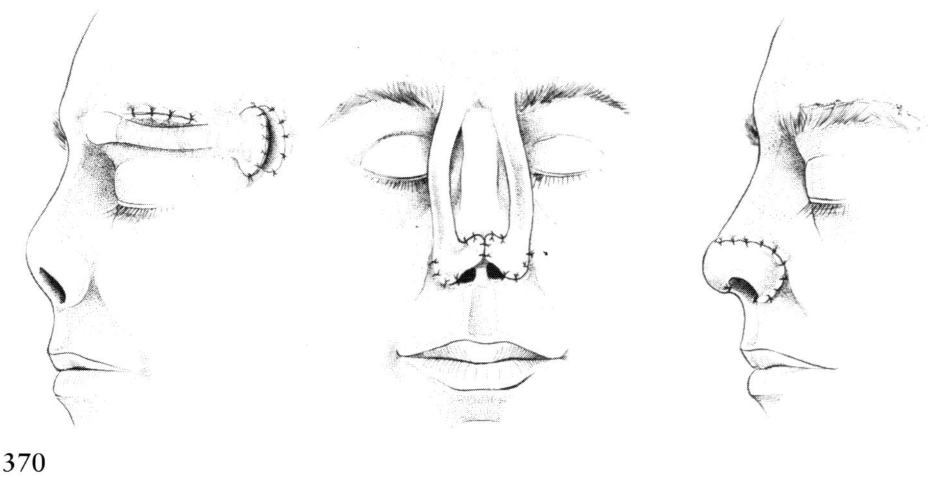

Fig. 28-8. Construction of a horizontal eye brow flap. (From Walter, C: Plast Chirugie im Kopf- und Halsbereich. Herausgegeben von J Berendes, R Link, F Zollner, 2 Band HNO-Heilkunde, Stuttgart, 2. neubearbeitete und erweiterte Auflage, 1977, Georg Thieme Verlag.)

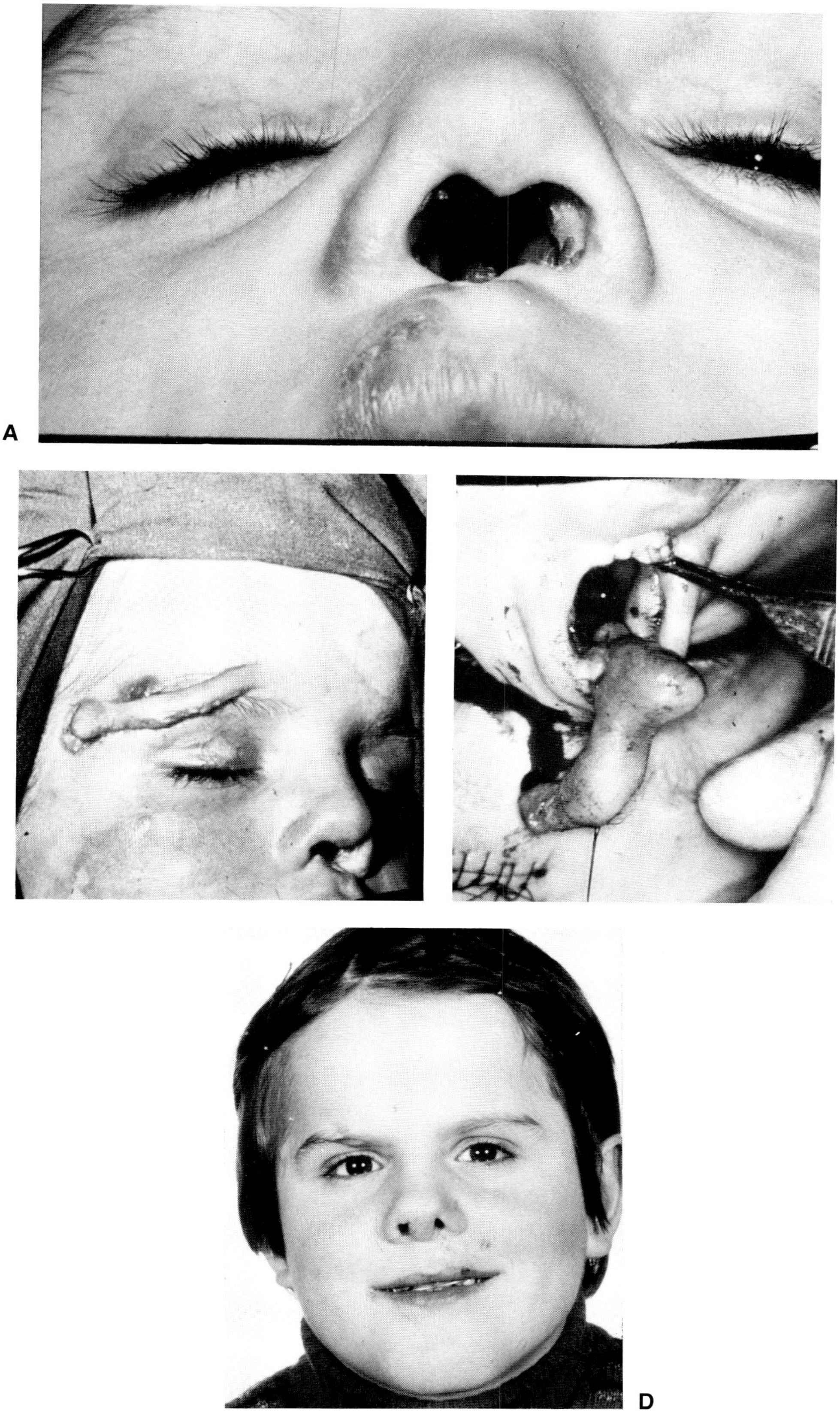

Fig. 28-9. **A,** Columella and septum loss due to infection. **B** and **C,** Reconstruction by a Schmid flap. **D,** Postoperatively.

Island Flaps

Next in the line of procedures in the coverage of nasal tissue defects is the island flap. This requires the shifting of skin based on a subcutaneous pedicle. Island flaps from the naso-labial fold or from the forehead can be used. Usually the forehead as well as the naso-labial area contains an excellent blood supply, which is mandatory for the survival of the transposed skin island. We know also of the VY advancement of skin for defect closure (Figs. 28-10, 28-11, 28-12 and 28-13, A-D). An extreme version of an island flap is a forehead skin island that is based on the subcutaneous vascular stem of the temporal artery and vein and is prepared and brought down underneath the cheek into the nose. The surgeon must decide which procedure should be used.

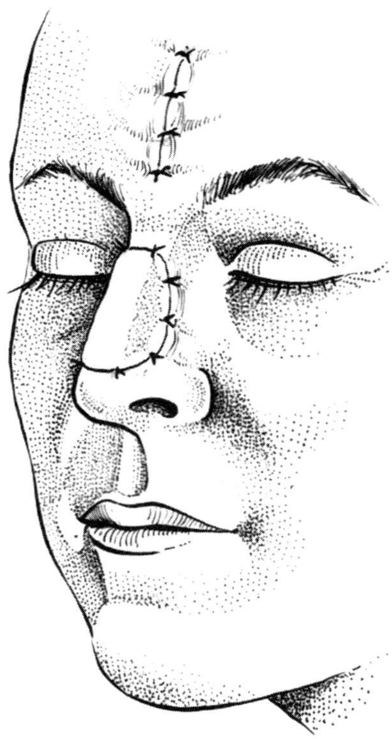

Fig. 28-10. Island flap. (From Plast Chirugie im Kopf-und Halsbereich. Herausgegeben von J Berendes, R Link, F Zollner, 2 Band HNO-Heilkunde, Stuttgart, 2. neubearbeitete und erweiterte Auflage, 1977, Georg Thieme Verlag.)

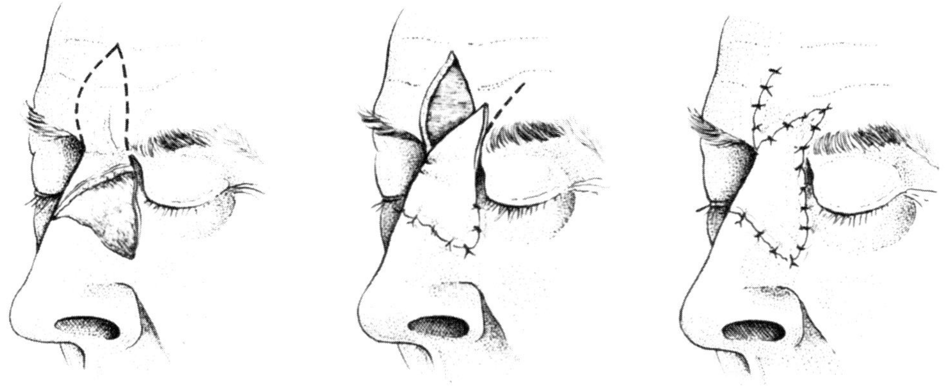

Fig. 28-11. V-Y type of flap. (From Plast Chirugie im Kopf-und Halsbereich. Herausgegeben von J Berendes, R Link, F Zollner, 2 Band HNO-Heilkunde, Stuttgart, 2. neubearbeitete und erweiterte Auflage. 1977, Georg Thieme Verlag.)

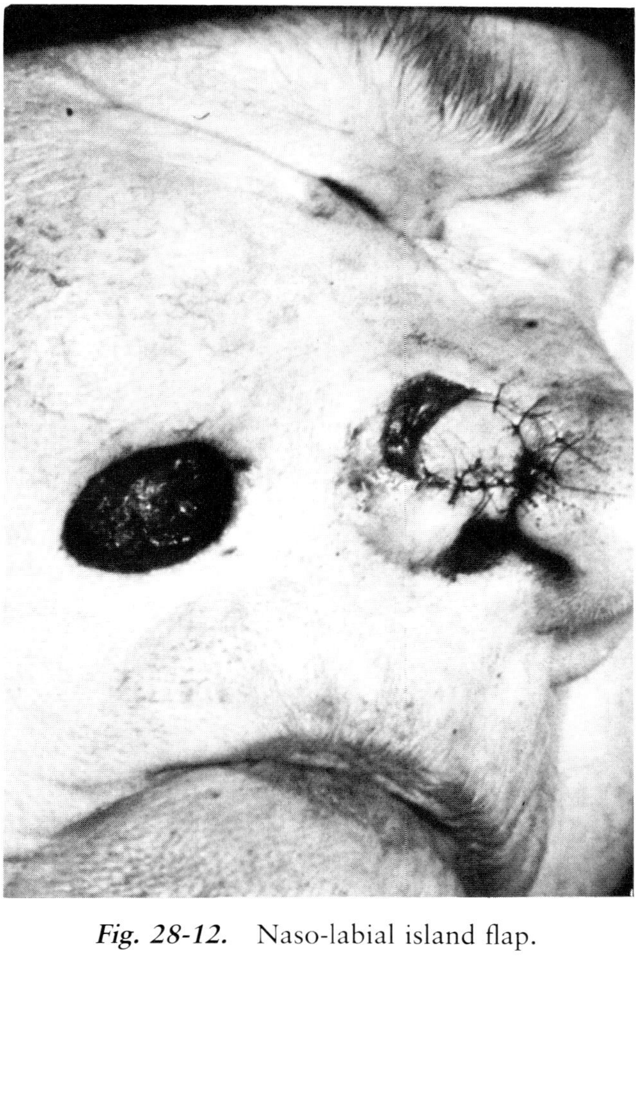

Fig. 28-12. Naso-labial island flap.

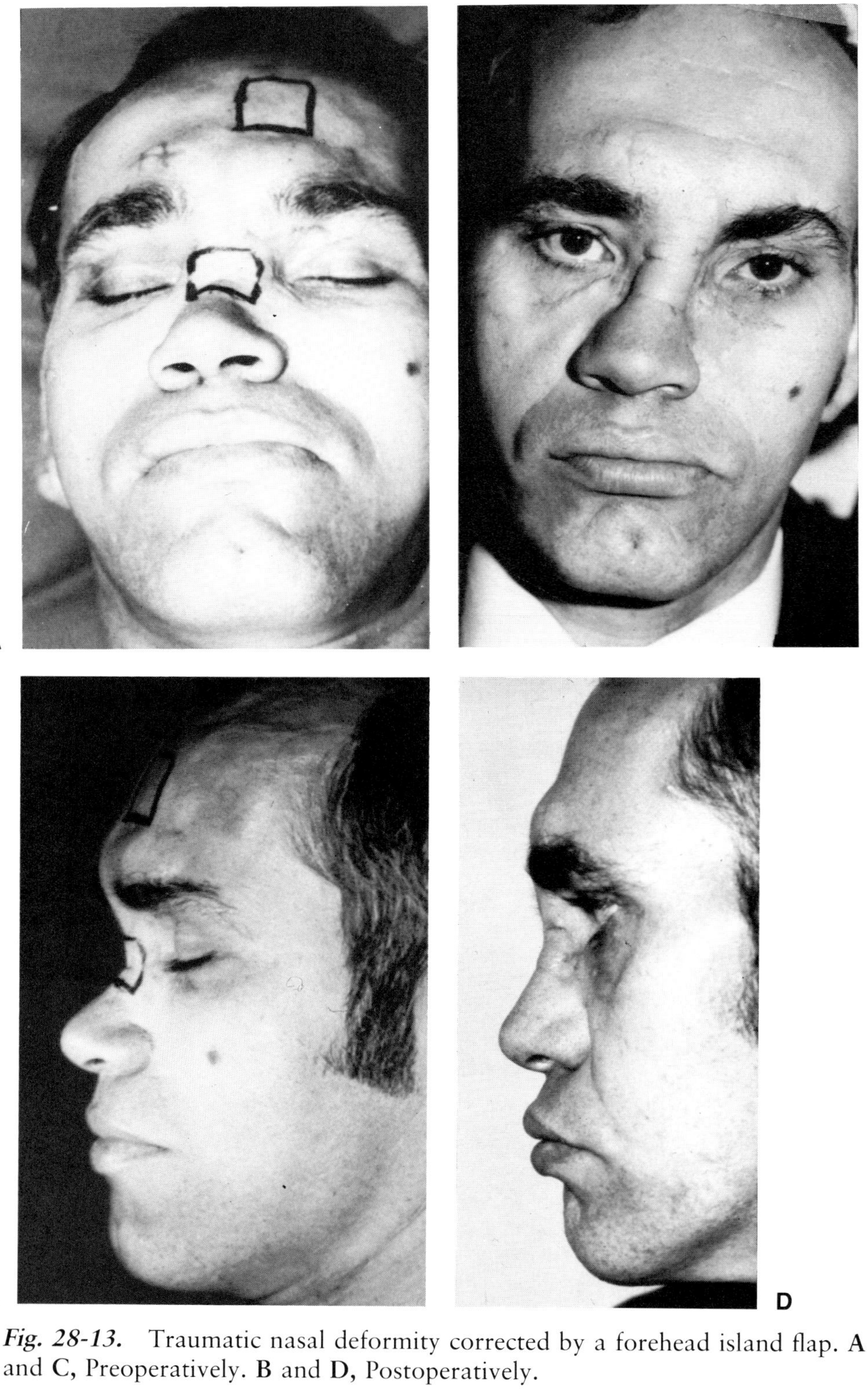

A B C D

Fig. 28-13. Traumatic nasal deformity corrected by a forehead island flap. **A** and **C**, Preoperatively. **B** and **D**, Postoperatively.

Median or Oblique Forehead Flap

Coming from India and first described by Susruta and later by Carpue, the midline or oblique forehead flap is one of the most widely used flaps for nasal reconstruction. It is based on the frontal artery and can be turned down 180 degrees. If the inner lining is missing as well, the flap can be folded inward at the distal portion if the forehead is high enough (Fig. 28-14, A & B).

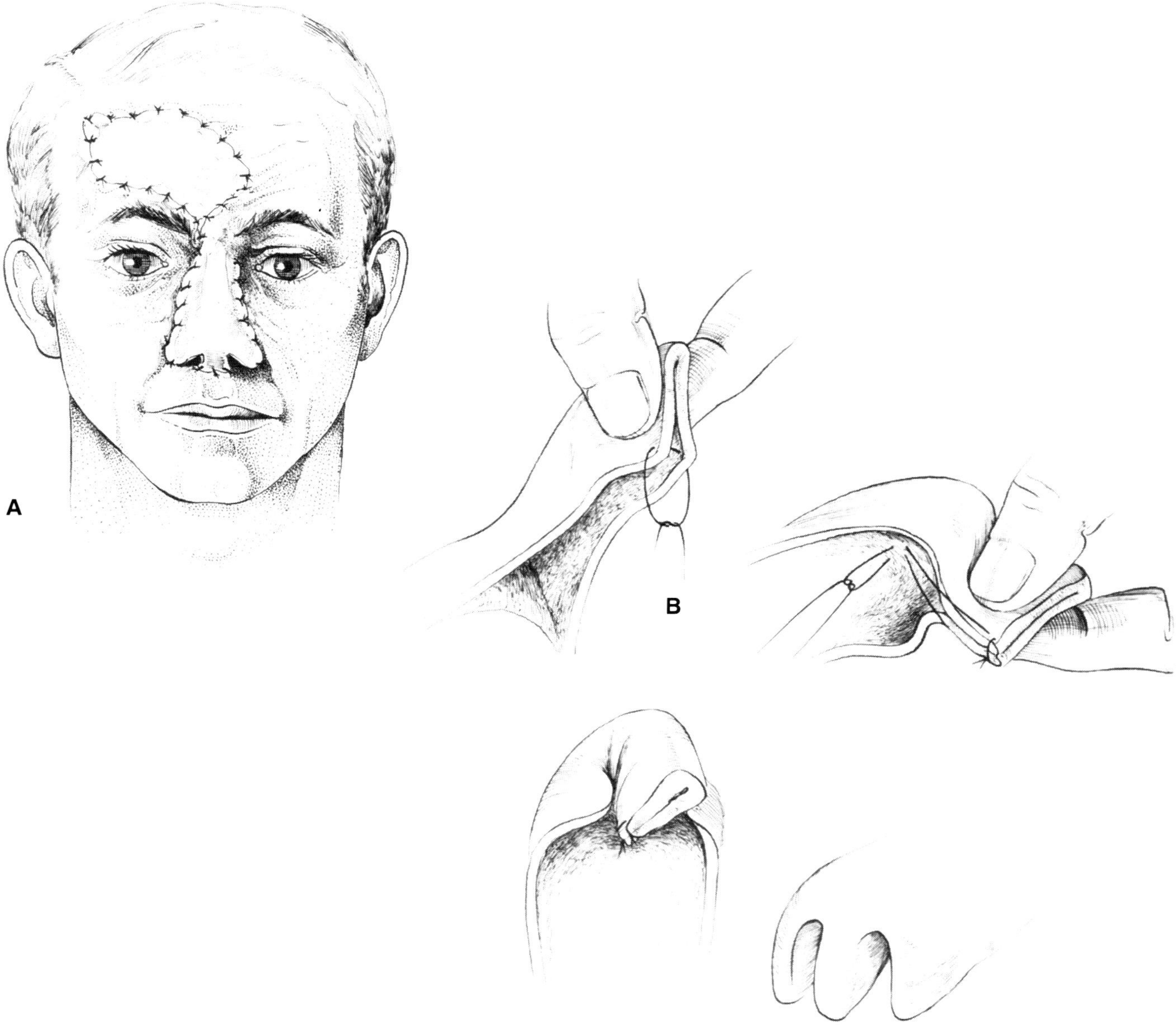

Fig. 28-14. **A,** Nasal reconstruction by a forehead flap. **B,** In-folding of the flap to produce the columnella and alae. (From Plast Chirugie im Kopf-und Halsbereich. Herausgegeben von J Berendes, R Link, F Zollner, 2 Band HNO-Heilkunde, Stuttgart, 2. neubearbeitete und erweiterte Auflage, 1977, Georg Thieme Verlag.)

If this does not seem feasible, additional cartilage and skin, in the form of a composite graft, can be implanted in the distal end. This will become the inner lining of the new nose. A very careful measurement is absolutely necessary to be certain that no tissue deficiency will be present when the flap is turned down. Because of its excellent blood supply there is no need for a delayed procedure (Figs. 28-15 and 28-16, A-D).

The forehead defect is closed directly if the flap is not more than 1.5 cm in width. If the area is wider, it is left uncovered to allow granulation tissue to develop and fill out the gap while pulling the wound edges closer together. By waiting it is usually the case that the granulation tissue will fill in the defect, making it easier afterwards to graft the skin portion without leaving indentations in the forehead surface. Split thickness skin grafts for coverage of facial areas are taken from either the buttocks or the inguinal area, and not from the thigh, which is more exposed (Figs. 28-17, A-E).

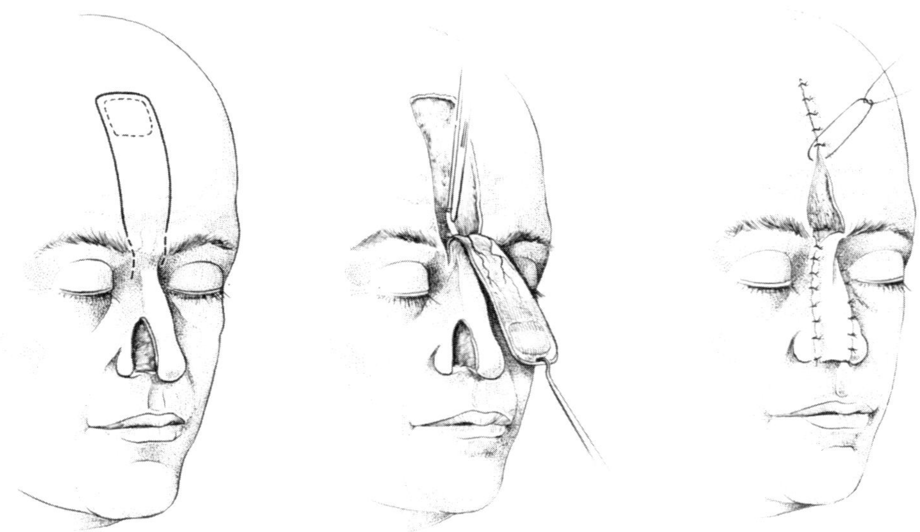

Fig. 28-15. Tip reconstruction by a midline forehead flap in combination with a composite graft. (From Plast Chirugie im Kopf-und Halsbereich. Herausgegeben von J Berendes, R Link, F Zollner, 2 Band HNO-Heilkunde, Stuttgart, 2. neubearbeitete und erweiterte Auflage, 1977, Georg Thieme Verlag.)

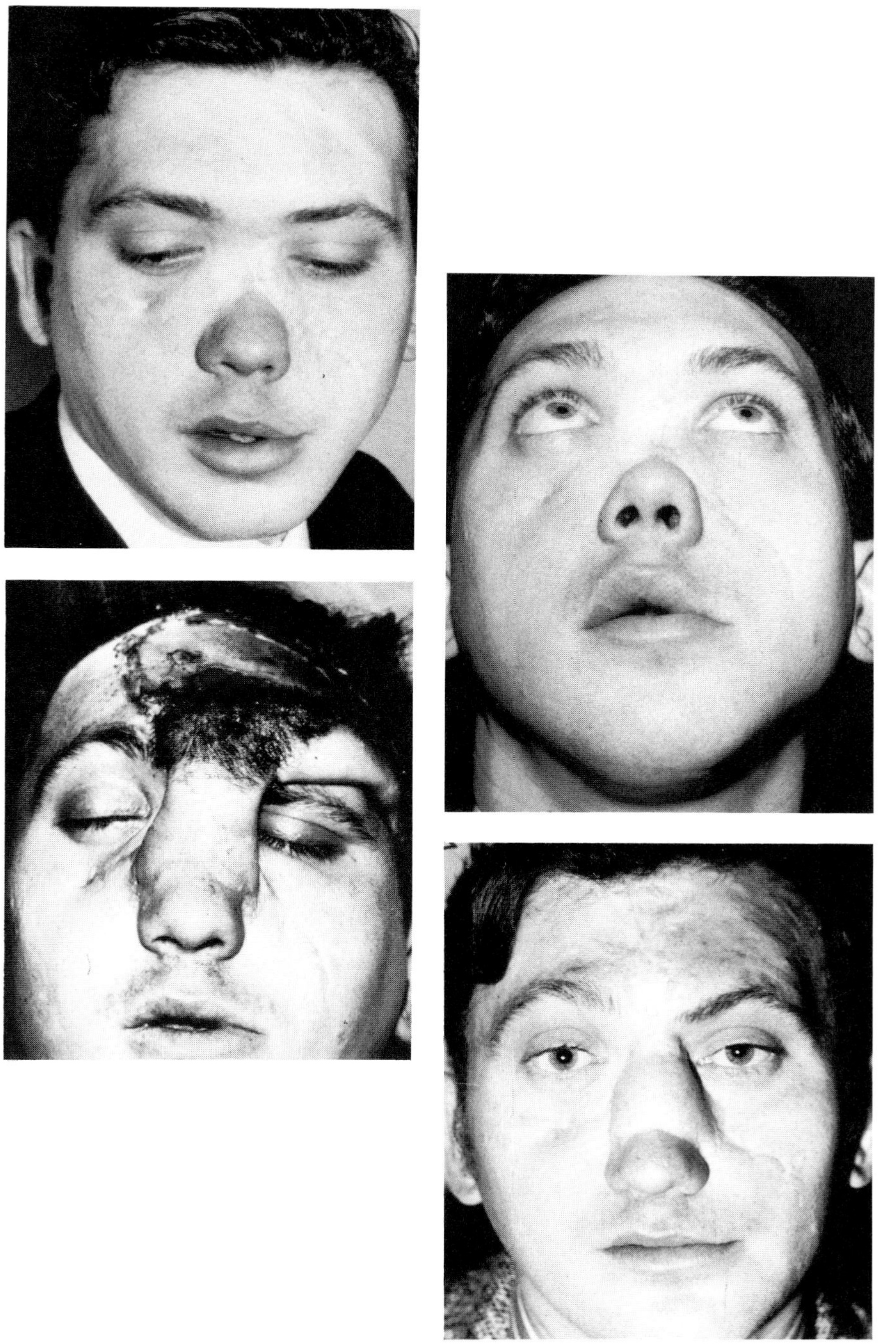

Fig. 28-16. A and B, Nasal reconstruction. C, By a forehead graft. D, Postoperatively.

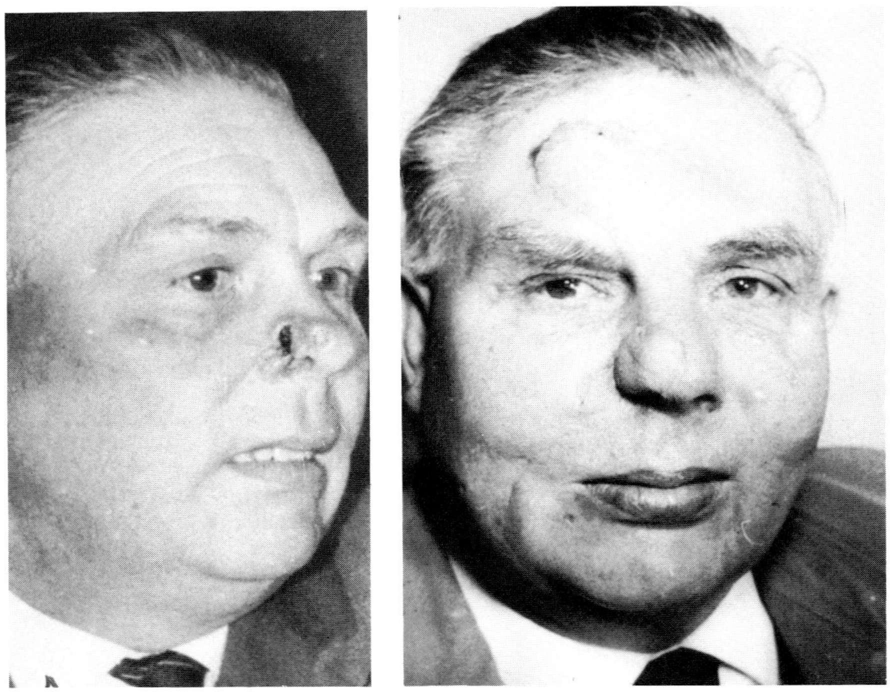

Fig. 28-17. **A**, Basal cell carcinoma. **B**, Treated by excision and reconstruction by a midline forehead flap in combination with a composite graft. **C-E**, Postoperatively.

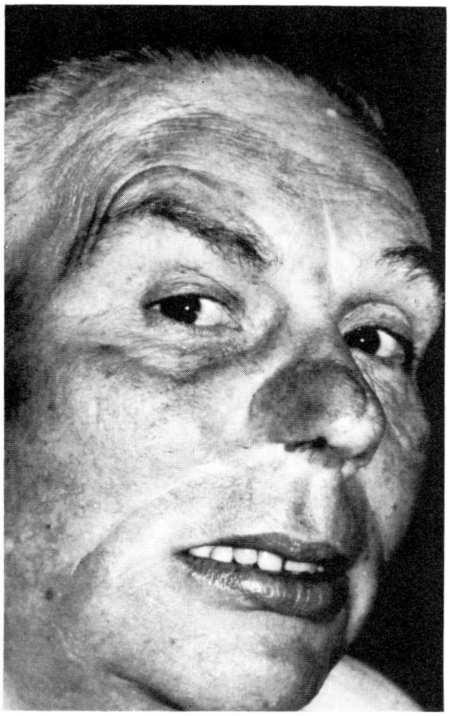

C

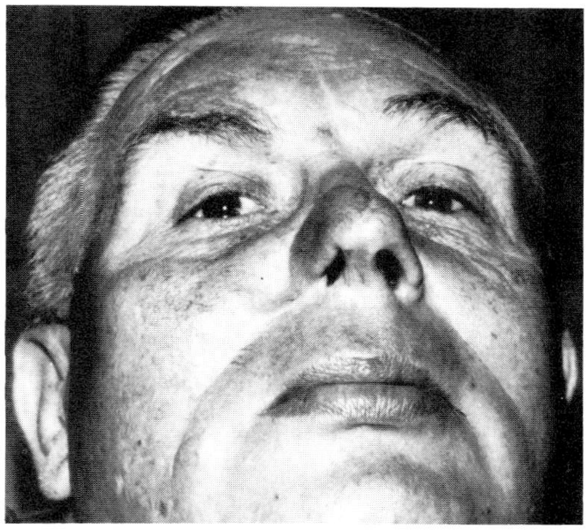

D

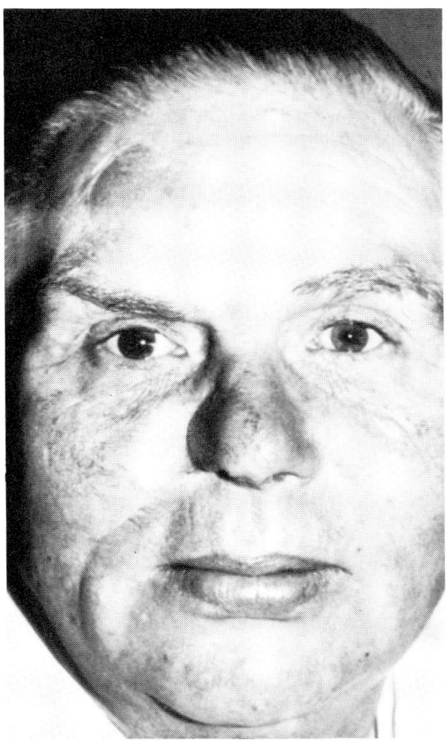

E

Converse Scalp Flap

The scalp rotation flap is the actual workhorse for nasal reconstruction. In this technique advocated by Converse, a lot of tissue with the excellent blood supply of the scalp is transposed into the nasal mid-facial region. Most of the incision lines are hidden in hair-bearing areas, and the dimensions of the tissues are determined only by the height of the forehead. In the horizontal dimension the entire forehead skin is available. That means that in nasal reconstruction we can infold the distal end of the flap like a glove and create a new nasal entrance together with the smooth dorsal lining, without distortion by scar tissue. The flap can also be underlined by a composite graft, as Gilles advocated in his original concept,[4] by using a small sickle flap from the scalp underlined by a composite graft for tip reconstruction. Harvesting the flap can be done without delay. The forehead skin is usually the best protected of all the facial tissues because hats are commonly worn for protection in outdoor sports and in professional life. That means the frequency of basal cell carcinomas with ensuing treatment or irradiation is usually not located in the forehead area and fresh, excellent skin is available (Figs. 28-18 and 28-19, A & B).

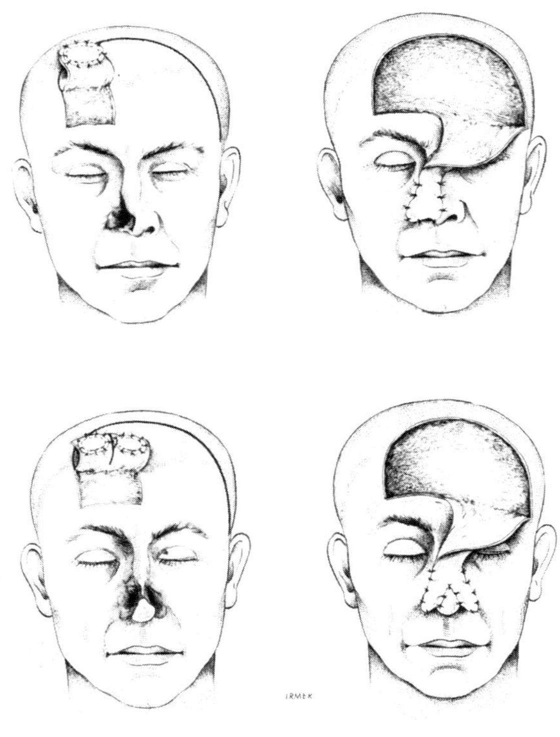

Fig. 28-18. Converse scalp flap underlined by a composite graft. By dividing the distal portion, it is possible to reconstruct both nasal passageways. (From Walter, C: Plast Chirugie im Kopf-und Halsbereich. Herausgegeben von J Berendes, R Link, F Zollner, 2 Band HNO-Heilkunde, Stuttgart, 2. neubearbeitete und erweiterte Auflage, 1977, Georg Thieme Verlag.)

It is possible to save the motion of the forehead by careful dissection of the skin from the frontalis muscles. This, of course, may diminish the blood supply, and a prolonged procedure that lasts for three or four days may be necessary. Again, the donor area is left open for granulation tissue to develop and is grafted in about 3 to 4 weeks when the base of the flap is returned to its original bed.

A 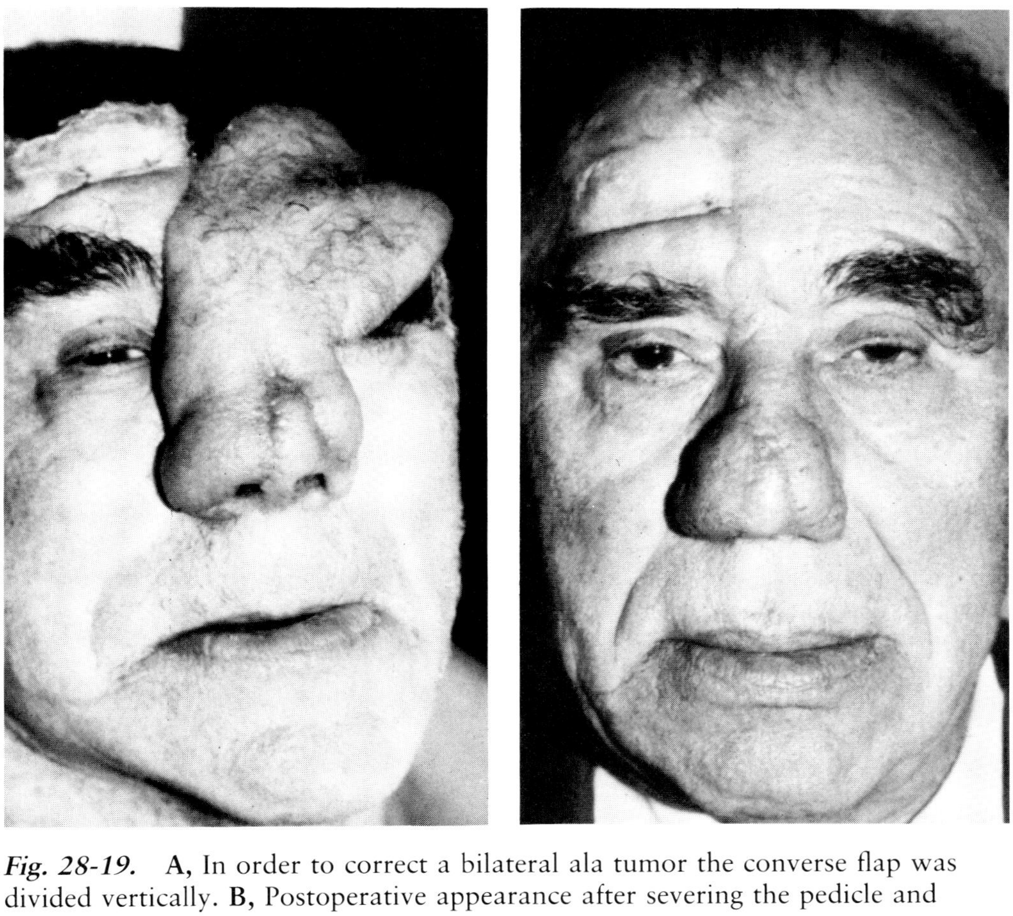 B

Fig. 28-19. **A,** In order to correct a bilateral ala tumor the converse flap was divided vertically. **B,** Postoperative appearance after severing the pedicle and redraping the scalp flap.

With the recent availability of artificial skin, the use of a donor site is avoided and the patient is made more comfortable. If enough skin is present on the stump of the nose, the remaining nasal skin is turned down to serve as inner lining (Fig. 28-20). To secure the skin and to prevent shrinkage, which does not happen too often when a scalp flap is used, rib cartilage is inserted for skeletal support. Cartilage can also be incorporated at the infolded skin edge and secured by mattress sutures. Preoperatively, at the initial incision a composite graft can be placed underneath the skin where the alar and tip area should be. Packing of the nose for 5 to 6 days is mandatory. After that an obturator is worn for at least three months. Additional procedures to shape the newly formed nose are delayed for at least 6 months. After that time, handling of the tissues is eased by the softening of the tissue (Fig. 28-21, A-F).

The Washio flap. A modification of a scalp flap, the so-called Washio flap has the advantage of avoiding any external visible scar except for that in the post-auricular region. Based on a rather small nutritional pedicle from the scalp, there have been reported disturbances in the vascular supply to the distal end, which is what is to become the new nose. Therefore this method needs careful delaying at least twice (Figs. 28-22 and 28-23).

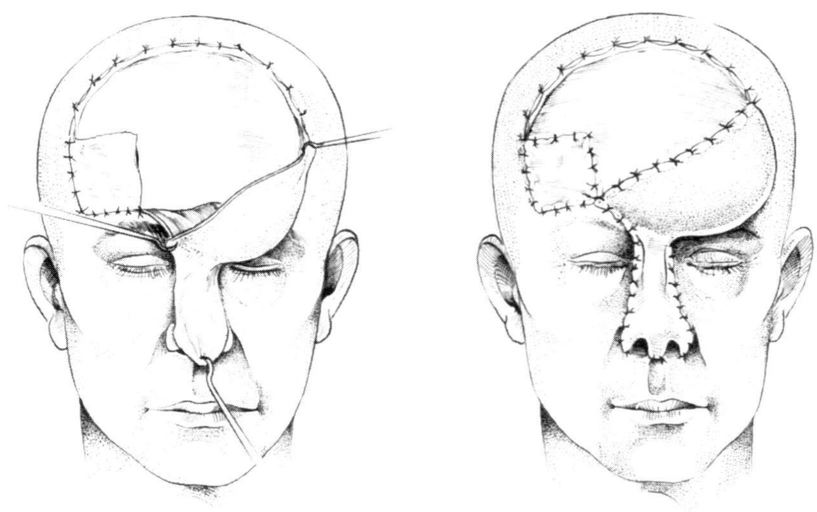

Fig. 28-20. Part of the remaining external nasal skin is turned down and serves as inner lining while the external coverage is achieved by the scalp flap. (From Walter C: Plast Chirurgie im Kopf-und Halsbereich, Herausgegeben von J Berendes, R Link, F Zollner, 2 Band HNO-Heilkunde, Stuttgart, 1966, Georg Thieme Verlag.)

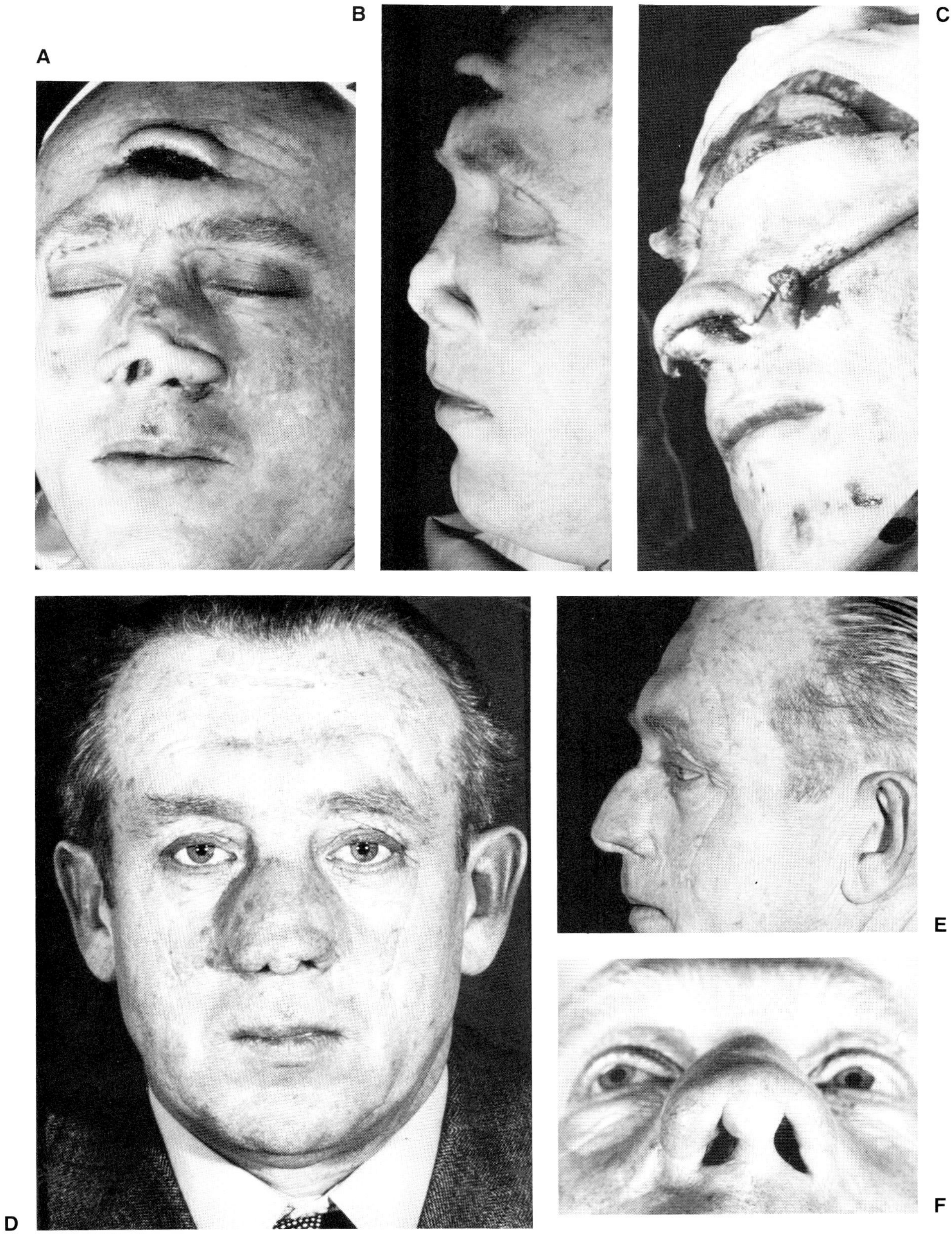

Fig. 28-21. **A-C,** Traumatic nasal deformity and several surgical procedures were corrected by a scalp flap underlined by a composite graft. **D-F,** Postoperatively.

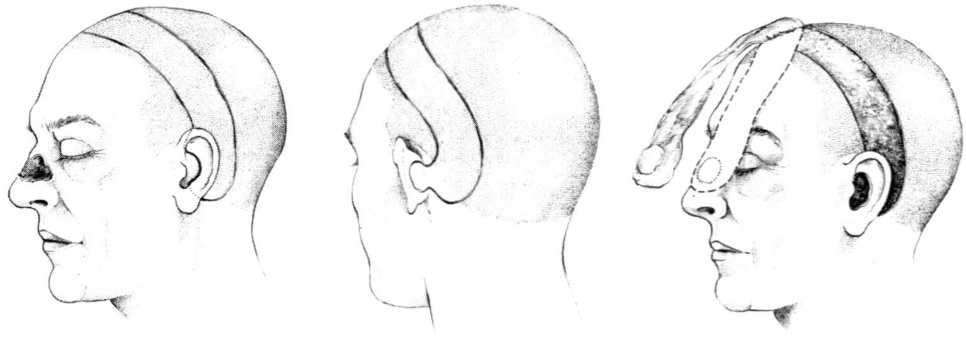

Fig. 28-22. Modified Washio sickle flap. (From Walter C: Plast Chirurgie im Kopf-und Halsbereich. Herausgegeben von J Berendes, R Link, F Zollner, 2 Band HNO-Heilkunde, Stuttgart, 2. neubearbeitete und erweiterte Auflage, 1977, Georg Thieme Verlag.)

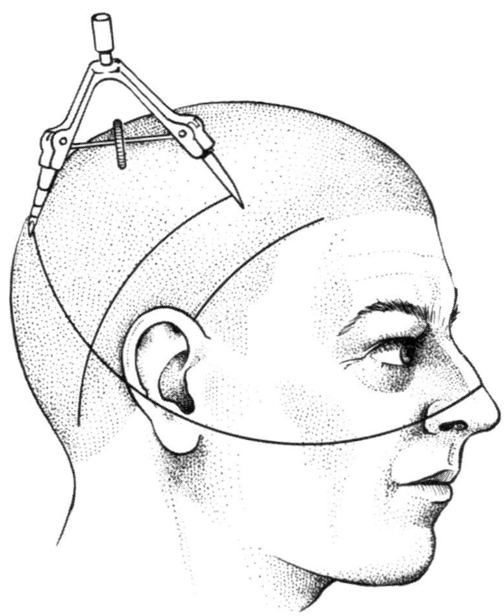

Fig. 28-23. The correct preoperative measurement is essential in order to be left with an adequate amount of tissue. (From Walter C: Plast Chirurgie im Kopf-und Halsbereich. Herausgegeben von J Berendes, R Link, F Zollner, 2 Band HNO-Heilkunde, Stuttgart, 2. neubearbeitete und erweiterte Auflage, 1977, Georg Thieme Verlag.)

Visor Flap

In mid-facial reconstruction, especially of the nose and the cheeks, the best suited material in the case of an intact forehead is the visor flap. It is based on the *A-temporalis* arteries bilaterally and can supply at least 100 cm2 of skin. This excellent blood supply ensures success in almost every case. The frontal area can keep its natural appearance and the surgeon is able to dissect the frontalis muscle off the skin flaps. However, when done, very careful separation of muscle and skin is necessary or the blood supply to the flap may be endangered. Over the bony forehead a delayed grafting leaves very little of a grafted area visible. The skin is draped over the nose and it is possible to cut a small pedicle into this big flap to achieve a nostril and a nasal tip. If that is not possible, then a small local flap can be turned into the nasal passageway to create the floor of the nostril. The cranial area of the nasal passageway can be reconstructed with a composite graft taken from the anterior part of the concha. The method of securing the graft has been described (Figs. 28-24, 28-25, 28-26, A-C, and 28-27, A-D). An obturator to prevent shrinkage is used for four months. It has to be taken out only for cleaning.

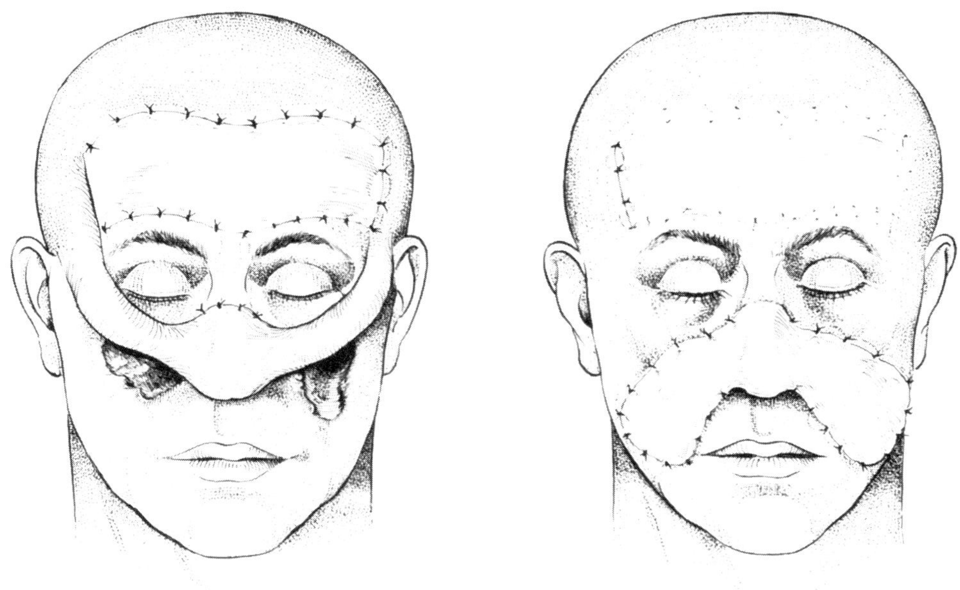

Fig. 28-24. Visor flap for mid-face reconstruction. (From Walter C: Plast Chirurgie im Kopf-und Halsbereich. Herausgegeben von J Berendes, R Link, F Zollner, 2 Band HNO-Heilkunde, Stuttgart, 2. neubearbeitete und erweiterte Auflage, 1977, Georg Thieme Verlag.)

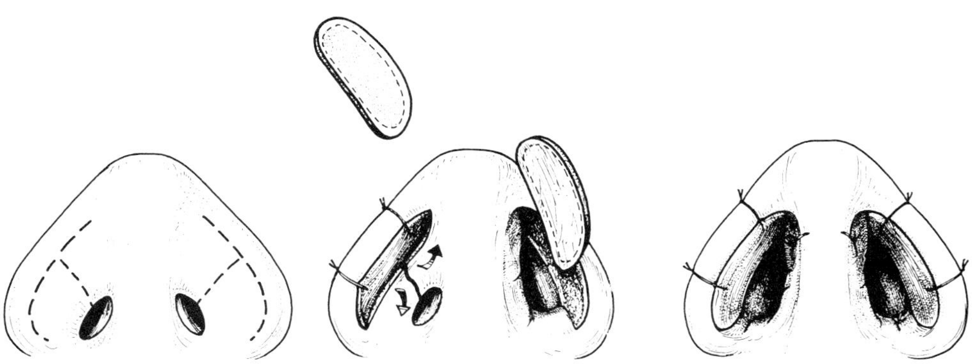

Fig. 28-25. Nasal entrance reconstruction is achieved by the insertion of composite grafts into the soft tissue in combination with small local flaps. Nasal obturators must be worn up to three months to prevent cicatricial restenosing. (From Walter, C Plast Chirurgie im Kopf-und Halsbereich. Herausgegeben von J Berendes, R Link, F Zollner, 2 Band HNO-Heilkunde, Stuttgart, 2. neubearbeitete und erweiterte Auflage, 1977, George Thieme Verlag.)

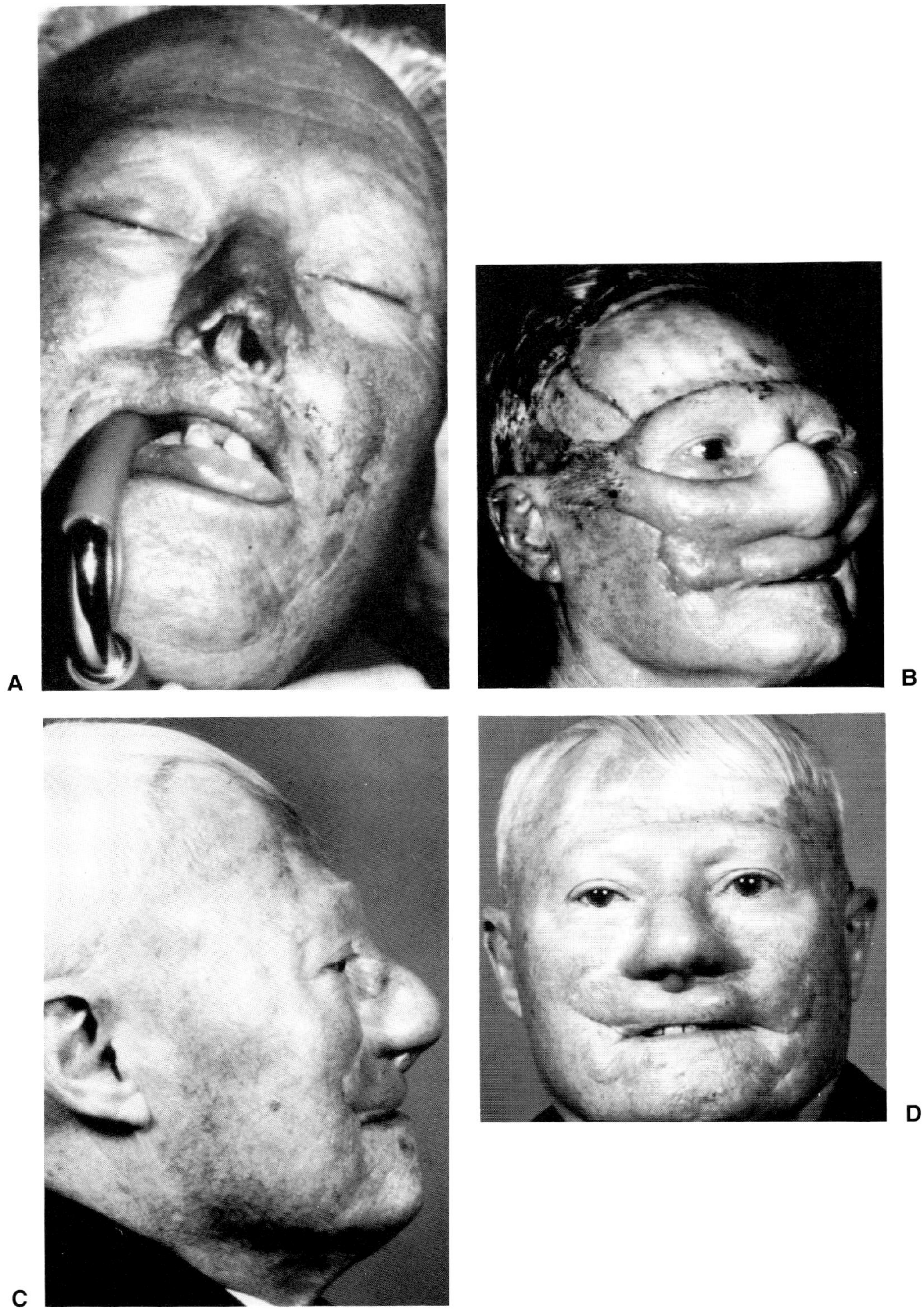

Fig. 28-26. Clinical case of nasal reconstruction after tumor removal. **A** and **B**, Preoperatively, **C-D**, Postoperatively.

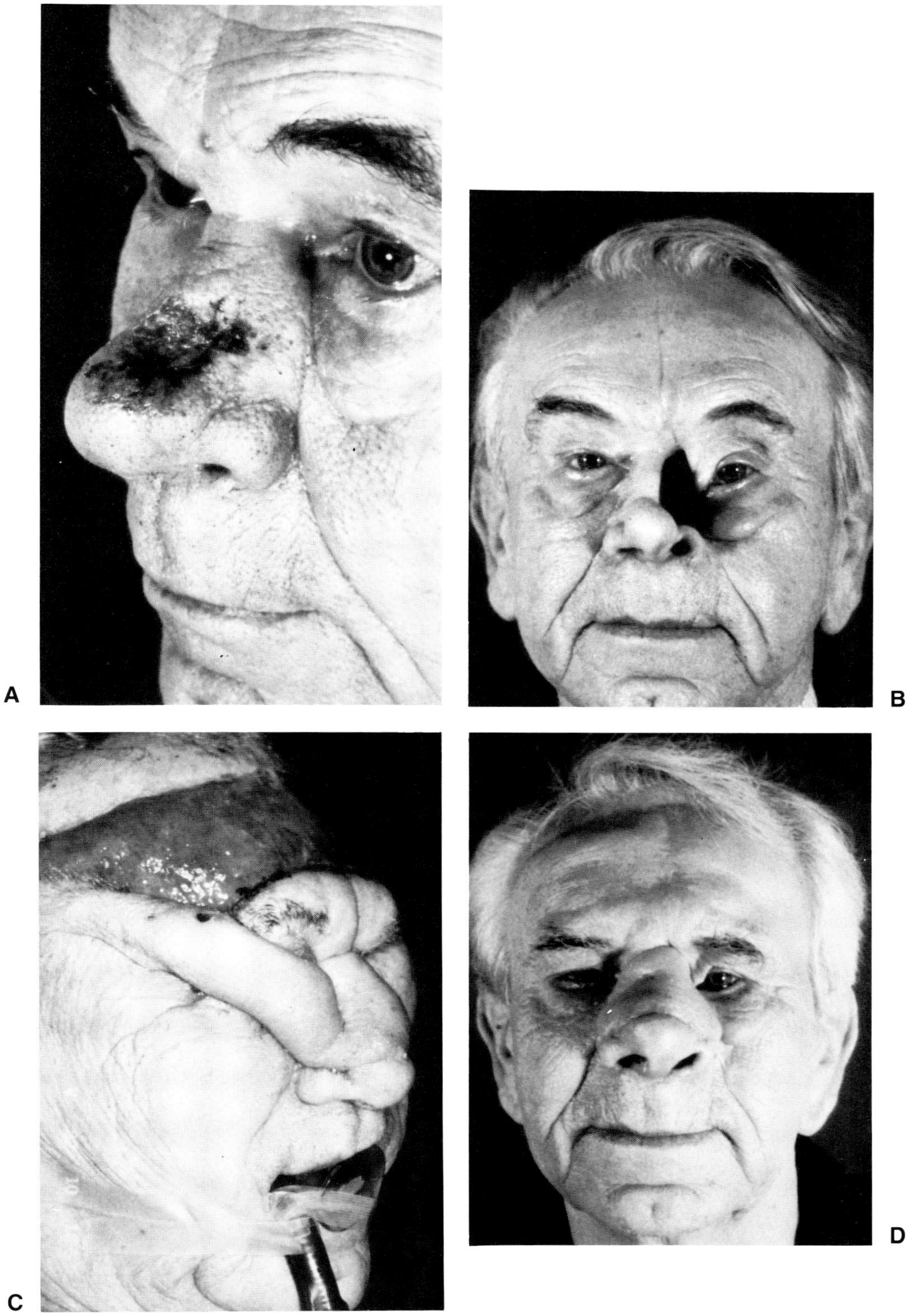

Fig. 28-27. Clinical case of nasal reconstruction after tumor removal. **A**, Basal tumor. **B**, Defect after cure of the tumor. **C**, Visor flap to close the defect. **D**, Postoperative picture after detachment of the flap.

Cheek Rotation Flap

Another useful flap for nasal reconstruction or upper lip and columella reconstruction is the horizontal cheek advancement flap advocated by Esser. The flap needs a totally intact cheek skin or a certain elasticity, which after mobilization can be advanced medially. The incision is carried out along the infraorbital rim and tragus upward to the temporal region. Anterior to the tragus the incision is carried down to the earlobe and to the neck. By small counter-incision it is also possible to advance the skin farther. The blood supply from the facial artery and vein must be kept intact. Careful dissection is therefore necessary to prevent injury to the facial nerve, but a certain thickness of the cheek flap is required to avoid skin necrosis (Fig. 28-28).

Usually there is only a small area to be grafted, but in the facial region a temporary grafting with a thin split skin is better than waiting for cicatrization. Later on, some of the skin grafts can be removed and replaced by full thickness skin grafts from the inguinal area. A light pressure packing is advantageous to minimize venous congestion (Figs. 28-29, A-C).

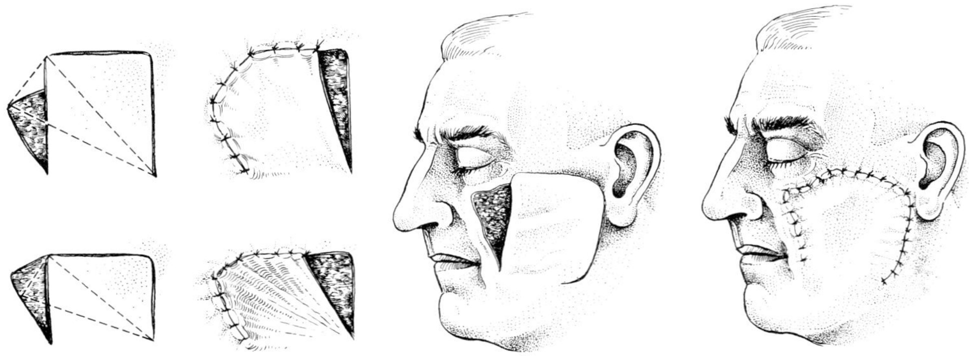

Fig. 28-28. Cheek rotation flap.

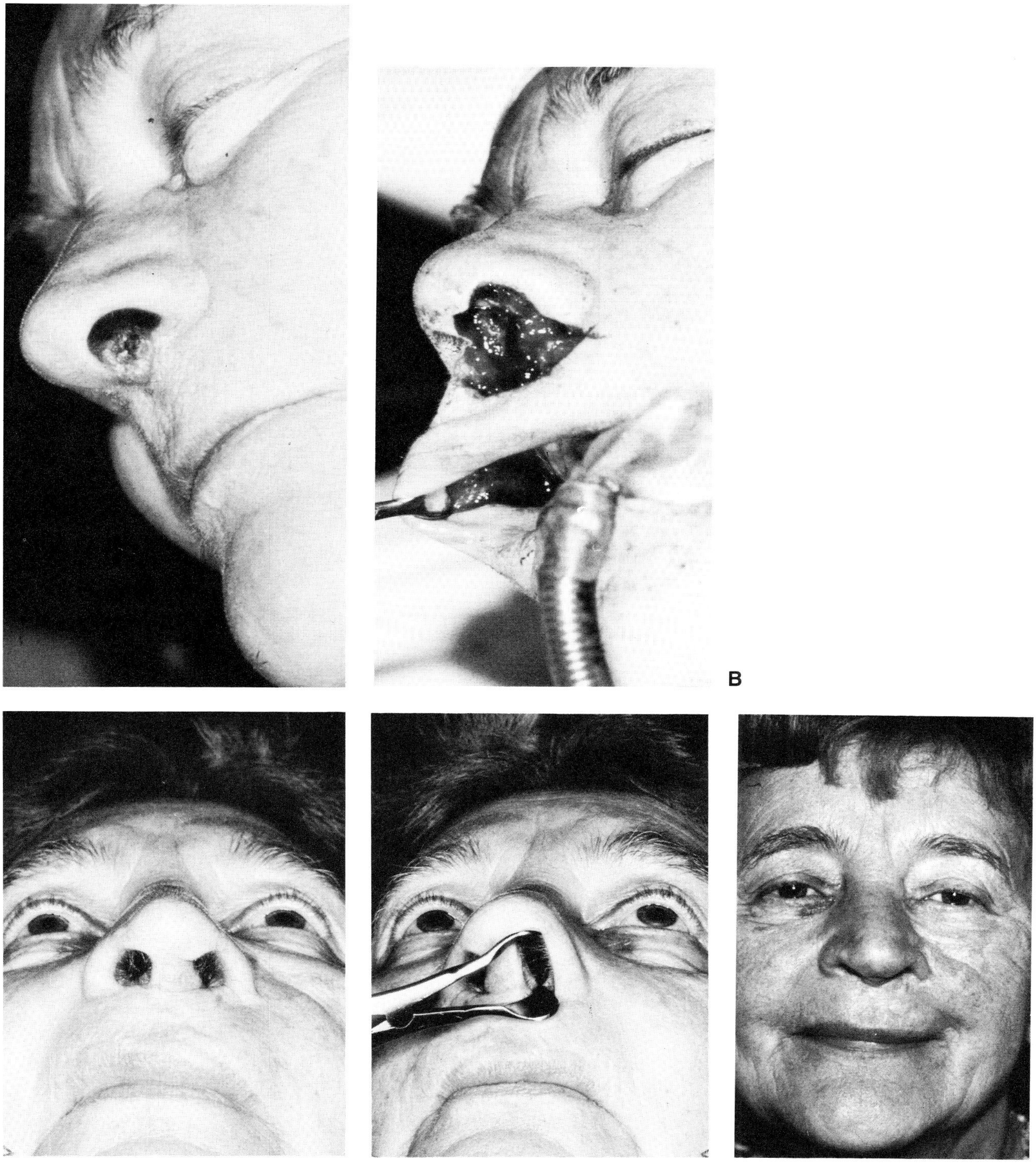

A B C D E

Fig. 28-29. **A,** Squamous cell carcinoma in the columella and floor of the nose. **B,** Corrected by excision enoral flaps for septal reconstruction and cheek rotation for nasal entrance and columella reconstruction. **C-E,** Postoperatively.

Small Flaps, Rhomboid or Bi-lobed

Small flaps are mainly used in the reconstruction of the ala. Rhomboid or bilobed flaps serve a similar purpose. They are an excellent alternative to grafts in treating small skin defects (Figs. 28-30, 28-31, 28-32, 28-33, 28-34, A,B, and 28-35, A-E).

Shoulder Flap

In very desperate cases as after severe burns in which no facial skin is available, another option is the horizontal shoulder flap,[1,5] which, delayed once, can be made long enough to reach the mid-face. However, such a flap can be used for total or partial facial and nasal tissue replacement. The skin is soft and pliable and can be molded according to the surgeon's ability. Once healed the color difference is hardly noticeable and this is a useful adjunct in nasal reconstruction when the surgeon is confronted with certain difficult problems.

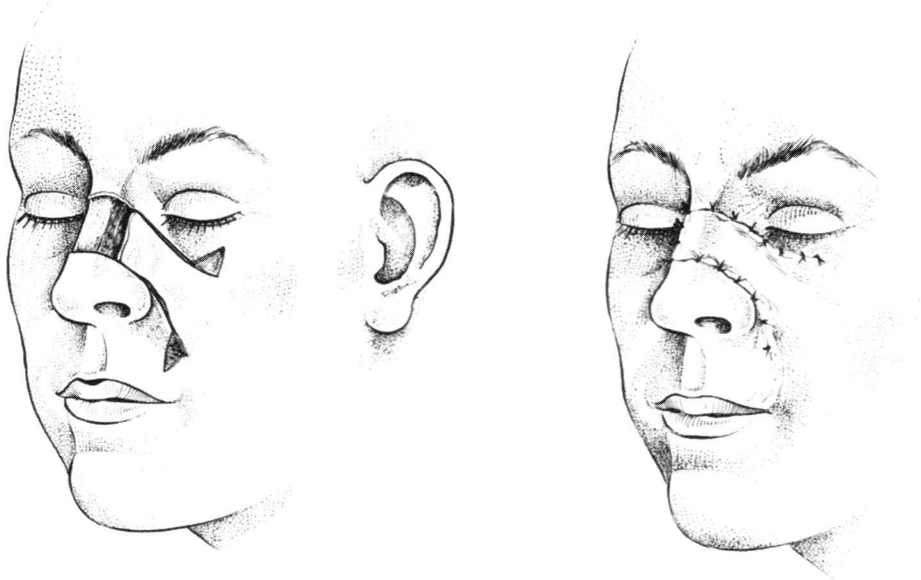

Fig. 28-30. Horizontal advancement flap. (From Walter C: Plast Chirurgie im Kofp-und Halsbereich. Herausgegeben von J Berendes, R Link, F Zollner, 2 Band HNO-Heilkunde, Stuttgart, 2. neubearbeitete und erweiterte Auflage, 1977, Georg Thieme Verlag.)

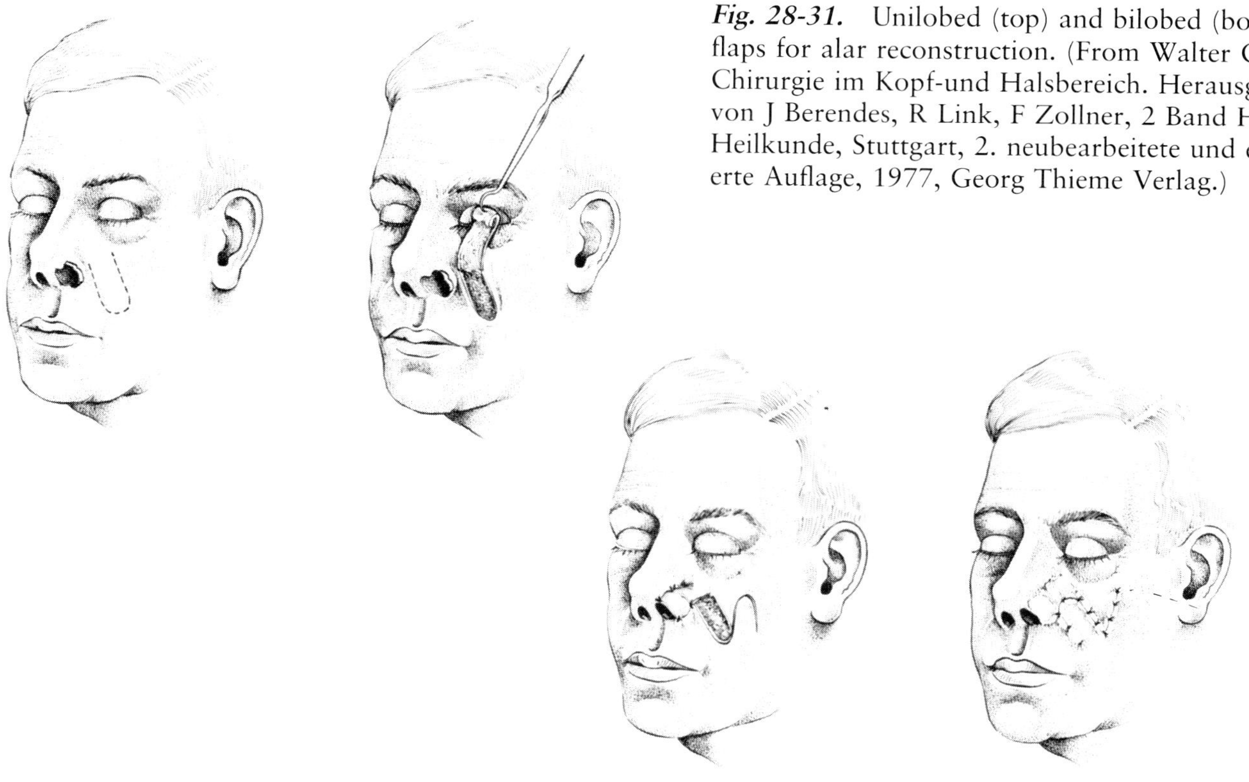

Fig. 28-31. Unilobed (top) and bilobed (bottom) flaps for alar reconstruction. (From Walter C: Plast Chirurgie im Kopf-und Halsbereich. Herausgegeben von J Berendes, R Link, F Zollner, 2 Band HNO-Heilkunde, Stuttgart, 2. neubearbeitete und erweiterte Auflage, 1977, Georg Thieme Verlag.)

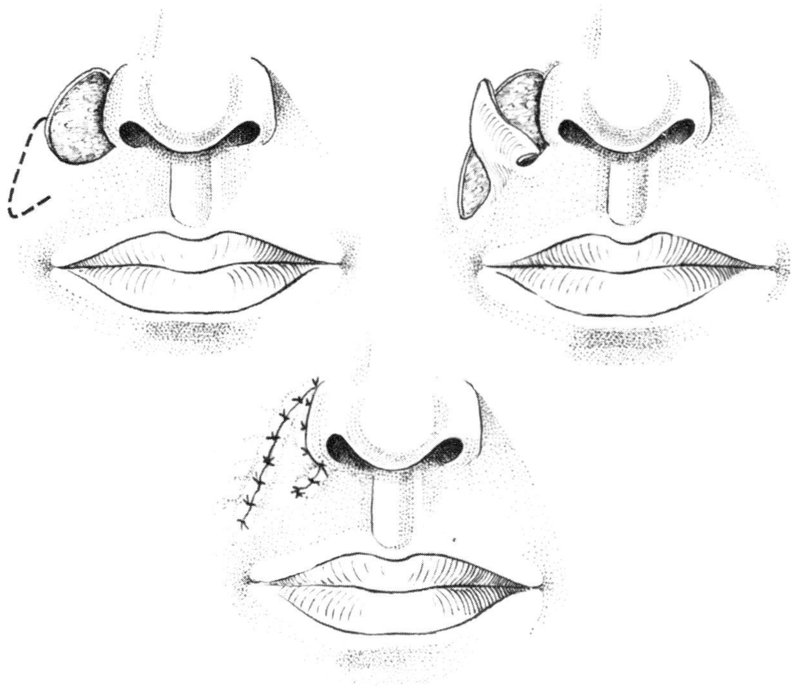

Fig. 28-32. Nasolabial flap. (From Walter C: Plast Chirurgie im Kopf-und Halsbereich. Herausgegeben von J Berendes, R Link, F Zollner, 2 Band HNO-Heilkunde, 1977, Georg Thieme Verlag, Stuttgart, 2. neubearbeitete und erweiterte Auflage.)

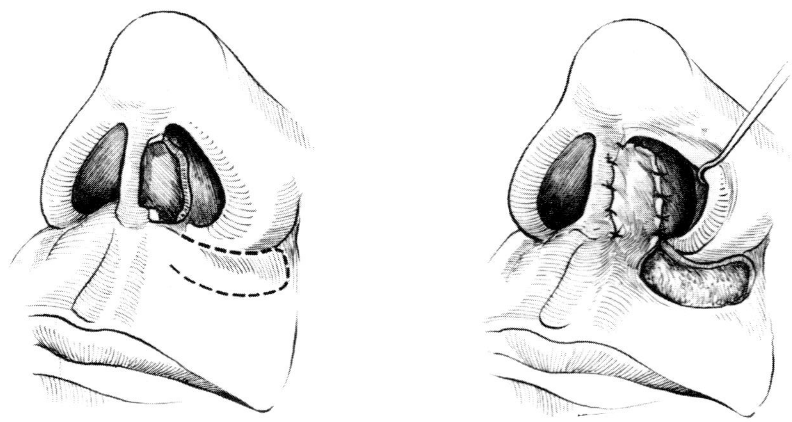

Fig. 28-33. Different flap planning for defect closure of the nose. (From Walter C: Plast Chirurgie im Kopf-und Halsbereich. Herausgegeben von J Berendes, R Link, F Zollner, 2 Band HNO-Heilkunde, Stuttgart, 2. neubearbeitete und erweiterte Auflage, 1977, Georg Thieme Verlag.)

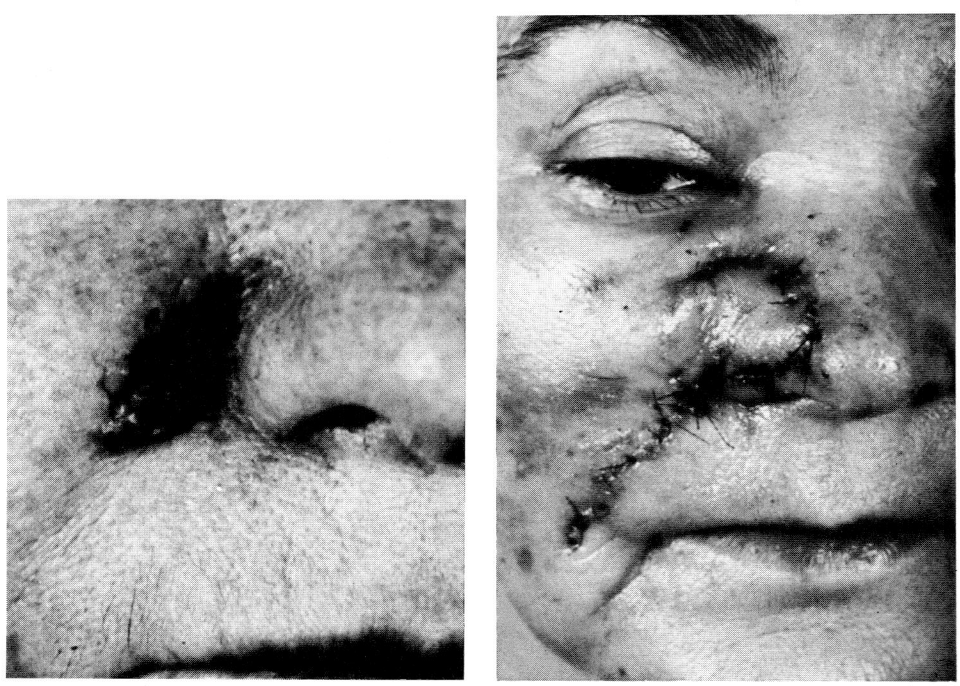

A B

Fig. 28-34. **A**, Basal cell carcinoma defect. **B**, Covered after excision by a naso-labial flap.

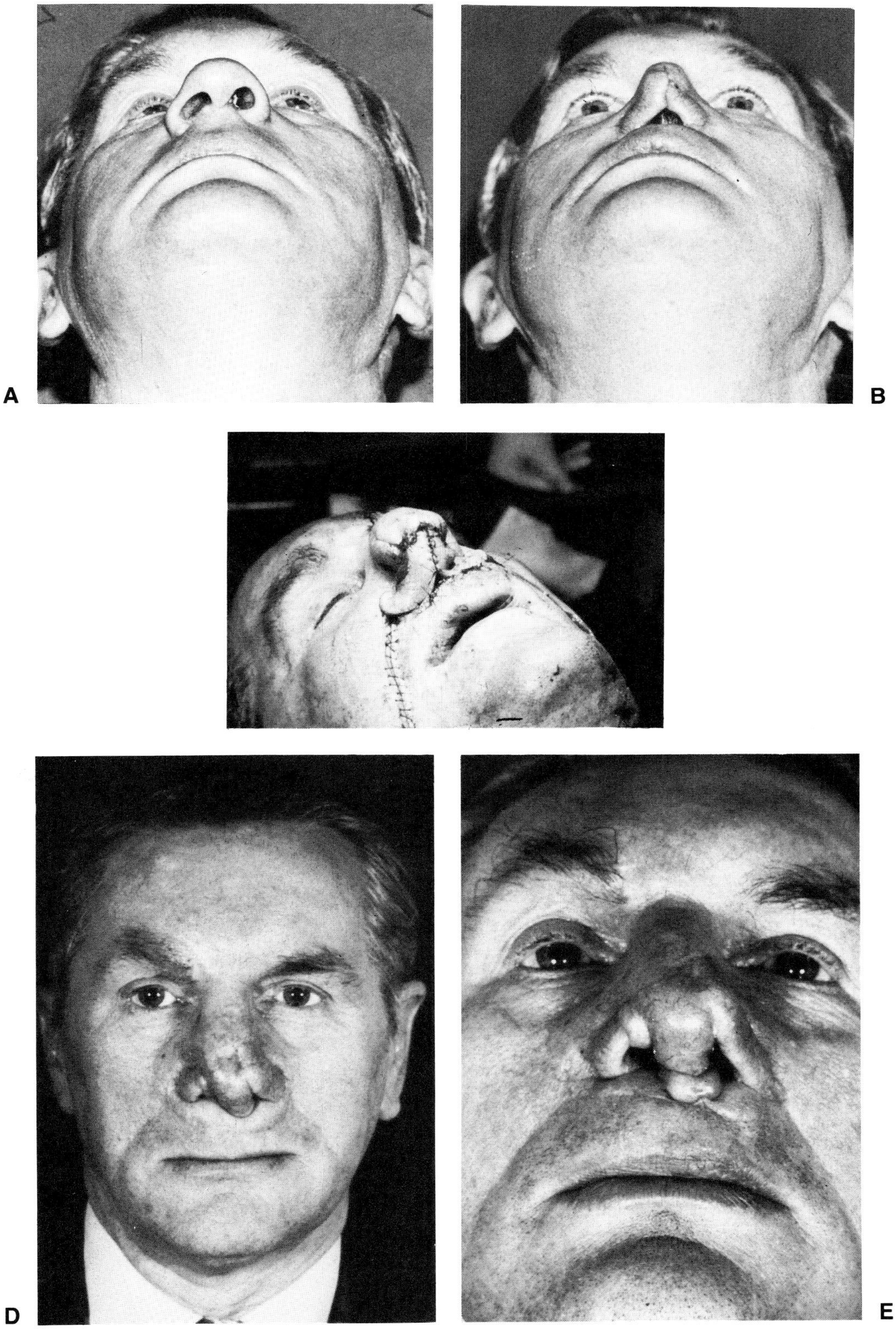

Fig. 28-35. A and B, Reconstruction of the columella after tumor resection. C, By two naso-labial flaps. D-E, Postoperatively.

Nasal Reconstruction Treatment Choices

In the discussion of methods of nasal reconstruction we have to differentiate between several choices of treatment:

1. Free grafts.
2. Local flaps within the nasal area.
3. Flaps from the adjacent facial parts.
4. Distant flaps like the upper arm tissue (Tagliacozzi) pedicles from distant areas like the abdomen, via the upper arm or lower wrist.
5. Free tissue transfer by micro-vascular anastomosis.

Free Grafts

If the tissue defect is not too large, the primary closure of the wound should be first attempted by free grafts either as skin grafts or as composite grafts, preferably using auricular tissue as a donor site. The only exception to this rule is the condition of the host tissue. If the host tissue is severely crushed or eradicated, it is less suitable for primary grafting.

We have many opportunities to use auricular composite grafts and have also learned to incorporate in our surgical armamentarium intranasal composite grafts, using turbinates or portions of the septum, where it seems feasible. The auricular grafts serve either as external coverage or as intranasal alignment. Cooling of the graft seems to increase the chances for a good take.[1] We have found lately that the local application of Heparin or cortisone ointment and cortisone systemically, seems to increase the chance for a good take.

It can be stated that the anterior portion of the avricular concha can and should be used exclusively for inner lining defect closures of the inner passageway because the curvature of the composite grafts blends very satisfactorily with the inner aspects of the vestibular skin and the cartilaginous structures. We can use the intranasal graft bilaterally, bridging the nasal septum in the form of a saddle, in which we just have to divide the midline section of the skin to attach the two skin halves to the appropriate host tissue areas and leave the cartilaginous strip intact to give support bilaterally in an umbrella or saddle fashion on top of the dorsum.

By the same token the floor of the nasal entrance can also be corrected by the implantation of such a graft into the inferior portion of the nasal passageway, tunneling the septum and the columella. Embedded in tissue, the blood supply is usually very good and the ingrowing vessels keep such grafts alive for a few days. It is advantageous to pack the nasal passageways with gauze for 5 days and let the patient wear or by silicone obturators over a period of 3 to 4 months to counteract a postoperative cicatricial narrowing.

Post-auricular composite grafts including skin and cartilage measured to the size of the nasal defect are used for external coverage. We have found that it is better to use two or three mattress sutures to bind the cartilaginous and skin portions closer together before suturing the graft into place. Careful measuring to avoid a greater distance from the center of the graft to the host edges should be done to avoid the center being away from the edges of the graft more than .75 cm.

Finally the helix rim of the ear, either in the cranial or anterior portion with larger skin portions attached, makes the reduplication of the nostril rim possible. The skin portion being larger, we can even gap quite large tissue defects on the external surface of the nose. The donor defect on the helix rim can easily be closed by additional excision of triangles to obtain a better tissue adaptation. This leaves a normal but smaller ear. We use a bolus technique as bandage on the nose, leaving everything untouched for about a week, and advise the patient to use ointment massages for two to three weeks and to cover the graft to prevent the transplanted tissue from drying out.

Local Flaps

For external coverage the unilobed or bilobed flap techniques, the Limberg-Dufour-Mentel flaps (rhomboid tissue excisions and flap closure) and the horizontal shifting of nasal skin alongside the dorsum of the nose are the methods of choice. In some cases a part of the nasal septum can be shifted sideways to serve as an inner lining for the alar reconstruction, but the disadvantage of such nasal treatment is the fact that it creates a septal perforation. In our opinion, therefore, all other methods should be given priority if one is able to obtain an almost identical postoperative result with different techniques rather than having to sacrifice a portion of the supporting septum. Local flaps can be obtained from the naso-labial region and used in combination with free grafts in nasal tip reconstruction.

Adjacent Flaps

I consider adjacent flaps, the oblique midline forehead flap, the scalp flap, the horizontal supra-eyebrow flap or the cheek advancement, and finally, the distant island flap from the forehead based on the temporal arterial stem.

Midline forehead flap. An easy flap to use is the midline forehead flap. We can incorporate part of the forehead bone, if used as a composite flap with the galea, and we can usually have a small pedicle and a wide distal portion on the border to the hairline. With such a flap to be turned almost 180 degrees downward, we can cover defects in the nose and reconstruct the nose very satisfactorily with it. There is also the possibility of lining the distal portion of the midline flap with a composite graft from the anterior concha of the ear to serve as the inner lining and cartilaginous structures. After three weeks such a composite flap is then turned downward, serving as a complete nasal tip, and only minor detailed reconstructive processes need to be done in the months to follow. Usually such pedicles can be severed about three months after the initial turn down.

Converse scalp flap.[2] The next in line to be considered is a large scalp flap, with which we can cover huge areas of the nose. With gloving techniques we can use such a large forehead flap for intranasal lining, and external coverage. Rib cartilage or auricular cartilage should be used in the same procedure to serve as the cartilaginous skeleton before tissue shrinkage can take place, which would ruin the initially good result.

Visor flap. The visor flap, based on both temporal arteries, is a huge flap that has the potential to reconstruct midline portions in toto. It is not only used for nasal reconstruction alone but for upper lip and cheek reconstruction grafts also. The reconstruction of the nasal apertures can be done at the later stage by inserting composite grafts into this soft tissue, opening up the nasal passageways.

Supra-orbital-temple-eyebrow pedicle. The supra-orbital-temple-eyebrow pedicle can be prepared in the temple region. We insert cartilage and skin to preform the nasal structures. It requires very tedious dissection to keep the vascular pedicle in the midline alive, and after the total preformation of the nasal tip or the alar or the columella, such a pedicle is turned down into the place and can also be used bilaterally in double alar tip reconstruction. The danger of this flap lies in its very small vascular pedicle for nutrition.

Washio flap. In an attempt to avoid external visible scarring in the facial region, the Washio flap has been designed, incorporating post-auricular skin and cartilage based on a pedicle in the scalp region. The danger is of a disturbance and renostasis developing in the distal portion of the pedicle, which makes careful preparation and staging of such a flap mandatory. It should, however, be considered in scarred faces and cases in which the patient prefers not to have an external visible scar.

Large island pedicles. Large island pedicles can be shifted over long distances from the mid-forehead by tunneling the cheek, based only on the temporalis artery and the vein, which need a careful dissection when preparing the island flap on the forehead.

Distant Flaps, Pedicles

The Indian classical method to form the nose from tissues of the upper arm has only a very limited field of application, because the immobilization of the arm causes constant shoulder pains and may lead to some impairment of function later on.

Free Tissue Transfer by Micro-Vascular Anastomosis

The inguinal free flap transfer depends for its nutrition on a correct micro-vascular connection between the vascular nutrition of the pedicle and either the temporalis artery and vein or the facial artery and vein. Some of the failures of nasal reconstruction result from impatience on the part of the surgeon and the patient and we recommend waiting several months in between stages to give the tissue time to adjust and make it more amenable to the next stage of surgery.

Summary

Congenital malformations, trauma, and benign and malignant tumors may call for reconstructive surgery procedures to cover defects. In order to establish proper diagnosis a careful examination including x-rays and biopsies is mandatory according to the case. A complete knowledge of the many possibilities in nasal reconstruction should prove beneficial to both patients and surgeons.

REFERENCES

1. Bakamjian VY: A two stage method for pharyngo-esophageal reconstruction with a primary pectoral skin flap, Plast Reconstr Surg 36:173, 1965.
2. Converse JM: Reconstructive plastic surgery, ed 2, Philadelphia, WB Saunders 1977.
3. Denecke HJ and Meyer R: Korrigierende und rekonstruktive Nasenplastik, Berlin Springer-Verlag, 1964.
4. Gillies H: New free graft (of skin and ear cartilage) applied to reconstruction of nostril, Br J Surg 30:305-307, 1943.
5. Joseph J: Nasenplastik und sonstige Gesichtsplastik, Leipzig, 1931, Kabitsch.
6. Walter C: Aesthetische Chirurgie der Nase, Gohrbrandt, Gabka, and Berndorfer, editors: Handbuch der Plastischen Chirurgie, vol 2, Berlin, 1966, Walter de Gruyer & Co.
7. Walter C: Die Anwendung der sog. Composite grafts in der plastischen Chirurgie, HNO, 14:200-206, 1966.
8. Walter C: Composite grafts in nasal surgery, Arch Otolaryngol 90:622-630, 1969.
9. Walter C: Plastische Chirurgie im Bereich des Gesichtes und des Halses, Kap. 25, Hals-, Nasen- Ohrenheilkunde in Praxis und Klinik J. Berendes, R. Link und F. Zöllner, 2. Aufl. Bd 2, Stuttgart, 1977, Georg Thieme Verlag.
10. Witwicka, Z: Reconstruction of nasal alae by means of a free implant from the aural concha, Otolaryngol Pol 20:537-539, 1966.

Appendix

Instruments for Rhinoplastic Surgeons

Walter E. Berman

Instruments are of great importance to surgeons in performing proper surgery. As a facial plastic surgeon, I have found some instruments of greater value to me in rhinoplastic surgery than others. The following instruments are the tools I find most useful, and these are the ones I have mentioned throughout the text. I have tried to make specific reference to the purpose for which an instrument is primarily used and have intentionally omitted the common tools such as scalpels, which every surgeon uses. These instruments can be obtained from most surgical supply houses.

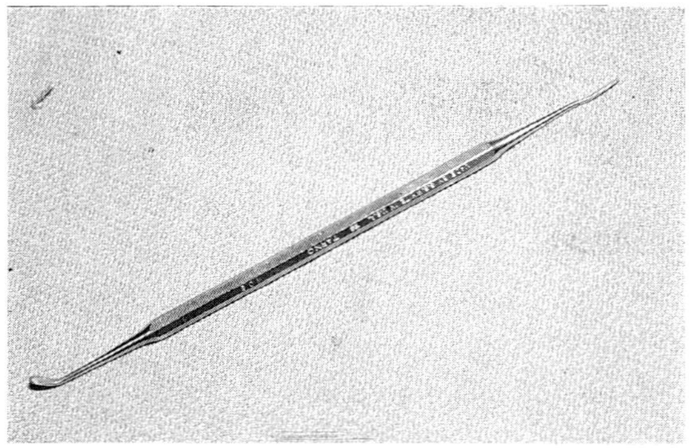

Fig. A-1. Cleoid discoid dental instrument has a straight end for elevating septal coverings and a curved end for dissecting out pieces of cartilage on the crest of the nasal septum.

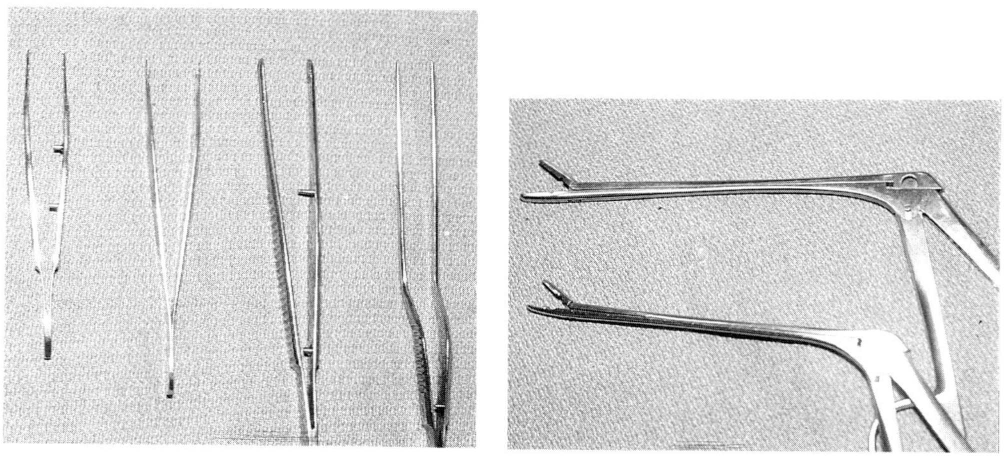

A B C D E

Fig. A-2. Forceps. **A**, The Castroviejo 2 mm toothed forceps is useful for more delicate procedures such as removing fibrofatty tissues off the delivered lower lateral cartilages. **B**, Brown Adson multiple toothed forceps is an all-purpose instrument. **C**, A six-inch thin straight forceps with teeth is used to place flex straws and telfa into each side of the nose for packing. **D**, A bayonet forceps is used for inserting and removing anesthetic packing. **E**, A Takahashi forceps, large and small, is used to remove segments of the nasal septum.

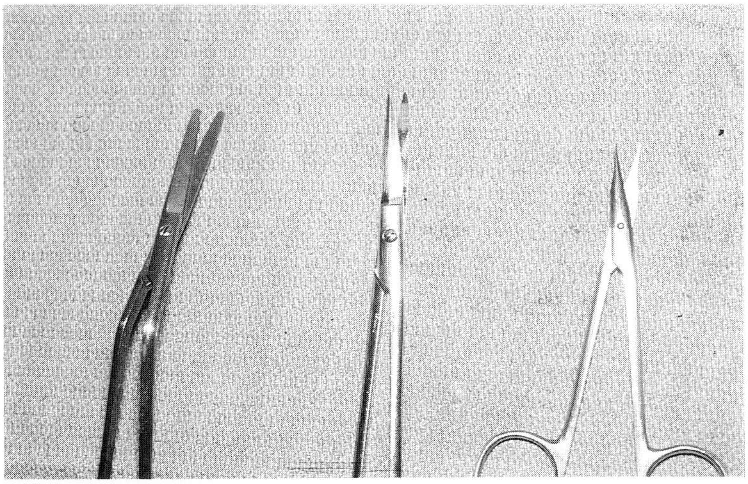

A B C

Fig. A-3. Scissors. **A,** An angled scissors is used to remove excessive anterior septal and upper lateral cartilages. **B,** A Foman scissors is used to undermine lower lateral cartilages and overlying skin on the nasal framework. **C,** A straight Stevens Iris Scissors is used to separate the lower lateral cartilage from the underlying vestibular skin.

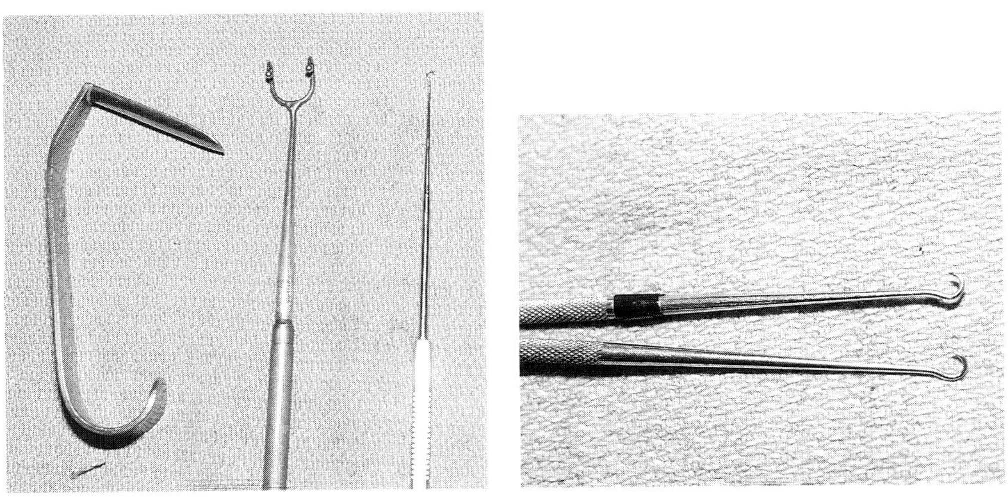

A B C D

Fig. A-4. Retractors. **A,** A Neivert retractor is used to hold anterior nasal skin. **B,** A Foman retractor is used to aid surgery on the lower third of the nose. **C,** A single hook is used to present the dissected lower lateral cartilage. **D,** A swivel retractor has two hooks and is adjustable to assist nasal tip surgery.

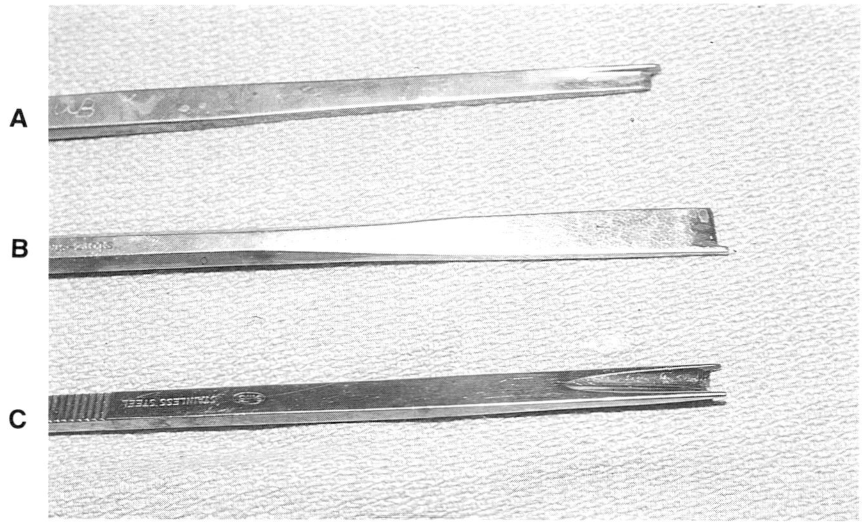

Fig. A-5. Bone cutters. **A,** Neivert lateral osteotome, 4 mm, with guard. **B,** Medial, 6 mm guarded osteotome. **C,** Anterior 6 mm nasal gouge to remove excess anterior nasal bone.

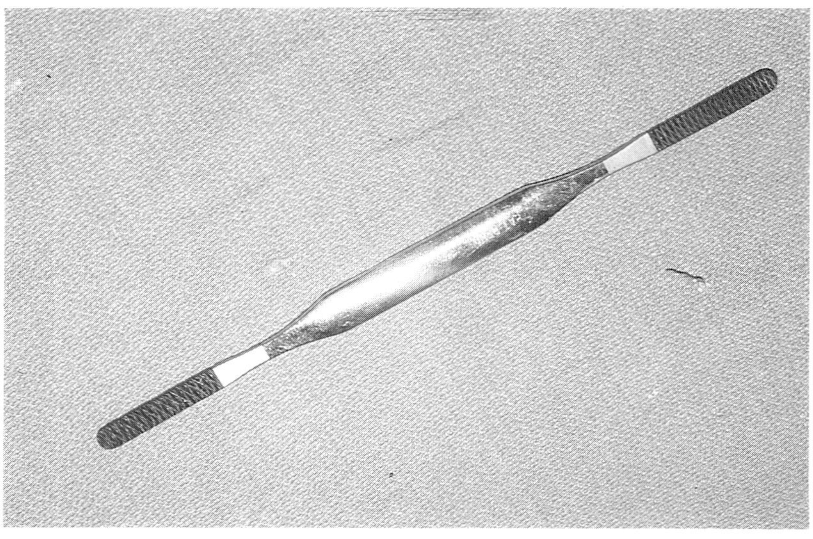

Fig. A-6. A Rees double-ended rasps.

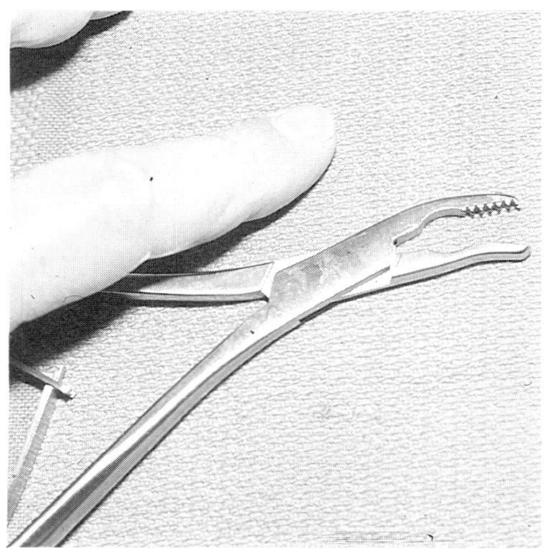

Fig. A-7. A Rubin tip morselizer for lower lateral cartilages.

Index